Postoperative Critical Care of the Massachusetts General Hospital

Postoperative Critical Care of the Massachusetts General Hospital

Second Edition

Department of Anesthesia
Massachusetts General Hospital

Editors

William J. Hoffman, M.D.
Instructor in Anaesthesia, Harvard Medical School; Assistant in Anesthesia, Massachusetts General Hospital, Boston

John D. Wasnick, M.D.
Assistant Professor of Anesthesiology, Cornell University Medical College; Assistant Attending Anesthesiologist, The New York Hospital, New York

Co-Editors

W. Andrew Kofke, M.D.
Associate Professor of Anesthesiology/CCM and Neurologic Surgery, and Director, Neurologic Anesthesia and Supportive Care Program, Department of Anesthesiology and Critical Care Medicine, University of Pittsburgh School of Medicine, Pittsburgh

Jerrold H. Levy, M.D.
Associate Professor of Anesthesiology, Emory University School of Medicine; Division of Cardiothoracic Anesthesia and Critical Care, Emory Clinic, Atlanta

Little, Brown and Company
Boston/Toronto/London

Second Edition

Second Printing

Library of Congress Cataloging-in-Publication Data

Postoperative critical care of the Massachusetts General Hospital/ Department of Anesthesia, Massachusetts General Hospital; editors, William J. Hoffman, John D. Wasnick; co-editors. W. Andrew Kofke,
p. cm.
rev. ed. of: postoperative critical care procedures of the Massachusetts General Hospital. 1st ed. c1986.
Includes bibliographical references and index.
ISBN 0-316-36838-5
1. Postoperative care—Handbooks, manuals, etc. 2. Critical care medicine—Handbooks, manuals, etc. I. Hoffman, William, 1959– II. Wasnick, John D. III. Massachusetts General Hospital. Dept. of Anesthesia. IV. Postoperative critical care procedures of the Massachusetts General Hospital.
[DNLM: 1. Critical Care—handbooks. 2. Postoperative Complications—handbooks. WO 39 P8585]
RD51.P66 1992
617′.919—dc20
DNLM/DLC
for Library of Congress 92-15625
CIP

Printed in the United States of America

SEM

Contents

Contributing Authors

Lee Adlestein, M.D.
Instructor in Anaesthesia, Harvard Medical School; Anesthesiologist, Brigham and Women's Hospital, Boston

James K. Alifimoff, M.D.
Anesthesiologist, Anesthesia Associates of Topeka, Topeka, Kansas

Michael Bannon, M.D.
Anesthesiologist, Anesthesia Medical Consultants, Albuquerque, New Mexico

Elizabeth C. Behringer, M.D.
Instructor in Anaesthesia, Harvard Medical School; Director, Postanesthesia Care Unit, and Assistant in Anesthesia, Massachusetts General Hospital, Boston

Bruce R. Bistrian, M.D., Ph.D.
Professor of Medicine, Harvard Medical School; Chief, Division of Clinical Nutrition, New England Deaconess Hospital, Boston

Albert T. Cheung, M.D.
Assistant Professor of Anesthesia, University of Pennsylvania School of Medicine and Hospital of the University of Pennsylvania, Philadelphia

Charles E. Cook, M.D.
Attending Anesthesiologist, Department of Anesthesiology, Miami Valley Hospital, Dayton, Ohio

Richard DeCesare, M.S.E.E., C.C.E.
Manager of Clinical Engineering, Department of Anesthesia, Massachusetts General Hospital, Boston

William F. Eckhardt, M.D.
Instructor in Anaesthesia, Harvard Medical School; Assistant in Anesthesia, Massachusetts General Hospital, Boston

Jean Elrick, M.D.
Instructor in Anaesthesia, Harvard Medical School; Assistant in Anesthesia, Massachusetts General Hospital, Boston

Richard Fine, M.D.
Assistant Professor of Anesthesiology, Cornell University Medical College; Assistant in Anesthesiology, The New York Hospital, New York

David J. Fish, M.D.
Assistant Professor of Anesthesiology and Surgery, Temple University School of Medicine; Codirector, Surgical Intensive Care Unit, Department of Anesthesia, Temple University Hospital, Philadelphia

William H. Frist, M.D.
Assistant Professor of Surgery, Department of Thoracic Surgery, Vanderbilt University School of Medicine; Surgical Director, the Vanderbilt Transplant Center, Vanderbilt University Medical Center, Nashville, Tennessee

Ronald I. Goldberg, M.D., Ph.D.
Resident, Department of Anesthesia, Massachusetts General Hospital, Boston

S. A. Grace, M.S.N., C.R.N.A.
C.R.N.A. Anesthesia Training, Columbia University College of Physicians and Surgeons; Staff Nurse Anesthetist, Anesthesia Department, New York Hospital-Cornell Medical Center, New York

William J. Hoffman, M.D.
Instructor in Anaesthesia, Harvard Medical School; Assistant in Anesthesia, Massachusetts General Hospital, Boston

Charles W. Hogue, Jr., M.D.
Instructor, Department of Anesthesiology, Washington University School of Medicine; Attending Anesthesiologist, Barnes Hospital, St. Louis

Phillipa J. Hore, M.D., F.F.A.R.C.S.
Instructor in Anaesthesia, Harvard Medical School; Senior Clinical Fellow, Department of Anesthesia, Massachusetts General Hospital, Boston

†Charles Huggins, M.D.
Associate Professor of Surgery, Harvard Medical School; Director of Blood Transfusion Service, Massachusetts General Hospital, Boston

Mitchell F. Keamy, M.D.
Chief, Department of Anesthesia, Humana Hospital-Sunrise, Las Vegas

W. Andrew Kofke, M.D.
Associate Professor of Anesthesiology/CCM and Neurologic Surgery and Director, Neurologic Anesthesia and Supportive Care Program, Department of Anesthesiology and Critical Care Medicine, University of Pittsburgh School of Medicine, Pittsburgh

Terry W. Latson, M.D.
Associate Professor of Anesthesiology, University of Texas Southwestern Medical Center at Dallas, Southwestern Medical School, Dallas

Jerrold H. Levy, M.D.
Associate Professor of Anesthesiology, Emory University School of Medicine; Division of Cardiothoracic Anesthesia and Critical Care, Emory Clinic, Atlanta

Alan Lichtenstein, M.D.
Chairman, Department of Anesthesia, Wright State University School of Medicine; Attending Anesthesiologist, Department of Anesthesia, Miami Valley Hospital, Dayton, Ohio

William J. Mazzei, M.D.
Vice Chairman, Department of Anesthesia, University of California, San Diego, School of Medicine; Medical Director of the Operating Rooms, UCSD Medical Center, San Diego

Lee Ann McGinnis, M.D.
Attending Anesthesiologist, Carolinas Medical Center, Charlotte, North Carolina

Alvin Morales, M.D.
Assistant Professor, Department of Anesthesiology, University of Puerto Rico Medical School, Rio Piedras, Puerto Rico

Krishna N. Nirmel, M.D.
Attending Neurosurgeon, University Hospital, Boston, Metrowest Medical Center, Boston, and Newton-Wellesley Hospital, Newton, Massachusetts

Christopher O'Connor, M.D.
Assistant Professor of Anesthesia, Rush Medical College of Rush University; Staff Anesthesiologist, Department of Anesthesiology, Rush-Presbyterian-St. Luke's Medical Center, Chicago

† Deceased

William Paganelli, M.D., Ph.D.
Assistant Professor of Anesthesiology, University of Vermont School of Medicine; Staff Anesthesiologist, Medical Center Hospital of Vermont, Burlington, Vermont

Debra Petrucci, M.D.
Neurosurgeon, Lahey Clinic Medical Center, Burlington, Massachusetts

Jesse D. Roberts, Jr., M.D.
Instructor in Anaesthesia, Harvard Medical School; Assistant in Pediatrics and Anesthesia, Massachusetts General Hospital, Boston

Allan H. Ropper, M.D.
Professor of Neurology, Tufts University School of Medicine; Chief of Neurology, St. Elizabeth's Hospital, Boston

Daniel Shapiro, M.D.
Fellow in Clinical Microbiology and Infectious Diseases, University of North Carolina at Chapel Hill School of Medicine; Attending Physician, University of North Carolina Hospitals, Chapel Hill, North Carolina

Leonard Soloniuk, M.D.
Anesthesiologist, Redding Anesthesia Associates, Redding, California

Regina K. Stuart, M.D.
Clinical Fellow in Surgery, Harvard Medical School; Chief Resident in Surgery, New England Deaconess Hospital, Boston

I. David Todres, M.D.
Associate Professor of Anaesthesia and Pediatrics, Harvard Medical School; Director, Neonatal and Pediatric Intensive Care, Massachusetts General Hospital, Boston

Gary J. Vorsanger, M.D., Ph.D.
Instructor in Anaesthesia, Harvard Medical School; Assistant in Anesthesia, Massachusetts General Hospital, Boston

John D. Wasnick, M.D.
Assistant Professor of Anesthesiology, Cornell University Medical College; Assistant Attending Anesthesiologist, The New York Hospital, New York

James Welch, B.S., C.C.E.
Vice President of Engineering, Protocol Systems Inc., Beaverton, Oregon

David Y. Williams, M.D., F.F.A.R.C.S.
Instructor in Anaesthesia, Harvard Medical School; Senior Clinical Fellow, Department of Anesthesia, Massachusetts General Hospital, Boston

Preface

The second edition of *Postoperative Critical Care of the Massachusetts General Hospital* continues the mission undertaken in the original version. Our purpose is to provide a guide to which the neophyte intensivist can readily refer. This is a handbook, designed to be used in the intensive care unit at all hours of the day and night.

This second edition updates appropriate topics and covers some new ground as well. Like the first edition, this manual is neither a cookbook of critical care medicine nor an exhaustive, annotated tome.

We hope this new edition will be used by students, residents, and attendings alike as a resource to assist in, but not to replace, the complex decision processes in postoperative critical care medicine.

The authors of these chapters have, in one way or another, spent all or part of their training within the Harvard Medical School system, mostly at the Massachusetts General Hospital. Now practitioners and faculty, the contributors have written on subjects of their subspeciality interests.

W.J.H.
J.D.W.

Acknowledgments

This second edition of *Postoperative Critical Care of the Massachusetts General Hospital* would not have been possible without the continual support of Drs. Richard Kitz and Henning Pontoppidan. The editors are equally grateful to the many anesthesiologists who contributed to their educations. Finally, we would like to thank Mary Jo Dwyer for her editorial assistance as well as her outstanding effort in producing the manuscript and coordinating this three-city effort.

Postoperative Critical Care of the Massachusetts General Hospital

Notice
The indications and dosages of all drugs in this book have been recommended in the medical literature and conform to the practices of the general medical community. The medications described do not necessarily have specific approval by the Food and Drug Administration for use in the diseases and dosages for which they are recommended. The package insert for each drug should be consulted for use and dosage as approved by the FDA. Because standards for usage change, it is advisable to keep abreast of revised recommendations, particularly those concerning new drugs.

1

Airway Management

Ronald I. Goldberg
Mitchell F. Keamy

- I. Evaluation for intubation
  - A. Normal respiratory function
  - B. Endotracheal intubation
  - C. Initial evaluation
- II. Intubation
  - A. Information
    - 1. Airway anatomy
    - 2. Medication allergies
    - 3. Aspiration risk
    - 4. Cardiovascular status
    - 5. Neurologic status
    - 6. Musculoskeletal status
    - 7. Coagulation status
    - 8. Past intubation problems
  - B. Additional considerations
  - C. Intubation method
    - 1. Orotracheal intubation
    - 2. Nasotracheal intubation
    - 3. Fiberoptic intubation
    - 4. Airway support devices
  - D. Thorough preparation for intubation
    - 1. The bed
    - 2. Ventilation
    - 3. Equipment
  - E. Monitoring during intubation
  - F. Endotracheal intubation techniques
    - 1. Oral intubation
      - a. Bed height
      - b. Head position
      - c. Laryngoscopy
      - d. The vocal cords
      - e. The ETT
      - f. Visualization of the cords
      - g. Impeded visualization
      - h. Following tube placement
      - i. Securing the ETT
      - j. Portable chest radiograph
    - 2. Nasotracheal intubation
      - a. Bed height
      - b. Nasal mucosal vasoconstriction and anesthesia
      - c. Endotracheal tube size
      - d. Preparations for emergency oral intubation
      - e. Nasal passage
      - f. Tracheal insertion
    - 3. Fiberoptic intubation
      - a. Equipment
      - b. Water-soluble lubricant
      - c. Oral intubation

d. Nasal intubation
e. Alternate nasal technique
4. Other techniques
a. Tactile intubation
b. Retrograde wire-guided intubation
c. The light wand
5. Cricothyrotomy
a. Equipment
b. Technique
c. Risk of tracheal laceration
d. Needle cricothyrotomy
e. Transtracheal jet ventilation
f. Tracheostomy
6. Complications of intubation
a. Sequelae of laryngoscopy
b. Endobronchial intubation
c. Tracheal tear
d. Esophageal intubation
e. Glottic and subglottic edema or tracheal mucosal necrosis
f. Complications of nasal intubation
III. Pharmacologic aids to intubation
A. Muscle relaxants
1. Succinylcholine
2. Nondepolarizing muscle relaxants
B. Sedative-hypnotics, analgesics, and amnestics
1. Barbiturates
2. Benzodiazepines
3. Narcotics
4. Ketamine
5. Etomidate
6. Propofol
C. Topical vasoconstrictors and anesthetics
D. Nerve blocks
E. Oropharyngeal topical anesthesia
F. Intravenous lidocaine
IV. Special intubation situations
A. Full stomach, vomiting or oral bleeding
B. Increased ICP
C. Coagulopathy
D. Myocardial ischemia
E. Neck injury
F. Oropharyngeal and facial trauma
G. Emergency pediatric intubations
H. Immunocompromised patients
V. Management of the chronically instrumented airway
A. Tracheal tube designs
1. Tube materials
a. Red rubber
b. Polyvinyl chloride (PVC)
c. Silicone
d. Armored or anode
2. Cuff designs
a. High-pressure, low-compliance
b. Low-pressure, high-compliance
c. Kamman-Wilkinson
d. Lanz cuffs
e. Prestretched cuff

- B. Maintenance of ETTs
  1. Suctioning
  2. Cuff pressures
  3. Tape changes
  4. Nasotracheal tubes
- C. Endotracheal and tracheostomy tube problems
  1. Tube leaks
     a. Prior cuff manipulation
     b. Supraglottic cuff position
     c. Damaged cuff system
  2. Obstruction
- D. Endotracheal tube changes
  1. Direct vision
  2. Bronchoscopic change
  3. A long malleable stylet
  4. When changing nasal tubes
- E. Tracheostomy
  1. Advantages
  2. Disadvantages
  3. Laryngotracheal injury from endotracheal intubation
  4. Tracheostomy appliances
     a. The Pittsburgh talking tracheostomy or Communitrach
     b. Fenestrated tracheostomy tubes
     c. Jackson tracheostomy tubes
     d. Extra length tracheostomy tubes
  5. Size
  6. Management of an indwelling tracheostomy
     a. Hygiene
     b. Replacement
- F. Airway bleeding
- G. Extubation
  1. Aspiration
     a. An imperfectly protected airway
     b. Neuromuscular or CNS dysfunction
     c. Vocal cord dysfunction
     d. Indwelling tracheostomy
     e. NG tube
  2. Suspected aspiration
  3. Partial airway protection devices
     a. Fenestrated tracheostomy tubes
     b. Tracheostomy buttons
     c. Jackson metal tracheostomy tubes
  4. Extubation or decannulation

The maintenance of respiratory gas exchange is fundamental to critical care. This goal is often accomplished by the augmentation of inspired oxygen concentration, chest physical therapy (CPT), and inhalation therapy. When these measures fail, definitive airway support is required in the form of endotracheal intubation or tracheostomy, usually in conjunction with mechanical ventilatory assistance. This chapter presents indications for intubation, intubation techniques, indications for tracheostomy, and tracheostomy management.

I. Evaluation for intubation

A. Normal respiratory function requires a patent airway, adequate respiratory drive, neuromuscular competence, intact thoracic anatomy, normal lung parenchyma, the ability to defend against aspiration, and the maintenance of alveolar patency by sigh and cough.

B. Endotracheal intubation will

1. Provide relative protection against pulmonary aspiration.
2. Maintain an adequate, low-resistance conduit for respiratory gas exchange.
3. Afford a means for coupling the lungs to ventilatory support devices and aerosol therapy.
4. Establish a route for secretion clearance.

C. Initial evaluation. A systematic assessment of the need for tracheal intubation is essential. The need for intubation can be immediate (cardiac arrest), emergent (impending respiratory failure), or urgent (decreased level of consciousness with inadequate airway control).

1. **Look at the patient.** If cardiopulmonary resuscitation is underway, bag-mask ventilation with 100% oxygen, followed by intubation, is required. Otherwise, perform evaluation rapidly to determine the urgency of the need for intubation. Assessment should include

   a. **Level of consciousness.** Obtundation, stupor, or coma may be of respiratory origin (e.g., hypoxemia or hypercapnia), as well as from metabolic, pharmacologic, or neurologic causes. Depressed consciousness from any cause can lead to airway obstruction, pulmonary aspiration, atelectasis, and pneumonia.

   b. **Integument.** Cyanosis is a sign of hemoglobin desaturation. Cyanosis is present when at least 5 g per deciliter of hemoglobin is desaturated. Thus, in anemia with low oxygen saturation, cyanosis may be absent. With polycythemia, small decreases in oxygen saturation may manifest as cyanosis. Cold diaphoretic skin suggests intense autonomic stress or circulatory failure.

   c. **Respiration**

      (1) Respiratory efforts should be noted, particularly the rate and depth of thoracic movements. Slow, deep respirations (<10/min) suggest narcotic depression or central nervous system (CNS) disorder. Tachypnea (>35/min) is a nonspecific finding that can be present with disorders that cause decreased respiratory system compliance (e.g., pulmonary edema, consolidation, adult respiratory distress syndrome [ARDS]) or increased respiratory load (e.g., increased dead space, fever). It is a common finding in pulmonary embolism and with respiratory muscle fatigue.

      (2) An absent gag reflex or the inability to maintain an adequate airway in all head positions, or both, indicate the need for intubation.

      (3) Evaluate respiratory flow by placing a hand in front of the patient's mouth and nose. If flow is not present but respiratory efforts are visible, clear the airway by extending the head, opening the mouth, pulling the jaw forward, and inserting an oral or nasal airway.

(4) Examine respiratory excursions for symmetry, timing, and coordination. Side-to-side asymmetry can be caused by pneumothorax, splinting, massive unilateral atelectasis, or large bronchial obstruction. Long inspiratory time suggests upper airway or other extrathoracic obstruction; long expiratory time suggests intrathoracic obstruction, bronchospasm, or both. Auscultation over the lungs and mouth or trachea can differentiate these pathologies. Discoordinate breathing efforts, such as inward abdominal motion or intercostal retraction during inspiration, or the use of abdominal wall muscles or neck muscles suggests respiratory muscle weakness or fatigue. Long inspiratory or expiratory pauses (e.g., Biot's, Cheyne-Stokes, or apneustic breathing) are caused by brainstem or metabolic abnormalities and/or depressant drugs.

(5) Briefly auscultate the chest for presence of symmetric breath sounds and bronchospasm and for coarse rhonchi or crackles indicative of pulmonary edema or secretions.

(6) **Apply oxygen by face mask** during the examination; the potential improvement in systemic oxygenation may allow more time to evaluate the patient and consider management options.

d. By the end of this brief examination, the decision should be made regarding the need for emergent intubation.

2. If it is determined that immediate or emergent intubation is not needed, a more thorough evaluation can be performed, which includes the following:

a. **Etiology.** The etiology of respiratory failure is usually known prior to evaluation for intubation. If time permits, readily reversible causes of respiratory failure should be considered prior to intubation. For example, rapid therapy for narcotic-induced respiratory depression, residual pharmacologic neuromuscular blockade, pneumothorax, acute pulmonary edema, or airway mucous plugging may circumvent the need for intubation.

b. **Arterial blood gases** (ABGs) are the best quantitative indicator of the need for urgent or semielective endotracheal intubation.

(1) Guidelines suggesting the need for intubation and respiratory support include:

(a) PaO_2 less than 50 mm Hg on 50% oxygen by mask. It is important to determine whether the patient is receiving the specified FIO_2. If time permits, give the patient oxygen, preferably by a nonrebreathing mask, with a repeat ABG. In patients with an isolated oxygenation defect, mask continuous positive airway pressure (CPAP) may be an appropriate alternative to intubation (see Chap. 2).

(b) A pHa less than 7.32, either from respiratory acidosis or uncompensated metabolic acidosis in patients without a history of chronic lung disease. Both conditions reflect the inability of the respiratory system to maintain acid-base homeostasis. In patients with acute exacerbation of chronic lung disease, direct initial efforts at conservative therapy to avoid intubation; low-dose oxygen supplementation, bronchodilator therapy, and CPT frequently result in improvements in respiratory status. During such therapy, the physician should be in continual attendance and must be prepared to intubate emergently in the event such therapy is unsuccessful.

(2) Three important points regarding hypoventilation
   (a) Evaluate readily reversible causes for hypoventilation, such as neuromuscular blockade or narcotic-induced central depression.
   (b) Hypercapnia in the absence of acidosis or obtundation is not a specific indication for intubation or ventilation.
   (c) Interpret arterial blood gases in the light of the patient's clinical appearance and trends. In equivocal situations, sequential measurements of vital capacity (VC) can be valuable in trend monitoring and in predicting failure. A VC of greater than or equal to 15 cc per kilogram of ideal body weight is a predictor of adequate, unassisted respiratory volume exchange; a progressive decrease in VC or a VC less than 12 cc per kilogram of ideal body weight should serve to alert the clinician to impending respiratory insufficiency.

II. Intubation

A. Information is needed to intubate a patient safely. Collect this while assembling the necessary equipment.

1. **Airway anatomy.** Receding mandible (micrognathia), small oropharynx, or a short, muscular "bull" neck is associated with difficult intubation. Temporomandibular joint or cervical spine immobility can make visualization of the glottis difficult.
2. **Medication allergies**
3. **Aspiration risk:** time since last gastric intake, recent vomiting, upper gastrointestinal (GI) bleeding, bowel obstruction, or a history of esophageal reflux.
4. **Cardiovascular status:** angina-ischemia, infarction, arrhythmias, aneurysms, or hypertension.
5. **Neurologic status:** increased intracranial pressure (ICP), ischemic symptoms, or intracranial aneurysm or hemorrhage.
6. **Musculoskeletal status:** neck and mandibular immobility or instability, neuromuscular disorders, especially recent cord denervation injuries, recent crush injuries, or burns.
7. **Coagulation status:** platelet count, anticoagulant therapy, or coagulopathy.
8. **Past intubation problems,** including history of periglottic or subglottic stenosis.

B. Additional considerations

1. Injuries or deformities of the chest wall, face, head, neck or abdomen
2. Obesity or edema
3. Presence of a nasogastric (NG) tube
4. Availability of an adequate IV
5. Availability of an ECG
6. The chest radiograph

C. Intubation method. In an emergency, options are limited by the requirements for experience, expedience, and availability of specialized equipment. The most useful techniques are the following

1. **Orotracheal intubation** is performed with direct laryngoscopy.
   a. **Advantages** include ease and minimal equipment needs. It is the most familiar technique, allowing endotracheal tube (ETT) placement under direct vision.
   b. **Disadvantages.** Adequate mandible and neck mobility are necessary to allow direct visualization. Topical, regional (block), or general anesthesia is often required. It is a significant hemodynamic stress if performed with inadequate anesthesia. Emesis may occur, with risk of pulmonary aspiration of gastric contents.
2. **Nasotracheal intubation** may be performed as a blind procedure guided by breath sounds or under direct vision with laryngoscope or fiberoptic bronchoscope.

a. **Advantages.** Blind placement can be performed in a neutral head and neck position without general anesthesia or muscle paralysis. Nasotracheal intubation can be performed in the noncooperative patient. Once the tube is in place, it is more comfortable and more easily secured than an orally placed tube.

b. **Disadvantages.** Severe nasal hemorrhage can be precipitated, which may further compromise the airway. It is more difficult to place the airway quickly. Spontaneous respiration must be present to guide the tube for blind placement. Placement by direct vision with laryngoscope and Magill forceps has the same disadvantages as oral intubation. Sinusitis or otitis can occur with prolonged nasal intubation. Nasal intubation should **not** be performed in the presence of suspected nasopharyngeal injury, basilar skull fracture, coagulopathy, or immunocompromise. Tube diameter is limited by choanal size.

3. **Fiberoptic intubation** may be performed orally or nasally. Pass the ETT over the fiberoptic bronchoscope. Under visual examination, the fiberscope is placed in the glottis.

a. **Advantages.** It is useful with disordered anatomy or in patients requiring maximal head-neck stability (i.e., unstable neck fractures).

b. **Disadvantages.** More skill is required than with other techniques. Fiberoptic intubation is best performed on cooperative patients. It is not the technique of choice for emergency intubation of apneic patients. In patients with upper airway bleeding or vomiting, visualizing hypopharyngeal anatomy is difficult because of the scope's small suction channel. A large tube (8.0-mm inner diameter [ID] or larger) must be used with the standard (6-mm) bronchoscope; otherwise, a pediatric (3.7-mm) bronchoscope must be used.

4. **Airway support devices** such as oral or nasal airways do not prevent aspiration or guarantee continuing airway patency; they should be used only as a temporary measure, with close patient observation.

D. **Make thorough preparation for intubation** prior to initial attempts in all but the most urgent cases.

1. Move the **bed** away from the wall and remove the headboard to allow access to the patient from above. If the headboard is fixed, move the patient diagonally in the bed to afford access to the airway.

2. **Ventilation** should first be assisted (or maintained) with 100% oxygen by mask and hand bag (e.g., Ambu or Laerdahl) unless the pharynx is obstructed with vomitus. In the obtunded or fatiguing patient, the airway can be assisted with gentle chin lift and the mask applied tightly over the patient's nose and mouth. Positive pressure ventilation, timed to coincide with spontaneous inspiratory efforts, will aid oxygenation and carbon dioxide elimination.

3. **Equipment** required for intubation is listed in Table 1-1. Minimal equipment includes suction with Yankauer tip, a laryngoscope with an appropriate blade (usually Macintosh 3 for adults and Miller 1 for small children), and an appropriately sized ETT with stylet inserted and the cuff checked. In adults, ETT size should be chosen to maximize the internal tube diameter short of exerting excessive pressure on the tracheal wall. In adult females, a 7.5- or 8.0-mm ID ETT is recommended, and in adult males, an 8.5- or 9.0-mm ID ETT is recommended. The absence of an air leak past the ETT during positive-pressure ventilation with the cuff down indicates too tight a fit at the laryngeal or tracheal level. For an emergent intubation with full stomach, a tube 0.5 mm smaller than usual will facilitate intubation. Suggested pediatric tube sizes are listed in Table 1-2 (see also Chap. 26).

Table 1-1. Equipment list for emergency intubation

Laryngoscope with working light
Endotracheal tubes of appropriate size
Malleable metal stylet
Plastic or fiber-silicone stylet
10-ml syringe
Oxygen supply; bag and mask ventilation
Suction with Yankauer tip
Stethoscope
Functioning IV
Blood pressure cuff
Resuscitation cart
Electrocardiogram
Suction catheters
Adjuvant drugs
- Atropine
- Lidocaine (IV)
- Ephedrine, phenylephrine
- Paralytics (succinylcholine, vecuronium)
- Sedative-hypnotics (thiopental, diazepam, etomidate, narcotics)
- Topical anesthetics

Table 1-2. Pediatric endotracheal tube sizes*

Age	Size
Premature infant	2.5 mm
Term infant	3.0 mm
1–4 mo	3.5 mm
4 mo–1 yr	4.0 mm
1.5–2.0 yr	4.5 mm
2.5–3.5 yr	5.0 mm
4–6 yr	5.5 mm
7–9 yr	6.0–7.0 mm

* Tube size should be adjusted to give airway leak pressures less than 25 cm H_2O; all tubes uncuffed.

E. **Monitoring during intubation** should include continuous ECG, pulse oximetry and frequent BP measurement, preferably automated. Pulse oximetry is particularly useful as a guide to the need for return to bag-mask ventilation and the commonly available saturation-dependent pitch tone signal allows auditory assessment of O_2 saturation without the need for the intubating physician to divert his/her gaze. In full cardiac arrest, pulse oximetry can be useful as a guide to adequate perfusion and ventilation during CPR.

F. **Endotracheal intubation techniques.** Experience is recommended before attempting an intubation in the ICU without skilled assistance.

1. **Oral intubation**

   a. Adjust **bed height** to bring the patient's head to a midabdominal height. Move the patient so the head is close to the top of the bed.

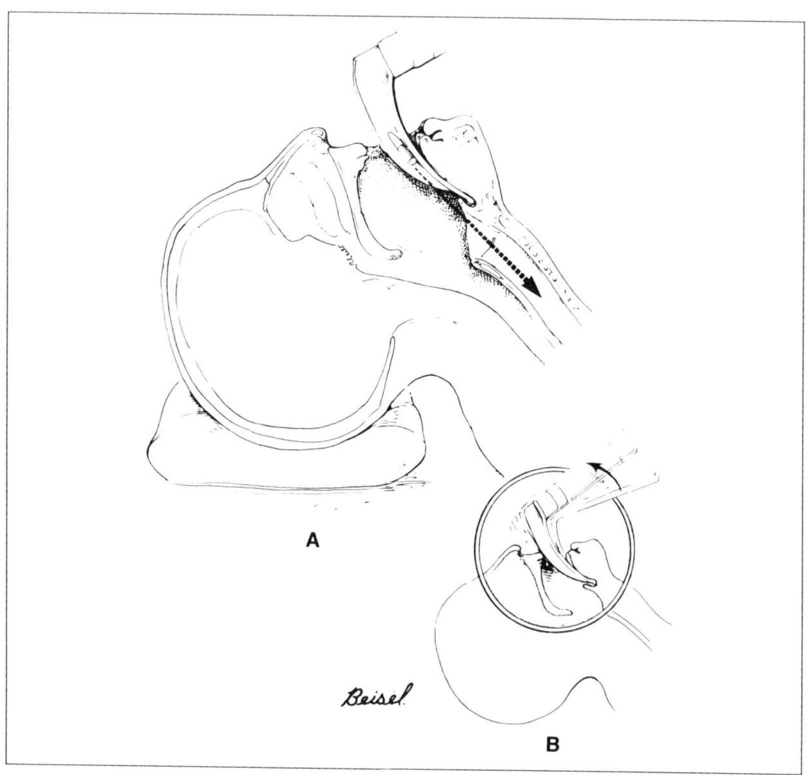

Fig. 1-1. A. For oral intubation in the absence of cervical spine injury or other serious neck pathology, the head should initially be placed in modified sniffing position, which optimizes the view of the larynx. B. Using the laryngoscope as a lever with the incisors acting as the fulcrum is improper technique.

b. **Head position.** Place the head in the "modified sniffing" position if there is no cervical spine injury or other neck pathology (Fig. 1-1). **This provides the most direct path for visualizing the larynx.**

c. **Laryngoscopy.** Hold the laryngoscope in the left hand, close to the junction of the blade and handle. Cross the right thumb and index finger, applying the thumb to the lower incisors and the index finger to the upper incisors, with an exaggeration of the finger-crossing the mouth opens. Insert the laryngoscope blade into the pharynx along with right side. Care should be taken to avoid pinching the lips between the blade and the teeth. In the adult, insert the Macintosh blade as far as possible without resistance along the curve of the anterior pharynx. Once the blade is inserted, move it anteriorly and to the midline, pushing the tongue to the patient's left and out of the field of vision. If the epiglottis and larynx are not visualized, lift the blade and handle anteriorly along the long axis of the handle, not twisted or levered (Fig. 1-2), and slowly withdraw them until the epiglottis drops into view. Then advance the blade into the vallecula and lift to expose the vocal cords and laryngeal structures (Fig. 1-2). If the cords cannot be visualized, do the following:

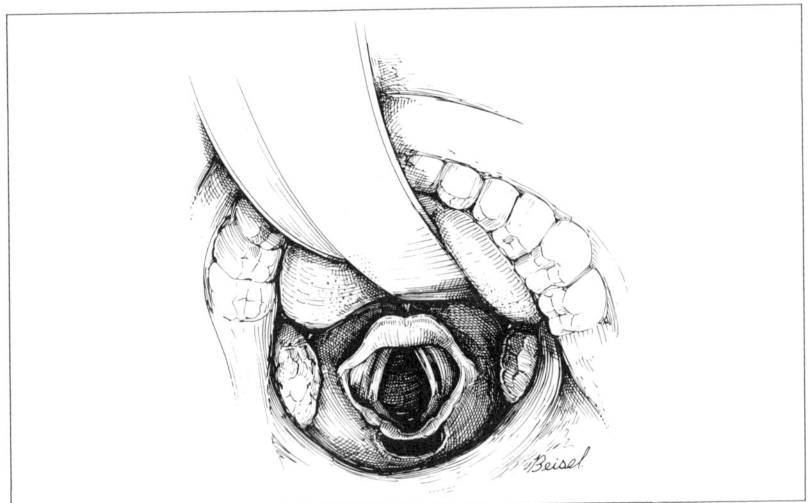

Fig. 1-2. View of the glottis by direct laryngoscopy with a Macintosh blade. Notice that the tip of the blade has been placed in the vallecula (the tip of a Miller blade is placed under the epiglottis, lifting it to view the glottis).

(1) If secondary to vomitus or foreign material, suctioning and manual extraction are required.
(2) If due to anterior position of the larynx, apply cricoid pressure or perform laryngoscopy with a straight blade.
(3) Increase head flexion to a steeply flexed position.
(4) After a 15- to 30-second intubation attempt, remove the laryngoscope, and ventilate the patient with bag and mask with cricoid pressure applied. **Do not allow hypoxemia to occur (or worsen) due to prolonged laryngoscopy in the patient who is easily mask ventilated.**

d. The **vocal cords** should be visualized prior to ETT placement. Posteriorly, the vocal cords terminate in the arytenoid cartilages; these should be visualized, along with a portion of the vocal cords. The tube should be seen to pass between the cords, anterior to the arytenoids.

e. Pass the **ETT** into the pharynx with the right hand from the right side of the mouth; it should pass without resistance through the vocal cords. Advance it until the tube cuff is seen to be beyond the vocal cords. If a stylet is in place, it should be removed by an assistant following vocal cord entry while tube position is observed.

f. If visualization of the cords or arytenoids is impossible on repeated attempts, insert a malleable stylet through the tracheal tube (without extending past the tube tip), and place a 40- to 80-degree anterior bend 2 to 3 inches from the tip of the tube ("hockey stick" configuration). This will allow passage of the tube tip along the posterior surface of the epiglottis, facilitating intubation. If the patient is breathing, amphoric breath sounds emanating from the proximal tube end suggest that the tube is being properly directed. The risk of esophageal intubation is increased if the tube is not seen to pass through the vocal cords. **Following placement,**

immediately verify ETT position by observing bilateral chest expansion and breath sounds and by noting the absence of sounds over the stomach.

g. Alternatively, if visualization of the cords is impossible with a Macintosh or straight blade, blades with a mirror (Siker) or a prism (Bellhouse) may help to view anterior structures.

h. **Following tube placement**

(1) Initially inflate the cuff with 3–5 cc of air. Adjust cuff volume once correct tube position is ensured.

(2) Fix the ETT in position by a hand resting on the face while positive-pressure breaths with 100% oxygen are attempted. Chest rise with ventilation, exhaled moisture condensation inside the tube, and bilateral breath sounds (auscultated in the axillae) should all be present. Auscultate the stomach. If tube position is uncertain despite these maneuvers, the tube should be held in position by an assistant and repeat laryngoscopy performed to confirm the position. If doubt still remains or the patient is deteriorating, remove the tube and reinstitute bag-mask ventilation prior to another intubation attempt. The only exception is full-stomach aspiration precautions, where some advocate leaving the (esophageal) tube in place with the cuff up to act as a conduit for vomitus. This is acceptable only if the tube does not interfere with repeat visualization of the cords.

(3) If the tube is advanced too far, the right mainstem bronchus will usually be selectively intubated, resulting in absence of breath sounds in the left lung field and at the right apex. Pull back the tube while ventilating and auscultating the left lung field until left breath sounds are heard.

(4) With the tube in good position, note the depth at the incisors. In adults, the usual depth is 20–23 cm. Record depth in the chart note describing the procedure.

i. **Securing the ETT** can be accomplished by a variety of techniques. The method used should be reliable and allow easy suctioning and tape changing.

j. **Obtain a portable chest radiograph** following intubation to confirm tube position and bilateral lung expansion. Neck flexion causes a 2-cm descent of the ETT tip from neutral; head extension or lateral rotation results in tube ascent of up to 2 cm. This relative mobility of tube position should be considered in evaluating tube position by chest radiograph.

2. **Nasotracheal intubation**

a. **Bed height** should be comfortable.

b. **Nasal mucosal vasoconstriction and anesthesia** are achieved with phenylephrine and lidocaine or with 4% cocaine sprayed intranasally (see **III.C**).

c. **Endotracheal tube size** is chosen (7.0–8.0 mm for adults).

d. **Preparations** are made as for emergency oral intubation (see **D**).

e. **Nasal passage** of the tube. Generously lubricate the nares and tube. Initially probe the nasopharynx with a rubber nasal airway to establish patency. Insert the ETT, applying firm, steady pressure posteriorly, aiming toward the ear. A loss of resistance marks entry into the oropharynx. An NG tube can be inserted through the tracheal tube prior to insertion to act as a guide stylet. This facilitates easy passage through the nasopharynx and may avoid tunneling of the tube into the mucosa.

f. **Tracheal insertion.** Three options are available.

(1) The laryngoscope and Magill forceps can be used to guide the tube into the trachea under direct vision. The laryngoscopic technique is the same as that used for oral intubation. Care must be taken to avoid tearing the ETT cuff with the jaws of the forceps. The forceps should be used to guide the tube direction rather than to advance the tube. An assistant should advance the tube on command as it is directed with the forceps.

(2) **Blind technique.** While listening for breath sounds at the proximal tube end, advance the tube during inspiration. A cough followed by a deep breath, condensation in the tube from exhaled moisture, and loss of voice suggest tracheal entry. Sudden loss of breath sounds suggests passage into the esophagus, piriform recess, or vallecula. Observation or palpation of the neck during tube advancement can often identify when a misdirected tube is advancing anteriorly into the vallecula or laterally into a piriform recess. Anterior flexion, extension, or lateral flexion of the neck may help to redirect the tube away from the vallecula, esophagus, or piriform recess, respectively

(3) The **Endotrol** tracheal tube (National Catheter, Argyle, NY) has a ring loop at the proximal end that, when pulled, causes anterior displacement of the tube tip away from the esophagus. It is sometimes useful for blind nasal intubation, especially when the neck cannot be manipulated.

(4) The usual distance of the tube tip from the nares is approximately 3 cm greater than from the incisors.

(5) A **fiberoptic bronchoscope** can be utilized to direct the tube into the trachea (see **3**).

3. **Fiberoptic intubation** can be performed orally or nasally, although the oral route is technically more difficult. Facility with a fiberoptic bronchoscope should be obtained prior to attempting emergency fiberoptic intubation.

a. **Equipment.** For an 8.0-mm ETT or larger, an adult (6-mm) bronchoscope is optimal. For smaller ETTs, use a pediatric (3.7-mm) bronchoscope. In addition to suction for a Yankauer tip sucker, separate wall suction for the bronchoscope port is desirable. Alternatively, oxygen may be insufflated through the bronchoscope port to blow secretions away from the lens and promote oxygenation of the patient. If oral intubation is planned, an ovassapian airway helps to protect the bronchoscope from the patient's teeth, prevent dorsal displacement of the tongue, and keep the instrument in the midline.

b. Lightly apply a **water-soluble lubricant** to the bronchoscope, and slip the chosen ETT over the scope. Pass the tube to and fro over the bronchoscope to ensure a relatively friction-free passage. If the fit is tight, select a larger tube, or apply silicone lubricant to the scope to avoid a jammed tube or damage to the scope.

c. For **oral intubation**, topical anesthesia is provided as outlined in **III**. An anticholinergic helps to dry secretions that may obscure the view. Pass the tip of the scope through the glottis under fiberoptic control, and visually maintain its intratracheal position while passing the ETT down the scope through the cords. Occasionally, the tracheal tube can be advanced to but not through the cords. This may respond to 90-degree counterclockwise rotation of the tube.

d. **Nasal intubation** can be effected in a similar manner. Anesthetize and vasoconstrict the nasal mucosa, as discussed for blind nasal

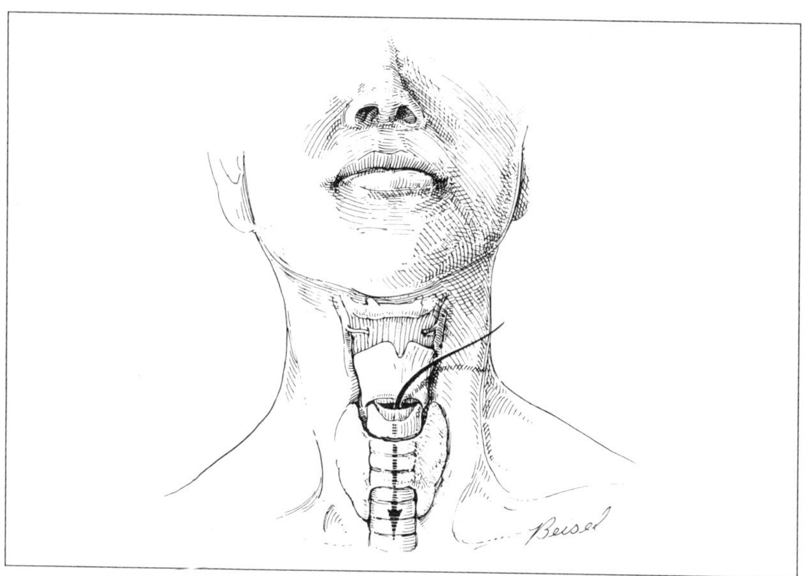

Fig. 1-3. The cricothyroid membrane is the entry point of an artificial airway during cricothyrotomy.

intubation (see **III.C, E**), and pass the scope, with ETT premounted, under direct vision through the nasopharynx into the trachea. Tongue retraction is not usually needed but is occasionally helpful. Maintain the scope's position in the trachea while an assistant passes the tube over the scope and through the nose. If difficulty is encountered passing the tube over the scope, rotate the scope 108 degrees to backflex it against its normal curvature.

e. An **alternate nasal technique** involves passage of the nasotracheal tube into the oropharynx as in the blind nasal intubation. Lubricate the scope and pass it through the tube into the pharynx. The remainder of the procedure is the same as in **d.**

4. **Other techniques** for intubation have been proposed.

   a. **Tactile intubation.** Manually palpate the epiglottis, and insert the tube under digital direction by the oral or nasal route.

   b. **Retrograde wire-guided intubation.** Place an IV catheter through the cricothyroid membrane, and pass a guide wire up into the pharynx. The wire is used as a means to pass a stiffer guide from above or is attached to the tube itself to act as a path for intubation.

   c. The **light wand** (Concept Inc., Largo, FL) is a malleable stylet with a light at the tip. Observation of the light's glow through the anterior neck helps to guide the tracheal tube into the trachea.

5. **Cricothyrotomy** is performed as an emergency procedure when the airway is compromised and intubation through the pharynx is impossible secondary to trauma or otherwise disordered anatomy.

   a. **Equipment.** Scalpel and a blunt dissecting instrument such as a Kelly clamp.

   b. **Technique.** Localize the cricothyroid notch (Fig. 1-3). Incise the skin and superficial subcutaneous tissues, and pierce the cricothyroid membrane. Expand the membrane opening bluntly or with a scalpel, and pass a small tracheostomy tube (No. 5 or No. 6) of ETT (6.0 or 6.5 mm) into the trachea.

c. Many of the commercially available devices for cricothyrotomy leave sharp blades or cannulas in the trachea. Because these devices pose the risk of tracheal laceration, their use is not recommended.

d. Alternatively, **needle cricothyrotomy** can be used quickly to provide life-saving **transtracheal jet ventilation** while other means are explored to secure the airway. A 14-g catheter-over-the-needle is used to puncture the cricothyroid membrane. An attached 10-ml syringe helps to confirm tracheal placement by aspiration of air. The catheter is directed toward the carina. Connecting the catheter to a source of 100% oxygen at 50 psi permits flows upward of 500 ml per second, sufficient for oxygenation and ventilation. Noncompliant oxygen supply tubing can be attached to the outlet of a standard wall oxygen flowmeter, which has been opened maximally to the flush position. A 1-ml syringe with the plunger removed and the top cut off is used intermittently to connect the tubing to the 14-g catheter, thus ventilating the patient. Alternatively, a side-hole cut in the tubing facilitates ventilation by intermittent occlusion of the hole with the thumb.

e. When transtracheal jet ventilation is employed, the chest should be observed to rise and fall with each jet; inadequate expiration can produce high airway pressures, leading to poor venous return and pneumothorax. Other complications of this technique are subcutaneous and mediastinal emphysema, tracheal mucosal trauma, bleeding, esophageal perforation, and arterial perforation.

f. Tracheostomy entails significant time and risk of bleeding that preclude its use as an emergency airway technique.

6. **Complications** of intubation

a. Sequelae of laryngoscopy

(1) Vomiting and pulmonary aspiration of gastric emesis can be precipitated by posterior pharyngeal stimulation with the laryngoscope blade.

(2) Laryngospasm secondary to glottic and hypopharyngeal irritation

(3) Hypertension and tachycardia may be poorly tolerated in patients with ventricular failure, tachyarrhythmias, coronary artery disease, or vascular aneurysms.

(4) Arrhythmias (bradycardia from vagal stimulation and ventricular ectopy from sympathetic stimulation)

(5) Intracranial hypertension

(6) Cervical spine or spinal cord injury

(7) Dental trauma or tooth aspiration

(8) Hypopharyngeal contusion or laceration

(9) Lip lacerations

b. Endobronchial intubation

c. Tracheal tear is more likely if a stylet is used inside the tube.

d. Esophageal intubation can produce esophageal or hypopharyngeal perforation. In addition, attempts to ventilate via an esophageally placed tube can produce gastric dilation or perforation, or both, as well as fatal anoxia if unrecognized.

e. Glottic and subglottic edema or tracheal mucosal necrosis with resulting scarring and stricture and vocal cord injury

f. Complications of nasal intubation

(1) Submucous dissection of the ETT

(2) Nasal hemorrhage

(3) Bacteremia
(4) Introduction of nasal bacteria into the lungs
(5) Sinusitis
(6) Otitis media

III. **Pharmacologic aids to intubation** include muscle relaxants, local anesthetics, amnestics, hypnotics, and analgesics (see Chap. 27).

A. **Muscle relaxants** induce complete respiratory arrest and abolish all protective airway reflexes. Because laryngoscopy and intubation can be extremely painful and distressing, **patients who are paralyzed and intubated must be obtunded or pharmacologically sedated.** The autonomic stress associated with awake paralysis and laryngoscopy can cause marked increases in ICP and exacerbate cardiovascular instability. At times, pharmacologic paralysis is required to effect emergency intubation. In these instances, **patient survival depends on rapid and skillful intubation.**

1. **Succinylcholine** is a depolarizing muscle relaxant with an onset time of 60 seconds and a clinical duration of 5–10 minutes. It is the relaxant of choice when rapid airway control is mandatory. It is not associated with significant first-dose hemodynamic changes, although repeat dosages in a short time span can cause bradycardia. Succinylcholine may cause massive potassium release in patients with large, acute burns, massive soft tissue injury, tetanus, upper and lower motor neuron disease, and muscular dystrophy. The degree of potassium release seems to correlate with the amount of muscle affected.

a. **Dose.** 1.0–1.5 mg per kilogram provides complete paralysis with rapid onset; 0.2 mg per kilogram is usually sufficient to break laryngospasm.

b. Contraindications

(1) **Burns and trauma.** No safe interval has been clearly established. Many clinicians avoid succinylcholine after 1 week postinjury and until healing is complete.

(2) **Neuromuscular disease.** The most vulnerable period for potassium release may be the first 6 months following nerve injury, or even longer in patients with progressive disease.

c. **Relative contraindications**

(1) **Peritonitis.** There exist isolated reports of hyperkalemic arrest occurring in patients with peritonitis.

(2) **Neuromuscular disease.** The most vulnerable period for potassium release may be the first 6 months following nerve injury, or even longer in patients with progressive disease.

(3) **Preexisting hyperkalemia**

(4) **Pseudocholinesterase deficiency**, either genetic or drug induced (e.g., echothiophate, neostigmine).

(5) **Penetrating eye injury.** Succinylcholine increases intraocular pressure. Its use is controversial. There are reports of safe usage especially with a defasciculating dose of a nondepolarizing relaxant (e.g., 0.05 mg/kg *d*-tubocurarine).

2. **Nondepolarizing muscle relaxants** include *d*-tubocurarine, pancuronium, metocurine, atracurium, and vecuronium. As a class, these drugs have a relatively long clinical duration of action (atracurium and vecuronium 35–45 min and the others approximately 90 min) and relatively slow onset (2–5 min with standard intubating doses). They may be useful, however, for reintubation in the patient with an airway already secured (e.g., ETT cuff leak or change from oral to nasal tube). *d*-Tubocurarine and metocurine are associated with hypotension (the former more strongly associated than the latter). Pancuronium can cause tachycardia. Metocurine and gallamine are ex-

clusively renally excreted and should not be used in anephric patients. Atracurium and vecuronium have few cardiovascular side effects. The elimination of atracurium is organ independent, and vecuronium is excreted in the bile.

a. **Intubating dosages**
   (1) Pancuronium: 0.10–0.15 mg per kilogram
   (2) *d*-tubocurarine: 0.6 mg per kilogram
   (3) Metocurine: 0.4 mg per kilogram
   (4) Atracurium: 0.4–0.5 mg per kilogram
   (5) Vecuronium: 0.10–0.15 mg per kilogram

b. **Contraindications**
   (1) Pancuronium: preexisting supraventricular tachyarrhythmias, myocardial ischemia
   (2) *d*-tubocurarine: hypotension
   (3) Metocurine: hypotension, renal failure
   (4) Atracurium: hypotension (with large dosages or rapid injection)
   (5) Vecuronium: hepatic failure

c. **Emergency intubation.** Occasionally, succinylcholine is contraindicated in situations where rapid airway control is needed. Speed of onset of nondepolarizing relaxants may be improved to 1–1.5 minutes if the intubating dose is increased (e.g., atracurium 1.5 mg/kg or vecuronium 0.25 mg/kg). The clinical duration is prolonged, and atracurium may cause hypotension with this approach. Alternatively, the usual intubating dose may be preceded by 4 minutes with a priming dose (approximately 10% of the intubating dose). It is important to evaluate the airway carefully for ease of intubation prior to administering nondepolarizing muscle relaxants.

B. **Sedative-hypnotics, analgesics, and amnestics.** These drugs are used during airway manipulation to blunt autonomic response and to obtund consciousness, pain, and recall.

1. **Barbiturates.** Sodium thiopental is the most commonly used IV barbiturate. Its brief hypnotic-amnestic action (3–4 min) is due to rapid redistribution. It is **not** analgesic but has profound vasodilatory and myocardial depressant properties that can blunt the cardiovascular stress response to intubation. In individuals who are hypovolemic or have preexisting myocardial dysfunction, sodium thiopental can cause lethal hypotension. It decreases ICP by decreasing cerebral metabolism and blood flow and has cerebral protective qualities, making it ideal as an adjunct to intubation in patients with increased ICP. The full dose for induction of anesthesia in healthy patients is 4 mg per kilogram. This dosage must be decreased (sometimes to as little as 50 mg total) depending on the cardiovascular status. Laryngospasm is easily precipitated, and the airway is unprotected (aspiration risk) with sodium thiopental administration.
2. **Benzodiazepines,** especially midazolam or diazepam, are frequently employed for IV sedation and amnesia during intubation. Onset is rapid (within 60–90 sec), and duration is brief (20–60 min) secondary to redistribution. Cardiovascular effects are minimal. For sedation, incremental doses of midazolam 0.5–1.0 mg or diazepam 2 mg may be repeated until the desired effect is achieved. The full dose for induction of anesthesia is midazolam 0.1–0.2 mg per kilogram and diazepam 0.3–0.5 mg per kilogram. As with any other cerebral depressant, aspiration risk increases as level of consciousness is blunted.
3. **Narcotics.** Fentanyl or morphine is commonly employed for analgesia, sedation, and cough suppression with intubation. Intravenous fentanyl has a rapid onset (1 min) and in usual doses (50–500 μg) has

a brief (1 h) duration of action. Intravenous morphine (2–10 mg) has a longer peak onset time (5–10 min), with a longer duration (1–3 h). Narcotics can slow the heart rate. Morphine is a venodilator and can cause hypotension in hypovolemic patients. Adjust dosages of fentanyl and morphine according to patient condition. Respiratory depression, obtundation, and blunting of protective airway reflexes are to be expected with narcotic administration.

4. **Ketamine** produces "dissociative anesthesia" by IV (1–3 mg/kg) or IM (5–8 mg/kg) administration. Pharmacologic effects include profound amnesia, analgesia, and sympathetic nervous system stimulation. Ketamine can be administered when sedation is required with hypovolemia, although in patients who are already sympathetically stressed, ketamine may cause hypotension by its direct myocardial depressive and vasodilatory properties. Ketamine increases cerebral metabolic rate and may aggravate intracranial hypertension.
5. **Etomidate** is an imidazole hypnotic agent with onset, duration, and CNS effects similar to thiopental but producing less respiratory and hemodynamic depression. Dose is 0.1–0.3 mg per kilogram IV. Etomidate may suppress adrenal function up to 2–4 hours after a single bolus.
6. **Propofol** is an alkyl phenol with sedative-hypnotic and amnestic properties. Onset of effects is similar to sodium thiopental, but recovery is faster. Cardiovascular depression is an important side effect. The full dose for induction of anesthesia in healthy patients is 1.5-2.5 mg per kilogram; infusions of 25–75 mcg/kg/min can be used to provide sedation.

C. **Topical vasoconstrictors and anesthetics.** Either cocaine or phenylephrine-lidocaine is used as a topical anesthetic and mucosal vasoconstrictor for nasal passage of ETTs. These agents are applied to the nasal mucosa using an atomizer aerosol or cotton-tipped applicators.

1. Cocaine, 4%, up to 2 mg per kilogram. It may produce systemic hypertension, tachycardia, or arrhythmias.
2. Lidocaine, 2–3%, up to 5–7 mg per kilogram, combined with phenylephrine, 0.25%. Dosage guidelines are approximate because the rate of systemic absorption is unpredictable.

D. **Nerve blocks** are performed with the amide local anesthetics (e.g., lidocaine, bupivacaine, mepivacaine). In general, these blocks diminish the ability to guard against aspiration. Do not perform the blocks in patients with coagulopathy. Commonly used blocks include the following (Cousins and Bridenbaugh, 1980; Moore, 1979):

1. Superior laryngeal nerve blocks
2. Piriform sinus block
3. Transtracheal block

E. **Oropharyngeal topical anesthesia** can be provided with viscous lidocaine or aerosol topical anesthetic sprays. It is also possible to blunt airway reflexes by topical anesthesia of the vocal cords through inhalation of aerosolized local anesthetic. Topical anesthetics in unmetered aerosol sprays pose greater risks of overdose and toxicity. In addition, topical anesthesia does little to block the pain of laryngoscopy in the muscles of the tongue.

F. **Intravenous lidocaine** may be useful to blunt the hemodynamic and intracranial hypertensive response to intubation. IV lidocaine, 1.0–1.5 mg per kilogram, should be administered when increased ICP or myocardial ischemia is of concern. It must be given 3 minutes prior to laryngoscopy to be maximally effective and has a brief duration (15 min) of action.

IV. Special intubation situations

A. **Full stomach, vomiting, or oral bleeding** increases the hazards of pulmonary aspiration during intubation. If intubation is anticipated, oral and NG tube feeding should be discontinued for 8 hours prior to intubation; however, this is seldom practical. If present, the NG tube should be placed on suction. The elective placement of an NG tube to drain the stomach prior to intubation may be effective for liquid gastric contents, but its presence is not a guarantee of an empty gastric fundus.

1. With obtundation, coma, or neuromuscular incompetence, the presence of oral foreign matter requires immediate oral intubation with laryngoscopic visualization. Suction with a Yankauer tip should be available. During intubation, estimate the severity of aspiration, and determine the pH of the suctioned material.
2. In the conscious patient, awake intubation is generally preferred unless contraindicated by cardiovascular or neurologic problems. Topical local anesthesia makes the procedure more comfortable, although its use decreases protective airway reflexes, increasing the risk of aspiration.
3. If general anesthesia must be performed, two individuals are required. The technique is similar to a rapid-sequence induction. Backup laryngoscope, tracheal tubes with malleable stylets, and suction should be available. Preoxygenation with 100% oxygen is undertaken for at least 10 breaths and IV sedation and paralysis accomplished rapidly after the placement of cricoid ring pressure (Sellick maneuver) by an assistant. Maintain cricoid pressure until breath sounds are auscultated and the ETT cuff is sealed. Use an ETT with stylet. Prior to attempting such an intubation, assess the patient's mandibular and neck anatomy. In the event of failure to accomplish intubation, ventilate the patient manually by bag mask with cricoid pressure maintained until consciousness and neuromuscular competence return.

B. **Increased ICP** (see Chap. 15). Pain or tracheal stimulation can produce a marked rise in ICP, even in comatose individuals. Intubation should be accomplished with minimal stimulation in any patient at risk for increased ICP. Several adjuncts can be used to facilitate intubation.

1. Local anesthetic block
2. General anesthesia, including barbiturates
3. Etomidate or narcotics if hemodynamic instability is present
4. Succinylcholine to obtain rapid paralysis, although its use may contribute to increases in ICP. Alternatively, in the patient who has been carefully evaluated for ease of intubation, paralysis can be obtained with a nondepolarizing relaxant (see **III.A.2**).
5. Intravenous lidocaine (1.5 mg/kg) may be administered to blunt hemodynamic response to intubation and to blunt the ICP increase induced by tracheal stimulation.

C. **Coagulopathy** or thrombocytopenia is a contraindication to nasal intubation because of the increased risk of nasal mucosal hemorrhage.

D. **Myocardial ischemia** or infarction imposes the need for a "minimal-stress" intubation. Unanesthetized intubation is usually associated with marked increases in arterial pressure and heart rate. Conversely, the anesthetic-sedative agents employed as adjuncts to intubation can result in hypotension. Either physiologic state may alter myocardial oxygen balance and threaten myocardial viability. A number of approaches are advocated for these intubations, including deep narcotic anesthesia, local anesthetic blockade of tracheal reflexes, and light anesthesia with the addition of sympathetic blockade and vasodilators. A full stomach and the potential risk of aspiration make the situation even more complex; clinical judgment must dictate the balance between the need for rapid intubation and the desirability of a gradual, nonstressful intubation sequence. Respiratory failure also represents a stress to the heart, and in the case of a patient with rapidly deteriorating respiratory function, intubation must not be inordinately delayed.

E. **Neck injury** with potentially unstable cervical vertebrae presents the risk of precipitating or aggravating spinal cord damage during intubation. Maintain a neutral head-neck-thorax relationship during intubation in all but the most dire emergencies. During a cardiac or respiratory arrest, the oral route for intubation is preferred and can often be accomplished with minimal neck movement. During intubation, a second experienced individual provides light traction (10–15 lbs) on the occiput, while carefully observing the head and neck for motion. Flexion and anterior head motion pose the greatest risks for cord injury. Extension is less of a hazard but should be minimized. If the intubation is difficult or the pharyngeal and vocal cord anatomy is not easily visualized, progressing to cricothyrotomy is prudent. In less emergent circumstances, nasal intubation, either blind or with fiberoptic guidance, is preferred. If available, fiberoptic stylet–guided oral intubation is a reasonable alternative.

F. **Oropharyngeal and facial trauma.** If any question of cranial vault disruption exists, the nasal route should be avoided for all catheters due to the risk of inadvertent penetration into the brain. In the case of a massively disrupted face, an immediate cricothyrotomy may otherwise be attempted, with adequate suction available. **Neuromuscular blockade should not be used due to the risk of losing remaining airway integrity and the danger of aspiration.**

G. **Emergency pediatric intubations** (see Chap. 26). Children are less cooperative than adults, making certain techniques (e.g., awake bronchoscopy or laryngoscopy) difficult. More rapid arterial oxygen desaturation occurs with apnea in children than in adults. In addition, the tracheal cartilage in prepubertal individuals is not fully developed, predisposing them to tracheal malacia and stenosis. Cuffed ETTs are usually avoided because the cuff material requires a smaller tube size in already narrow airways and because of the risk of tracheal damage from overdistention of the trachea. Tubes placed in pediatric patients should have a leak of air regurgitating back around the tube into the pharynx with positive-pressure ventilation. A leak at 15–25 cm H_2O of positive airway pressure is optimal. A greater leak makes ventilation more difficult, and a lesser leak is likely to cause tracheal edema on extubation and to increase the risk of tracheal damage.

H. **Immunocompromised patients** require intubation with a technique that will minimize tracheal soiling. Aspiration is disastrous in this population, and nasal intubation should be avoided because of the risks of sinusitis and airway contamination with nasopharyngeal pathogens. Perform intubation under direct vision, with care taken to avoid contact of the tube with the oral mucosa prior to passage through the cords.

V. **Management of the chronically instrumented airway**

A. **Tracheal tube designs.** Variation exists in tube material and cuff design.

1. **Tube materials**

a. **Red rubber** tubes are nondisposable and are relatively rigid, usually with a high-pressure cuff. They are not used in the ICU.

b. **Polyvinyl chloride (PVC)** tubes are disposable, flexible, and transparent and are the current standard tube. They can kink or occlude with compression (e.g., biting) or with acute bends.

c. **Silicone** is softer than PVC and more likely to kink.

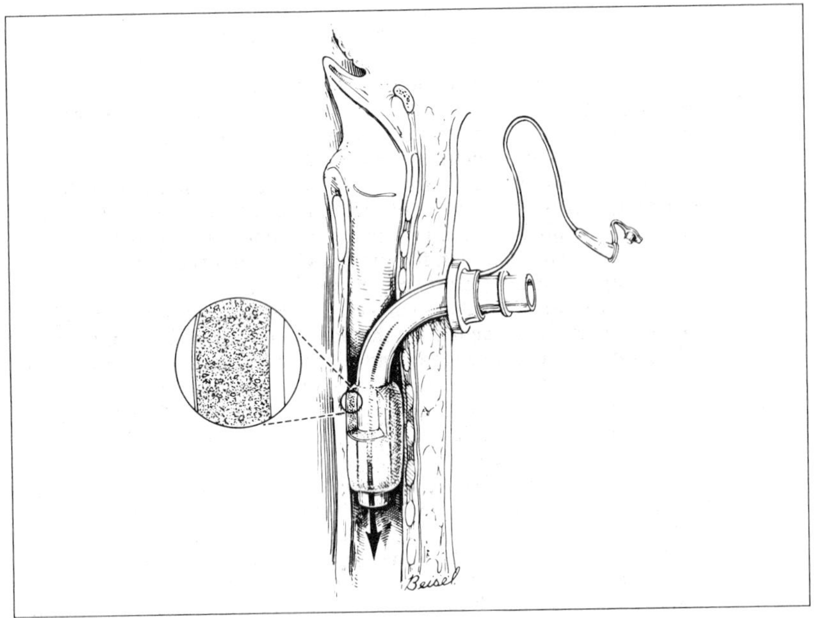

Fig. 1-4. Kamman-Wilkinson tube (Bivona, Fome Cuff).

d. **Armored or anode** tubes are metal-coiled tubes with a rubber, silicone, or PVC coating. They are less likely to kink in situ but are floppier than PVC, requiring a stylet for placement. They are expensive.

2. **Cuff designs**
   a. **High-pressure, low-compliance** cuffs are mounted on red rubber tubes and can produce tracheal damage.
   b. **Low-pressure, high-compliance** cuffs are found on standard disposable ETTs. They present a high surface area for tracheal contact at relatively low pressures to preserve tracheal mucosal blood flow.
   c. **Kamman-Wilkinson** tubes, which have a foam-filled cuff, are employed in patients with tracheal dilatation or those requiring excessive cuff pressure to seal (Fig. 1-4). **The cuff is deflated for insertion** and allowed to inflate passively in the trachea, the cuff then being left open to air. The air is aspirated from the cuff periodically; a minimal cuff volume is required to ensure acceptable lateral wall pressures. If air is inserted into the cuff, the tube takes on the characteristics of the standard high-compliance tube.
   d. **Lanz cuffs** have a balloon-with-a-shield pilot system to buffer the cuff pressure. The pilot system has a thick plastic guard for a highly compliant inner balloon that distends with pressures above 28 cm H_2O, relieving high tracheal cuff pressure. The tracheal cuff characteristics are similar to the standard low-pressure, high-compliance cuffs found on other disposable tubes. In patients with high airway pressures, creating a tracheal seal during positive-pressure ventilation can be difficult.
   e. A **prestretched** cuff can be made by inflating a Portex tracheal

tube cuff with 50 cc of air while it is submerged in warm water. It is cooled in tapwater while still inflated. This produces a very high-volume, high-compliance, low-pressure cuff. The risk of tube obstruction secondary to cuff evagination over the tip must be consid-
Maintenance of **ETTs**

1. **Suctioning.** The pharynx and trachea require frequent suctioning in intubated patients. (Tracheal suctioning is described in Chap. 2.)
2. **Cuff pressures.** Maintain pressures in the tracheal tube cuff at 25 cm H_2O or less. If higher cuff pressures are required, changing the tube to a foam-cuffed tube should be considered.
3. **Tape changes.** Reapply the tape used to secure the tube at regular intervals. In the case of an oral tube, change the tube position from one side of the mouth to the other, being careful not to apply excessive pressure on the corner of the mouth. In addition, take care to avoid pinching the lips between the tape and the tube.
4. Periodically assess **nasotracheal tubes** for sinusitis, otitis media, and necrosis of the nares.

C. **Promptly evaluate endotracheal and tracheostomy tube problems.** The problems usually take the form of gas leaks on ventilation, with obstruction to ventilatory gas flow occurring less commonly but more urgently.

1. **Tube leaks** manifest as a loss of delivered tidal volume, usually with an audible pharyngeal leak on mechanical inspiration. Commence evaluation with an assessment of respiration adequacy by chest auscultation and observation during manual ventilation with 100% oxygen. This allows rapid diagnosis of mechanical obstruction to gas flow or massive leak, in which case urgent reintubation may be required. If positive pressure ventilation or positive end-expiratory pressure (PEEP) is required, temporarily seal the trachea by placing a posterior pharyngeal pack under direct vision. The usual causes of tube leaks include the following:
   a. **Prior cuff manipulation.** Be sure that the cuff has not been inadvertently left in the deflated state.
   b. **Supraglottic cuff position.** A cuff that holds air but does not seal the airway or seals only with large air volumes (>10–20 cc) may be above the vocal cords. Positioning can be evaluated by chest radiograph, laryngoscopic examination, or asking the patient to talk. Deflate the cuff and advance the tube. Then confirm intratracheal placement.
   c. **Damaged cuff system**
      (1) The inability of the cuff system to hold any air is an indication, in most instances, for tube replacement. Temporary seal can be obtained by packing the hypopharynx, thereby allowing time for careful preparation.
      (2) A slow leak from the cuff can be managed more deliberately. Usual leak sites are
         (a) **The self-sealing valve.** This leak can be diagnosed and managed by inserting a three-way stopcock into the valve, inflating the cuff, and closing the system with the stopcock. Alternately, the cuff tubing can be clamped ahead of the valve.
         (b) **The seal between pilot balloon and small-bore inflation tubing.** This leak can be diagnosed and managed by cutting off the pilot balloon, inserting a small-bore catheter (e.g., 20- or 22-gauge) or blunt needle into the inflation tubing, and using a three-way stopcock to open and close the system.

(c) **The cuff or cuff-tube seal.** This leak is assumed when the pilot balloon tubing is intact as demonstrated by continued leak despite the maneuvers in (**a**), (**b**). In this case, the tube must be changed.

(d) **Tracheal dilation.** This leak is best evaluated with a chest radiograph that is compared to old films. The inflated cuff provides a tissue-air interface that usually allows radiographic evaluation of tracheal widening. Tracheal dilation precedes tracheomalacia, which can produce chronic respiratory problems. It is best managed by changing to a low-pressure distensible appliance, such as a Kamman-Wilkinson foam cuff tube or a prestretched Portex tube, which offers less lateral distending pressure to the trachea while simultaneously filling a larger volume.

2. **Obstruction** (see Chap. 2). Airway appliance obstruction is an emergency, recognized early as ventilator overpressure ("pop-off"). In patients with intact respiratory drive and strength, it is often difficult to distinguish among severe bronchospasm, the patient's "fighting" the ventilator, and airway occlusion. As with any other emergency, quickly evaluate the airway, accomplished most conveniently by hand-bagging with simultaneous auscultation. The inability to ventilate should immediately prompt passage of a suction catheter to probe the tube for patency. If an obstruction is present, it will be obvious and should prompt an immediate tube change.

D. **Endotracheal tube changes** are indicated for mechanical tube failure, local infection, or tissue damage from the tube. The goal during ETT change is the maintenance of a secure airway during the entire procedure. If feasible, the stomach should be emptied prior to a tube change. A number of techniques have been utilized; the most common follow.

1. **Direct vision.** The tube is changed with laryngoscopy. Following preoxygenation, appropriate sedation, and analgesia, laryngoscopy is performed with an assistant's maintaining the position of the old tube. Continue mechanical ventilation during this maneuver. If patient resistance or muscle tone hinders adequate visualization, administer a muscle relaxant, although if tube position is lost, subsequent risk increases. Visualize the tube to be replaced as it passes through the vocal cords. Bring the tip of the new ETT to the epiglottis, and position it next to the old tube. Following adequate suctioning, the assistant deflates the cuff on the old tube and removes it, with immediate placement of the new tube into the trachea. The procedure should be performed without losing sight of the vocal cords.

2. **Bronchoscopic change.** A bronchoscope, preferably 3.7 mm (pediatric), is used. Pass the new tube over the scope to the handle, and, using standard technique, place the scope tip at the cords. After visually ascertaining that the pharynx and supraglottic are suctioned clear, an assistant deflates the cuff on the indwelling tube, and the scope is advanced through the larynx beside that tube, until tracheal mucosa and cartilages are clearly visualized. While the endoscopist maintains intratracheal visualization of the scope position, the assistant slowly withdraws the old scope, and the new tube is advanced over the scope into the trachea. Prior to removing the old tube, slide the new tube almost to the scope tip in order to ensure its free passage over the scope and into the trachea. This technique is particularly well suited for patients in whom direct laryngoscopy would be contraindicated or technically difficult.

3. **A long malleable stylet,** such as an NG tube or any of a number of other commercially available devices, can be used to perform blind tube changes. Pass the stylet through the tube already in place and

remove the tube, being careful not to dislodge the stylet. Then slip the new tube into position over the guide. This technique allows tube change when visualization is impossible.

4. **When changing nasal tubes,** change to an oral tube as an intermediate step rather than attempt a bilateral nasal tube placement.

E. **Tracheostomy.** Elective tracheostomy is performed in the operating theater.

1. **Advantages** of tracheostomy over nasal or oral intubation
   a. More comfortable
   b. Eliminates the risk of direct laryngeal damage and dysfunction (see **3**)
   c. Allows more thorough mouth care, which may decrease pulmonary infection risk by decreasing mouth flora
   d. Allows phonation with special appliances or ventilation techniques that allow a deflated cuff
2. **Disadvantages** of tracheostomy
   a. Loss of tracheostomy tube position prior to tract maturation (4–14 d) can result in a fatal airway loss.
   b. The neck becomes relatively unavailable for venous access due to the contamination risk from secretions.
   c. Erosion into neighboring vascular structures can occur with life-threatening hemorrhage.
   d. Stenosis at the tracheostomy site can occur.
   e. The tracheostomy site can become infected and secondarily infect nearby open skin areas. This is especially problematic in burn patients or after recent midline sternotomy.
   f. Tracheoesophageal fistula formation, especially with chronic indwelling NG tube
3. **Laryngotracheal injury from endotracheal intubation** and ascertaining the appropriate time for conversion from ETT to tracheostomy is a controversial issue. There is evidence, although it has not been universally confirmed, that incidence and severity of glottic damage are related to duration of intubation.
   a. The most common acute sequela to long-term (>24 h) endotracheal intubation is stridor, usually secondary to periarytenoid edema, which compromises abduction of the cords. The incidence is 1–6%, depending on the series and the duration of intubation. In addition, bowing of the cords and transient incompetence of adduction can lead to postextubation aspiration, especially in the first day postextubation (see **G.1.c**). Postextubation hoarseness is almost universal and may be of long duration.
   b. Chronic complications include encroachment of granulation tissue into the airway, intercord scarring, and stenosis at the level of the cords and the cuff site. The incidence of chronic complications is reported at 0–11%.
   c. Elective tracheostomy should be considered after 5–10 days of chronic intubation, although given the unpredictability of ETT-related damage, it should be delayed if weaning and extubation appear imminent.
4. **Tracheostomy appliances.** In addition to the usual appliances and styles discussed in **A**, a number of special devices are commercially available.
   a. The Pittsburgh **talking tracheostomy** or Communitrach (Fig. 1-5). A separate lumen for retrograde gas flow through the glottis and pharynx is provided just proximal to the tracheal cuff. This lumen has a fingertip control and, when connected to a 10–12 liter gas-flow source, allows phonation.

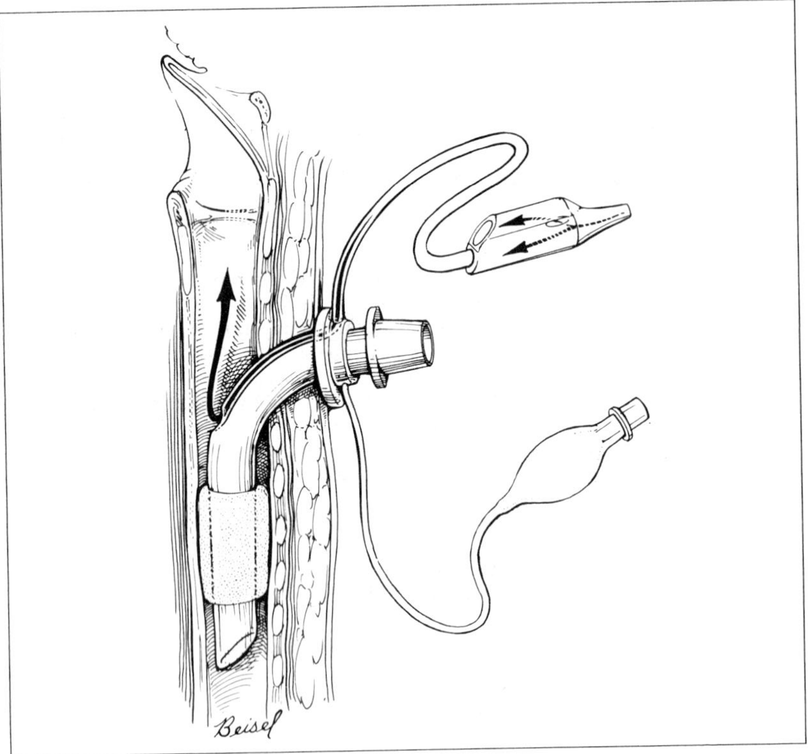

Fig. 1-5. Talking tracheostomy.

b. **Fenestrated tracheostomy** tubes (Fig. 1-6) are employed during weaning (see **G.3**). The fenestration, or window, in the tube allows gas flow from the trachea through the pharynx. The tubes are available with or without an inflatable cuff.

c. **Jackson tracheostomy** tubes are metal, with an inner cannula and no cuff. They are occasionally used following ventilator weaning as an intermediate step in the decannulation process (see **G.3**).

d. **Extra-length tracheostomy** tubes are available from a number of manufacturers for use in obese patients or those with massive edema. For the most extreme cases, a fastening flange is available that attaches to various-sized ETTs and provides a fixation point at the neck. Tube length can be adjustable to as much as the full length of the tube.

5. **Size** designations of tracheostomy tubes and ETTs vary, depending on the style (Table 1-3).

6. **Management of an indwelling tracheostomy**

a. **Hygiene.** Clean the tracheostomy site daily with a cotton swab moistened in diluted peroxide. Subsequently, rinse the site with saline. Change tracheostomy tapes when they are dirty. For tubes with an inner cannula, remove and clean the cannula daily.

b. **Replacement**

(1) **Changing an "immature" tracheostomy tube.** Do not perform tracheostomy tube changes in a stoma less than 5–7 days

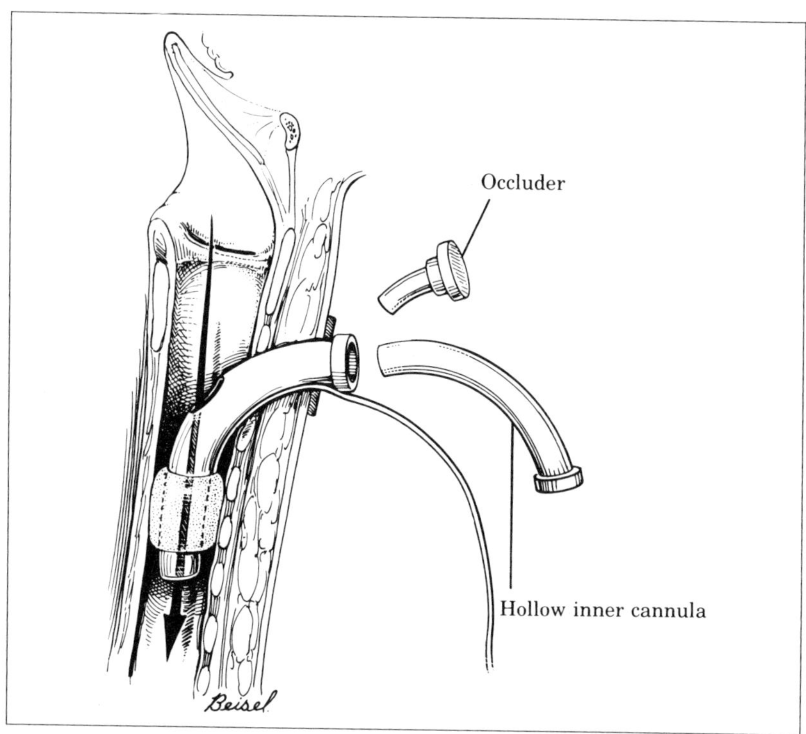

Fig. 1-6. Fenestrated tracheostomy tube. With the cuff inflated and the long, hollow inner cannula in place, function is similar to a standard cuffed tracheostomy tube. With the inner cannula removed, the cuff deflated, and the occluder in place, gas flow is routed through the glottis and pharynx.

old. If an earlier tube change is required, change the tracheostomy tube over a malleable stylet or Foley catheter. Prior to such a tube change, however, make full preparation for emergency oral intubation; the surgeon who performed the tracheostomy should be present. If inadvertent decannulation occurs and there is no clear tract to reinsert the tube, intubate the patient orally. The stoma tract can then be carefully reestablished with the airway secure.

(2) **Routine tracheostomy tube changes** should be done weekly or bimonthly to ensure appliance mobility, cleanliness, and function.

(a) Suction the patient and clean the tracheostomy site.

(b) Administer 100% oxygen.

(c) Have emergency airway equipment readily available.

(d) Perform the procedure with sterile technique. Check the appliance to be inserted for completeness and cuff integrity. Tracheostomy tubes are provided with obturators to present a smooth surface for insertion; these obturators should be in place.

(e) Evaluate breath sounds and air flow following placement, suction the airway, and obtain a chest radiograph.

Table 1-3. Size designations of tracheostomy and endotracheal tubes

ETT (ID mm)	Jackson tracheostomy tube no.	Olympic button size (OD mm)*	French size	Suction catheter size (French)
2.5	00		13	4
3.0	0		15	6
3.5	1		16.5	8
4.0	2		18	
4.5			21	
5.0	3	9		10
5.5	4	9	24	
6.0			27	
6.5	5	10		12
7.0	6		30	14
7.5		11	33	
8.0	7			
8.5	8	12	36	
9.0	9	13	39	
9.5				
10.0	10	14	42	

*OD = outer diameter.

(f) The airway mucosa can be anesthetized with 3 or 4 ml of 2% lidocaine sprayed into the airway for tracheostomy tube changes in the coughing patient with a reactive airway.

F. Airway bleeding. Suctioning of blood from the airway requires prompt evaluation. Most commonly, this bleeding represents mucosal erosion from the repeated trauma of suctioning. Fiberoptic bronchoscopy is the most direct means of assessment; if the source is not obvious, pull back the tube with the bronchoscope in place to view the trachea underlying the cuff. If, after examination, any doubt remains as to the etiology of persistent bleeding, obtain a repeat examination by an ears, nose, and throat consultant. With tracheostomy, the risk of erosion into mediastinal blood vessels exists. If this occurs, exsanguination or suffocation can result. If bleeding continues and is of sufficient quantity, there is a risk of clotting within the ETT and airway obstruction. If bleeding is not significant and suctioning is not mandatory, a period of healing without irritation is warranted; unfortunately, this is seldom the case. Another alternative is to attempt to advance the tube past the area of erosion; in the case of tracheostomy, a long (or adjustable) tracheostomy tube can be employed.

G. Extubation. Following a period of respiratory stability, a decision is made that the patient is ready for extubation or, in the case of tracheostomy, decannulation. The original indications for airway support should have resolved. The patient should be able to oxygenate adequately, ventilate, clear secretions, and protect the lungs from aspiration.

1. Aspiration can occur at any time due to the following:
   a. An **imperfectly protected airway.** Aspiration can occur despite an indwelling cuffed tracheal tube.
   b. **Neuromuscular or CNS dysfunction.** An adequate gag should be present, and the VC should be adequate (>15 cc/kg ideal body weight) to cough effectively. Airway protection should be main-

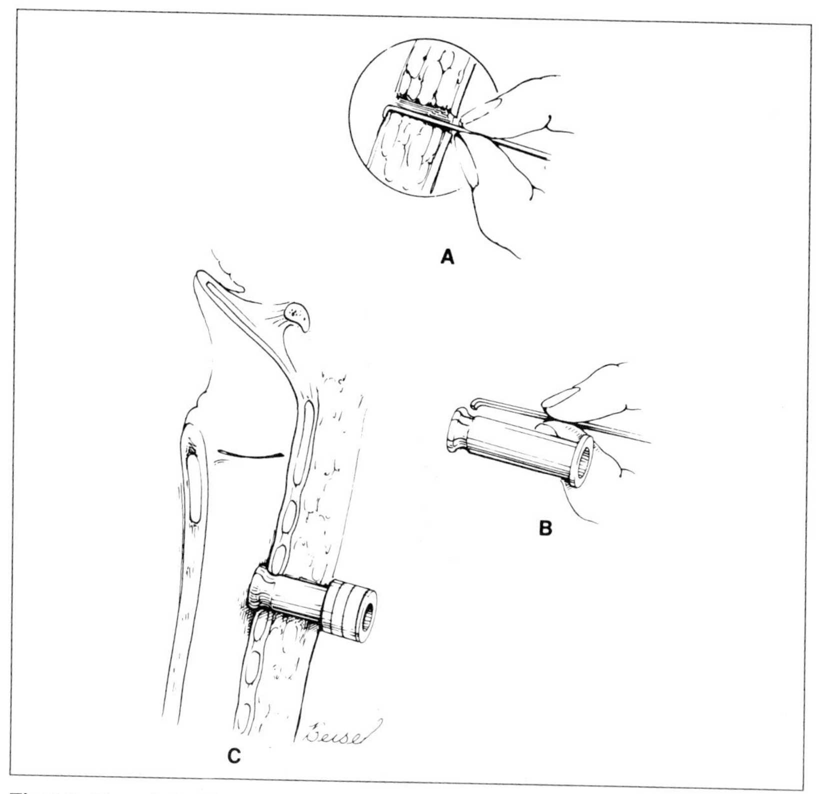

Fig. 1-7. Olympic tracheostomy button. A. A sterile pipe cleaner is used to measure the distance from the anterior tracheal wall to the skin. B. This distance is measured on the tracheostomy button. C. Spacers are placed to ensure a firm fit.

tained until these problems resolve. With depressed mentation, it is important to assess the ability to maintain airway patency postextubation. Airway obstruction provoked by flexing the patient's neck and head indicates the need for continued airway support. However, the opposite does not hold; maintenance of the airway on flexion does not ensure continued patency or adequate aspiration defense.

c. **Vocal cord dysfunction** secondary to prolonged oral-nasal intubation. Frequently such dysfunction resolves over days to weeks after extubation. Approaches to this problem include the following:
   (1) Performance of a tracheostomy, leaving a cuffed tracheostomy tube in place (to prevent aspiration) until cord function returns
   (2) Extubation, leaving the patient NPO, with enteral or parenteral feeding until the patient is no longer at risk. If the patient is fed enterally, the tube must be located in the duodenum to guard against reflux and aspiration.

d. **Indwelling tracheostomy** can cause aspiration by mechanically interfering with coordinated swallowing. Approaches to this problem include the following:
   (1) Insert a tracheostomy button, followed by serial assessment of swallowing with methylene blue tests (see **2.d**)

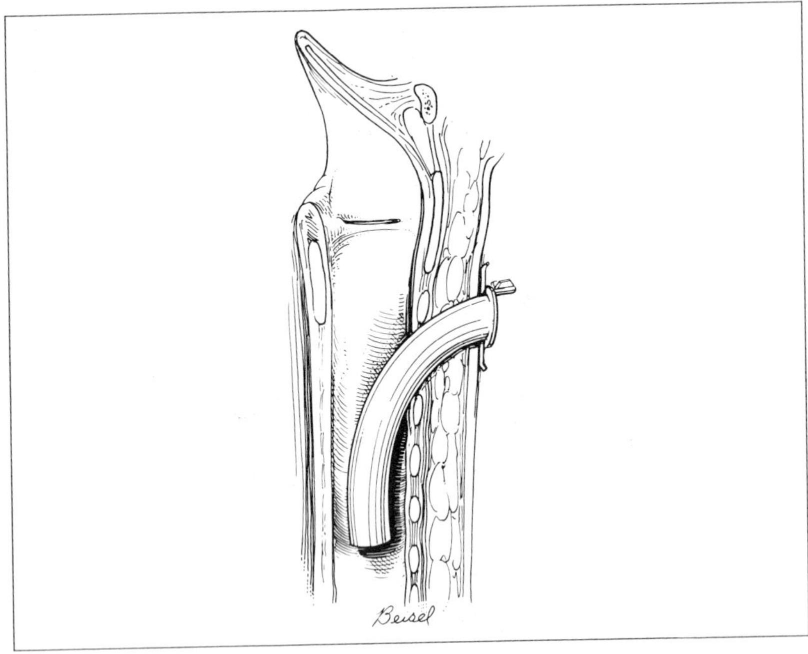

Fig. 1-8. Jackson metal tracheostomy tube.

(2) Decannulate the patient and keep him or her NPO, using enteral tube or parenteral feeding until swallowing function returns. If adequate swallowing does not return, the patient may have to undergo tracheostomy again.

e. An **NG tube** can produce pharyngeal discoordination.

2. Aspiration should be suspected in these cases:
   a. Persistent lobar infiltrates are present.
   b. Paroxysms of coughing, hypoxemia, or bronchospasm occur, especially with oral intake.
   c. Suspicious (gastric-appearing) secretions are suctioned from the tracheal tube.
   d. The **methylene blue** test is positive. It is performed as follows: Feedings (usually liquids) are tinted with methylene blue (0.5 ml in 10.0 ml of fluid provides intense color). If an airway tube is present, its cuff is deflated. If blue material is suctioned from the tracheal tube following ingestion, the test is positive. Alternately, brightly colored food (e.g., grape juice) can be used. Occasionally the test will be positive with swallowed liquids and negative for semisolids.
3. If recurrent suctioning, intermittent ventilation, or airway protection while eating is required, the following appliances can be used to provide partial airway protection as the patient progresses:
   a. **Fenestrated tracheostomy tubes** (Fig. 1-6) allow breathing through the tracheostomy or the natural airway.
      (1) With the cuff inflated and the inner cannula in place, tube function is similar to a standard tracheostomy tube.

(2) With the inner cannula removed and the tube occluded, gas flow is routed through the fenestration to the glottis and pharynx. **The cuff must be deflated when the tube is occluded** to avoid total airway obstruction should the fenestration shift in the trachea or obstruct.

b. **Tracheostomy buttons** (Fig. 1-7) are employed to maintain a stoma without an appliance occupying the airway.

(1) A standard intermittent positive-pressure breathing adapter is provided with the button to provide a stoma for suctioning or emergency ventilation (although retrograde pharyngeal flow will occur).

(2) Fasten the button with tracheostomy tape in a fashion similar to a tracheostomy tube.

(3) Rotate the button in place every day.

c. **Jackson metal tracheostomy tubes** (Fig. 1-8) have no cuff and can be utilized, gradually decreasing tube size until decannulation is feasible. Fenestrated metal tubes can also be used.

4. Extubation or decannulation should be preceded by oxygen administration and suctioning of the airway and mouth. Humidified mask oxygen should be available. Hold gastric feeding for 8 hours prior to extubation.

a. An ETT should be removed during exhalation. Alternatively, the patient can be given a positive-pressure breath as the tube is removed. Provide mask oxygen, and assess the patient for upper airway obstruction. If obstruction occurs, it can be due to laryngospasm, laryngeal edema, or glottic injury. If stridor occurs, administer racemic epinephrine by aerosol, and prepare in advance to reintubate if acute deterioration occurs. Place the patient head up (i.e., Fowler's position), and administer mist-humidified oxygen.

b. Remove a tracheostomy or tracheostomy button in similar fashion during exhalation. Place a dry, sterile gauze pad over the stoma, which spontaneously closes over days. Provide oxygen, and assess the patient for airway obstruction.

c. After prolonged intubation, closely observe the patient for signs of aspiration (see **2**).

Selected References

Bellhouse, C. P. An angulated laryngoscope for routine and difficult tracheal intubation. *Anesthesiology* 69:126, 1988.

Benumof, J. L., and Scheller, M. S. The importance of transtracheal jet ventilation in the management of the difficult airway. *Anesthesiology* 71:769, 1989.

Bishop, M. J., Weymuller, E. A., Jr., and Fink, B. R. Laryngeal effects of prolonged intubation. *Anesth. Analg.* 63:335, 1984.

Caldwell, S. L., and Sullivan, K. N. Artificial airways. In G. C. Burton and J. E. Hodgkin (eds.), *Respiratory Care: A Guide to Clinical Practice* (2nd ed.). Philadelphia: Lippincott, 1984.

Cooperman, L. H. Succinylcholine-induced hyperkalemia in neuromuscular disease. *J.A.M.A.* 213:1867, 1970.

Cousins, M. J., and Bridenbaugh, P. O. *Neural Blockade in Clinical Anesthesia and Management of Pain.* Philadelphia: Lippincott, 1980.

Dorsch, J. A., and Dorsch, S. E. Endotracheal tubes. In *Understanding Anesthesia Equipment* (2nd ed.). Baltimore: Williams & Wilkins, 1984.

Goodman, L. R. Pulmonary support and monitoring apparatus. In L. R. Goodman (ed.) *Intensive Care Radiology: Imaging of the Critically Ill.* Philadelphia: Saunders, 1983.

Greenway, R. E. Tracheostomy: Surgical problems and complications. *Int. Anesthesiol. Clin.* 19:151, 1972.
Lennon, R. L., Olson, R. A., and Gronert, G. A. Atracurium or vecuronium for rapid sequence endotracheal intubation. *Anesthesiology* 64:510, 1986.
Levinson, M. D., Scuderi, P. E., Gibson, R. L., and Comer, P. B. Emergency percutaneous transtracheal ventilation. *J. Am. Coll. Emerg. Physicians* 8:396, 1979.
Moore, D. C. *Regional Block* (4th ed.). Springfield, IL: Thomas, 1979.
Roberts, J. *Fundamentals of Tracheal Intubation.* New York: Grune & Stratton, 1983.
Stoelting, R. K. Endotracheal intubation. In R. D. Miller (ed.), *Anesthesia.* New York: Churchill Livingstone, 1981.
Weis, F. R., and Hatton, M. N. Intubation by use of the light wand: Experience in 253 patients. *J. Oral Maxillofac. Surg.* 47:577, 1989.
Whited, R. E. A prospective study of laryngotracheal sequelae in long-term intubation. *Laryngoscope* 94:367, 1984.
Wilson, R. S. Tracheostomy and tracheal reconstruction. In J. A. Kaplan (ed.), *Thoracic Anesthesia.* New York: Churchill Livingstone, 1983.

2

Postoperative Techniques of Mechanical Ventilation and Respiratory Care

Elizabeth C. Behringer

- I. Respiratory adjunct therapy
  - A. Aerosolized therapy
    - 1. Rationale
    - 2. Complications
    - 3. Modes of delivery
    - 4. Types of aerosols
      - a. Bland
      - b. Mucolytic
      - c. Racemic epinephrine (Vaponefrin)
      - d. Selective B2 sympathomimetic agonists
      - e. Anticholinergic agents
  - B. Techniques of lung expansion
    - 1. Purpose
    - 2. Techniques
      - a. Breathing exercises
      - b. Ambulation
      - c. Mask CPAP
      - d. IPPB
  - C. Techniques to improve mucociliary clearance
    - 1. Pharmacologic augmentation
    - 2. Mechanical augmentation
      - a. Chest physical therapy
      - b. Tracheal suctioning
      - c. Therapeutic bronchoscopy
- II. Oxygen therapy
  - A. Rationale
  - B. Complications
  - C. Modes of administration
    - 1. Variable performance devices
    - 2. Fixed performance devices
    - 3. Intermediate devices
- III. Mechanical ventilation
  - A. Basics
  - B. Modes of mechanical ventilation
- IV. Weaning from mechanical ventilation
  - A. Definition
  - B. Indications
  - C. General principles
  - D. Techniques
  - E. Evaluation for endotracheal extubation
  - F. Failure to wean

Pulmonary dysfunction is ubiquitous postoperatively. Patients with existing lung disease undergoing upper abdominal or thoracic surgery are clearly at risk for further deterioration of their marginal preoperative pulmonary function. Upper abdominal, thoracotomy, and median sternotomy incisions can cause significant reductions in several lung volumes and capacities, such as functional residual capacity, expiratory reserve volume, inspiratory reserve, forced vital capacity, and maximal expiratory flow. Atelectasis, impaired mucociliary clearance of secretions, hypoxemia, hypercarbia, and decreased lung compliance may ensue. This chapter reviews the postoperative techniques of respiratory care in practice at the Massachusetts General Hospital. Aerosolized therapy, techniques of lung expansion, and methods to improve mucociliary clearance are outlined. Modes of oxygen administration are reviewed as well. The final sections contain an overview of the predominant methods of mechanical ventilation and discuss methods of weaning from mechanical ventilation.

I. Respiratory adjunct therapy

A. Aerosolized therapy

1. Rationale. Postoperatively all therapeutic gases must be humidified for several reasons:

a. Normal methods of humidification, the upper airway and nasopharynx, are bypassed in patients who remain intubated or tracheostomized or who are status postlaryngectomy.

b. The systemic administration of drugs, such as atropine, with significant anticholinergic effects may cause the drying of secretions.

c. A goal of therapy is to expectorate secretions, overcoming atelectasis and preventing pneumonia. Viscous secretions are difficult to clear. Humidification of all therapeutic vapors helps to thin secretions for easier clearance.

d. Ciliary function may be depressed by the administration of dry gases.

e. Humidification adds water vapor to therapeutic gases.

(1) Humidity of inspired gases: 80–100% relative humidity for all intubated patients

(2) Temperature of inspired gases: 32–37°C

(3) Heated humidifiers allow rain out of water into ventilator tubing or the endotracheal tube (ETT) as the gases cool. Keep the humidifier and its tubing at a level below the patient to prevent water from occluding the airway.

(4) Monitor airway temperature to prevent burns to the airway.

f. Aerosolized therapy adds water particles to therapeutic gases. Particles less than 8 μg can deliver water at the level of the bronchiole.

2. Complications of aerosol use: bronchospasm; overhydration, which occurs with continuous use of the hydrosphere or the ultrasonic nebulizers; bacterial contamination.

3. Modes of delivery

a. Hand-held, metered dose inhalers

b. Intermittent positive pressure breathing devices

c. Jet nebulizers

d. Hydrosphere or Babbington nebulizer

e. Ultrasonic nebulizer

4. Types of aerosols

a. Bland. Bland aerosols serve to humidify inspired gases, hydrate mucosal surfaces, and induce the expectoration of sputum. They are inert in the therapy of respiratory tract diseases. Two types are used:

(1) Water
(2) Saline: hypotonic, isotonic, hypertonic

b. **Mucolytic.** Acetylcysteine (Mucomyst)
(1) Dose: 2–5 ml of 5–20% solution in 2 ml NS q4–8h via jet nebulizer; 1–2 ml of 10–20% solution may be instilled directly into the ETT.
(2) Purpose: Liquefies inspissated mucous plugs
(3) Side effects: Bronchospasm: it is advisable to administer in conjunction with a bronchodilator; mucosal irritation; nausea and vomiting.
(4) When administered to nonintubated patients, the drug does not reach the level of the small airways.

c. **Racemic epinephrine (Vaponefrin)**
(1) Dose: 0.5 ml of a 2.25% solution diluted in 2.5–3.5 ml NS q4–6h
(2) Purpose: A vasoconstrictor efficacious in the treatment of laryngeal edema
(3) Side effects: rebound edema; tachycardia—use caution in administering to patients with coronary artery disease.

d. **Selective B2 sympathomimetic agonists**
(1) Purpose: dilatation of bronchioles, facilitation of mucus clearance, treatment and prevention of bronchospasm
(2) Types
(a) Metaproterenol (Alupent): B2 effects predominate. Dose: 0.2–0.3 ml of 5% solution in 2–3 ml of NS q4–6h via nebulizer
(b) Albuterol (Ventolin): B2 effects predominate. Dose: 0.5 ml of the 0.5% solution in 2–3 ml of NS q6–8h via nebulizer.
(c) Isoetharine (Bronkosol): B1 and B2 effects. The routine use of this agent has fallen out of favor due to the efficacy and availability of the selective B2 agonists.

e. **Anticholinergic agents.** These agents cause bronchodilatation through a vagolytic mechanism. When administered prior to tracheal suctioning, these agents combat bradycardia and are devoid of significant systemic cardiovascular effects.
The **types** used are:
(1) Ipratropium (Atrovent): a derivative of methylatropine supplied as a metered dose inhaler. Dose: 2 puffs qid.
(2) Glycopyrrolate (Robinul). Dose: 0.4 mg in 2–3 ml of NS
(3) Atropine. Dose: 0.4 mg in 2 ml NS

B. **Techniques of lung expansion**

1. **Purpose.** The normal sigh maneuver is reproduced by any lung expansion technique. The sigh maneuver to near total lung capacity reverses microatelectasis. Thus, any lung expansion technique increases lung volume and is designed to prevent atelectasis and pneumonia. The techniques are particularly useful in patients who cannot sigh—for example, patients with upper abdominal or thoracic incisions or those with neurologic or neuromuscular disorders.
2. **Techniques**

a. **Breathing exercises**
(1) It is important to teach these to patients **preoperatively.**
(2) Exercises: diaphragmatic breathing, pursed-lip breathing, deep breathing, costal excursion exercises, sustained maximal inspiration with cough, incentive spirometry

b. **Ambulation**
(1) Immobilization of the patient serves to decrease lung volumes further and promote retention of secretions and atelectasis. Prolonged immobilization fosters venous stasis and the formation of contractures as well.

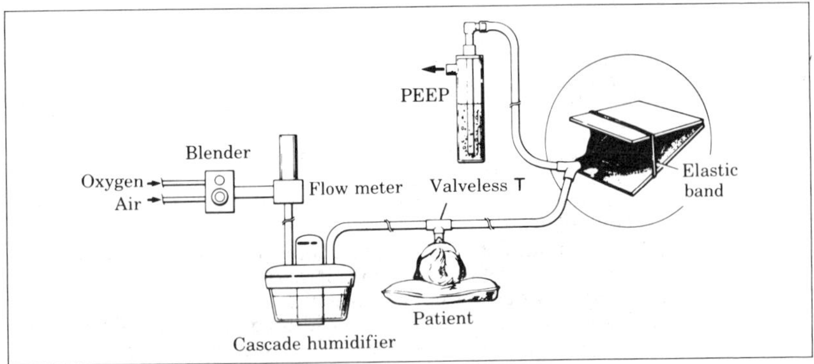

Fig. 2-1. Valveless CPAP circuit. (From M. A. Rie and R. F. Wilson. Acute Respiratory Failure. In J. Tinker and M. Rapin (eds.), *Care of the Critically Ill Patient.* New York: Springer-Verlag, 1983. P. 335. With permission.)

(2) Passive mobilization: passive range-of-motion exercises turning and changing position in bed

(3) Active mobilization: sitting in bed, dangling over the edge of the bed, out of bed to chair, walking, physical therapy. Active mobilization requires that patients be stable from a respiratory and hemodynamic standpoint. Caution must be used to avoid accidental extubation or vascular decannulation. Several medical personnel must be available to help patients with their initial attempts at active mobilization.

c. Mask CPAP (Fig. 2-1)

(1) Continuous positive airway pressure (CPAP) serves to maintain positive airway pressure throughout the respiratory cycle; it prevents and reverses airway closure, increases functional residual capacity (FRC), and aids in overcoming hypoxemia. CPAP can be used in intubated or extubated patients with low lung volumes, a state common after major abdominal or thoracic surgery or trauma **(Table 2-1).**

(2) The respiratory and hemodynamic effects of CPAP are similar to the effects of positive end-expiratory pressure (PEEP) (see **III.C**)

(3) Considerations for mask CPAP

(a) Used in extubated patients

(b) Used in awake and alert patients with intact airway reflexes

(c) Used in patients with adequate respiratory muscle strength

(d) Used in patients who are not hypercarbic

(e) Used in patients who are cardiovascularly stable

(f) Administer mask CPAP by a tight-fitting, clear mask for 10–15 min at 2–10 cm H_2O pressure q1–4h. The duration of use is limited by patient discomfort. Mask CPAP is not a substitute for endotracheal intubation. If hypoxemia progresses or hypercarbia, tachypnea, or impending acute respiratory failure exists, intubate and mechanically ventilate the patient.

(4) Complications of mask CPAP

(a) **Trauma** to the facial skin from the tight-fitting mask

(b) **Aspiration** of gastric contents. Gastric distension occurs easily. Do not use mask CPAP in patients with recent esoph-

Table 2-1. Secretion and atelectasis management continuum*

	Chest physical therapy		Humidity/aerosol	Pharmacologic aids	Aids to chest expansion	
Level of therapy	Intubated	Nonintubated	Intubated or nonintubated	Intubated or nonintubated	Intubated	Nonintubated
Basic	Large breaths Suction prn (or q2–4h) Turn q2–4h Gentle percussion-vibration q6–8h (while awake) Ambulation as tolerated	Large breaths Coughing prn Gentle percussion-vibration q6–8h (while awake) Ambulation as tolerated	Humidified therapeutic gases Systemic hydration	Bronchodilator aerosol q6–8h	CPAP 5 cm H_2O	Incentive spirometry
More vigorous	Large breaths Suction q1–2h and prn Turn q1–2h Postural drainage Vigorous percussion-vibration q2–4h Ambulation as tolerated Fiberoptic bronchoscopy	Large breaths Coughing q1–4h Turn q1–2h Postural drainage Vigorous percussion-vibration q2–4h Ambulation as tolerated Fiberoptic bronchoscopy	Heated humidification Systemic hydration USN or hydrosphere with normal saline solution q4–6h	Bronchodilator aerosol q4h Parenteral bronchodilators Acetylcystein aerosol q4–8h Acetylcysteine instillation (in ETT) q1–4h	CPAP 5–10 cm H_2O IMV + PEEP	Incentive spirometry IPPB q4–6h Facemask CPAP 2–10 cm H_2O 10–15 min q1–4h

* A number of techniques are available to manage postoperative problems with secretions, atelectasis, or both. The variable intensity with which each can be applied suggests a clinical continuum of maneuvers that can be individualized for a particular patient.

ageal or gastric surgery to avoid anastomotic breakdown. Nausea and vomiting is another complication. It is imperative that the patient have an intact mental status and protective airway reflexes. Patients with indwelling nasogastric tubes should have them suctioned prior to the institution of mask CPAP.

(5) Patients require coaching in order to accept mask CPAP. Patients with claustrophobia will not accept this method readily.

d. Intermittent positive pressure breathing (IPPB)

(1) Purpose: to provide passive lung expansion to extubated patients. A pressure-limited ventilator with a mouthpiece adapter provides 10–15 minutes of therapy.

(2) The efficacy of IPPB is questionable. Patient teaching is mandatory. IPPB against a closed glottis or in the face of decreased lung compliance is ineffective.

(3) IPPB may be useful in patients who are unable to take deep breaths. The overall efficacy of IPPB is unclear.

(4) Contraindications: recent pulmonary, tracheal, upper gastrointestinal, or esophageal surgery

(5) IPPB can be administered q4–6h in conjunction with a nebulized bronchodilator or saline. Exhaled volumes should be measured.

C. Techniques to improve mucociliary clearance. Tracheobronchial secretions are retained when the normal mechanisms for clearance are depressed. Retained secretions can elicit atelectasis and hypoxemia. Causes are depressed normal clearance mechanisms and excessive mucus production.

Patients at risk for poor clearance and excess production of mucus are smokers and asthmatics. Patients at risk for poor clearance of mucus are those with cystic fibrosis, emphysema, bronchiectasis, or viral upper respiratory infections and those undergoing general anesthesia, prolonged intubation, suction trauma, or high levels of inspired oxygen. The first technique to improve mucociliary clearance is to remove the inciting cause whenever possible.

1. Pharmacologic augmentation. Several commonly used drugs have the potential to increase mucus transport, including isoproterenol, terbutaline, epinephrine, and aminophylline. The dose range to improve mucociliary function is the same as the dose used for bronchodilatation.

2. Mechanical augmentation

a. Chest physical therapy (CPT)

(1) Purpose: To promote increased lung volumes and the clearance of secretions

(2) Indications

(a) Therapy of several acute lung diseases characterized by the inadequate clearance of secretions or low lung volumes

(b) Preventing complications in patients with a depressed level of consciousness, a depressed gag or cough reflex, obesity, quadriplegia, or chronic sputum production.

(3) **Components of CPT**

(a) Postural drainage. Mobilizes secretions with the aid of gravity. The lung segments to be drained are placed in an upright position, perpendicular to the ground. Coughing and tracheal suctioning remove secretions from the larger airways subsequently. Postural drainage is useful in postoperative patients at bed rest. Patient positioning for postural drainage may result in accidental extubation, vascular decannulation, hypoxemia, or a rise in intracranial pressure. Patients with known or suspected spinal cord or vertebral injury should be log-rolled at neurosurgeon's or orthopedic surgeon's discretion.

(b) Percussion and vibration

(i) Percussion: Performed over the affected lung segment, during inspiration as well as expiration

(ii) Vibration: Occurs over the involved lung segments during exhalation

(c) Coughing. This is an important portion of CPT in all patients. In the patient who is unable to cough and clear secretions spontaneously, other methods must be used: blind nasotracheal suctioning, pharyngeal stimulation with a catheter, or use of a minitracheostomy.

(d) Percussion, vibration, and postural drainage are most effective when performed by informed nurses and respiratory therapists. It is important to notify all involved personnel of the following:

(i) The location of the affected lung segments by physical examination or chest x ray

(ii) Complications of CPT: massive pulmonary hemorrhage, hypoxemia, causing or exacerbating preexisting rib fractures, increased intracranial pressure, exacerbation of myocardial ischemia, coagulopathies, or bronchospasm

b. Tracheal suctioning

(1) Purpose: to clear secretions mechanically

(2) Methods

(a) In intubated patients: Manually ventilate with 100% oxygen. Sterile saline may be instilled into the ETT. Insert a sterile suction catheter into the ETT to induce coughing and the clearance of sputum. Manually ventilate the patient with 100% oxygen. Repeat the sequence as needed to loosen and clear secretions.

(b) In extubated patients: Preoxygenate the patient. The following methods can be used:

(i) Blind nasotracheal suctioning. This technique is performed by well-trained personnel. Frequent blind nasotracheal suctioning indicates that the patient requires further ICU care and should be evaluated for reintubation or minitracheostomy and a source of increased sputum production.

(ii) Minitracheostomy is a 4.0 cuffless ET tube that is placed by a trained surgeon. Minitracheostomies are placed by making a horizontal incision with a guarded scalpel through the cricoid membrane. The minitracheostomy is placed over a stylet and secured. Minitracheostomies help to clear secretions in patients with present but ineffectual coughs and the presence of a mild to moderate amount of secretions. **Minitracheostomies do not replace reintubation.** If the amount of secretions causes hypoxia, hypercarbia, tachypnea, and signs of respiratory distress, intubate the patient. Minitracheostomies are contraindicated in patients who do not consent to the procedure or have a coagulopathy or difficult airway anatomy. Complications include the need for urgent reintubation, airway bleeding, pretracheal placement, and laryngospasm.

(c) Precautions. Any form of tracheal suctioning can cause hypoxia, arrhythmias, vomiting, increased intracranial pressure, airway trauma, or bacterial contamination of the airway.

c. **Therapeutic bronchoscopy.** The fiberoptic bronchoscope (FOB) is useful in the diagnosis and therapy of a myriad of pulmonary disorders. It can be used to visualize affected lung segments, as well as remove secretions throughout the suction channel and collect diagnostic specimens. The appropriate use of the FOB requires training and practice. It is particularly helpful in patients who are resistant to CPT or who have preexisting conditions that may preclude vigorous CPT, such as cervical spine or chest wall trauma, recent airway surgery, or multiple orthopedic appliances. **Complications of fiberoptic bronchoscopy**: hypoxemia, bronchospasm, arrhythmias, hypertension, hemoptysis, laryngospasm pneumothorax.

II. Oxygen therapy

A. Rationale. Supplemental oxygen administration is indicated in a variety of disease states to assist in the prevention and treatment of hypoxemia. Supplemental oxygen does not reverse or treat underlying airspace abnormalities; it serves to maximize the level of arterial oxygenation. A variety of oxygen administration devices are available. Thus, oxygen may be delivered in a manner appropriate to the particular disease states of the individual patient (Table 2-2).

B. Complications

1. **Absorption atelectasis.** This phenomenon occurs with the administration of 100% oxygen.
2. **Flammability.** Oxygen is combustible. It is vital to avoid the hazard of fire in any setting in which oxygen is administered through careful and appropriate handling of related equipment.
3. **Hypoventilation.** Patients who depend on hypoxic ventilatory drive may become hypercarbic in the face of an aerobic environment.
4. **Mucociliary clearance.** Oxygen delivered at levels greater than 50% for moderate amounts of time will decrease mucociliary clearance. When a patient inhales 75% oxygen for 9 hours, mucociliary clearance is diminished by 40%. When 50% oxygen is inhaled for 30 hours, mucociliary clearance is diminished by approximately 50%.
5. **Tracheobronchitis.** May become symptomatic when high concentrations of oxygen are inhaled over a period greater than 12 hours. Symptoms are cough, substernal pain, and dyspnea.
6. **Bronchopulmonary dysplasia and retrolental fibroplasia,** seen in the neonatal population
7. **Central nervous dysfunction.** Myoclonus, nausea, paresthesias, unconsciousness, and seizures may result as a complication of hyperbaric oxygen therapy at pressures in excess of 2 atmospheres.
8. **Pulmonary oxygen toxicity.** Pulmonary oxygen toxicity may be fatal from progressive and severe hypoxemia due to interstitial fibrosis. The effects of oxygen toxicity are prevented by an understanding of the syndrome, in addition to the cautious restriction of oxygen delivery to the lowest concentration and shortest duration of oxygen therapy compatible with a satisfactory PAO_2. Clinically significant oxygen toxicity may occur when concentrations of greater than 50% are administered for periods over 48 hours. PEEP is a particularly useful means in which to maximize oxygenation while reducing the level of inspired oxygen.

C. Modes of administration

1. **Variable performance devices** allow the entrainment of room air. The concentration of oxygen in the airway will approach that of the

Table 2-2. FIO_2 of oxygen administration devices

Device	Oxygen flow	FIO_2[a]
Nasal cannula	1–6 L/min	0.25–0.45
Simple face mask	6–15 L/min	0.35–0.65
Aerosol facemask[b]	6–15 L/min	0.40–0.70
Aerosol face tent[b]	15 L/min	0.30–0.45
Partial rebreathing mask	So reservoir bag does not collapse	0.6 –0.8
Nonrebreathing mask	So reservoir bag does not collapse	0.85–0.95

[a] If air entrainment occurs, FIO_2 will decrease with higher peak inspiratory flow and increase with lower inspiratory flow. There is disparity in the literature regarding FIO_2s attained with these devices. Thus, the noted FIO_2s are approximate.
[b] Nebulizer oxygen concentration is 30–100%.

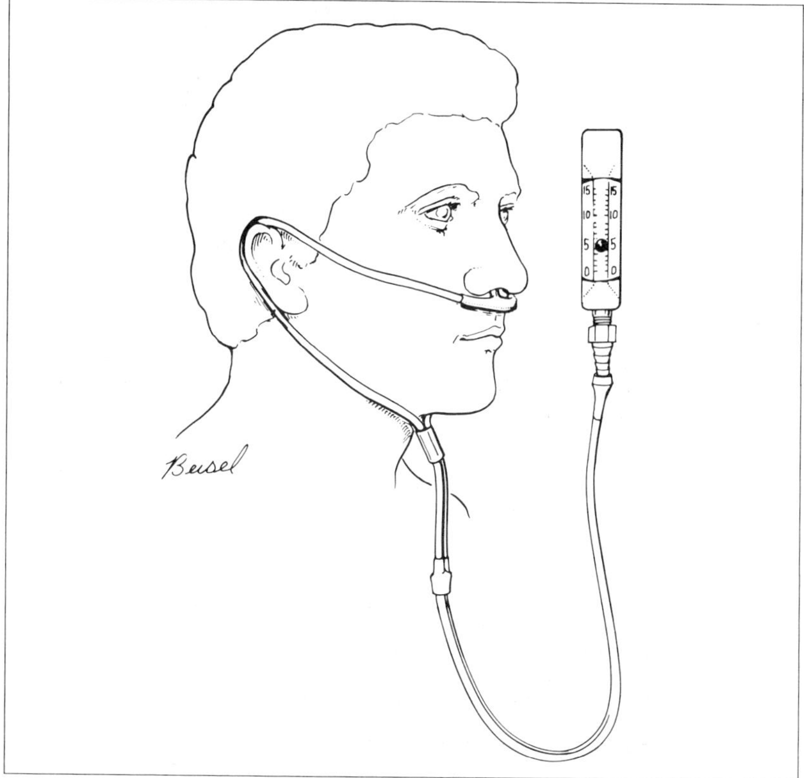

Fig. 2-2. Nasal cannulas.

delivered gas when gas flow increases, tidal volume decreases, or inspiratory flow rate decreases.

a. **Nasal cannula (Fig. 2-2).** Plastic prongs are inserted into the nares. The nasopharynx is then insufflated with 100% unhumidified oxygen. Varying the flow rate of oxygen will change the FIO_2. Nasal cannula are notable for patient comfort. Drying of the

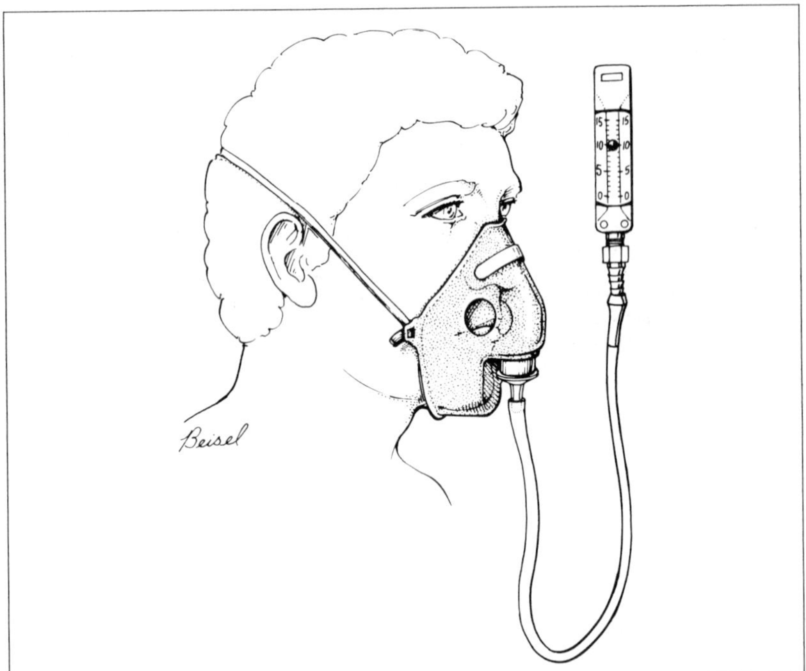

Fig. 2-3. Simple mask.

nasal mucosa can occur when the flow rate rises above 6 liters per minute. Note that the $F_{I}O_2$ will increase only 4% above room air with each liter per minute increase in the oxygen flow rate.

b. **Simple mask (Fig 2-3).** Disposable plastic masks connected to 100% unhumidified oxygen by plastic tubing constitute simple masks. A change in the oxygen flow rate will vary the $F_{I}O_2$. Simple masks may deliver oxygen flow rates from 6–15 liters per minute, providing $F_{I}O_2$ of 0.35–0.65.

c. **Partial rebreathing mask (Fig. 2-4).** This is a simple mask with a valveless reservoir bag and exhalation ports; 100% unhumidified oxygen is delivered by plastic tubing to the device. The inhaled gas is thus a combination of oxygen from the reservoir bag and entrained room air. This device delivers $F_{I}O_2$ between 0.6–0.8. The mask must fit snugly in order to ensure motion of the reservoir bag. Then the oxygen flow rate is adjusted to keep the reservoir bag distended.

d. **Nonrebreathing mask (Fig. 2-5).** This device is a simple mask with a reservoir bag and two one-way valves. A one-way valve is positioned between the reservoir and the mask. 100% unhumidified oxygen is delivered to this device via plastic tubing. The inhaled gas comprises reservoir bag oxygen and a small amount of room air. Oxygen flow rate must be adjusted to ensure distension of the reservoir bag. A tight-fitting mask is required as well. This device can deliver $F_{I}O_2$ between 0.85 and 0.95.

e. **Aerosol face tent (Fig. 2-6).** This device delivers oxygen from a variable oxygen nebulizer over the mouth and nose. It delivers only modest amounts of oxygen.

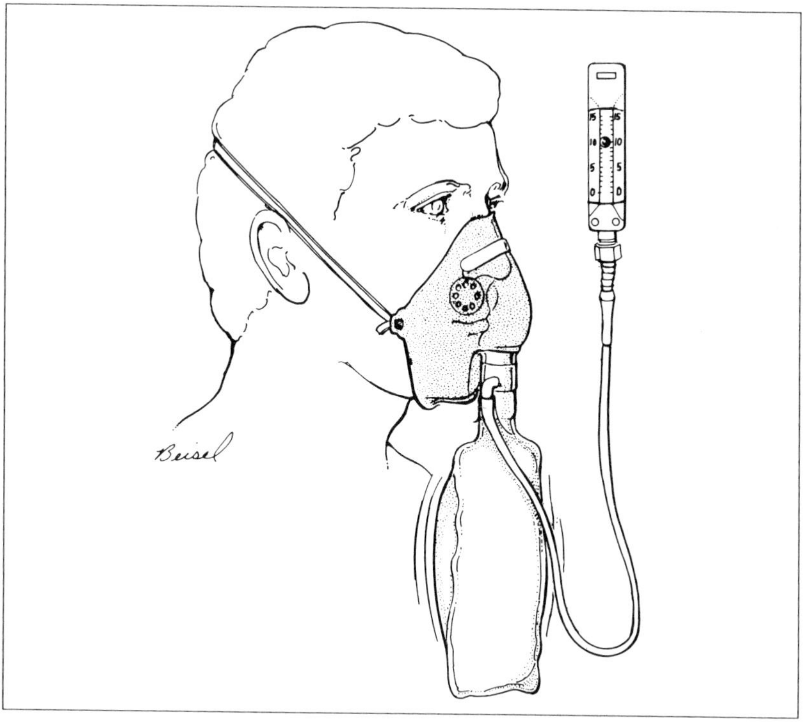

Fig. 2-4. Partial rebreathing mask.

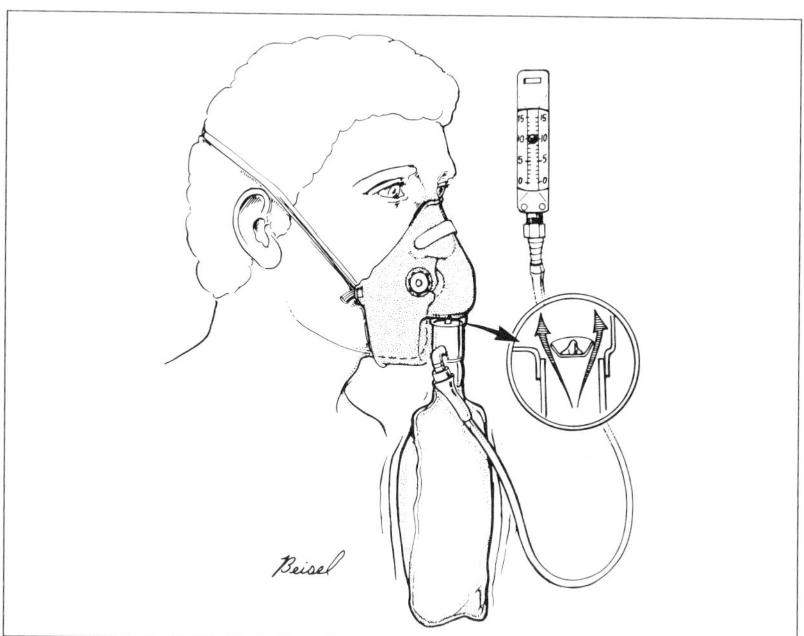

Fig. 2-5. Disposable nonrebreathing mask.

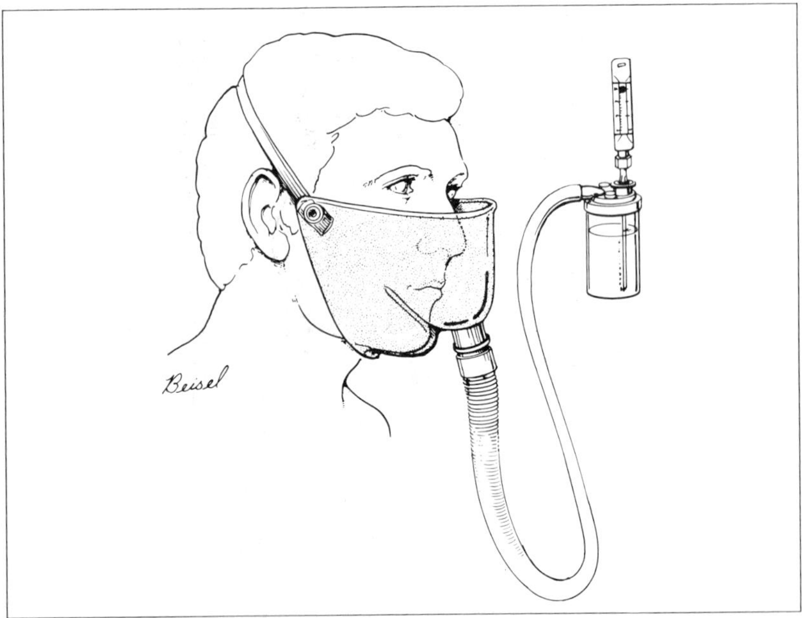

Fig. 2-6. Aerosol face tent.

2. **Fixed performance devices,** which utilize high oxygen flow rates for all inspired gases. Therefore, the fraction of inspired oxygen is independent of the ventilatory pattern.
   a. **Tight-fitting nonrebreathing device.** This device delivers 100% oxygen through a tight-fitting facemask with one-way valves and a nonemptying reservoir bag. It is most often used as a temporizing maneuver prior to more advanced airway management in the form of intubation.
   b. **Venturi mask (Fig. 2-7).** This device combines room air with unhumidified oxygen to deliver a F_IO_2 between 24 and 40% with accuracy. The flow rates of oxygen are therefore high.
3. **Intermediate devices,** either variable or fixed in function based on the oxygen flow rate, deliver humidified oxygen through a nebulizer and large-bore tubing at concentrations of oxygen between 30 and 100%. These devices behave as fixed performance devices as the total gas flow rate is increased.
   a. **Aerosol facemask (Fig. 2-8)**
   b. **Aerosol tracheostomy mask (Fig. 2-9).** Both of these devices are modifications of the simple face mask with the aforementioned changes allowing for humidification of oxygen.
   c. **T piece (Fig. 2-10),** a device used in conjunction with an indwelling ETT. The patient must be breathing spontaneously with adequate tidal volume and respiratory rate while on a T piece. A T piece may be used as part of a regimen of weaning from mechanical ventilation or as a temporizing measure in a postoperative patient prior to extubation in the recovery room.

III. Mechanical ventilation

A. Basics

1. **Definition.** Mechanical ventilation: any method in which a mechani-

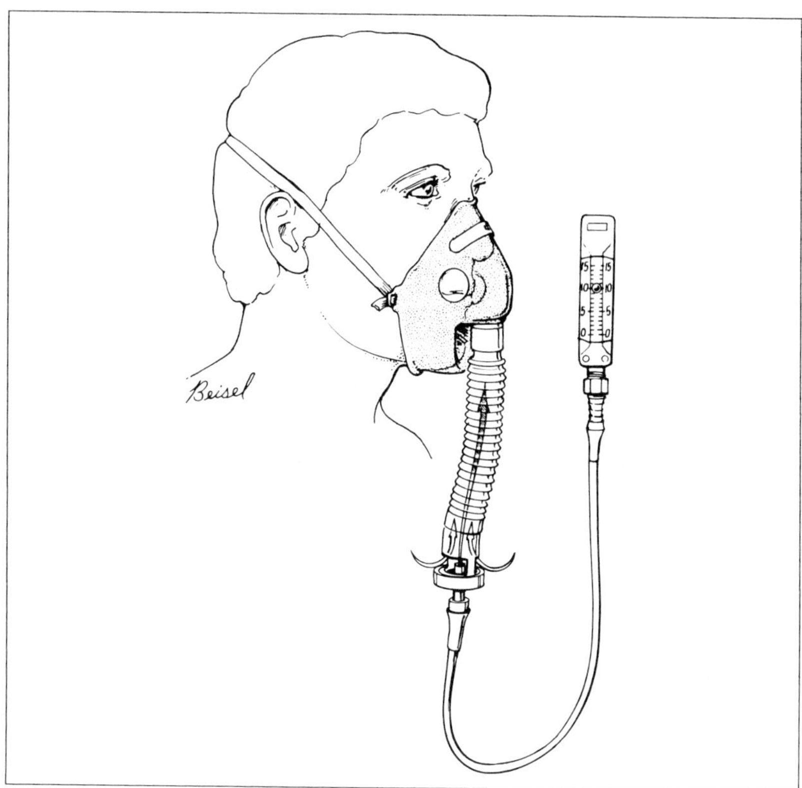

Fig. 2-7. Air entrainment (Venturi) mask.

cal device is used to supplement or provide the patient's requirements for breathing

2. **Classification.** Mechanical ventilators may be classified according to the method in which tidal volume is delivered.
   a. Time cycled: The tidal volume is delivered and inspiration ends after a preset time interval.
   b. Volume cycled: The tidal volume is delivered and inspiration ends after a preset volume is delivered.
   c. Pressure cycled: The tidal volume is delivered and inspiration ends when a preset pressure is reached.
3. **Indications for mechanical ventilation.** The process of mechanical ventilation can be used therapeutically or prophylactically.
   a. **Etiologies of therapeutic mechanical ventilation.** Many disease processes can cause respiratory failure as defined by Pontoppidan et al. 1972 (Table 2-3). Examples of these processes include:
      (1) Intubation and mechanical ventilation following cardiac arrest
      (2) Hypoventilation due to:
         (a) Residual general anesthesia
         (b) CNS depressant drug overdose
         (c) Residual neuromuscular blockade
         (d) CNS dysfunction due to myasthenic syndromes, Guillain-Barré syndrome, stroke, polio, and others

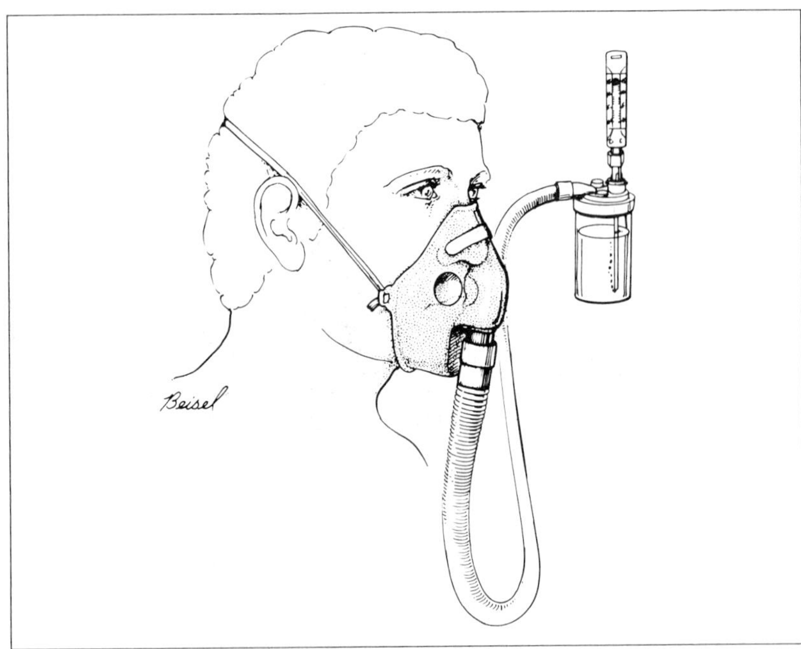

Fig. 2-8. Aerosol facemask.

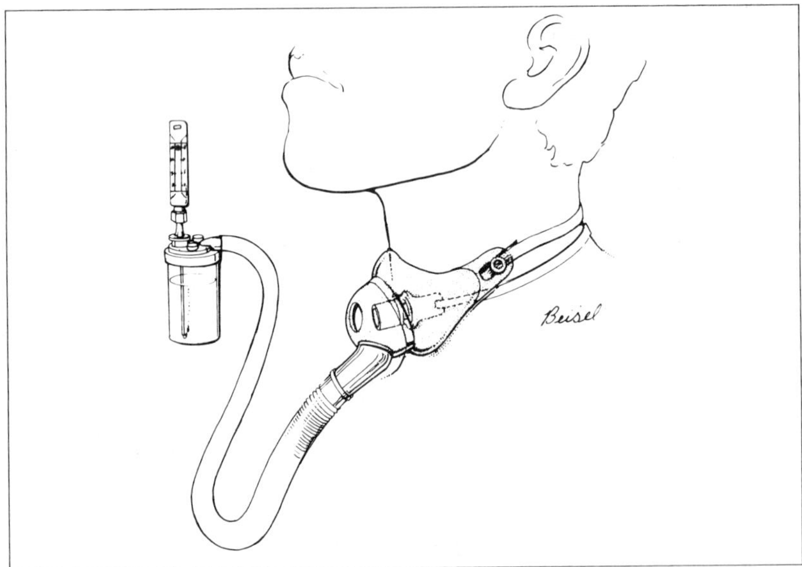

Fig. 2-9. Aerosol tracheostomy mask.

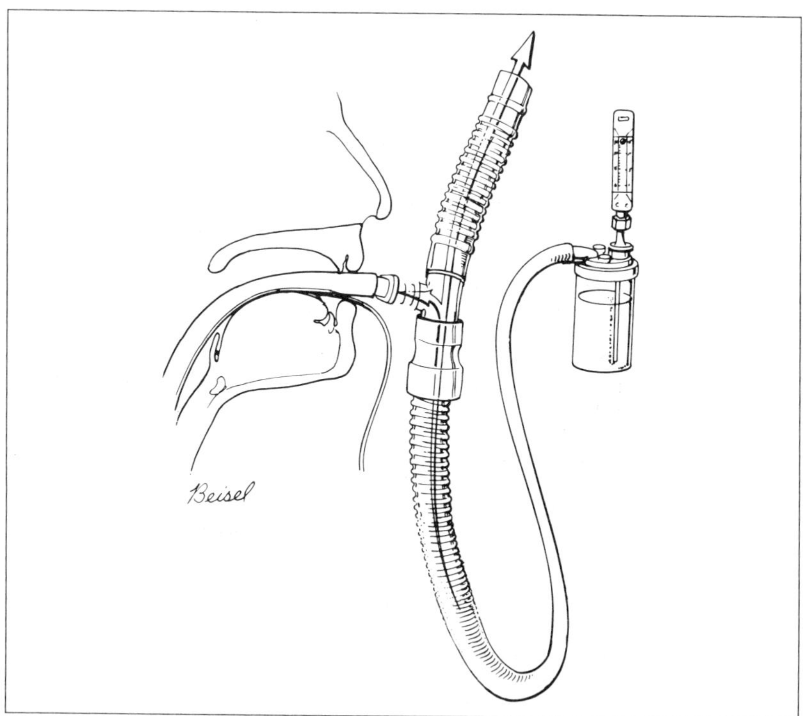

Fig. 2-10. Briggs T piece.

Table 2-3. Bedside tests of pulmonary function

Test	Norm	Intubate/ventilate
Respiratory rate	12–20	>35
Vital capacity (cc/kg)	65–75	<15
Negative IF (cm H_2O)	75–100	<25
FEV_1 (cc/kg)	50–60	<10
PaO_2 (mm Hg)	75–100 (room air)	<70 (mask oxygen)
$PaCO_2$ (mm Hg)	35–45	>55*
V_D/V_T	0.25–0.40	>0.60

*Except with chronic hypercapnia.
Modified from H. Pontoppidan, B. Geffin, and E. Lowenstein. Acute respiratory failure in the adult. *N. Engl. J. Med.* 287:690, 1972.

(3) Hypoxemia
  (a) Adult respiratory distress syndrome (ARDS)
  (b) Pulmonary edema
  (c) Pulmonary embolus
  (d) Pneumonia
  (e) Atelectasis or lobar collapse
(4) Trauma
  (a) Flail chest
  (b) Ruptured diaphragm

b. Etiologies requiring prophylactic mechanical ventilation
(1) Hemodynamic instability
(2) Postoperative recovery
(3) Cachexia and malnutrition in the face of a concurrent major physiological insult
(4) High risk of aspiration of gastric contents (for example, massive upper GI hemorrhage, probable aspiration of acid or particulate stomach contents)

4. Institution of mechanical ventilation

a. Ventilator orders (Table 2-4)
(1) Mode of ventilation: See **B.**
(2) Fraction of inspired oxygen (FIO_2): The prescribed FIO_2 must be kept at a minimum to avoid the ill effects of oxygen therapy. When initiating ventilator therapy on a critically ill patient with an unknown oxygen demand, the safest initial setting is 90–100% FIO_2. This should be weaned readily based on the patient's clinical appearance, oxygen saturation by pulse oximetry, and arterial blood gas data. A postoperative patient whose oxygen requirement is known intraoperatively may be initiated on a lower FIO_2 in the recovery room if this is deemed prudent by the delivering anesthetist.
(3) Respiratory rate
(4) Tidal volume. Minute ventilation comprises respiratory rate × tidal volume. In adults, the approximate minute ventilation is body weight in kilograms × 100. Increases in minute ventilation are seen with increases in either carbon dioxide production or dead space. Initial settings for minute ventilation may be determined as follows:
  (a) Respiratory rate: 8–12 breaths per minute in patients with a normal minute ventilation
  (b) Tidal volume: In adults, a tidal volume of 10–15 cc per kilogram of body weight is sufficient.
(5) Positive end-expiratory pressure (see **C**)
(6) Other parameters that may be specified
  (a) Inspiratory: expiratory (I-E) ratio. This determines the period of time spent in the inspiratory and expiratory phases of the respiratory cycle. In patients without significant pulmonary disease, the initial setting is 1 : 2. Patients with significant lung disease, such as asthma, may require a more prolonged expiratory phase—for example, 1 : 3. Mean airway pressures can be increased in states of severe respiratory dysfunction by prolonging the inspiratory time. Occasionally this maneuver can be used to increase a marginal PaO_2. The proper way in which to set the I-E ratio includes inspection and auscultation over the chest to ensure that the expiratory phase of the respiratory cycle is complete prior to

Table 2-4. Respiratory care orders in postoperative ventilated patients

Ventilator orders on arrival to the ICU*	
Mode	IMV
FIO_2	90–100% initially
Rate	8–12 breaths/min
Tidal volume	10–15 cc/kg
PEEP	2–5 cm H_2O
I:E Ratio	1:2
Adjunctive orders	
CPT	
Types of CPT: turning, postural drainage, vibration, percussion, etc.	
Frequency	
Cautions to therapist or nurse	
Aerosol medications	
Device (nebulizer, USN, hydrosphere)	
Dose	
Dilution and diluent	
Frequency	
When to withhold	
Chest radiograph	
Frequency	
Special views	
Weaning orders	
All types of weaning	
FIO_2	
PEEP	
Timing of measurements: ABG, VC, IF	
When to call physician (e.g., BP >200 systolic, RR >35, diaphoresis)	
IMV weaning	
IMV respiratory rate	
Conventional weaning	
T piece or CPAP	
How long off ventilator	
How often off ventilator	
Earliest and latest time of day for weaning	
Posture	

RR = respiratory rate.
*These are ventilator settings commonly used in the usual postoperative, anesthetized adult patient on arrival in the ICU. Exceptions certainly occur.

the start of the inspiratory phase. This helps to avoid "stacking of breaths" on the ventilator, which will increase airway pressures as well.

(b) Type of ventilator (Table 2-5)

(c) Ventilator sensitivity. The sensitivity determines the negative pressure required to draw a mechanical breath in an assisted mode. The sensitivity should be adjusted for each individual. A high setting may initiate a breath with nonrespiratory sources of airway pressure. A low setting would not allow the patient to initiate a breath, therefore converting the mode to a controlled mechanical ventilation type.

Table 2-5. Volume-limited ventilators[a]

Ventilator	Emerson IMV & 3PV	Bournes Bear-1	Bournes Bear-2	Bennett MA-1	Bennett MA-2	Puritan Bennett 7200	Engstrom Erica	Siemens 900b	Siemens 900c
Mechanism of V_T delivery	Piston driven by rotating cam	Pneumatic flow generator	Pneumatic flow generator	Compressor-powered bellows	Compressor-powered bellows	Micro-processor-controlled pneumatic flow generator	Micro-processor-controlled pneumatic flow generator	Micro-processor-controlled pneumatic flow generator	Micro-processor-controlled pneumatic flow generator
Modes	IMV, CMV, CPAP	IMV, CMV, A/C, CPAP	SIMV, CPAP, CMV, A/C	CMV, A/C, IMV, CPAP with modification	SIMV, IMV, CMV, A/C, CPAP	SIMV, CMV, A/C, CPAP	SIMV, CMV, A/C, EMMV[d], CPAP	SIMV, A/C, CPAP	SIMV, A/C, CPAP, PC[b], PS[c]

Rate (breath/min)	0.2–25.0 (IMV) 0.2–50.0 (3PV)	0.5–60.0	0.5–60.0	1–60 (>100 without calibration)	3–60 (CMV) 0.33–30.00 (IMV)	0.5–70.0	0.4–40.0 (150 with EMMV & uncalibrated V_T)	6–60 (A/C) 0.6–60.0 (SIMV)	0.5–120.0
PEEP (cm H_2O)	0–25	0–30	0–50	0–15	0–45	0–45	0–30	0–50	0–50
Pressure limit (cm H_2O)	150	100	120	80	120	120	100	100	120

EMMV = extended mandatory minute volume; PC = pressure control; PS = pressure support.

[a] This table summarizes characteristics of a number of volume-limited ventilators. They are not all in use at Massachusetts General Hospital. Characteristics do tend to change somewhat from year to year.

[b] Pressure control allows pressure-limited ventilation.

[c] Pressure support allows application of a preset pressure throughout spontaneous inspiration.

[d] EMMV ensures that a minimum ventilation will occur. No mechanical inspirations occur if spontaneous minute volume exceeds the set minute volume.

b. Ventilator alarms

(1) **Apnea alarm,** indicating absence of a breath after a predetermined time period has elapsed. Appropriate investigatory measures include the following:

(a) Assess the patient's level of consciousness. Have drugs that depress respiration been administered recently? Is the patient profoundly hypercarbic as a cause of obtundation?

(b) Manually ventilate and oxygenate the patient on 100% FIO_2 and assess for possible airway obstruction.

(2) **Disconnect alarm,** indicating that the patient has been disconnected from the ventilator and low airway pressures are present. Appropriate investigatory measures include:

(a) Look quickly for the source of an obvious disconnection. If a source is not readily seen, manually ventilate and oxygenate the patient with 100% FIO_2.

(b) Inspect the circuitry of the ventilator for large leaks, and assess the prescribed amount of PEEP with a manometer.

(3) **High airway pressure,** signifying that the preset maximum airway pressure has been exceeded. Causes of a sudden increase in airway pressure include:

(a) Airway obstruction: kinking of the ETT, plugging of the ETT with secretions or blood, accidental extubation or malposition of the ETT

(b) Decreased pulmonary compliance: Sudden and severe bronchospasm, pulmonary edema, and tension pneumothorax are common possibilities.

(4) **Low FIO_2,** indicating that the delivered FIO_2 is less than the preset level. Appropriate investigatory measures include:

(a) Check the oxygen analyzer reading on the ventilator. If the reading is lower than the preset level, increase the FIO_2 immediately. Call respiratory therapy to check the ventilator.

(b) If in doubt about oxygen delivery of a particular ventilator, the safest maneuver is manually to ventilate and oxygenate the patient on 100% FIO_2 until a replacement ventilator is set up or the source of the error is discovered.

(5) **High airway temperature,** indicating that the inspired humidified gases have been overheated. If the temperature of the inspired gases exceeds 105°F, manually ventilate and oxygenate the patient with 100% FIO_2 at ambient temperature while the ventilator is being serviced or replaced.

(6) **Low exhaled tidal volume,** signifying that the preset tidal volume is not being delivered. Proper steps include:

—Examine the circuit for leaks and disconnections.

B. Modes of mechanical ventilation. Following is a partial list of the most commonly utilized methods of mechanical ventilation.

1. Intermittent positive-pressure ventilatory modes (IPPV)

a. Definition: IPPV mode will deliver intermittent cyclic positive pressure breaths during inspiration.

b. Controlled mechanical ventilation (CMV). Mechanical breaths are delivered at a preset rate and tidal volume regardless of the patient's effort. This mode is useful in the following cases:

(1) Patients with periods of apnea from drug overdose or CNS pathology

(2) Patients requiring neuromuscular blockade or heavy sedation to maximize gas exchange

c. **Assist-control ventilation.** This mode has two capabilities. A preset minute ventilation will be delivered regardless of patient effort. Additionally, the ventilator senses each patient-initiated spontaneous breath and delivers a preset tidal volume as well.

d. **Intermittent mandatory ventilation (IMV).** This mode combines spontaneous and controlled methods of ventilation. A preset tidal volume and rate are delivered. Between controlled breaths, the patient may spontaneously breathe warmed, humidified oxygen. It is indicated in a patient who can provide a portion of the work of breathing.

   (1) **Synchronized IMV** (SIMV), a combination of assisted and spontaneous ventilation. The preset minute ventilation will be triggered by the patient's negative inspiratory effort, and the mechanical-assisted breath will be delivered. The patient continues to breathe spontaneously between assisted cycles. If the patient fails to initiate a breath during the assisted period of ventilation, the ventilator reverts to a conventional IMV mode and delivers the preset breath. The major advantage of the SIMV mode over the IMV mode is patient comfort.

e. **Continuous positive airway pressure (CPAP).** The patient is breathing spontaneously, and no mechanical breaths are delivered. A preset level of positive airway pressure is maintained throughout the respiratory cycle. The respiratory and hemodynamic effects of CPAP are similar to PEEP. (See **III.B.**)

f. **Assisted ventilation.** A preset tidal volume is delivered when the patient initiates a negative inspiratory effort. The patient determines the respiratory rate given his or her current minute ventilation and preset tidal volume.

g. **Inspiratory pressure support ventilation (IPS).** IPS requires a pressure-cycled ventilator. A preset pressure is obtained when the patient initiates an inspiratory effort. Thus, it requires the patient to be able to initiate spontaneous breaths. The preset pressure delivers a tidal volume that varies from patient to patient based on the individual's lung compliance. If lung compliance increases (as a pneumonia clears, for example), the generated tidal volume will increase, although the preset pressure has not varied.

h. The modes of IPS, assisted ventilation, assist control, and SIMV require a modest inspiratory effort to trigger the ventilator. Thus, at least theoretically, these modes of ventilation are the least likely to precipitate respiratory muscle disuse atrophy because they allow the respiratory muscles to exercise.

i. **Complications associated with IPPV**

   (1) Complications associated with intubation and extubation. See Chap. 1.

   (2) Complications associated with endotracheal and tracheostomy tubes. See Chap. 1.

   (3) Complications associated with ventilator malfunction. This series of complications can be kept to a minimum with knowledgeable physician and respiratory therapy staff. Ventilators must be checked on a regular basis and infection control standards strictly enforced. Problems and questions must be dealt with promptly. Several important complications include: bacterial contamination of components of the ventilator, machine failure, alarm failure, disabling alarms unintentionally, inadequate humidification or nebulization of inspired gases, excessive heating of inspired gases.

   (4) Physiologic complications of mechanical ventilation. These

medical complications of mechanical ventilation are numerous and include:

(a) Barotrauma, manifested by several routes, including pneumomediastinum, subcutaneous emphysema, pneumoperitoneum, and pneumothorax
(b) Massive gastric distension
(c) Atelectasis
(d) Pneumonia
(e) Inadvertent hypoventilation or hyperventilation
(f) Reduction in venous return with concomitant decrease in cardiac output (CO) and hypotension. In patients with underlying atherosclerotic disease, vascular insufficiency may occur due to decreased CO as well.
(g) Decreases in left atrial volume with positive pressure may lead to increased circulating antidiuretic hormone. Water retention will result.

2. Positive end-expiratory pressure (PEEP)

a. Definition. PEEP is a means to maintain superatmospheric pressure artificially once the expiratory phase of respiration is complete. PEEP requires that the patient be intubated and placed on a positive-pressure ventilator. PEEP serves to increase alveolar pressure, and therefore FRC will increase as well. Since an increase in FRC will increase lung volume, PaO_2 will improve.

b. Uses

(1) Augmentation of the PaO_2 when hypoxemia is severe
(2) Treatment of pulmonary edema. PEEP used in this situation will decrease intrapulmonary shunting and attempt to match perfusion with ventilation. Note that interalveolar fluid is only redistributed.
(3) Improvement of oxygenation while allowing for the use of lower nontoxic levels of inspired oxygen
(4) Prevention of atelectasis in patients following thoracic, cardiac, or abdominal surgery. Although this is a common use of PEEP, there is little supporting evidence.

c. Cautions: PEEP should be withheld or titrated with caution in the following circumstances:

(1) Decreased CO
(2) Hypotension
(3) Hypovolemia
(4) Presence of a tension pneumothorax
(5) Presence of known increased intracranial pressure without the benefit of an intracranial pressure monitor

d. Complications. The adverse effects of PEEP may be categorized by system:

(1) **Cardiovascular**
(a) Decreased CO secondary to reduce preload. This may be exacerbated by hypovolemia and result in hypotension.
(b) Increased lung water secondary to increased antidiuretic hormone (ADH) secretion. This is due to decreased left atrial volume.

(2) **Pulmonary**
(a) Barotrauma
(b) Increased work of breathing

(3) **Neurologic.** Cerebral perfusion pressure (CPP) may decrease as mean arterial pressure (MAP) falls due to a decrease in CO. Remember that CPP = MAP − ICP. Intracranial pressure

(ICP) may increase as well due to increased cerebral blood volume.

(4) **Renal.** ADH levels may increase with concomitant fall in urine output.

e. **Determination of "best" PEEP**

(1) PEEP affects the cardiovascular and respiratory systems. Thus, the "best" PEEP should maximize the pulmonary benefits while minimizing the cardiac complications. The goal is to provide optimal tissue oxygenation.

(2) PEEP will increase FRC due to the recruitment of alveolar units that were previously perfused but not ventilated. Patent alveolar units will be further distended. Static compliance will increase in the newly expanded alveolar lung units and will decrease in the overdistended units. Thus, static compliance may be plotted as PEEP is increased until a maximum is reached.

(3) CO is reduced by PEEP due to impaired venous return. Left ventricular (LV) function is also impaired at higher levels of PEEP such as 15 cm H_2O or greater.

(4) It is important to measure CO serially as PEEP is increased to determine the point at which additional increments of PEEP will diminish CO and, thus, reduce tissue oxygen delivery.

(5) The diminution in CO seen with the augmentation of PEEP may be initially managed with volume loading or inotropic agents. If these measures fail, the level of PEEP must be reduced to previous levels.

f. **Effects of PEEP on pulmonary vascular pressure data**

(1) As noted, PEEP may alter LV compliance and intrathoracic pressure, which is transmitted to the heart.

(2) Pulmonary capillary wedge pressure (PCWP) may not reflect changes in left ventricular end diastolic pressure (LVEDP).

(3) If the catheter is in West's zone 1 of the lung, then pulmonary capillary wedge pressure may not reflect intravascular pressure. Instead it may reflect the alveolar pressure.

(4) When possible, keep the catheter below the level of the left atrium.

(5) An echocardiogram or gated blood pool scan is helpful in the determination of LV volume and ejection fraction in confounding clinical cases.

IV. Weaning from mechanical ventilation

A. **Definition:** Weaning is the process of discontinuing a patient from mechanical ventilatory support.

B. **Indications.** Once a patient has stabilized and is improving from the initial insult that mandated intubation and mechanical ventilation, he or she should be considered for weaning. Criteria to initiate the weaning process include:

1. The patient should be able to initiate spontaneous breaths.
2. **Respiratory mechanics**

a. **Inspiratory force.** The patient is able to generate a negative inspiratory force of greater than 20 cm H_2O.

b. **Vital capacity.** The patient's vital capacity is equal to or in excess of 10 ml per kilogram of ideal body weight. Performance of this maneuver requires that the patient be cooperative.

c. **Minute ventilation and maximum voluntary ventilation.** Resting minute ventilation should be less than 10 liters per minute. Ideally, patients should be able to double their minute ventilation voluntarily.

d. **Tidal volume.** The patient should have a normal spontaneous tidal volume of at least 500 cc.

3. **Observation of breathing pattern and respiratory muscles.** It is vitally important to assess the pattern and quality of breathing and respiratory muscle function serially during the process of weaning. Signs of impending failure from weaning include:
   a. Increased respiratory rate and decreased tidal volume
   b. Paradoxical inward motion of the abdomen during inspiration, indicating diaphragmatic dysfunction
   c. Excessive use of the accessory muscles of respiration
4. The patient should be in stable condition, free from any ongoing cardiovascular instability.

C. **General principles**

1. **Pain control.** The patient should be comfortable and pain free if possible. Judicious use of intravenous narcotics, analgesics such as ketorolac, or use of epidural analgesia should be established prior to weaning.
2. **Treatment of acute metabolic alkalosis** should be considered. The timing and initiation of therapy remains controversial. If the patient has a chloride-responsive metabolic alkalosis, treatment may be started with sodium chloride, potassium chloride, and, in severe cases, hydrochloric acid. Acetazolamide (Diamox) will cause renal loss of bicarbonate through inhibition of carbonic anhydrase.
3. The patient should require chest physical therapy and suctioning at reasonable intervals of every 3–4 hours. The patient should have a good cough and ability to clear secretions during CPT.
4. The nursing staff, respiratory therapy staff, and the patient should understand the weaning plan.
5. The patient should be on a relatively low level of oxygen and PEEP/CPAP (40% FIO_2 and PEEP 5) prior to extubation.
6. Weaning from mechanical ventilation should be stopped when the patient is distressed from a respiratory or cardiovascular standpoint.
7. The timing and duration of the weaning process is closely tied to the preoperative physical status, the operative intervention, and the perioperative course of the patient.

D. **Techniques**

1. **T piece wean.** The patient is discontinued from mechanical ventilatory support and placed on a Briggs T piece. Thus, the patient assumes all the work of breathing during the T piece trial. The frequency and duration of the trials are gradually increased given the patient's progress. A general rule in all trials of weaning is to avoid pushing the patient to the point of exhaustion. Serial assessment of the patient's vital signs, oxygen saturation by pulse oximetry, arterial blood gas determinations, and pattern of breathing is necessary. Once the patient tolerates long periods of weaning on a Briggs T piece with maintenance of stable vital signs and arterial blood gas determinations, he or she may be evaluated for extubation.
2. **Intermittent mandatory ventilation (IMV) wean (Fig 2-11).** The patient gradually assumes the entire work of spontaneous breathing as the mandatory ventilator breaths are reduced successively. The advantages of IMV weaning include a graded exercise for the muscles of respiration and a gradual process of weaning in patients in whom a rapid descent from mechanical ventilation is unlikely. The precise method of decreasing the IMV breaths and evaluating for extubation will vary from patient to patient. The general guidelines of monitoring and patient evaluation during the process of weaning apply in this setting as well.

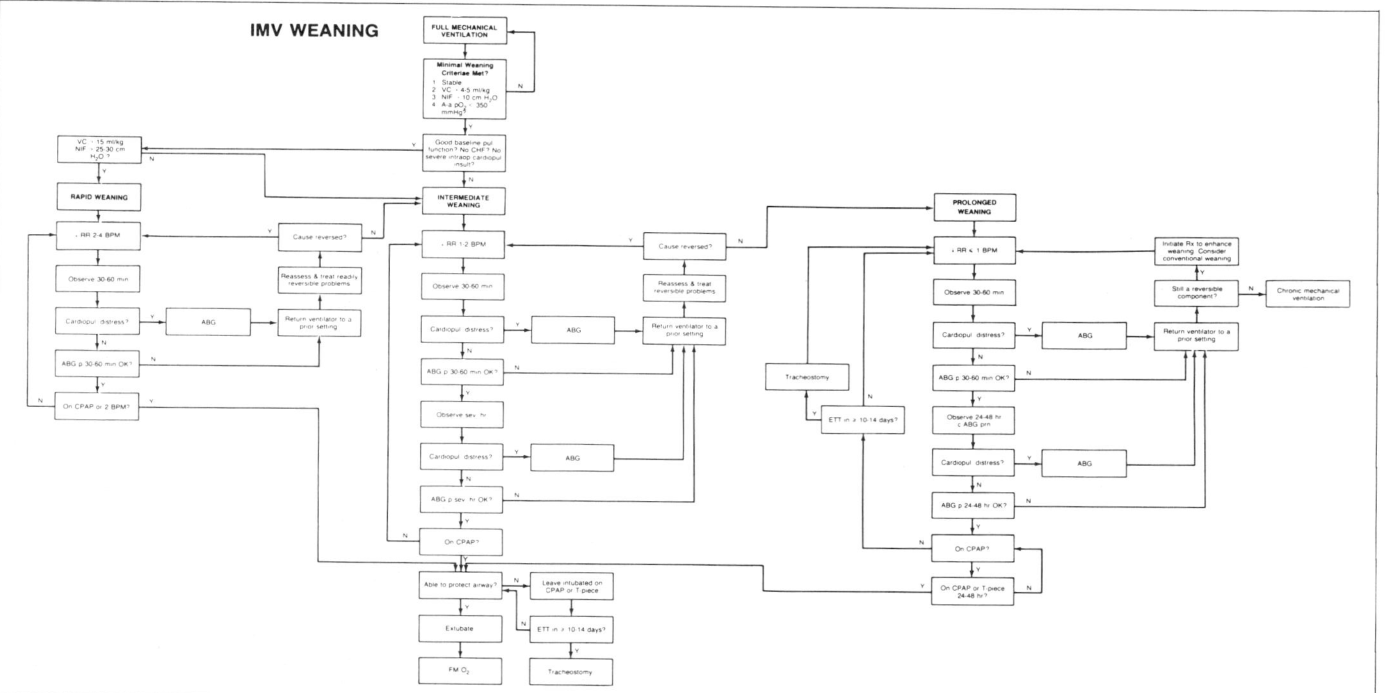

Fig. 2-11. Intermittent mandatory ventilation—weaning algorithm. Depending on patient status, rapid, intermediate, or prolonged weaning can be anticipated. This algorithm depicts as discrete what is actually a continuum of severity of patient illness and duration of IMV weaning. It is a general approach to IMV weaning and is no substitute for individualized, titrated bedside care. *BPM* = breaths per minute; *N* = no; *NIF* = negative inspiratory force; *RR* = respiratory rate; *Y* = yes.

3. **CPAP wean.** In this process, the patient assumes the entire work of spontaneous breathing during graded trials on CPAP. The frequency and duration of the CPAP trials are gradually increased based on the patient's clinical picture. Once the patient can maintain stable vital signs, oxygen saturation, arterial blood gases, and comfortable pattern of breathing for a long time period, he or she may be evaluated for extubation. Initial weaning trials on CPAP may be of short duration, such as 5 minutes or 1 hour. The time intervals are set based on the patient's clinical status.
4. **Inspiratory pressure support (IPS) wean.** A spontaneously breathing patient on the IPS mode of ventilatory support is gradually dropped to a low-level of support. For example, an IPS of 5 will serve to overcome the work of breathing through the ETT. When stable on an appropriate trial of low-level IPS, the patient may be evaluated for extubation.

E. **Evaluation for endotracheal extubation.** A patient weaned successfully from mechanical ventilation should be evaluated for extubation. Several important guidelines in evaluation follow:

1. Ideally, the patient should be awake, alert, cooperative, and able to protect his or her airway.
2. Cardiopulmonary stability should reign.
3. The patient's respiratory mechanics should be adequate.
4. The patient should be able to cough well and clear a modest amount of secretions readily. The patient should not require frequent chest physical therapy and endotracheal suctioning.
5. The patient should ideally require a modest level of oxygen and PEEP (FIO_2 40% and PEEP 5).
6. The patient should be comfortable and free of anxiety and pain. Excessive use of analgesics and sedatives should be avoided prior to extubation.
7. Residual neuromuscular blockade should be fully reversed.
8. Tube feedings should be held prior to extubation in patients at high risk for aspiration or in patients with high gastric residuals.
9. The patient should undergo CPT and endotracheal suctioning at an appropriate interval prior to extubation.
10. Patients at risk for laryngeal edema should be evaluated for a cuff leak prior to extubation. The ETT cuff is deflated, and the patient is asked to attempt to phonate or is ambued, listening for a characteristic leak. If any questions concerning the anatomic patency of the airway exist, the patient should be extubated under direct vision of a fiberoptic bronchoscope. If warranted, the patient should be taken to the operating room and extubated in a controlled setting.

F. **Failure to wean.** It is an essential part of the weaning process to examine reasons for weaning failure. Several etiologies exist that may precipitate a failed attempt at weaning.

1. **Hypoxemia**
   a. Low CO. The weaning process may induce ischemia in patients with significant coronary artery disease. Congestive heart failure (CHF) may be precipitated by ischemia or by increased preload during the weaning process especially in patients with marginal left ventricular function.
   b. Hypoventilation
   c. Ventilation-perfusion mismatch
   d. Anatomic right-to-left shunts
2. **Increased ventilatory requirements**
   a. Increased carbon dioxide production
      (1) Hypermetabolic states

(2) Carbohydrate overfeeding

b. High physiologic dead space

3. **Increased work of breathing**
   a. Small ETT size
   b. High-resistance ventilator
   c. Chest wall bony abnormalities
   d. Decreased lung compliance
   e. Bronchospasm
4. **Decreased drive to breathe**
   a. Drug induced
   b. Central nervous system disorders
   c. Metabolic alkalosis
5. **Psychological disorders.** Anxiety and/or agitation will impair the weaning process. Once an organic cause is eliminated, the judicious use of anxiolytics can facilitate weaning in certain patients.
6. **Respiratory muscle dysfunction or fatigue.** Measures to increase the efficiency of the respiratory muscles include:
   a. Improvement of the patient's nutritional status
   b. Correct any underlying metabolic derangements that may contribute to muscle dysfunction, such as decreased phosphorous, calcium, or magnesium.

Selected References

Ashbaugh, D. G., and Petty, T. L. Positive end-expiratory pressure physiology. Indications and contraindications. *J. Thorac. Cardiovasc. Surg.* 65:165, 1973.

Cohen, C. A., Zagelbaum, G., Gross, D., et al. Clinical manifestations of inspiratory muscle fatigue. *Am. J. Med.* 73:308, 1982.

Covelli, H. D., Black, J. W., Olsen, M. S., et al. Respiratory failure precipitated by high carbohydrate loads. *Ann. Intern. Med.* 95:579, 1981.

Demers R. R. Complications of endotracheal suctioning procedures. *Respir. Care* 27:453, 1982.

Deneke, S. M., and Fanburg, B. L. Normobaric oxygen toxicity of the lung. *N. Engl. J. Med.* 303:76, 1980.

Ditchey, R. V. Volume-dependent effects of positive airway pressure on intracavitary left ventricular end-diastolic pressure. *Circulation* 69:815, 1984.

Dulfano, M. J., Adler, K., and Wooten, O. Physical properties of sputum. IV. Effects of 100 per cent humidity and water mist. *Am. Rev. Respir. Dis.* 107:130, 1973.

Fiastro, J. F., Habib, M. P., and Quan, S. F. Pressure support compensation for inspiratory work due to endotracheal tubes and demand continuous positive airway pressure. *Chest* 93:499, 1988.

Gibney, R. T. N., Wilson, R. S., and Pontoppidan, H. Comparison of work of breathing on high gas flow and demand valve continuous positive airway pressure systems. *Chest* 82:692, 1982.

Graham, W. G. B., and Bradley, D. A. Efficacy of chest physiotherapy and intermittent positive-pressure breathing in the resolution of pneumonia. *N. Engl. J. Med.* 299:624, 1978.

Hotchkiss, R. S., and Wilson, R. S. Mechanical ventilatory support. *Surg. Clin. North Am.* 63:417, 1983.

Ingram, R. H., Jr. Mechanical aids to lung expansion. *Am. Rev. Respir. Dis.* 122 (suppl.):23, 1980.

Irwin, R. S., and Demers, R. R. Mechanical Ventilation in Intensive Care Medicine. In J. M. Rippe, R. S. Irwin, J. S. Alpert, and J. E. Daler (eds.), *Intensive Care Medicine*. Boston: Little, Brown, 1985.

Irwin, R. S., and Demers, R. R. Respiratory Adjunct Therapy. In J. M. Rippe, R. S. Irwin, J. S. Alpert, and J. E. Daler (eds.), *Intensive Care Medicine*. Boston: Little, Brown, 1985.

Irwin, R. S., Rosen, M. J., and Bramans, S. Cough. A comprehensive review. *Arch. Intern. Med.* 137:1186, 1977.

Kacmarek, R. M., Dimas, S., Reynolds, J., et al. Technical aspects of positive end-expiratory pressure (PEEP): I. Physics of PEEP devices. *Respir. Care* 27:1478, 1982.

Kacmarek, R. M., Dimas, S., Reynolds, J., et al. Technical aspects of positive end-expiratory pressure (PEEP): II. PEEP with positive-pressure ventilation. *Respir. Care* 27:1490, 1982.

Larca, L., and Greenbaum, D. M. Effectiveness of intensive nutritional regimens in patients who fail to wean from mechanical ventilation. *Crit. Care Med.* 10:297, 1982.

Lourenço, R. V., and Cotromanes, E. Clinical aerosols. I. Characterization of aerosols and their diagnostic uses. *Arch. Intern. Med.* 142:2163, 1982.

MacIntyre, N. R. Respiratory function during pressure support ventilation. *Chest* 89:677, 1986.

Marini, J. J., Pierson, D. J., and Hudson, L. D. Acute labor atelectasis: A prospective comparison of fiberoptic bronchoscopy and respiratory therapy. *Am. Rev. Respir. Dis.* 119:971, 1979.

Millbern, S. M., Downs, J. B., Jumper, L. C., and Modell, J. H. Evaluation of criteria for discontinuing mechanical ventilatory support. *Arch. Surg.* 113:1441, 1978.

Morganroth, M. L., Morganroth, J. L., Nett, L. M., and Petty, T. L. Criteria for weaning from prolonged mechanical ventilation. *Arch. Intern. Med.* 144:1012, 1984.

Murphy, D. F., and Dobb, G. D. Effect of pressure support of spontaneous breathing during intermittent mandatory ventilation. *Crit. Care Med.* 15:612, 1987.

Perel, A. Newer ventilation modes—Temptations and pitfalls. *Crit. Care Med.* 15:707, 1987.

Pontoppidan, H. Mechanical aids to lung expansion in nonintubated surgical patients. *Am. Rev. Respir. Dis.* 122 (suppl.):109, 1980.

Pontoppidan, H., Geffin, B., and Lowenstein, E. Acute respiratory failure in the adult. *N. Engl. J. Med.* 287:690, 1972.

Pontoppidan, H., Wilson, R. S., Rie, M. A., and Schneider, R. S. Respiratory intensive care. *Anesthesiology* 47:96, 1977.

Roussos, C., and Macklem, P. T. The respiratory muscles. *N. Engl. J. Med.* 307:786, 1982.

Sahn, S. A., Lakshminarayan, S., and Petty, T. L. Weaning from mechanical ventilation. *J.A.M.A.* 235:2208, 1976.

Schiff, M. M., and Massaro, D. Effect of oxygen administration by a Venturi apparatus on arterial blood gas valves in patients with respiratory failure. *N. Engl. J. Med.* 277:950, 1967.

Sladen, A., Laver, M. B., and Pontoppidan, H. Pulmonary complications and water retention in prolonged mechanical ventilation. *N. Engl. J. Med.* 279:448, 1968.

Sleigh, M. A., Blake, J. R., and Liron, N. The propulsion of mucus by cilia. *Am. Rev. Respir. Dis.* 137:726, 1988.

Suter, P. M., Fairley, H. B., and Isenberg, M. D. Optimum end-expiratory airway pressure in patients with acute pulmonary failure. *N. Engl. J. Med.* 292:284, 1975.

Tahvanainen, J., Salmerpera, J., and Nikki, P. Extubation criteria after weaning from intermittent mandatory ventilation and continuous positive airway pressure. *Crit. Care Med.* 11:702, 1983.

Tyler, D. C. Positive end-expiratory pressure: A review. *Crit. Care Med.* 11:300, 1983.

Wanner, A. Clinical aspects of mucociliary transport. *Am. Rev. Respir. Dis.* 116:73, 1977.

Wanner, A., and Rao, A. Clinical indications for and effects of bland, mucolytic, and antimicrobial aerosols. *Am. Rev. Respir. Dis.* 122 (suppl.):79, 1980.

Weisman, I. M., Rinaldo, J. E., Rogers, R. M., and Sanders, M. H. Intermittent mandatory ventilation. *Am. Rev. Respir. Dis.* 127:641, 1983.

3

Acute Respiratory Failure

Leonard Soloniuk

- I. Initial approach to patients with respiratory failure
  - A. Initial assessment
    1. Airway patency
    2. Adequacy of respiratory effort
    3. Level of consciousness
    4. Arterial blood gas (ABG) determination
    5. Presence of cyanosis or evidence of arterial desaturation
    6. Auscultation of the chest
  - B. Maintenance of a patent airway
  - C. Supplemental oxygen therapy
  - D. Mechanical ventilation
    1. Bag-and-mask ventilation
    2. Ventilator orders for intubated patients
  - E. Treatment for bronchospasm
- II. Definitions, pathophysiology, and classification of respiratory failure
  - A. Definitions
    1. Arterial hypoxemia
    2. Hypoventilation
  - B. Pathophysiology
    1. Hypoventilation
    2. Ventilation-perfusion (V/Q) mismatch
    3. Shunting
    4. Diffusion impairment
    5. Nonrespiratory causes of hypoxemia
       - a. Decreased FIO_2
       - b. Hemodynamic instability
       - c. Metabolic disturbances
       - d. Extrapulmonary shunting
  - C. Functional classification
    1. Ventilatory failure
       - a. Respiratory muscle fatigue
       - b. Decreased ventilatory drive
       - c. Neuromuscular disorders
       - d. Mechanical defects
    2. Gas exchange failure
       - a. Airway abnormalities
       - b. Pulmonary vascular abnormalities
- III. Evaluation and monitoring of patients with respiratory failure
  - A. History
    1. Preoperative medical history and status
    2. Surgical events
       - a. Area of surgery
       - b. Facial and neck surgery
    3. Anesthetic events
  - B. Subjective complaints
  - C. Physical examination
  - D. Evaluation of oxygenation
    1. ABG determinations
    2. Pulse oximetry
    3. Mixed venous oxygen tension (P_vO_2)
    4. Oxygen transport variables

- **E. Respiratory function tests**
  - **1. The right-to-left-shunt (Q_S/Q_T)**
  - **2. Dead space to tidal volume ratio (V_D/V_T), carbon dioxide production (VCO_2)**
- **F. Chest radiography**
- **G. ECG**
- **H. Pulmonary artery catherization**
- **I. Assessment of other organ systems**

IV. Early postoperative pulmonary complications

- **A. Upper airway obstruction**
  - **1. Foreign matter**
  - **2. Soft-tissue obstruction**
  - **3. Upper airway edema**
  - **4. Extrinsic masses compressing the airway**
  - **5. Acute hypocalcemia**
- **B. Respiratory center depression**
  - **1. Mechanical ventilation with continued endotracheal intubation**
  - **2. Naloxone (Narcan) IV administration**
  - **3. Nalbuphine (Nubain)**
- **C. Persistent neuromuscular blockade from nondepolarizing muscle relaxants**
- **D. Endotracheal tube misplacement**
- **E. Low functional residual capacity states**
  - **1. Adequate pain control**
  - **2. Chest physical therapy**
  - **3. Humidification of inhaled gases**
  - **4. Bronchodilators**
  - **5. Positioning of the patient**
  - **6. Mechanical suctioning of the airway**
  - **7. Positive airway pressure**
- **F. Pneumothorax**
- **G. Aspiration**
- **H. Pulmonary edema**
  - **1. Bronchospasm**
  - **2. B-adrenergic agonists**
    - **a. Beta-1 selective agents**
    - **b. Nonselective agents**
  - **3. Aminophylline**
  - **4. Anticholinergic agents**
    - **a. Glycopyrrolate (Robinul)**
    - **b. Ipratropium (Atrovent)**
  - **5. Glucocorticoids**
  - **6. Volatile anesthesia**

V. Delayed pulmonary complications

- **A. Pneumonia**
- **B. Pulmonary embolism (PE)**
  - **1. Risk factors**
  - **2. Diagnosis of pulmonary embolism is difficult**
    - **a. Evidence of DVT**
    - **b. A normal radionuclide pulmonary perfusion scan**
    - **c. Pulmonary angiography**
  - **3. Treatment**
    - **a. Heparin anticoagulation**
    - **b. Thrombolytic therapy**
    - **c. Surgical embolectomy**
    - **d. Inferior venal caval interruption**

Respiratory failure exists when arterial oxygen saturation or carbon dioxide elimination is inadequate. It is the final common pathway for many disease processes and is a common occurrence in the postoperative intensive care unit. Treatment involves maintenance of adequate oxygen delivery to vital organs with supportive therapy of respiratory function, as well as specific therapy directed toward the underlying condition. This chapter discusses the diagnosis and management of respiratory failure in adults during the postoperative period.

I. Initial approach to patients with respiratory failure

A. Initial assessment of the patient with suspected respiratory failure consists of a rapid initial examination of the patient's distress. Immediate intervention takes priority over all other patient management considerations. Once the patient is more stable, perform a more leisurely and thorough evaluation of the patient to provide a database for more definitive intervention and management of the respiratory failure (see **III**). The initial assessment includes evaluation of:

1. **Airway patency.** Inability of the patient to maintain a patent upper airway or inability to protect the airway from aspiration and clear secretions are indications for immediate placement of an artificial airway.
2. **Adequacy of respiratory effort.** Evaluate respiratory rate, coordination of respiratory muscles, and patient fatigue. A respiratory rate less than 6 per minute or greater than 30 per minute, paradoxical diaphragmatic movement, recruitment of accessory muscles of respiration, and a patient's subjective feeling of dyspnea and fatigue are signs of impending respiratory failure and indications for intervention.
3. **Level of consciousness.** Obtundation or agitation may be signs of hypoxemia or hypercapnia.
4. **Arterial blood gas (ABG) determination.** If the arterial oxygen tension (PaO_2) is less than 50 mm Hg or if the arterial carbon dioxide tension ($PaCO_2$) is greater than 50 mm Hg with an associated acidemia (pH less than 7.30), respiratory failure is present and warrants immediate treatment. Do not delay intervention to wait for ABG results if clinical signs indicate impending respiratory failure.
5. The presence of cyanosis or the evidence of arterial desaturation on pulse oximetry may be helpful in the initial assessment of the patient.
6. Auscultate the chest to ensure bilaterality of breath sounds and adequacy of air movement. Suspicion of a pneumothorax in a patient with evidence of impending respiratory failure or severe hemodynamic deterioration necessitates immediate drainage. This can be accomplished with a 14- or 16-gauge needle-catheter placed in the second intercostal space in the midclavicular line. If time and expertise permit, a chest tube (tube thoracostomy) can be placed. (See chapter on invasive procedures).

B. **Maintenance of a patent airway** (see Appendix). Soft tissue obstruction of the upper airway can be managed by pulling the jaw forward and placing the patient in an upright or lateral position or by the temporary insertion of an oro- or nasopharyngeal airway. Excessive narcotic effect can be reversed by incremental doses of naloxone (Narcan). If these maneuvers are inappropriate or insufficient to restore a patent airway, insertion of an endotracheal tube (ETT) should be performed. Treat stridor and upper airway edema as outlined in **IV.A.3.**

C. **Supplemental oxygen therapy is the next step if hypoxia is present.**

1. The wisest course in treating the patient with impending respiratory failure is administering the highest possible inspired concentration of oxygen (FIO_2). Once arterial desaturation is reversed, the FIO_2 can be

incrementally decreased based on serial ABGs or pulse oximetry. There is concern on the part of many clinicians about administrating a high FIO_2 to patients with chronic lung disease who are carbon dioxide retainers because of the potential of decreasing alveolar ventilation. Hypoxemia must be corrected nevertheless. If hypoventilation occurs with relief of hypoxia, intubation and mechanical ventilation is necessary.

2. **Mask administration of O_2** (with a reservoir bag if available) is appropriate if the patient is not intubated.

D. **Mechanical ventilation.** If there is evidence of hypoventilation or refractory hypoxemia, the patient's ventilation should be mechanically assisted or, if necessary, controlled.

1. **Bag-and-mask ventilation** is often the appropriate initial means of providing assisted ventilation to hypercapnic patients who are not intubated. Even in patients who will need intubation and mechanical ventilation, a period of assisted ventilation with bag and mask can provide a greater margin of safety during attempts at intubation.
2. **For intubated patients,** typical initial ventilator orders are:
   - **a.** Mode: intermittent mandatory ventilation (IMV)
   - **b.** FIO_2: 90–100%
   - **c.** Rate: 8–12 breaths per minute
   - **d.** Tidal volume: 10–15 cc per kilogram (600–1,200 cc)
   - **e.** Inspiratory: expiratory (I-E) ratio: 1:2
   - **f.** Positive end-expiratory pressure (PEEP): 0–5 cm H_2O. PEEP is not routinely used in patients with small airways obstruction (e.g., chronic obstructive pulmonary disease [COPD], asthma or bronchospasm) or increased intracranial pressure (ICP).

E. **Treatment for bronchospasm should be initiated** as outlined in **IV.I.**

II. **Definitions, pathophysiology, and classification of respiratory failure**

A. **Definitions.** Respiratory failure can be defined as gas exchange inadequate to meet metabolic needs. The exchange of oxygen or carbon dioxide, or both, may be impaired, leading to an abnormally low PaO_2 with or without an abnormally elevated $PaCO_2$.

1. **Arterial hypoxemia.** A PaO_2 of less than 60 mm Hg on room air indicates respiratory failure (in the absence of extrapulmonary shunting). The normal PaO_2 varies with age and ambient barometric pressure.
2. Hypoventilation may be associated with hypoxemia and is synonymous with an elevated $PaCO_2$.

B. **Pathophysiology**

1. **Hypoventilation** implies that alveolar ventilation is reduced relative to total body carbon dioxide production, leading to carbon dioxide retention and an elevated $PaCO_2$. Unless oxygen consumption is reduced proportionately to the reduction of alveolar ventilation (an unlikely occurrence), hypoxemia will accompany the carbon dioxide elevation.
2. **Ventilation-perfusion (V/Q) mismatch** is the most common cause of hypoxemia. It is the mechanism of hypoxemia in airway disease (e.g., COPD and asthma) and in pulmonary vascular disease (e.g., pulmonary edema, acute respiratory distress syndrome [ARDS]).
3. **Shunting** can cause severe hypoxemia that is refractory to a high FIO_2 (Fig. 3-1). Arteriovenous fistulas can cause intrapulmonary shunts, but more commonly shunting results from an area of lung that is perfused but completely unventilated. This can occur because of atelectasis or consolidation. The magnitude of shunting can be quantified by measuring the PaO_2 on an FIO_2 of 1.0 (usually impracti-

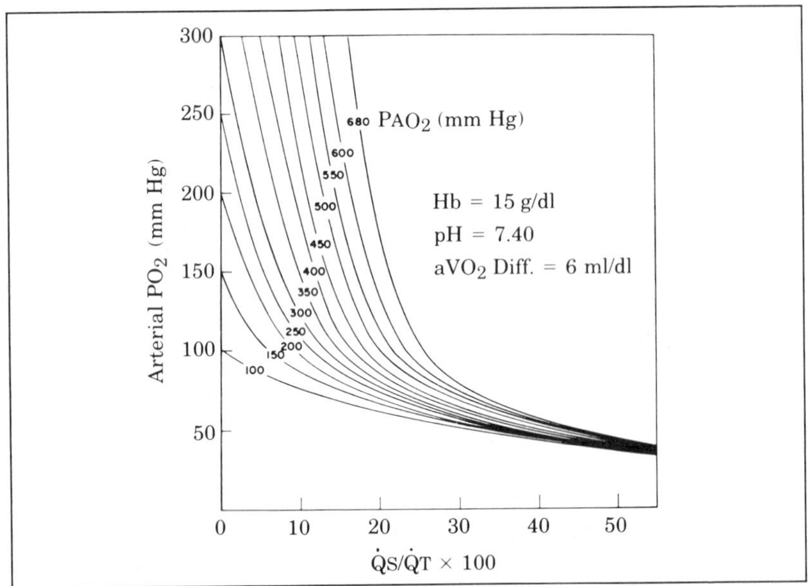

Fig. 3-1. Relationship between percent, right-to-left shunt ($\dot{Q}s/\dot{Q}_T \times 100$), PaO_2, and inspired O_2 or alveolar O_2 tension (P_AO_2). Note that below a $\dot{Q}s/\dot{Q}_T$ of 30, small changes in $\dot{Q}s/\dot{Q}_T$ can produce drastic alterations in PaO_2, particularly when breathing high oxygen concentrations, and that at a $\dot{Q}s/\dot{Q}_T$ above 30, PaO_2 changes little with large changes in inspired oxygen concentration. (From H. Pontoppidan, M. B. Laver, and B. Geffin. Acute respiratory failure in the surgical patient. *Adv. Surg.* 4:163, 1970. With permission.)

cal in critically ill patients) or by using the shunt equation (see **III.E.1**).

4. **Diffusion impairment** implies that the pulmonary capillary blood does not reach equilibration with the PaO_2 of the alveolar gas. It may be significant in patients with interstitial lung disease but is probably much less significant than ventilation-perfusion mismatching as a cause of hypoxemia.
5. **Nonrespiratory causes of hypoxemia**
   a. **Decreased F_IO_2,** a rare iatrogenic cause of hypoxemia in mechanically ventilated patients; must be ruled out as a possible cause of hypoxemia
   b. **Hemodynamic instability,** with a decreased CO or anemia, can lead to decreased tissue oxygen delivery and increased tissue oxygen extraction, causing a decreased mixed venous oxygen tension ($P\bar{v}O_2$ and a resultant decrease in PaO_2).
   c. **Metabolic disturbances** such as fever, sepsis, or thyrotoxicosis can lead to an increased tissue oxygen extraction and a decreased $P\bar{v}O_2$.
   d. **Extrapulmonary shunting** has the same effect as intrapulmonary shunting, with venous admixture leading to arterial hypoxemia.

C. **Functional classification.** Acute respiratory failure can be functionally divided into two categories: failure of ventilatory exchange and gas exchange. These categories are not mutually exclusive and frequently overlap.

1. **Ventilatory failure** (respiratory pump failure, hypercapnic failure) is the failure to maintain adequate alveolar ventilation, due to either a decrease in minute ventilation or an increased dead space. Its presence is established by the presence of an elevated $PaCO_2$ on ABG analysis. The site of failure can be in the CNS control of ventilation, in the efferent and afferent nervous pathways, at the neuromuscular junction, with primary respiratory muscle dysfunction, or in loss of integrity of the thorax and pleura.
   a. **Respiratory muscle fatigue** is an important cause of ventilatory failure. It is frequently present in the later stages of diseases with a primary failure of gas exchange; the large minute ventilation and increased work of breathing leads to inspiratory muscle fatigue with a characteristic sequence of events (Cohen, 1982). Respiratory rate increases, followed by alternation between abdominal and rib cage breathing (respiratory alternans), paradoxical inward abdominal motion during inspiration (abdominal paradox), and, finally, $PaCO_2$ increases associated with decreased minute ventilation and respiratory rate. Respiratory muscle fatigue is treated with mechanical support of ventilation.
   b. **Decreased ventilatory drive** can result from CNS depression from drugs (e.g., anesthetic agents and narcotics) or head injury, myxedema, or central sleep apnea syndrome.
   c. **Neuromuscular disorders** that can cause ventilatory failure include myasthenia gravis, polyneuritis, residual neuromuscular blockade, phrenic nerve palsy, and severe electrolyte disorders (hypophosphatemia, hypomagnesemia).
   d. **Mechanical defects** leading to ventilatory failure can include upper airway obstruction, flail chest, kyphoscoliosis, massive obesity, pneumothorax, pleural effusion, and ascites.
2. **Gas exchange failure** (nonventilatory or normocapnic respiratory failure) is the failure of the pulmonary parenchyma leading to an abnormally low PaO_2. The $PaCO_2$ is initially low or normal but can be elevated in later stages of the disease. Causes of gas exchange failure include:
   a. **Airway abnormalities,** such as COPD (with irreversible small airways obstruction) and asthma
   b. **Pulmonary vascular abnormalities**
      (1) Cardiogenic pulmonary edema from congestive heart failure, caused by increased hydrostatic forces in the pulmonary capillary, is identifiable by the presence of a high pulmonary capillary wedge pressure or elevated left ventricular end-diastolic pressure.
      (2) Noncardiogenic pulmonary edema from increased pulmonary capillary leak occurs in ARDS. It is distinguished from cardiogenic pulmonary edema by the presence of a compatible clinical picture, although pulmonary artery catheterization (showing a pulmonary artery occlusion pressure (PAOP) less than 15–18 mm Hg) is often necessary to make an accurate distinction.
      (3) Increased pulmonary vascular resistance with pulmonary artery hypertension can be primary or associated with thromboembolism, vasoconstriction (from vasoactive mediators, acidosis, or hypoxemia), or compression of pulmonary vessels.

III. **Evaluation and monitoring of patients with respiratory failure.** Postoperative patients with respiratory failure need an initial evaluation to determine preoperative respiratory status, potential etiologies of the respiratory failure, and the severity of respiratory impairment. Based on this evaluation, therapeutic interventions are initiated and repeated evaluations periodically performed to evaluate response to therapy and monitor for potential complications.

A. **History.** The medical history can indicate which patients are at increased risk for postoperative respiratory failure and what disease processes may be contributing to the episode of respiratory failure. Three specific areas should be evaluated:

1. **Preoperative medical history and status**
   a. Prior history of **respiratory disease,** including small airways disease (chronic bronchitis or emphysema), bronchospastic disease, recent respiratory infections, restrictive disease, and neuromuscular disorders
   b. **History of smoking,** including when last smoked and total exposure (in pack-years of cigarettes)
   c. Preoperative **exercise tolerance**
   d. **Use of respiratory medicines,** including corticosteroids, bronchodilators, and oxygen therapy
   e. Preoperative values of **ABGs**
   f. Preoperative **pulmonary function tests (PFTs)**
   g. **Pulmonary course following prior surgeries**
   h. **History of cough or sputum production**
   i. **Upper airway problems** in the past, including prior tracheotomies and symptoms suggestive of sleep-apnea syndrome
2. **Surgical events**
   a. **Area of surgery.** The risk of postoperative respiratory complications varies with the site of surgery, with thoracic and upper abdominal surgery associated with the greatest risk, lower abdominal surgery associated with an intermediate risk, and surgery on the extremities associated with the lowest risk.
   b. **Facial and neck surgery** should alert one to the possibility of airway compromise from direct obstruction (blood or pus in the airway), compression due to a tumor or hematoma, hypocalcemic tetany, or impairment of the recurrent laryngeal nerves causing vocal cord paralysis.
3. **Anesthetic events.** Review the anesthetic record to determine:
   a. Any difficulties in managing the airway
   b. Anesthetic agents that could contribute to postoperative respiratory depression: the total amount of narcotics and the last dose, the use of neuromuscular blockers and reversal agents, the use of intrathecal or epidural opioids that could be causing respiratory depression, or the possibility of a high level of spinal or epidural anesthesia that could be impairing respiratory muscle function
   c. The possibility of excessive fluid administration

B. **Subjective complaints.** Directly inquiring of a patient of his or her breathing can be quite helpful in assessing the degree and sometimes the cause of respiratory distress.

1. A patient who reports trouble breathing and being fatigued almost certainly needs endotracheal intubation and mechanically assisted ventilation.
2. A tachypneic patient who is not dyspneic may require no respiratory intervention, as in the case of a patient compensating for a metabolic acidosis from diabetic ketoacidosis.
3. Occasionally, one is tempted to dismiss a patient's complaints of dyspnea as being secondary to anxiety and to administer a sedative to the patient. Unless the patient is already on full mechanical ventilation, THIS SHOULD NOT BE DONE. If, after a thorough evaluation, no obvious cause of the dyspnea is found, closely monitor and periodically reevaluate the patient.

C. **Physical examination**

1. Level of consciousness

2. Airway patency and gag reflex
3. Respiratory effort and coordination
4. Vital signs
5. Presence of cyanosis, pallor, or diaphoresis
6. Breath sounds: bilaterality, presence of wheezing or stridor
7. Percussion: dullness, hyperresonance
8. Chest wall disease: obesity, kyphoscoliosis, circumferential eschar, flail chest

D. **Evaluation of oxygenation**

1. **Arterial blood gas (ABG) determinations** are the sine qua non for determination of adequate oxygenation. Each ABG should be evaluated in three different aspects:

   a. **Oxygenation (PaO_2).** Normal PaO_2 with room air breathing ranges from 75 mm Hg (in the elderly) to 100 mm Hg (in the young). A rapid way of estimating the expected PaO_2 at sea level is

   $$\text{Expected } PaO_2 = 110 - (0.5 \times \text{age in years})$$

   The PaO_2 should be maintained above 60 mm Hg; a PaO_2 of 50 mm Hg or less requires urgent intervention. Usually, in the acutely ill patient, a margin of safety is desired, and the PaO_2 is maintained above 80 mm Hg.

   The alveolar gas equation may be used to evaluate the efficiency of gas exchange when the patient is not breathing room air. In simplified form,

   $$PaO_2 = (P_B - P_{H2}O) \times FIO_2 - PaCO_2/RQ$$

   P_B = barometric (ambient) pressure
   PH_2O = water vapor pressure at body temperature (47 mm Hg at 37°C)
   FIO_2 = the fractional concentration of inspired O_2
   $PaCO_2$ = the arterial CO_2 tension
   RQ = the respiratory quotient (usually about 0.8)

   From this, the alveolar-to-arterial O_2 gradient can be calculated. With normal lungs, it is 0–10 mm Hg at room air and increases with increasing FIO_2 up to 25–50 mm Hg.

   b. **Ventilation ($PaCO_2$).** Arterial carbon dioxide tension ($PaCO_2$) is essentially equivalent to alveolar carbon dioxide tension ($PACO_2$). It is directly proportional to alveolar ventilation and inversely proportional to total body carbon dioxide production.

   Normal $PaCO_2$ is 36–45 mm Hg. Lower values represent alveolar hyperventilation; higher values represent alveolar hypoventilation. Unless the patient has a chronic, compensated respiratory acidosis with a preexisting elevated $PaCO_2$, the goal should be normocapnia.

   c. **Acid-base status** (see Chap. 26). The arterial pH is normally in the 7.38–7.45 range. The therapeutic goal is to maintain a normal pH. A pH of less than 7.30 requires immediate intervention. If the patient's respiratory status is unstable and requires frequent arterial access (more than 4 ABGs in a 24-hour period), an arterial cannula can be placed (see Chap. 4). This provides ready access to samples or arterial blood, as well as beat-to-beat blood pressure monitoring, which can be most useful in hemodynamically unstable patients.

2. **Pulse oximetry** has become increasingly useful in monitoring postoperative intensive care patients with respiratory failure. It can noninvasively detect arterial desaturation and is especially useful during patient transport and in rapidly assessing the effects on patient oxy-

genation of various maneuvers (e.g., a decrease in FIO_2, suctioning, position changes). The goal is usually to maintain arterial saturation above 90%. Oximetry suffers from being expensive, subject to motion artifact, and less reliable in low flow states such as in patients who are hypoperfused because of cold extremities or hypotension.

3. **Mixed venous oxygen tension (P_vO_2).** The P_vO_2, sampled via a pulmonary artery catheter, is normally about 40 mm Hg. A fall in P_vO_2 generally indicates an increase in tissue oxygen extraction because of a decrease in oxygen delivery relative to tissue oxygen demands. A P_vO_2 of 30 mm Hg or less generally indicates significant tissue hypoxia with anaerobic cellular metabolism. However, the use of P_vO_2 does not necessarily indicate adequate tissue oxygenation; the P_vO_2 does not reflect regional blood flow to critical organs (brain, kidneys, heart) but a global average of oxygenation.
4. **Oxygen transport variables** can be calculated to evaluate the adequacy of tissue oxygen supply.
   a. Oxygen content of blood cannot be measured directly but can be calculated from the oxygen saturation (usually measured directly with a co-oximeter or, less accurately, calculated from tables using the PaO_2) and the hemoglobin concentration.

   $$CaO_2 = (1.39\text{ cc }O_2/\text{g Hgb})(\text{g Hgb/dl blood})(SO_2) + (PO_2)(0.003\text{ ml }O_2/\text{mm Hg/dl blood})$$

   where the second term is the amount of dissolved O_2.

   b. Tissue oxygen delivery can be calculated from the arterial oxygen content and the CO

   $$\text{Oxygen delivery} = (CO)(CaO_2)$$

   c. Oxygen consumption is calculated with the modified Fick equation, using the arterial oxygen content, the mixed venous oxygen content, and the CO:

   $$VO_2 = (CO)(CaO_2 - C_vO_2)$$

   Oxygen consumption normally is 304 ml/min/kg or 140–170 ml per square meter of body surface area.

E. **Respiratory function tests** to assess pulmonary function

1. **The right-to-left-shunt ($\dot{Q}S/\dot{Q}T$)** is the fraction of total blood flow shunted from the right to the left side of the cardiac circulation without being oxygenated. It is an index of overall inefficiency of oxygenation and is affected by anatomic shunting, ventilation-perfusion mismatching, and diffusion defects. It is calculated with the shunt equation

   $$\dot{Q}S/\dot{Q}T = \frac{CcO_2 - CaO_2}{CcO_2 - CvO_2}$$

   where CcO_2 = pulmonary oxygen content (using calculated alveolar oxygen tension from alveolar gas equation)

   CaO_2 = arterial oxygen content
   CvO_2 = mixed venous oxygen content

   Normal resting $\dot{Q}S/\dot{Q}T$ is 2–5%. In the presence of an elevated shunt fraction (e.g., > 30%), increments in FIO_2 have a diminishing effect on PaO_2. Conversely, at low shunt fractions, with high FIO_2, small changes in shunt fraction produce large changes in PaO_2 (Fig. 3-1).
2. **Tests of lung mechanics are reviewed in Chapter 2.**

F. **Chest radiography.** Initial and serial chest radiograph findings are important in diagnosis and management. Findings that may suggest factors contributing to respiratory failure include consolidation (pneumonia or ARDS), pulmonary edema, accidental endobronchial intubation, pneumothorax, atelectasis, or hyperexpansion (with increased lucency).

G. The **ECG** may be helpful in diagnosing associated myocardial ischemia and rhythm disturbances. There may be changes suggestive of cor pulmonale or pulmonary embolism, but these are nonspecific and are rarely helpful.

H. **Pulmonary artery catherization** is useful when intravascular volume status is unclear, myocardial dysfunction is possible, renal function is deteriorating, or high levels of PEEP (10 cm of H_2O or greater) are required to maintain adequate oxygenation. With a catheter in place, PCWP and cardiac output (CO) can be measured, and derived variables such as stroke volume, systemic vascular resistance (SVR), and pulmonary vascular resistance (PVR) can be calculated. Although it is not the practice at the Massachusetts General Hospital, mixed venous blood saturation can be continuously monitored with oximetric catheters or samples can be drawn through the proximal port of the catheter and oxygen transport variables calculated.

I. **Assessment of other organ systems.** Assessment of the function of other vital organs is essential in evaluating patients with respiratory failure. Rather than guiding therapy solely on measurements of total CO or total oxygen transport, evaluate the adequacy of regional distribution of cardiac output and oxygen transport by determining the adequate function of other organ systems. Mentation, urine output, peripheral blood flow, blood-urea nitrogen, serum creatinine, and liver function tests are indicators of adequacy of regional oxygen delivery.

IV. **Early postoperative pulmonary complications**

A. **Upper airway obstruction** in unintubated patients is not a rare postoperative occurrence. Examination of the patient may reveal a "tracheal tug" (suprasternal notch retraction of airway and soft tissue) or a rocking motion of the abdomen with respiration. The presence of snoring suggests loss of pharyngeal muscle tone, whereas stridor suggests glottic edema.

1. Remove any **obstructive foreign matter** from the airway, and suction out blood and sputum from the pharynx.
2. Manage **soft-tissue obstruction** of the upper airway by applying jaw lift, placing the patient in a lateral position, sitting the patient up, or inserting a temporary oral airway or a nasopharyngeal airway (see Chap. 1).
3. **Upper airway edema** can be managed with
   a. Upright posture
   b. Inhalation of cool, humidified mist at high FIO_2
   c. **Nebulized racemic epinephrine,** 0.25–0.5 ml of 1 : 200 solution (2.25%) in 3 ml saline, administered q1–4h PRN
   d. **Inhalation of metered aerosolized corticosteroids** such as dexamethasone (Decadron Respihaler) or beclomethasone, 2–3 puffs q6h
   e. **Parenteral corticosteroids,** such as dexamethasone 1–4 mg IV q6h for up to 12 doses
   f. **Endotracheal intubation** may be required if the edema will be prolonged, as in the case of an airway burn or massive facial trauma.
4. **Extrinsic masses compressing the airway,** such as a hematoma following neck surgery, require emergency surgical treatment.
5. **Acute hypocalcemia** following parathyroid surgery may cause stridor and is readily treated by intravenous calcium chloride, 300–500 mg.

B. **Respiratory center depression** may be caused by narcotics, residual anesthetic agents, or underlying preoperative abnormalities in the control of respiration. Residual narcotic effect should be suspected in the patient with a decreased respiratory rate (rate < 12/min) and pinpoint pupils.

1. **Mechanical ventilation with continued endotracheal intubation** is the treatment of choice until the residual effects of the medications are abated.
2. **Naloxone (Narcan) IV administration** in incremental doses of 20–40 μg may be appropriate to attempt to reverse suspected narcotic respiratory depression. If it is used, monitor the patient closely to detect recurrent respiratory depression occurring 15–30 minutes after the last dose of naloxone. Administering an IM dose equal to the total IV dose of naloxone used may prevent the recurrent depression. The use of naloxone, especially in excessive doses, risks producing pain, agitation, hypertension, myocardial ischemia, or pulmonary edema.
3. **Nalbuphine (Nubain)** in incremental 2–5 mg doses, and butorphanol (Stadol) in doses of 0.5–1 mg, may be used in an attempt to reverse respiratory depression without producing excessive pain. There is, however, the potential of precipitating an acute withdrawal syndrome in patients tolerant to narcotics.

C. **Persistent neuromuscular blockade from nondepolarizing muscle relaxants** should be suspected in a "floppy" patient or in the presence of respiratory muscle weakness or fatigue. It can be confirmed with a peripheral nerve stimulator showing lack of sustained tetany in response to a tetanic stimulus or fade with a train-of-four stimulus. Alternatively, ask the patient to raise his or her head from the bed. Ability to sustain a head lift for 5 seconds makes persistent neuromuscular blockade unlikely. If persistent blockade is likely, an anticholinesterase can be administered with an anticholinergic (see Chap. 29). If this is unsuccessful in reversing the residual blockade, mechanical ventilation is indicated until the neuromuscular block spontaneously resolves.

D. **Endotracheal tube misplacement.** If there is a possibility that an ETT has become dislodged, perform direct laryngoscopy to confirm the tube position. An x ray can also verify the position of the ETT, but there is no time for this if the patient has an obstructed airway. Endobronchial intubation will present with a large $P(A\text{-}a)O_2$. Breath sounds may be unilaterally decreased and possibly associated with coughing or wheezing (from carinal stimulation). Supraglottic tube position is suggested by the patient's ability to phonate or the need for a very large amount of air (> 30 ml) in the tube cuff to effect a seal.

E. **Low functional residual capacity (FRC) states** are common following abdominal and thoracic surgery and in patients whose preoperative state puts them at additional risk: the obese, the elderly, and patients with COPD or ascites. Pathogenesis and treatment of states with a low FRC are discussed more fully in Chapter 2. Briefly, the respiratory pattern tends to be rapid, with shallow breaths at low lung volumes and inadequate sighing and coughing. Consequently, lung volumes are reduced, and FRC falls below closing capacity, so that alveolar closure occurs during tidal volume respiration. Atelectasis results, producing ventilation-perfusion abnormalities and intrapulmonary shunting, leading to hypoxemia. Additionally, the failure to clear secretions and the presence of collapsed airways predispose the patient to the development of respiratory infections. Major therapeutic goals are to expand lung volumes and remove pulmonary secretions.

1. **Adequate pain control.** The use of opioids and local anesthetics with regional anesthetic techniques for postoperative pain control is a major advance in the prevention and treatment of low FRC states

following abdominal or thoracic surgery in high-risk patients (see Chap. 12). They allow the patient to breath comfortably, without splinting and without the respiratory depression from systemic narcotics.

2. **Chest physical therapy** (see Chap. 2)
3. **Humidification of inhaled gases**
4. **Bronchodilators** (see **IV.I**)
5. **Positioning of the patient.** Sitting a patient up removes the weight of intraabdominal contents from the diaphragm, allowing increased lung expansion. Frequent changes in patient position may aid in the mobilization of secretions.
6. **Mechanical suctioning of the airway** to remove secretions and stimulate coughing. In difficult cases, fiberoptic bronchoscopy may be useful.
7. **Positive airway pressure** by means of mask continuous positive airway pressure (CPAP) or PEEP (see Chap. 2)

F. **Pneumothorax** must be considered with any sudden respiratory or cardiovascular deterioration.

1. Recent placement of a central venous catheter, asthma, bullous emphysema, cavitary pneumonia, ARDS, and high peak inspiratory pressures with mechanical ventilation place patients at increased risk for barotrauma.
2. Physical examination may reveal unilateral hyperresonance with percussion or unilaterally diminished breath sound. Tracheal deviation may be present with tension pneumothorax.
3. Chest radiography establishes the diagnosis, but hemodynamic deterioration with clinical evidence for a pneumothorax requires immediate treatment without delaying for radiographic confirmation.
4. With severe hemodynamic deterioration, a large (14- or 16-gauge) IV catheter can be quickly inserted in the second intercostal space in the midclavicular line. Chest tube placement is the definitive treatment (see Appendix).

G. **Aspiration** is generally suggested by a history of unconsciousness with an unprotected airway or difficulty with maintenance of an intact airway on induction of or emergence from anesthesia. A gastric fluid pH less than 2.5, a large volume of aspirated fluid, and particulate matter in the aspirate increase the extent of lung injury.

1. Treatment is primarily supportive. Intubate the patient until the conditions that predisposed to aspiration (e.g., diminished gag reflex, obtundation) have resolved. Administer oxygen therapy and positive airway pressure as needed to treat hypoxemia. Treat associated bronchospasm as detailed in **IV.G.**
2. Remove particulate matter with tracheal suctioning. Large particles or the presence of regional loss of lung volume on clinical examination or chest x ray indicate the need for bronchoscopy.
3. Prophylactic antibiotics and corticosteroids have no role in the treatment of aspiration syndrome.

H. **Pulmonary edema** refers to the presence of greater-than-normal quantities of lung water. It presents with rales and tachypnea on physical examination and pulmonary capillary pressure (cardiogenic pulmonary edema) or increased pulmonary vascular permeability (ARDS). Undertake a vigorous search for the etiology of the pulmonary edema. Manage cardiogenic pulmonary edema by manipulation of preload, afterload, and contractility (as discussed in Chap. 8). With noncardiogenic pulmonary edema, maintain PCWP as low as is consistent with an adequate CO with fluid restriction, diuresis, vasodilators (e.g., nitroglycerin), or a combination. For both types of pulmonary edema, PEEP or CPAP can be used effectively.

1. **Bronchospasm** can arise as an exacerbation of an underlying disorder. In addition, it should prompt consideration of pulmonary edema, pulmonary embolism, anaphylaxis, or upper airway obstruction. Occasionally, bronchospasm can be precipitated or exacerbated by an indwelling ETT, especially if it is in contact with the carina. These potentially reversible causes should be sought and treated. Otherwise, oxygen therapy, humidification of inspired gases, and bronchodilators are the mainstays of therapy.
2. **Beta-adrenergic agonists** are the first-line agents for treatment of acute bronchospasm. Agents with predominant beta-2 activity are preferred to minimize the undesirable beta-1 effects of tachycardia, arrhythmias, and hypertension. Central nervous system stimulation is also a potential side effect. Administration is usually via nebulization, although an IV infusion (usually of epinephrine) is an excellent alternative in unintubated patients too dyspneic to tolerate inhalation therapy or in refractory patients with severe bronchospasm. In refractory bronchospasm, the doses that follow can be increased in the drug administered more frequently, with the presence of beta-1 side effects usually being the limiting factor.
   a. **Beta-2 selective agents** produce predominantly beta-2 effects, although beta-1 effects can occur. Available agents include:
      (1) **Albuterol (Proventil, Ventolin)** is commonly used. The dose is 0.5 ml of a 0.5% solution (2.5 mg) in 2–3 ml of NS inhaled via nebulizer q4–6h.
      (2) **Metaproterenol (Alupent).** Dose is 0.2–0.3 ml of 5% solution in 2–3 ml of NS inhaled via nebulizer q3–4h.
      (3) **Terbutaline (Brethine, Bricanyl)** can be administered via nebulizer with a dose of 1–2 mg in 2–3 ml of NS q4–6h. It can be administered subcutaneously with a dose of 0.25–0.5 mg SQ q4–6h.
      (4) **Bitolterol (Tornalate) and pirbuterol (Maxair)** are available only as metered dose inhalers, making administration via ETT difficult. An adapter that facilitates administration to an intubated patient is available.
   b. **Nonselective agents** produce both beta-1 and beta-2 effects. They include:
      (1) **Isoetharine (Bronkosol).** Dose is 0.25–0.5 ml of 0.5–1.0T solution in 2–3 ml or NS inhaled via nebulizer q4–6h.
      (2) **Racemic epinephrine** produces both alpha-adrenergic and beta-adrenergic effects, leading to mucosal vasoconstriction, making it advantageous in situations where mucosal edema is (or may be) present. Dose is 0.5 ml of 2.25% solution in 2.5–3.5 ml of NS inhaled via nebulizer q1–4h.
      (3) **Epinephrine** produces potent alpha and beta effects. It is the drug of choice for bronchospasm secondary to anaphylaxis.
         (a) **Subcutaneous administration** requires adequate skin blood flow, which may not be present in postoperative or critically ill patients. Dose is 0.3 ml of 1 : 1,000 solution SQ q20min for three doses.
         (b) **Given by IV,** it has a fast onset and offset, facilitating bedside titration. An IV infusion (1 mg in 250 ml 5% D/W) starting 0.5–1.0 μg/min, can be titrated to effect.
      (4) **Isoproterenol** can be used for refractory bronchospasm. Via IV infusion (1 mg in 250 ml 5% D/W), the dose starts at 1–5 μg/min, titrated to effect. Tachycardia, arrhythmias, and hypotension are the principal adverse effects.
3. **Aminophylline.** This agent can be readily administered as an IV infusion and has been widely used to treat bronchospasm. Its significant disadvantages include unpredictable kinetics, frequent drug

interactions, and a narrow therapeutic-to-toxic ratio with frequent side effects.

a. A **loading dose** should be administered to patients who have not been receiving aminophylline or a theophylline preparation. The dose is 6 mg per kilogram of lean body weight infused over 20 to 30 minutes.

b. **Maintenance dose**

(1) **Young, healthy patients:** 0.7 mg/kg/h for 12 hours; then 0.5 mg/kg/h

(2) **Elderly, healthy patients:** 0.5–0.7 mg/kg/h for 12 hours, then 0.3 mg/kg/h

(3) Congestive heart failure patients and patients with liver disease require smaller doses than healthy patients.

c. Measure **blood levels** frequently in unstable patients.

4. **Anticholingeric agents** may be helpful for patients with bronchospasm, especially in combination with B-adrenergic agonists.

a. **Glycopyrrolate (Robinul)** can be nebulized in a dose of 0.2–0.4 mg in 2–3 ml of NS q2–8h.

b. **Ipratropium (Atrovent)** is available only with a metered dose inhaler, making it less useful for critically ill patients. The dose is two inhalations (36 μg) q6h.

5. Administer **glucocorticoids** for refractory bronchospasm. Methylprednisolone (SoluMedrol) 0.5 mg/kg IV q6h or hydrocortisone (SoluCortef) 100–150 mg IV q6h are typical dosages. The effect of the glucocorticoids may take several hours to be manifest.

6. **Volatile anesthesia** may have a role in the most refractory cases. Halothane has been used in this setting.

V. **Delayed pulmonary complications.** Postoperative causes of respiratory failure that are usually delayed include the following:

A. **Pneumonia** (see Chap. 25) is a significant cause of respiratory deterioration. The diagnosis is suggested by the presence of one or more of the following: fever, leukocytosis, purulent sputum, and roentgenographic infiltrates. After sputum and blood cultures are planted, initiate empiric broad-spectrum antimicrobial therapy based on the suspected pathogens (see Chap. 25). The goals of treatment are defervescence, reduction in leukocytosis, reduction in radiographic infiltrates, and clearing of purulence and pathogenic organisms from the sputum. Patients who do not respond to initial therapy should have a reassessment of antimicrobial therapy and a vigorous search for the etiology of the infection.

B. **Pulmonary embolism (PE)** continues to be a significant cause of postoperative morbidity and mortality. Consider it when sudden, quantal respiratory deterioration occurs in patients at risk.

1. **Risk factors.** More than 95% of pulmonary emboli arise from lower-extremity deep venous thrombosis (DVT). Factors that predispose to DVT include hip and pelvic surgery, prolonged bed rest, the postpartum period, right ventricular failure, carcinoma, obesity, and estrogen use. Also at risk is the rare "hypercoagulable" patient with antithrombin III, protein C, protein S deficiency, or homocystinuria.

2. **Diagnosis of pulmonary embolism is difficult.** Symptoms, signs, ECGs, ABGs, laboratory studies, and routine chest roentgenograms are nonspecific and insensitive.

a. **Evidence of DVT** on venography or noninvasive studies necessitates treatment with anticoagulation or inferior venal caval interruption. However, more than 20% of patients with PE have no evidence of DVT, and the presence of DVT does not definitely answer the question of the cause of the respiratory deterioration.

b. **A normal radionuclide pulmonary perfusion scan** eliminates the possibility of clinically significant PE. In patients with existing parenchymal lung disease (COPD, pneumonia, ARDS), the perfusion scan is nonspecific unless normal. A ventilation scan may add specificity if the chest x ray is clear and the perfusion defects are segmental or larger.
c. **Pulmonary angiography** remains the standard for detection of PE. In patients with nondiagnostic perfusion scans, in the presence of severe respiratory deterioration, and in patients with contraindications for anticoagulation (e.g., recent neurosurgery), undertake angiography to demonstrate the presence of PE before proceeding with anticoagulant therapy, thrombolytic therapy, embolectomy, or interruption of the inferior vena cava.

3. **Treatment**
   a. **Heparin anticoagulation** is the standard therapy for PE. Unless contraindicated, initiate it immediately in the presence of a strong clinical suspicion of PE without waiting for confirmatory tests.
   b. **Thrombolytic therapy** may be considered in patients with massive embolism and resultant arterial hypotension (see Chap. 20). It is usually contraindicated in postoperative patients because of the hemorrhagic risk.
   c. **Surgical embolectomy** is indicated for massive embolism and systemic hypotension when facilities and personnel for cardiopulmonary bypass are immediately available.
   d. **Inferior venal caval interruption** is required in patients with documented PE who have a contraindication to anticoagulation. Placement of a filter or clip or placation of the venal lava is indicated on an urgent basis in these patients.

C. **The adult respiratory distress syndrome (ARDS)** is a syndrome of diffuse alveolar capillary membrane injury resulting in noncardiogenic pulmonary edema and respiratory failure. It is an important and frequent cause of respiratory deterioration in the postoperative period.

1. **Diagnosis of ARDS** depends on the recognition of profound respiratory failure with severe hypoxemia associated with:
   a. The presence of a compatible clinical condition that can initiate the alveolar damage. Table 3-1 lists conditions that are recognized to be associated with ARDS.
   b. Diffuse infiltrates on chest radiogram, with at least multilobar involvement
   c. Exclusion of other diagnoses, specifically left ventricular failure, chronic pulmonary disease, atelectasis, and pulmonary embolism
2. **Pathophysiology**
   a. The specific mechanism of the diffuse alveolar capillary membrane injury in ARDS is unknown. A large number of potential mediators of the acute lung injury have been proposed, but none has been satisfactorily established as the cause of the syndrome. Whatever the mediator(s), the result is increased alveolar permeability and interstitial edema, leading to decreased pulmonary compliance. Progression leads to alveolar edema and collapse.
   b. V/Q mismatching and intrapulmonary shunting occur, with the shunt fraction usually increased to greater than 15%.
   c. Lung volumes are reduced, including significant reductions in functional residual capacity (FRC), because of the alveolar edema and collapse.
   d. These factors cause a profound hypoxemia, which, because of the shunting, is resistant to correction by a high FIO_2.
3. **Clinical course.** Initially after the alveolar injury, no clinical or radiographic signs may be present. In the following 12–24 hours,

Table 3-1. Causes of adult respiratory distress syndrome (ARDS)

Infectious causes
Gram-negative sepsis
Bacterial pneumonia
Fungal and pneumocystic carinii pneumonia
Tuberculosis
Viral pneumonia
Trauma
Burns
Fat embolism
Fractures
Lung contusion
Nonthoracic trauma
Shock of any etiology
Aspiration
Gastric contents
Near drowning
Drug related
Chlordiazepoxide (Librium)
Colchicine
Dextran 40
Ethchlorvynol (Placidyl)
Fluorescein
Leukoagglutinin reaction
Narcotics (heroin, methadone, propoxyphene)
Salicylates
Thiazides
Metabolic disorders
Diabetic ketoacidosis
Uremia
Histiochemical
Dextran
Inhaled toxin (NO_2, NH, CL_2, cadmium phosgene, smoke, oxygen)
Pancreatitis
Smoke inhalation
Miscellaneous
Amniotic fluid embolism
Bowel infarction
Carcinomatosis
Consumptive coagulopathy
Dead fetus
Eclampsia

Adapted from Bone, R. C., George, R. B., and Hudson, L. D. (eds.). *Acute Respiratory Failure*. New York: Churchill Livingstone, 1987.

there is deterioration with the onset of tachypnea and crackles, progressive hypoxemia refractory to supplemental oxygen, carbon dioxide retention, and the development of interstitial, and then alveolar, infiltrates diffusely on chest roentgenograms. The initial lung injury may resolve within several days, or it may progress to a more indolent stage. This more advanced stage of ARDS is characterized by progressive pulmonary fibrosis with decreased functional residual capacity and compliance, increased dead space (V_D/V_T), and elevated pulmonary vascular resistance. Recovery is possible, even in the advanced stages, but many patients die of septic complications or multisystem organ failure.

4. **Therapy for ARDS** is directed toward control of the initiating disorder and supportive care aimed at maintaining adequate tissue oxygenation of vital organs. Although numerous specific therapies for ARDS have been proposed, none has been adequately demonstrated to be beneficial; specifically, corticosteroids are not indicated in the treatment of ARDS. The cornerstones of therapy remain:
   a. **Ventilator support** with reduction of F_{IO_2} to minimal levels
   b. **PEEP** to open all recitable small airways and alveoli
   c. **Minimize transvascular plasma leakage** (keep pulmonary artery occlusion pressure (PAOP) low)
   d. Find and treat **sepsis**
   e. Maintain adequate **cardiac output** and **renal blood flow**
   f. Careful attention to **support of other organ systems**

VI. **Chronic respiratory failure.** One of the more challenging problems in the postoperative ICU is the care of patients with chronic respiratory failure. These patients include previously normal patients with ARDS, as well as patients with preexisting chronic respiratory failure with superimposed acute respiratory failure. These patients require support of ventilation and oxygenation while meticulously managing complications and keeping the risk of iatrogenic problems as low as possible. Ultimate recovery depends on the patient's overcoming the cause of the respiratory failure.

A. **Ventilator support**

1. Basic principles and techniques remain important: chest physical therapy, bronchodilation, and humidification of administered gases. In addition, scrupulous system-by-system attention to classically nonrespiratory aspects of care (e.g., cardiovascular system, central nervous system, metabolism, kidneys) is essential, as is an ongoing search for sepsis.
2. Reducing the F_{IO_2} to less than 50–60% with adequate oxygenation is a major therapeutic goal in the treatment of chronic respiratory failure. The F_{IO_2} in humans at which oxygen toxicity can occur has not been determined and may be influenced by a number of factors. F_{IO_2} levels less than 50–60% seem to be tolerated for prolonged periods without overt evidence of oxygen toxicity.
3. PEEP (see Chap. 2). The application of PEEP recruits airspaces, which increases functional residual capacity and improves gas exchange. PEEP may thereby allow administration of a lower oxygen concentration. The inability to maintain PaO_2 above 60 mm Hg at a F_{IO_2} greater than or equal to 50% is, in general, a valid indication for a PEEP trial. In applying PEEP, weigh its benefits of reducing venous admixture and increasing PaO_2 against the potential detriments of barotrauma, reduction of CO and BP, and increased intracranial pressure (ICP).
   a. **PEEP is increased** incrementally in steps of 3–5 cm H_2O, and ABGs are drawn after the patient stabilizes (in hemodynamics and in ventilator pressures), usually 15–30 minutes, although the full effect may take longer to be manifest.

b. **Reversal of arterial desaturation** is the usual end point for application of PEEP. The lowest level of PEEP is chosen that will allow reduction of FIO_2 to less than, or equal to, 50–60% while maintaining PaO_2 at greater than 60 mm Hg. Rarely is it necessary to increase PEEP above 15–20 cm H_2O.

c. Other criteria for determining the level of PEEP to administer have been proposed: **maximal lung compliance, minimal shunt fraction, greatest level of oxygen delivery, and lowest dead space.** However, if reversal of arterial hypoxemia occurs before fulfilling one of these criteria, further PEEP increases are probably not warranted. On the other hand, if a patient should fulfill one of these criteria and is still hypoxemic, further PEEP increments may be beneficial.

d. **A continuous-flow, nondemand valve system** should be used, and circuit pressures should be observed to ensure that the positive pressures prescribed are not lost with efforts to breathe spontaneously.

e. **Airflow obstruction (asthma, COPD)** is a relative contraindication to the use of PEEP. The hypoxia is usually easily treated with an increased FIO_2, and there is usually an associated pulmonary hyperinflation that can be made worse with PEEP (Tuxen, 1989). In the case of dynamic airway collapse, PEEP in low levels may be beneficial in maintaining open airways. The ventilator cycling pressure should be observed as PEEP is added. If the peak pressures do not rise with the PEEP, low levels of PEEP may be helpful in preventing dynamic airway collapse.

f. **Barotrauma** is a risk of PEEP therapy, especially if the patient is suffering from a pulmonary parenchymal destructive process such as ARDS, staphylococcal pneumonia, or emphysema. Appropriate adjustments in tidal volume and rate can decrease peak inspiratory pressure and prevent air trapping, possibly lessening the risk of barotrauma.

g. **Cardiovascular function may be compromised** by the use of PEEP (see **D**). The effects of PEEP can be monitored by examining the changes in heart rate, CO, and pulmonary and systemic pressures, as well as monitoring RRV function if available. There are several means by which PEEP can affect CO:

(1) The predominant effect of PEEP is to decrease venous return to the heart. The decrease in CO that results can be treated with IV fluid infusion, inotropic support, or both.

(2) At higher levels of PEEP, pulmonary vascular resistance (PVC) may increase. The resultant right ventricular overload may cause leftward septal shift and decreased ventricular compliance, leading to compromise of left ventricular function, as well as right ventricular ischemia.

4. **Respiratory muscle oxygen consumption.** The oxygen consumption of the respiratory muscles can be increased with a reduced compliance, or increase in airway resistance. In these situations, it may be advisable to provide enough mechanical ventilator assistance to meet the patient's minute ventilator requirements entirely. By providing full ventilator support, the oxygen consumption of the respiratory muscles may be decreased, thus providing more oxygen to other tissue beds. On the other hand, maintenance of some respiratory muscle effort may contribute to diaphragmatic muscle strength and facilitate subsequent weaning. A reasonable approach in patients who have been placed on mechanical ventilation after a protracted period of respiratory failure is to "rest" the respiratory muscles with full ventilator support along with adequate sedation for 24–48 hours, and then to lessen support to allow some respiratory muscle effort.

B. Adequacy of tissue oxygenation. A major goal in managing patients with respiratory failure is the maintenance of vital organ function, which includes ensuring adequate tissue oxygenation. Judging adequate tissue oxygen delivery can be difficult.

1. The best evidence of adequate tissue oxygen delivery is adequate organ function (good urine output, normal mentation, warm well-perfused extremities).
2. One potential measure of adequate tissue oxygen delivery is mixed venous oxygen tension (PO_2). A normal or increased PO_2 (> 40 mm Hg) does not ensure that oxygen delivery is adequate, but a decreased PO_2 (< 25 mm Hg) is suggestive of tissue hypoxia in this setting.
3. The presence of a metabolic acidosis or increase serum lactate is suggestive of tissue hypoxia.
4. Cardiac index generally should be maintained at greater than 2.0–2.5 L/min/m^2.
5. The optimal level of hemoglobin (or hematocrit) is not well established. Most clinicians keep the hematocrit around 30–35%.

C. Cardiovascular support. Hemodynamic and respiratory function are complexly intertwined in respiratory failure and especially in ARDS. Cardiovascular function must be carefully monitored from the standpoint of effects on hemodynamics, respiratory function, and systemic function in general.

1. **Ventricular preload** should be maintained with adequate volume replacement. If large amounts of PEEP are applied (and transmitted to the great vessels), venous return will be compromised. Consequent decreases in CO generally can be treated with IV fluid infusion, inotropic support, or both.
2. **Right ventricular distention** may occur if PVR is greatly elevated. In such situations, consider inotropic support earlier because intravascular volume replacement may further increase right ventricular distention. Right ventricular distention will diminish left ventricular function by causing septal shift into the left ventricular cavity. Left ventricular compliance will decrease, and left ventricular filling will be impaired. Second, coronary perfusion of the right ventricle will suffer secondary to the rise in right ventricular systolic and diastolic pressures. Right ventricular ischemia with further right ventricular dysfunction can follow.
3. In an attempt to minimize lung water, keep hydrostatic pressure in the pulmonary circulation low. However, maintain adequate intravascular volume to preserve systemic organ perfusion. Monitor patients carefully when intravascular volume is decreased to minimize pulmonary hydrostatic pressures:
   a. With a decrease in intravascular volume, there will be less tolerance to PEEP since decreased CO with positive airway pressure is largely due to changes in preload.
   b. Right ventricular ejection may already be impeded (by increased PVR). Thus, an adequate right ventricular preload is required.
   c. With multiple organ system failure, tissue oxygen needs may be greatly increased. Consequently, a high CO may be necessary.
   d. Decreased renal perfusion may lead to renal failure, which in turn increases mortality.
   e. There is no evidence that increased lung water is an important factor in further progression of lung injury.
4. **PaO_2, cardiovascular function, and oxygen consumption.** The interplay of the many factors that affect PaO_2 is complex. Changes in CO, oxygen delivery, tissue oxygen extraction, or any combination of these may have significant effects on PaO_2. Acute changes in PaO_2 may be due to changes in CO or tissue oxygen consumption and may

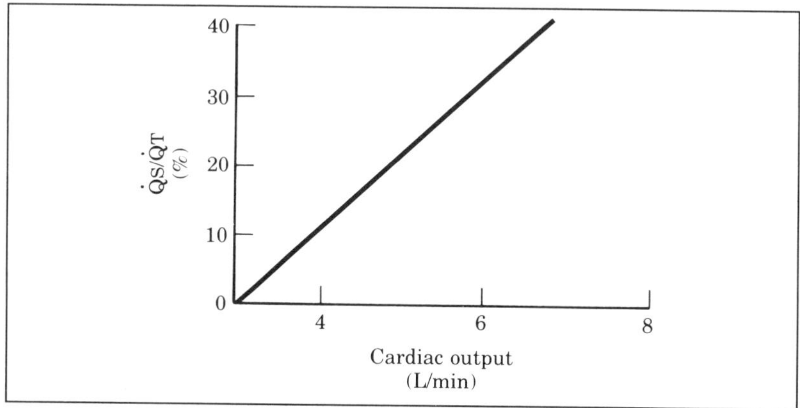

Fig. 3-2. Effects of CO changes on $\dot{Q}S/\dot{Q}T$. Increases in CO can produce a detrimental increase in $\dot{Q}S/\dot{Q}T$, whereas decreased CO can decrease $\dot{Q}S/\dot{Q}T$. Opposing effects of CO changes on $P\bar{v}O_2$ make effects on PAO_2 unpredictable.

not reflect progressive reversal of lung injury. A direct positive correlation between CO and shunt fraction has been observed in patients with ARDS (Fig. 3-2). An increase in CO may therefore cause the PaO_2 to decrease independent of any changes in pulmonary structure or function. Opposing this, however, is the tendency for an increase in CO to increase oxygen delivery, which tends to increase PaO_2. The net effect of CO changes on PaO_2 in a given patient is unpredictable. The following manipulations (which have not been tested in randomized studies) may be done in an attempt to increase PaO_2. The effect on PaO_2 and oxygen transport variables must be monitored because the effect in a given patient cannot be predicted.

a. **Decrease cardiac output.** In some individuals, CO may be excessively elevated (e.g., the febrile or septic patient), and it may be advisable to lower CO and thus decrease shunt fraction. Decreases in CO may be achieved by cooling a hyperthermic patient or administering appropriate sedation. Deliberate hypothermia has not been demonstrated to be useful.
b. **Increase cardiac output.** The aim is to increase oxygen delivery in the hope that it will outweigh the increased shunt fraction (QS/QT) and potential decrease in PaO_2. CO can be increased with fluid infusion, inotropes, or both.
c. **Decrease oxygen consumption.** This can be accomplished with sedation, neuromuscular blockade (in the ventilated patient), and prevention and treatment of fever.

D. **Nutritional support** (see Chap. 18). Adequate nutrition is essential to recovery from prolonged respiratory failure. Inadequate nutrition slows recovery, whereas excessive nutritional support may increase ventilator demands. The previously healthy patient may require only maintenance nutritional support, but many surgical patients with postoperative respiratory failure have preexisting deficits that require repletion for optimal recovery.

1. **Respiratory quotient.** The respiratory quotient (VCO_2/VO_2) normally is 1.0 for a glucose energy source and 0.7 for fat energy source. Glucose administered in excess of metabolic needs leads to fat synthesis resulting in an RQ greater than 1.0, due to increased $\dot{V}CO_2$ leading to increased ventilator requirements to maintain normocap-

nia. This can be a significant factor in patients with a high VD/VT. In patients with high mechanical ventilator requirements or difficulty weaning from the ventilator, the RQ can be measured or the caloric intake can be empirically reduced. If a high RQ is demonstrated, the amount of glucose infused can be decreased to lessen VCO_2.

2. **Intravenous lipid infusions** can be utilized to deliver substantial caloric intake. Although this is not the general practice at the Massachusetts General Hospital, many clinicians use lipid infusions to provide 50% of the calories for patients in respiratory failure.
3. Nutrition during active weaning from mechanical ventilation should be altered to avoid excessive carbon dioxide production or increased respiratory drive. Administration of calories and nitrogen at maintenance levels and not attempting nutritional repletion is appropriate during this period.

E. **Sepsis** (see Chap. 19). Although sepsis is often the precipitating event for respiratory failure, especially in ARDS, it can also develop later and must be constantly monitored for and treated early. It is the most common cause of death in patients with ARDS. Nosocomial infections, particularly pneumonias, are frequent complications of respiratory failure and must be treated aggressively. Vigorous evaluation and treatment of infection in patients with ARDS may improve survival.

1. **Periodic monitoring** of the patient with respiratory failure should include:
   a. **Sputum appearance and Gram's stain**
   b. **White blood count and blood smear**
   c. **Culture of sputum, urine, and wound drainage**
2. **Respiratory tract colonization** of patients with respiratory failure is expected and must be distinguished from infection, an often difficult distinction. An increase in sputum production, leukocytosis, changing radiographic infiltrates, physical findings of pneumonia, pleuritic pain, cough, or nonspecific clinical deterioration can be clues to an active infection. Some important clinical signs and symptoms of sepsis include:
   a. Sudden onset of dyspnea, tachypnea, agitation, or confusion
   b. Hypothermia or hyperthermia
   c. A high CO state with low systemic vascular resistance and an elevated PO_2
   d. Hyperglycemia
   e. Thrombocytopenia
   f. Hypoxemia and respiratory alkalosis
3. Patients in the ICU have several unique causes of fever and sepsis:
   a. **Sinusitis and otitis media secondary to nasotracheal or nasogastric tubes** (20–30% of patients with nasotracheal tubes in some series)
   b. **Sepsis secondary to invasive catheters** (e.g., PA catheters, hyperalimentation lines, urinary catheters)
   c. **Drug fever**
   d. **Cholecystitis**
   e. **Deep venous thrombosis**
   f. **Pulmonary emboli**
4. **If sepsis is suspected,** begin a thorough search for the possible source. A review of the history, a thorough examination, appropriate cultures, and Gram's stains are indicated. If there is no identifiable focus, roll-plate and change all invasive intravascular catheters. Abdominal and thoracic computerized topographic scans, ultrasonic scans, and other noninvasive tests may be necessary if no source is located. Broad-spectrum antibiotic therapy (and possibly antifungal therapy) may be necessary.

F. **Prophylaxis for upper gastrointestinal hemorrhage.** Patients with respiratory failure should receive prophylaxis against gastrointestinal hemorrhage. Although vigorous-use antacids or histamine-2 (H-2) antagonists is effective, sucralfate (Carafe), 1 tablet qid, may be the agent of choice because some studies suggest it may markedly reduce the incidence of nosocomial pneumonias compared to the use of antacids or H-2 antagonists. If antacids or H-2 antagonists are used, monitor gastric pH to ensure that it is maintained greater than 4.0. If the patient is being fed by an enteral route, prophylaxis is probably not necessary.

G. **Hematological complications.** There is a high incidence of disseminated intravascular coagulation (DIC) in patients with ARDS. Thus, prothrombin time, partial thromboplastin time, and platelet count should be monitored periodically. (Management of DIC is outlined in Chap. 20.)

Selected References

Bell, R. C., Coalson, J. J., Smith, J. D., et al. Multiple organ system failure and infection in adult respiratory distress syndrome. *Ann. Intern. Med.* 99:293, 1983.

Bone, R. C., George, R. B., and Hudson, L. D. (eds.). *Acute Respiratory Failure.* New York: Churchill Livingstone, 1987.

Cohen, C. A., Zagelbaum, G., Gross, D., et al. Clinical manifestations of inspiratory muscle fatigue. *Am. J. Med.* 73:308, 1982.

Danek, S. J., Lynch, J. P., Weg, E. G., et al. The dependence of oxygen uptake on oxygen delivery in the adult respiratory distress syndrome. *Am. Rev. Respir. Dis.* 122:387, 1980.

Marini, J. J. Should PEEP be used in airway obstruction? *Am. Rev. Respir. Dis.* 140:1, 1989.

Raffin, T. A. ARDS: Mechanisms and management. *Hosp. Practice* 22:65, 1987 (Nov. 15).

Schmidt, G. A., and Hall, J. B. Acute or chronic respiratory failure. Assessment and management of patients with COPD in the emergent setting. *J.A.M.A.* 261:3444, 1989.

Tuxen, D. V. Detrimental effects of positive end-expiratory pressure during controlled mechanical ventilation of patients with severe airflow obstruction. *Am. Rev. Respir. Dis.* 140:5, 1989.

West, J. B. (ed.). *Pulmonary Pathophysiology: The Essentials* (3d ed.). Baltimore: Williams & Wilkins, 1987.

4

Vascular Cannulation

Michael Bannon

- I. Venous cannulation
  - A. Peripheral venous access
    1. Veins
    2. Cannula size
    3. Techniques for locating and distending peripheral veins
    4. Technique for peripheral venous cannulation
    5. Emergency peripheral venous access during resuscitation
  - B. Central venous access
    1. General guidelines and precautions
    2. Indications for central venous access
    3. Choice of access site
    4. External jugular vein cannulation
    5. Internal jugular vein cannulation
    6. Subclavian vein cannulation
    7. Antecubital vein cannulation with long catheter
    8. Femoral vein cannulation
  - C. Care of indwelling venous catheters
    1. Infection
    2. Thrombosis
    3. Infiltration
- II. Pulmonary artery catheterization
  - A. Indications
  - B. Standard French catheter
  - C. Preferred insertion site
  - D. Preparation for insertion
  - E. Technique for insertion
  - F. Complications and care of PA catheters
    1. Pulmonary infarction
    2. Pulmonary artery rupture
- III. Arterial cannulation
  - A. Indications
  - B. Radial artery
  - C. Collateral circulation
  - D. Technique for radial artery cannulation
  - E. Complications of arterial cannulation

In the postoperative patient, vascular cannulation is essential. Vascular cannulation provides the ability to measure pressures which help guide medical therapy and provide a route for administration of medications.

I. Venous cannulation

A. Peripheral venous access

1. Although any palpable or visible vein can be used, the veins of the hand and forearm are preferable due to ease of access and stability. Other considerations for access sites are:
   - **a.** Ideally, cannulation attempts should begin distally on the extremity. In the event of vein infection, thrombosis, perforation, or extravasation, subsequent cannulation can be performed more proximally.
   - **b.** Patient comfort can be enhanced by avoiding veins near joints or in the dominant arm.
   - **c.** Leg veins provide adequate access sites but are less desirable due to the risk of deep vein thrombosis.
2. Cannula size should be appropriate for the intended purpose. For volume infusion in adults, use a cannula that is 16 gauge or larger and 3 inches or less in length. Resistance to flow is inversely proportional to the fourth power of the conduit radius and directly proportional to catheter length. Blood infusion cannulas should be 18 gauge or larger.
3. Techniques for locating and distending peripheral veins include using a tourniquet to obstruct venous return, exercising the extremity, maintaining the extremity in a dependent position, applying warm compresses, vasodilating with nitroglycerin, and utilizing venous distension devices.
4. Technique for peripheral venous cannulation with catheter over a needle
   - **a.** Apply a tourniquet proximal to the IV site and cleanse the overlying skin with alcohol or povidone-iodine solution.
   - **b.** Anesthetize the skin with 1% lidocaine or procaine in the awake patient.
   - **c.** Stabilize the skin and vein with one hand; then puncture the skin with the needle bevel upward held in the other hand.
   - **d.** Enter the vein 5–10 mm from the skin insertion site, approaching from above or from the side. After blood return is noted in the needle hub, advance the needle another 1 mm into the vein (farther for larger-gauge catheters) to ensure that the needle tip and catheter tip are fully inside the vein.
   - **e.** Holding the needle and skin firmly in place, slide the catheter off the needle into the vein. Compress the vein proximally, remove the needle, attach IV tubing, and document free backflow of blood and forward flow of IV fluid without extravasation.
5. Emergency peripheral venous access during resuscitation or for the patient in shock can be obtained in several ways:
   - **a.** The **external jugular vein** may remain visible after the extremity veins have constricted.
   - **b.** The **saphenous vein** can be cannulated percutaneously or via surgical cut down where it crosses immediately anterior to the medial malleolus. The cephalic, basilic, and brachial veins in the arm are also amenable to surgical cutdown.
   - **c.** The **femoral vein** is identified by its position in the femoral sheath immediately below the inguinal ligament and medial to the femoral artery pulsation. Cannulation can be performed percutaneously with a 6-inch or longer catheter-over-needle, as already described. Alternatively, a 2-inch, 18-gauge catheter-over-needle can be placed first, as above, and then changed over a guidewire to a longer catheter.

d. As a last resort, a rigid-styletted needle (such as a 22-gauge spinal needle) can be inserted into the marrow space of the **tibia**, via the midportion of its antero-medial (flat) surface. Intracostal and intrasternal venous access can be obtained by needle insertion into the marrow of the ribs at the lateral aspect of the sixth to ninth ribs, or the body of the sternum just above the xiphoid.

e. Lower extremity volume infusion might be unreliable in patients with intraabdominal trauma due to possible inferior venal caval interruption.

B. Central venous access

1. General guidelines and precautions

a. A thorough knowledge of anatomy, technique, and possible complications in order to choose the appropriate access site and perform cannulation safely is essential.

b. Rigid adherence to sterile technique

c. Guidewires should always be in view to avoid inadvertent embolization of the wire into the circulation.

d. To avoid vessel damage or perforation, never force a catheter, guidewire, or dilator.

e. Always check the compatibility of catheters and guidewires beforehand. Ensure that guidewires fit through and are at least 2 inches longer than their associated catheters.

f. Never withdraw a catheter or guidewire that has been inserted through a needle; the tip of the catheter or wire could be sheared off, embolizing into the circulation.

g. Confirm correct catheter placement by chest radiograph.

h. Avoid air embolism by utilizing maneuvers that maintain central venous pressure higher than ambient atmospheric pressure: Valsalva maneuver, positive airway pressure, and insertion site located below the level of the heart (i.e., Trendelenburg position for subclavian and jugular vein cannulation). Keep occlusive caps on all catheter ports and eliminate air from all IV bags and tubing.

i. Continue to monitor the patient during all cannulation procedures. ECG monitoring may reveal atrial or ventricular dysrhythmias from a guidewire inserted too far. Provide supplemental oxygen to patients with drapes covering the face. Watch for airway obstruction in sedated patients and airway disconnection in mechanically ventilated patients. Continuous monitoring of hemoglobin oxygen saturation via pulse oximetry is strongly recommended.

2. Indications for central venous access include central venous or pulmonary artery pressure measurements, infusion of nonisotonic or irritative solutions (e.g., hyperalimentation), infusion of vasoactive drugs, hemodialysis, transvenous pacemaker insertion, and absence of accessible peripheral veins.

3. Choice of access site (Fig. 4-1) depends on the indication for central venous access and knowledge of potential complications. For example, pulmonary artery catheters are more easily passed from the subclavian or neck veins than the groin or arm veins. Subclavian cannulation is not advised in patients with bleeding diathesis due to difficulty compressing a punctured subclavian artery. Right internal jugular cannulation carries a higher risk of pneumothorax than the left due to the higher position of the right pleural dome; left internal jugular cannulation can cause injury to the thoracic duct, which lies in the left chest.

4. External jugular vein cannulation

a. Advantages: low risk of pneumothorax and hemorrhage, relative ease of controlling bleeding by compression, and usually easy to see

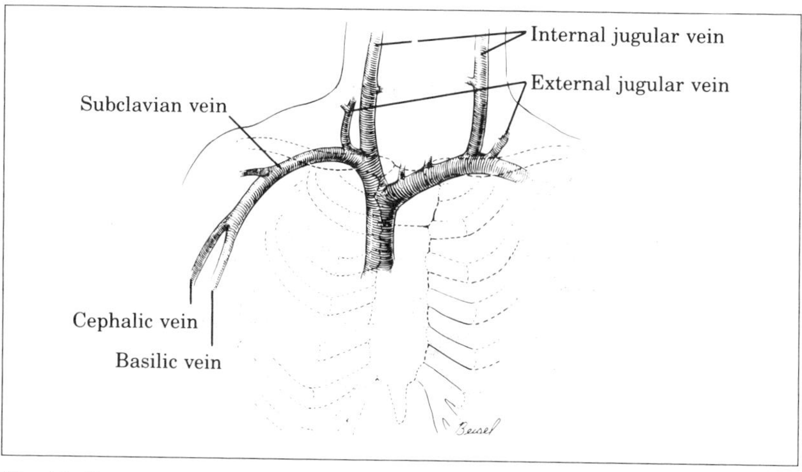

Fig. 4-1. Common routes for central venous access.

b. Disadvantages: Due to the presence of venous valves and the near 90-degree angle at which the external jugular joins the subclavian vein, it can be difficult to pass a catheter into the central circulation. The catheter may become kinked by changes in head position.

c. Technique

(1) After sterile preparation and draping of the neck, infiltrate local anesthetic over the vein. Visualization can be enhanced by manual compression of the vein at the clavicle.

(2) Cannulate the external jugular vein with a short catheter-over-needle assembly as already described (**I.A.**).

(3) Once free flow of blood through the catheter has been demonstrated, advance a flexible J-tip guidewire through the catheter. Manual pressure over the clavicle sometimes helps to guide the wire intrathoracically.

(4) After removing the introducing catheter, insert the central venous catheter of desired length over the wire, and remove the guidewire.

5. Internal jugular vein cannulation

a. Advantages: ideal location for patients requiring surgical access to the chest, lower risk of pneumothorax than subclavian, relative ease of controlling bleeding by direct compression, and relative ease of passing catheter into the superior vena cava due to lack of sharp angles

b. Disadvantages: possibility of injury to other structures in the neck (carotid artery, vagus nerve, brachial plexus, lymphatic channels), difficult to maintain sterility in presence of tracheostomy, and difficult placement in patients with neck injury. The internal jugular approach is relatively contraindicated in patients with known carotid disease because inadvertent carotid puncture can lead to stroke due to thrombotic embolus or decreased cerebral perfusion from compression of the artery.

c. The internal jugular vein lies lateral to the carotid artery. There are three primary approaches for cannulating the internal jugular: anterior, middle, and posterior (named by their relationship to the

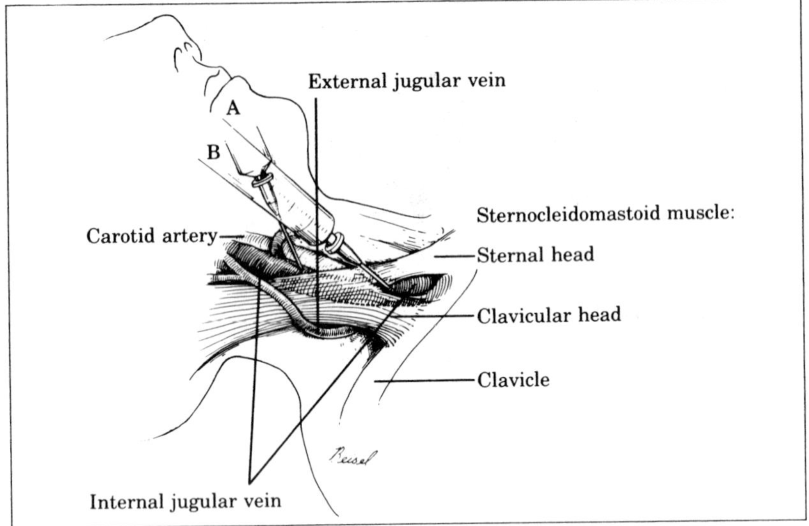

Fig. 4-2. Two approaches to internal jugular venous cannulation. With approach A, the carotid artery is palpated, and the needle is directed laterally toward the ipsilateral nipple or hip. With approach B, the apex of the triangle formed by the heads of the sternocleidomastoid muscle is palpated, and the needle is directed approximately toward the ipsilateral hip.

sternocleidomastoid muscle (Fig. 4-2)). The **anterior approach** is described in detail:

(1) The right internal jugular vein is preferred due to its shorter and more direct route to the superior vena cava. The patient's head is flat on the bed and turned away from the side to be used. Administer supplemental oxygen to ensure adequate oxygen delivery under drapes and increase arterial saturation, thereby facilitating comparison of arterial and venous blood color.

(2) Widely prepare and drape the neck in the usual sterile fashion, and place the patient in the Trendelenburg position.

(3) Locate the carotid artery with gentle palpation to avoid carotid sinus stimulation and resultant bradycardia. Carotid location can be facilitated by placing the fifth finger of the left hand in the patient's sternal notch (for right IJ cannulation) and the thumb along the angle of the mandible, at which point the index and middle fingers should fall over the carotid.

(4) Infiltrate 1% lidocaine via a 22-gauge locater needle just lateral to the arterial pulsation, midway between the sternal notch and the mastoid process. Evacuate all local anesthetic from the syringe to avoid change in color of the venous blood.

(5) Advance the locater needle with the right hand at an angle of 30–45 degrees to the skin toward the ipsilateral nipple (away from the carotid), aspirating gently. If blood return is not obtained, slowly withdraw the needle while aspirating (it is possible to collapse the vein on insertion, passing through it without aspirating blood).

(6) If still unsuccessful, withdraw the needle and reinsert it in a

slightly different position, starting laterally and moving medially toward the artery with successive attempts.

(7) When the vein is located with the 22-gauge finder needle, compare the blood color to an arterial sample if available.

(8) Remove the 22-gauge needle, and similarly insert either a short catheter-over-needle assembly or an 18-gauge thin-walled introducer needle into the vein at the same angle and depth. The position of the left hand or the neck can be utilized to ensure identical orientation of the introducer assembly.

(9) Insert a 0.035-inch J-tipped guidewire through the introducer catheter or needle, remove the introducer, and insert the desired central venous catheter over the wire (modified Seldinger technique). One advantage of the catheter-over-needle over the thin-wall needle is that the guidewire can be withdrawn through the catheter, if necessary, but not through the thin-wall needle.

d. If the anterior approach is unsuccessful, one of the alternative approaches for cannulation of the internal jugular vein can be attempted:

(1) With the **middle approach** to the internal jugular vein (Fig. 4-2), insert the needle at the apex of the triangle formed by sternal and clavicular heads of the sternocleidomastoid muscle and the clavicle at an angle of 45–60 degrees to the skin, aiming toward the ipsilateral nipple.

(2) With the **posterior approach** to the internal jugular vein, insert the needle at the posterior border of the sternocleidomastoid muscle midway along its length (at the point where the external jugular vein crosses the muscle). Pass the needle underneath the sternocleidomastoid muscle almost parallel to the skin, aiming toward the sternal notch.

6. Subclavian vein cannulation

a. Advantages: avoids risk of carotid artery puncture and damage to other neck structures

b. Disadvantages: risk of pneumothorax, chylothorax, subclavian artery puncture, subclavian vein thrombosis, and injury to the brachial plexus, phrenic nerve, and recurrent laryngeal nerve. Bleeding may be difficult to control from the subclavian vessels.

c. Technique

(1) Place the patient in the supine, Trendelenburg position with the head turned away, and place a roll between the scapulae to allow the shoulder to fall posteriorly.

(2) Widely prepare and drape the clavicle area in the usual sterile fashion.

(3) Infiltrate the skin and subcutaneous tissue under the medial half of the clavicle with 1% lidocaine via a 22-gauge needle.

(4) Advance the needle just under the clavicle, aiming 1–2 cm above the sternal notch, parallel to the medial clavicle. The vein lies between the first rib and the clavicle. Do not aim the needle posteriorly toward the subclavian artery or below the first rib where the apical pleura lies.

(5) After locating the subclavian vein, proceed with cannulation with the introducer needle, guidewire, and catheter as described in **B.4.c.**

7. Antecubital vein cannulation with long catheter (Fig. 4-3)

a. Advantages: ease of controlling bleeding and lack of nearby critical structures

b. Disadvantages: difficulty passing into the central circulation and

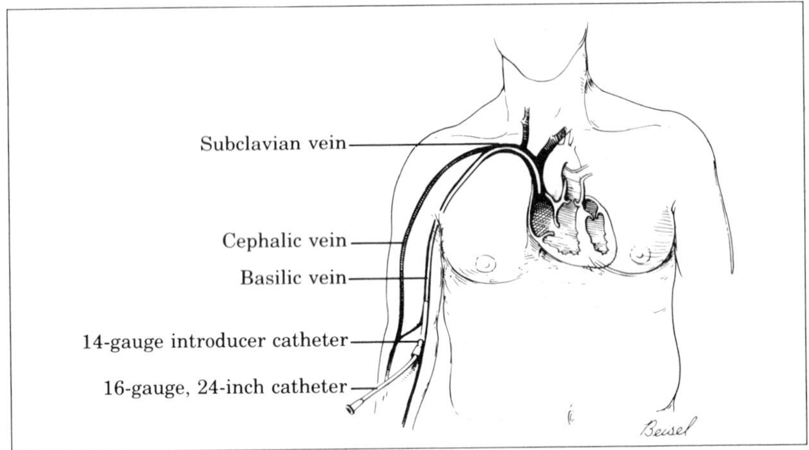

Fig. 4-3. The antecubital approach to central venous catheter placement.

limited longevity as thrombosis and phlebitis develop more readily in smaller veins with lower blood flow

c. **Technique**

(1) The median basilic vein generally provides an easier route to the central circulation than the cephalic vein and is therefore preferable.

(2) After tourniquet placement, sterilely prepare, drape, and infiltrate the antecubital fossa with 1% lidocaine subcutaneously.

(3) Use a 24-inch, 16-gauge catheter in a sterile plastic sheath through an attached 14-gauge introducing needle assembly (Intracath). After entering the vein with the 14-gauge needle, remove the tourniquet, and thread the catheter through the needle.

(4) Withdraw the introducing needle, and retain it over the catheter. A folding needle guard prevents subsequent shearing of the catheter.

(5) Cannulating the vein first with a standard 3-inch, 14-gauge catheter-over-needle offers the advantage of threading the 24-inch catheter through an introducer catheter rather than a needle and the presence of a large-bore IV should the long line be removed.

8. **Femoral vein cannulation**

a. The technique for femoral vein cannulation is described under **A.5.c.**

b. Relative contraindications to elective femoral vein cannulation include absent femoral pulses, groin or peritoneal infection, obstruction or trauma of the inferior vena cava, hypercoagulability, and pulmonary thromboembolism.

c. The catheter should be long enough to reach the inferior vena cava. If used for central pressure monitoring, the catheter should reach the diaphragm.

C. **Care of indwelling venous catheters** is directed toward preventing, detecting, and treating potential complications.

1. **Infection** remains the most common significant complication of venous catheters. Ongoing surveillance for signs of local and systemic

infection will aid in determining the time for removing or changing catheters. Since infection rates climb significantly after 72 hours, all catheters should ideally be changed every 3 days. However, mandatory line changes are necessary only when signs of infection occur. Although the infectious implication of changing central venous catheters over a guidewire is controversial, central lines should probably be changed via a fresh insertion site if possible. Other methods for decreasing infection rates include using catheters with fewer lumens, attaching antimicrobial-impregnated subcutaneous cuffs to catheters, or applying sterile films or antimicrobial ointments to the skin insertion site.

2. **Thrombosis** of the vein occurs more frequently with larger catheter size relative to vein size, prolonged cannulation, lower extremity insertion site, intermittent rather than continuous flushing of the catheter, and with certain catheter compositions. Teflon coating and heparin bonding of catheters can decrease the incidence of thrombus formation on catheters (especially pulmonary artery [PA] catheters). Once formed, thrombi can embolize into the pulmonary circulation, especially on removal of central venous and PA catheters. Thrombus formation and intraluminal clotting can reduce venous flow, causing distal stasis and swelling. In addition, drug infusion and pressure monitoring may no longer be feasible.
3. **Infiltration** and extravasation into the extravascular space can occur at any time, especially in peripheral veins. Partially withdrawing multiport catheters (such as pulling a PA catheter back to the right atrial position) can lead to the inadvertent subcutaneous or peripheral administration of solutions meant for the central circulation.

II. Pulmonary artery catheterization

A. **Indications** for PA catheterization include measurement of right atrial (RA), pulmonary arterial (PA), and pulmonary artery occlusion (PAO) pressures and measurement of cardiac output (CO) by thermodilution and sampling of pulmonary arterial (mixed venous) blood. Evaluation of right and left ventricular function, pulmonary processes, shunts, shock, and metabolic processes can be made with data derived from these measurements.

B. The standard 110 cm-long, 7.0 French catheter contains a distal lumen at the tip for measurement of PA and PAO pressures; a proximal lumen ends 30 mm from the tip for measurement of RA pressure, administration of fluid and drugs, and injection of the thermal bolus for CO determination. The catheter also contains a lumen for inflating the balloon at the tip and a wire for thermodilution and temperature monitoring. Larger (7.5 French) catheters are available with an additional central infusion port (VIP catheter), a lumen for passage of cardiac pacing wires, or a fiberoptic channel for determination of continuous mixed venous oxygen saturation.

C. The preferred **insertion site** is via the right internal jugular vein, which provides the straightest and shortest course to the right heart. The subclavian veins, the left internal jugular vein, and the external jugular veins also provide adequate access. Use of the antecubital and femoral veins frequently requires fluoroscopic guidance.

D. **Preparation for insertion**

1. Ensure that appropriate resuscitation supplies and personnel for complete airway, breathing, and circulatory support are immediately available. Supplies include a temporary transvenous pacing wire and an external pacemaker in patients with preexisting left bundle branch block because the PA catheter tip may cause a transient right bundle branch block (3% incidence) as it passes through the right ventricle, resulting in complete heart block.

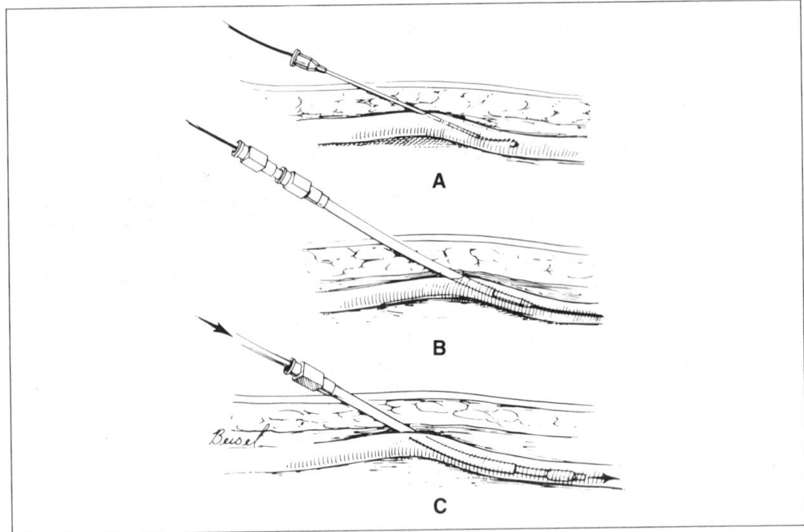

Fig. 4-4. Pulmonary artery catheter venous insertion. A. After the vein is cannulated with a short catheter, a 0.035-inch wire is inserted, and the short catheter is removed. B. An introducer-dilator assembly is then passed over the wire (the initial puncture usually needs to be enlarged somewhat with a scalpel). C. The dilator and wire are removed, after which the PA catheter is passed through the introducer.

2. Continuous blood pressure (BP) and ECG monitoring is required. Flush catheter ports with heparinized saline, and connect the distal (PA) port to a properly calibrated pressure transducer and monitor.
3. Test the balloon by inflating with 1.5 cc of air after the protective sheath has been placed over the catheter. In patients with right-to-left shunt, use carbon dioxide to avoid the possibility of systemic air embolus from a ruptured balloon. The catheter introducer should be a full French size larger than the catheter (8.0 French introducer for a 7.0 French catheter).

E. Technique for insertion (Fig. 4-4)

1. After successful insertion of the guidewire into an appropriate central vein (as described under **B.4.c.**, make a small skin incision over the guidewire to facilitate insertion of the introducer.
2. Pass the introducer/dilator assembly over the guidewire; then remove the dilator and guidewire together, leaving the introducer in place. Aspirate back on the sidearm lumen of the introducer to ensure intravenous placement and to evacuate intracatheter air. Flush the sidearm with heparinized saline solution (or connect a continuous IV solution) to prevent clotting.
3. Thread the PA catheter through the introducer, oriented so the natural curve in the catheter corresponds with the direction of the right ventricular outflow tract. Inflate the balloon with 1.0–1.5 cc air after the catheter tip has reached the right atrium (20 cm from the right internal jugular vein). Substantial resistance to inflation indicates malposition of the catheter. Complete lack of resistance to inflation or an inability to withdraw the air may indicate balloon rupture. Do not advance the catheter any farther without the balloon inflated to avoid vessel damage. Never withdraw a catheter with an inflated balloon.
4. Continuous monitoring of the distal (PA) port pressure as the catheter

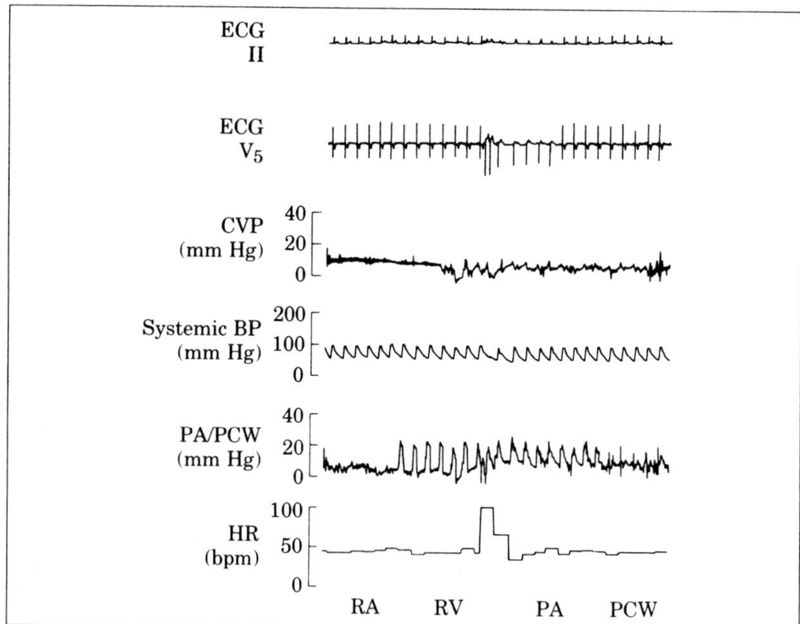

Fig. 4-5. Waveforms on insertion of a PA catheter. Note ventricular ectopy as the catheter transverses the right ventricular outflow tract, abrupt step-up in diastolic pressure heralding entry into the PA, loss of pulse pressure, and decrease in mean pressure indicative of PCW position. *bpm* = beats per minute; *HR* = heart rate; *RA* = right atrium; *RV* = right ventricle.

is advanced will reveal the characteristic waveforms of the right atrial (RA), right ventricle (RV), pulmonary artery (PA), and pulmonary artery occlusion (PAO) pressures (Fig. 4-5). A central venous pressure (CVP) trace will be noted as the catheter enters the RA. An abrupt increase in systolic pressure that falls rapidly toward zero indicates entry into the RV. Passage into the PA is heralded by a step up in the diastolic pressure and presence of a dicrotic notch in the waveform. With entry into the PAO position, a and v waves will appear in the dampened trace, and the mean pressure should be less than or equal to the PA diastolic pressure. The balloon is then deflated, and the waveform should revert to that of the PA pressure.

5. If an RV trace is not observed after inserting the catheter 30–40 cm (from the right internal jugular or subclavian veins) or a PA trace is not observed after 40–50 cm, deflate the balloon, withdraw the catheter, and repeat the insertion attempt. Otherwise, coiling and knotting of the catheter can result.
6. Although ventricular dysrhythmias commonly occur as the catheter passes through the RV outflow tract, they are rarely sustained or hemodynamically significant. The incidence can be decreased by ensuring full inflation of the balloon and passing rapidly through the RV into the PA. For serious dysrhythmias, deflate the balloon, and quickly pull back the catheter to the RA position.
7. Once the PA catheter is in the desired position, extend the sterile protective plastic sheath over the catheter and securely fasten it to

the introducer. This sheath maintains a portion of the PA catheter sterile, thus allowing further manipulation of the catheter position in a sterile fashion. Securely suture the introducer in place.

F. **Complications and care of PA catheters** are the same as described for any central venous catheter (**C. 1–3**). There are additional concerns related specifically to the care of PA catheters.

1. **Pulmonary infarction** can occur if the catheter migrates distally into the wedge or occlusion position and is not promptly detected. For this reason, continuous monitoring of the PA waveform is necessary.
2. **Pulmonary artery rupture** can be caused by overinflation of the balloon, balloon inflation in a catheter already in the wedge position, permanent wedge position with resultant pulmonary infarction, advancing a catheter with a deflated balloon, and vigorous flushing. Although the reported 0.2% incidence is low, the consequences can be severe. Hemoptysis in a patient with a PA catheter indicates a possible pulmonary infarction or pulmonary artery rupture. If the hemoptysis is severe, rapid intubation of the contralateral lung can be lifesaving. The risk of pulmonary artery rupture is increased in patients with pulmonary hypertension or mitral valve disease and anticoagulated patients.

III. Arterial cannulation

A. **Indications** for an intraarterial cannula are the need for frequent arterial blood sampling (for blood gas analysis) and the need for BP monitoring. Direct arterial pressure monitoring may be required in patients with unreliable indirect BP monitoring, in hemodynamically unstable patients, or in any patient benefiting from continuous, beat-to-beat monitoring of the arterial pressure waveform.

B. The radial artery is the most commonly used site for arterial cannulation. Advantages of the site include an easily documented collateral circulation, easy access to it, large enough size to measure pressure accurately without occluding the artery, and location in an area not prone to infection. Other sites are the dorsalis pedis, femoral, axillary, ulnar, posterior tibial, temporal, and brachial arteries. In general, it is preferable to avoid end arteries with poor collateral circulation, such as the brachial artery. Also, axillary artery cannulas have an increased risk of cerebral air emboli, and femoral artery cannulas have an increased risk of lower extremity vascular compromise. Cannulation of the arteries in the foot should be avoided in diabetic patients.

C. Whenever possible, test the collateral circulation prior to arterial cannulation. The Allen's test is used for the radial artery, although several studies have questioned the usefulness of the test due to a significant number of false-positives and false-negatives. The Allen's test is performed by having the patient make a tight fist, thereby exsanguinating the hand. The radial and ulnar arteries are digitally compressed; then the patient opens the hand. The ulnar artery compression is released, and with normal ulnar collateral blood flow, a pinkish color should return to the hand within 15 seconds. A positive Allen's test indicates poor ulnar collateral flow, relatively contraindicating cannulation of that wrist. Other tests, such as the postocclusive reactive circulatory, hyperemia (PORCH) test may prove more useful. (Vaghadia et al. 1988)

D. **Technique for radial artery cannulation**

1. Perform evaluation of adequate ulnar collateral circulation as described in **C**.
2. Secure the hand on an armboard in 60 degrees of dorsiflexion by placing a roll of gauze under the wrist (Fig. 4-6).
3. Locate the radial artery just proximal to the head of the radius. Beginning distally on the artery allows one to move more proximally

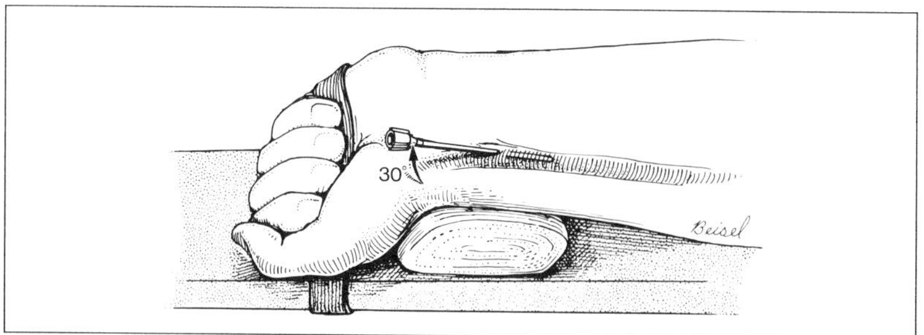

Fig. 4-6. Hand and wrist positioned on a small armboard for radial artery cannulation.

should arterial spasm or hematoma formation occur. Prepare and drape the area in the usual sterile fashion; then infiltrate the skin over and beside the artery with 1% plain lidocaine.

4. Insert an 18- or 20-gauge, 2-inch catheter-over-needle device at a 30-degree angle to the skin. Advance the catheter and needle together until blood appears in the hub of the needle (or until blood pulsates out of the capless needle).
5. While holding the needle in the fixed position, advance the catheter off the end of the needle as described for peripheral venous cannulation (**I.A.4**). Remove the needle, and document pulsatile flow.
6. Alternatively, the artery can be intentionally transfixed by the catheter-over-needle assembly (Fig. 4-7). Remove the needle, and slowly withdraw the catheter until pulsatile flow is observed. Then advance the catheter into the artery. If the catheter will not advance, try flattening the angle of the catheter to the skin or passing a guidewire through the catheter.
7. The modified Seldinger technique is sometimes used (especially for larger arteries) where the artery is first entered with an introducer needle. A guidewire is then passed through the needle, the needle removed, and an appropriately sized catheter passed over the guidewire. One-piece kits, with the needle, catheter, and guidewire all in one device, are available (Arrow).
8. Secure the arterial cannula in place, preferably by suturing (especially if not at the radial artery site). Check connections to avoid inadvertent disconnects. Continuous monitoring of the waveform is suggested for early detection of disconnects when the site is obscured under drapes.

E. **Complications** of arterial cannulation include thrombosis, infection, embolism, skin necrosis, fistula and aneurysm formation, and possible exsanguination from a disconnected line.

1. The risk of thrombosis, the most common complication, is increased by prolonged duration of catheterization, larger-size catheters, tapered catheters, and an intermittent rather than a continuous heparin flush. Provided that cannulas are promptly removed with signs of distal ischemia, thrombosis is rarely associated with permanent adverse sequelae.
2. The risk of infection is increased in catheters placed by surgical cutdown as compared to those inserted percutaneously. The risk of infection is also increased with catheters' remaining in place for longer than 72 hours. However, catheters can remain for up to several weeks with proper care and surveillance for signs of infection.

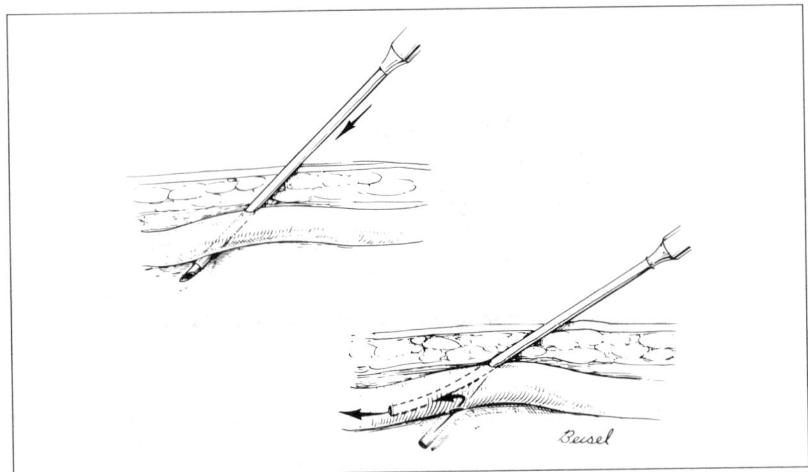

Fig. 4-7. Technique for radial artery cannulation. The vessel is transfixed, the needle removed, and the cannula withdrawn until blood pulses out freely, at which time the cannula is gently advanced.

3. Cerebral air embolism is possible with vigorous intermittent flushing of arterial cannulas, especially in children and conditions of low BP.

Selected References

Hoar, P. F., Wilson, R. M., and Mangano, D. T., et al. Heparin bonding reduces thrombogenicity of pulmonary-artery catheters. *N. Engl. J. Med.* 305:993, 1981.

Matthay, M. A., and Chatterjee, K. Bedside catheterization of the pulmonary artery: Risks compared with benefits. *Ann. Intern. Med.* 109:826, 1988.

Scott, W. L. Complications associated with central venous catheters. A survey. *Chest* 94:1221, 1988.

Sprung, C. L., Elser, B., Schein, M. H., et al. Risk of right bundle-branch block and complete heart block during pulmonary artery catheterization. *Crit. Care Med.* 17:1, 1989.

Vaghadia, H., Schechter, M. T., Sheps, S. B., and Jenkins, L. C. Evaluation of a postocclusive reactive circulatory hyperaemia (PORCH) test for the assessment of ulnar collateral circulation. *Can. J. Anaes.* 35:591, 1988.

5

Bedside Vital Signs Monitoring

James Welch and Richard DeCesare

The measurement of physiologic parameters is central to the diagnosis and management of critically ill patients. Advances in electronic and sensor technology have automated many of these measurements, providing continuous display of vital signs and alarms when parameters exceed acceptable ranges. The performance of these devices is limited by the sensor. When measurements disagree with clinical assessment, an understanding of the principles and causes for error in the measurement is essential to appropriate patient management.

I. Methods and principles of ECG measurements

A. Electrodes and leads. Continuous ECG is the oldest and most common continuous vital signs measurement. In the simplest form, a pair of electrodes is placed on the patient's chest. The depolarization of the heart creates a potential (voltage) gradient of approximately 1 millivolt between the electrode pair. Unfortunately, electrical noise radiating from the electrical power distribution system is also present on the surface of the patient. This 60-cycle interference signal is approximately 1 volt, or 1,000 times the strength of the patient ECG signal. The effects of this interference can be significantly reduced by placing a third "driven" electrode on the patient. The driven electrode senses the electrical interference signal common to both electrodes and drives an opposing signal onto the patient through the driven lead, canceling the interference signal. The effectiveness of the driven electrode depends on the quality of the electrode and skin preparation. Any difference in electrode contact results in an electrode imbalance, allowing interference to mix with the differential ECG signal. Electrode quality is important in determining the quality of the waveform. Only silver/silver chloride electrodes should be used in critical care settings because they provide a low contact impedance and a quality trace. Avoid lower-cost stainless steel electrodes, since they will not allow a quick waveform recovery after defibrillation.

The simplest ECG monitors measure a single lead (usually lead II) through a three-lead cable, with the right leg electrode used as the driven electrode. Full lead selection (I, II, III, aVr, aVl, aVf, C) is more commonly found in critical care. Recently, multichannel ECG monitoring has emerged as the standard critical care ECG monitoring strategy. These devices employ two or three individual channels, which can display simultaneously all seven leads by combining channels. For example, summing lead I and III yields lead II. Proper skin preparation and the use of quality electrodes, lead wires, and cables are the most important factors in obtaining and maintaining quality ECG waveforms. Compromising any of these elements results in noisy traces, wandering baselines, and the generation of avoidable false alarms.

B. Filtering. All ECG amplifiers employ electronic filters to reduce artifact. Two filter modes are found in bedside monitors: diagnostic and monitor. The diagnostic mode is defined by performance standards set by the American Heart Association (AHA). The bandwidth is set at 0.05–100 hz. This mode should be used for all diagnostic ECG measurements, especially the measurements of ST elevation. The monitoring mode has a more restrictive bandwidth—usually 0.5–100 hz. The rise in the lower end is implemented to stabilize baseline wander in the ECG due to respiratory artifact. Unfortunately, this can also cause waveform distortion, resulting in a false ST elevation.

C. Beat detection. The measurement and display of heart rate is determined by a beat detector. Early beat detectors were implemented in electronic components. Today beat detectors are determined by digital algorithms that sense the dominant shape of the QRS complex. Beat detectors must distinguish artifact from true ECG beats of various morphologies. They must also separate pacemaker spikes from the subsequent beats. Pacemaker spikes are commonly "stripped" out of the waveform by electronic components before beat detection and then added back to the waveform for display. Design limitations can make these detector circuits sensitive to electrical noise, resulting in false heart rate displays. Many different strategies are used in modern digital beat detectors. Failure of the beat detector usually results in false-positive high heart rate alarms generated by artifacts such as patient movement, loose lead wires, and poor electrode contact. Changing electrodes, lead wires, and cables usually produces dramatic improvement in the reduction of false alarms.

D. **Arrhythmia analysis.** Arrhythmia analysis is based on the classification of detected QRS complexes. All bedside systems available today are oriented toward ventricular arrhythmias. The low amplitude of the P wave makes it impractical to detect atrial arrhythmias except as determined by R to R intervals. Most systems require a learning time where the dominant QRS shape (assumed to be normal sinus rhythm) is identified. As with beat detection, a number of different strategies are used in QRS shape classification. Abnormal complexes are typically stored in the bedside monitor for review by the clinician to confirm the classification. Most systems allow the clinician to redefine misclassified complexes. Recently simultaneous multilead analysis has been employed to improve performance by reducing false-positives produced by artifact. Most manufacturers publish the performance of their analysis packages using either the AHA or MIT-BIH published waveform databases. Although these data may seem impressive, actual performance is usually lower due to the nonideal circumstances of the critical care unit. Proper electrode preparation, placement, and high-quality lead wires and cables optimize system performance.

II. **Pulse oximetry.** During the 1980s, pulse oximeters went from introduction to a standard of care in anesthesia, recovery, and ICU faster than any other medical device in history. The ability to measure arterial oxygen saturation noninvasively is "arguably the most significant technological advance ever made in monitoring the well-being and safety of patients during anesthesia, recovery, and critical care" (Severinghaus).

A. **Methods and principles of measurement. Pulse oximeters** measure continuous noninvasive arterial oxygen saturation by measuring the absorption of light passing through a pulsating vascular bed. All pulse oximeters shine two wavelengths of light through the tissue, red and infrared. Oxygenated hemoglobin (HbO_2) and reduced hemoglobin (RHb) absorb varying amounts of light depending on their concentrations. This is detected by the pulse oximeter and the ratio of $HbO_2/(HbO_2 + Hb)$ gives the SaO_2 in percentage saturated Hb. Various tissues absorb light in varying amounts, but only arterial blood absorbs in a pulsatile fashion. This pulsatile portion of the absorption signal is used to determine the saturation of the arterial blood only. Pulse oximeters, like all other patient monitors, have their limitations. Typically, if the sensor is applied correctly and there is a steady pulse rate from the oximeter that agrees with the ECG heart rate, the pulse oximeter numbers can be trusted.

B. **Accuracy.** The gold standard of oximetry is the laboratory co-oximeter, which uses 4 wavelengths of light to measure Hb, HbO_2, HbCO, HbMet in a sample of hemolyzed blood. All pulse oximeters are empirically calibrated against a co-oximeter using a population of healthy volunteers. Readings may differ by 2–3% among manufacturers. In comparison studies with co-oximeters, pulse oximeter accuracy has been within 2% with saturations between 70% and 100% and within 3% with saturations between 50% and 70%. Below saturations of 50%, the accuracy deteriorates significantly.

C. **Limitations**

1. **Motion artifact.** The most common source of interference is motion artifact. The amplitude of the detected pulse is extremely small, and movement of the sensor causes erratic pulse detections and saturation numbers. Performance can be improved by moving the sensor to a different site (fifth digit or nose or ear), using an adhesive type of sensor as opposed to a finger clip, and taping the cable to the limb to relieve stress on the sensor.
2. **Low perfusion states.** Pulse oximeters require the detection of a pulse to determine saturation; therefore, factors that compromise the pulse strength interfere with SaO_2 readings. The most common cause is cold, vasoconstricted fingers. Wrapping the hand or using an alternate site (nose, ear) should help. Performance will degrade during cardiac arrest or cardiac bypass and when the sensor is placed distal to an inflated blood pressure cuff.
3. **Ambient light interference.** Light interference can cause erroneous readings even though the pulse rate may be accurate. This occurs because of an incorrectly applied sensor. The detector in the sensor must be covered by skin; otherwise, light from the room or from the sensor emitter (reflected around the finger) will alter the readings. Wrapping the sensor and finger with an optically opaque material will reduce the effects of ambient light interference.
4. **Electrosurgical interference.** Electrosurgical devices can interfere with pulse oximeters. The effects can be minimized by placing the sensor and its cables as far from the electrostatic unit generator and cables as possible.
5. **Nail polish.** Certain nail polishes affect saturation readings because of their color and opacity. Remove nail polish before applying the sensor.
6. **Dyshemoglobins.** Pulse oximeters function based on the assumption that only two species of hemoglobin are present. If other species are present, i.e., MetHb or COHb, the saturation reading will be invalid. Carboxyhemoglobin absorbs infrared light similar to oxyhemoglobin, resulting in false high saturation values. Methemoglobin absorbs red light similar to reduced hemoglobin, resulting in false low values.
7. **Dyes.** Intravascular dyes will interfere with pulse oximeter readings if they absorb light at either the red or infrared wavelength. The effects are usually transient (minutes) but can be dramatic. Saturations readings as low as 1% have been reported with methylene blue. Indocyanine green and indigo carmine have also caused spurious low saturation readings.
8. **Skin necrosis.** There have been a few reported cases of skin erosion from long-term use (> 1 day) of reusable "clip" sensors. The manufacturers recommend checking the sensor site at least every 4 hours.

III. **Methods and principles of pressure measurement.** The systemic BP is uniformly recognized as a prime indicator of patient well-being. Yet clinicians are often confronted with conflicting data obtained from indirect (cuff) and direct (transduced) measurements. Indirect and direct BP determinations are measurements of different manifestations of the same basic phenomenon. Although indirect measurement with a sphygmomanometer has gained widespread acceptance in health care, it lacks the beat-to-beat accuracy and intravascular access necessary for care of critically ill patients. However, both techniques have the potential for inaccuracy and misuse. When measurements disagree, choosing which measurement technique is better for determining the course of care can be a problem. An understanding of the fundamental principles and limitations of these measurement techniques provides the insight necessary to make the right decision.

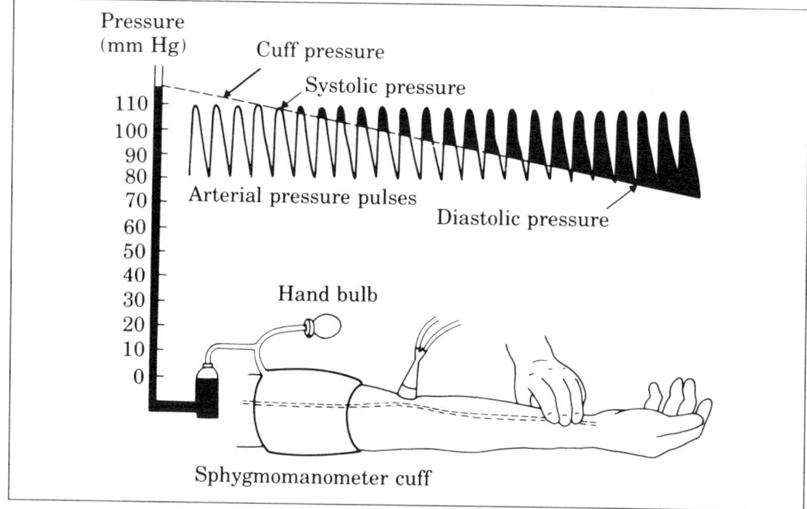

Fig. 5-1. Indirect BP determinations utilizing an occlusion cuff and distal-flow sensing will slightly underestimate systolic pressure. Diastolic determination is less well defined. (From R. F. Rushmer, *Cardiovascular Dynamics.* Philadelphia: Saunders, 1961. With permission.)

A. Indirect BP measurement techniques

1. Indirect BP determinations are based on a balance of forces between the occlusion pressure exerted by an external cuff and the intravascular pressures opposing occlusion. The basic assumption is that these forces are directly coupled to each other (i.e., there are no pressure losses in the intervening tissue). When the cuff is placed around the extremity, its external circumference becomes fixed. Increasing the cuff volume through a squeeze bulb and one-way valve compresses the surrounding tissue, producing a collapsing force on the arterial wall. Whenever cuff pressure exceeds arterial pressure, the artery collapses, obliterating distal blood flow (Fig. 5-1). Arterial pressure is indirectly estimated by measuring declining cuff pressure while detecting the beginning of distal pulsed flow (systole) and the cessation of interrupted flow (diastole).
2. Flow distal to the cuff can be detected by several methods.
   - **a.** Auscultation over the artery distal to the cuff with a stethoscope is the most commonly used detection method. At cuff pressures slightly below systolic levels, the intravascular pressure forces the collapsed artery open. A jet of blood is ejected, resulting in arterial wall vibration and turbulent flow. The energy produced by this disturbance is audible as Korotkov sounds (Fig. 5-2).
   - **b.** Palpation of the radial (or distal) artery can be used where a stethoscope is not available or practical. Only systolic pressures can be determined by this detection method.
   - **c.** Ultrasonic Doppler echocardiography can be used to detect arterial wall motion distal to the occlusion cuff. An ultrasonic signal is directed against the arterial wall. Vessel wall motion produced by blood ejections changes the frequency of the reflected beam (Doppler principle), which is detected and amplified. This method is particularly useful in hypotensive patients, low cardiac output (CO) conditions, and pediatric patients.

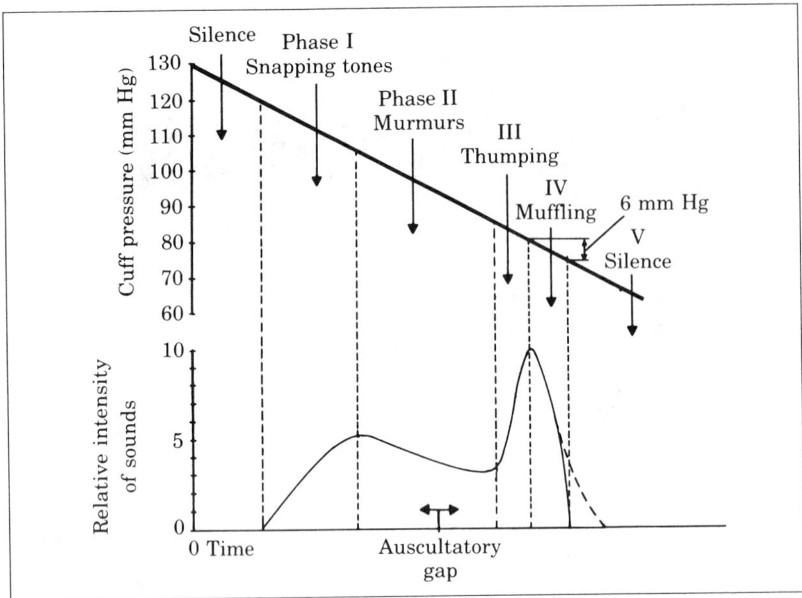

Fig. 5-2. Korotkov sounds are so characteristic that they have been separated into five phases. Snapping tones occur at cuff pressures slightly below intravascular systolic pressure. As the cuff is deflated, intermittent flow occurs for longer periods of the pressure pulse cycle (phases II and III). The sounds change from the snapping staccato pitch (phase I) to a muffled tone (phase IV) and finally silence (phase V). In some patients, phase IV may persist at cuff pressures well below intravascular diastolic pressure. Both phases IV and V should be recorded for consistent diastolic determinations. (From L. A. Geddes, *The Direct and Indirect Measurement of Blood Pressure.* Chicago: Year Book Medical, 1970. P. 111. With permission.)

3. Oscillotonometry is a cuff-based technique that does not require the sensing of distal flow. The measurement is based on changes in the volume of the occlusion cuff caused by the opening of the artery that it surrounds. This change in volume produces a similar change in the cuff pressure. As a result, pressure swings occur in the cuff that correspond to arterial pressure oscillations above the cuff pressure. Although maximum cuff oscillations correlate with intravascular mean pressure, oscillatory criteria for systolic and diastolic pressure determination are unclear.
4. Sources of error
   a. **Improper cuff size.** Cuff width should be about 1.2 times the diameter of the limb or 0.4 times the limb circumference. Marks on the inside of the cuff indicate the acceptable range of arm circumferences. Too wide a cuff will produce artificially low BP readings; too narrow a cuff will give artificially high readings. The air bladder of the cuff should be positioned over the medial aspect of the limb. Herniation of the cuff bladder will produce measurement errors.
   b. **Stethoscope application.** Excessive pressure applied to the artery by a stethoscope, especially in children, can result in artificially low BP readings by interfering with distal flow.
   c. **Deflation rate.** The amount of pressure deflation between heart beats determines the minimum error of the indirect method. The

faster the deflation rate, the greater the error. A deflation rate of 3 mm Hg per beat is recommended to ensure only minimal error. Lower heart rates require deflation rates to maintain measurement accuracy.

d. **Detection sensitivity.** The ability to detect Korotkov sounds is dependent on the energy available in the distal flow and the quality of the sensing system. Hypotension, low CO, or both produce lower signal energy levels, weaker Korotkov sounds, and potentially artificially low systolic and uncertain diastolic measurements. A poor-quality stethoscope will attenuate the Korotkov sounds, producing similar results. The sensitivity of the observer's hearing will also affect the measurement.

e. **Detection end points** (Fig. 5-2)

(1) **Systole.** Distal flow occurs only when cuff pressure is below arterial pressure. Therefore, indirect systolic readings are usually below intravascular systolic pressure. The difference is typically about 3 mm Hg for normotensive patients.

(2) **Diastole.** The detection criterion for diastolic pressure is less well defined. Phase IV, the beginning of the muffled sound, occurs 3–8 mm Hg above true diastolic pressure. The muffled sound, however, can persist well below intravascular diastolic pressure.

f. **Hydraulic effects.** The cuff must be on the same horizontal plane as the left ventricle. If it is not, a hydraulic fluid column will sum with the central pressure, casing a measurement error. The error (in mm Hg) is equivalent to 1.86 times the distance in inches from the correct horizontal position. A high cuff position will result in a false-low measurement, whereas a low cuff position will produce a false-high reading.

g. **Respiratory variations.** Respiratory effects on the cardiovascular system can cause cyclic variations in the arterial pressure waveform. These effects can result in periodic changes in the arterial pulse. Variations in sequential indirect determinations can be the result of measurements taken at different times in the respiratory cycle. Measurement consistency can be improved by synchronizing the indirect measurement with the respiratory cycle.

5. Automated methods

a. **Advantages.** Automating the indirect method can reduce measurement errors. Cuff deflation rate, detector sensitivity, and detection criteria are controlled by the machine. Controlling these parameters improves the consistency of the measurement. Automation also frees the observer to perform other tasks.

b. **Disadvantages.** The observer is removed from frequent patient contact and loses the ability to filter information obtained during the measurement. Respiratory variation, premature ventricular contractions, and other abnormal cardiac rhythms may cause inconsistent readings. Accuracy at hypotensive and hypertensive levels is also questionable. Motion and electrosurgical interference cause signal artifacts. When an artifact is detected, the cuff pressure may be held by the instrument until a true signal is sensed. This prolongs the overall cuff inflation time, which can cause venous congestion if the measurement is repeated too frequently. Cycle times shorter than 2 minutes should be used with caution in order to avoid limb ischemia, venous congestion, or both.

B. Invasive pressure-measurement techniques

1. **A complex waveform** is produced by ventricular contraction that is the result of the characteristics of both the ventricle and the vascula-

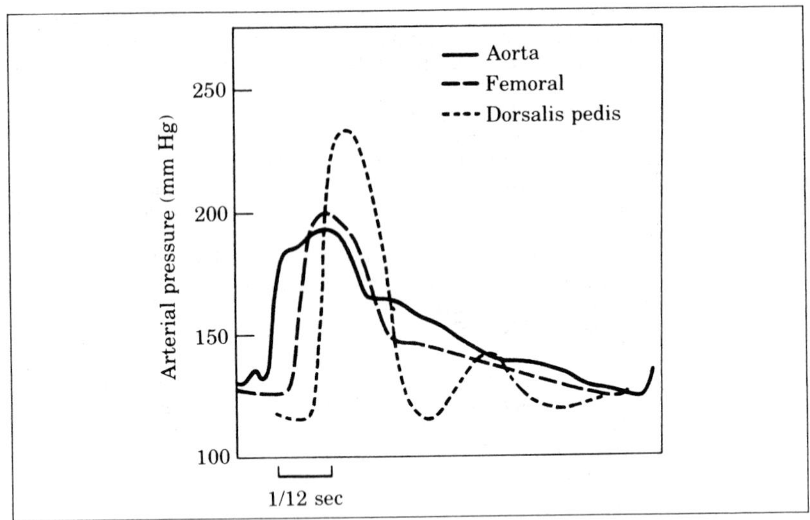

Fig. 5-3. In comparison to central BP pulses, peripheral pulses are narrower, with generally higher systolic pressures and dicrotic notches occurring later in the pulse. Peripheral pulse diastolic and mean pressures are approximately equal to or slightly lower than central measurements.

ture. Measurement at a remote location (e.g., radial artery) does not necessarily reflect the central arterial waveform (Fig. 5-3). Systolic pressure is particularly affected by vascular conditions. Diastolic pressure is less affected by the vascular characteristics and therefore is a reasonable indicator of the central diastolic pressure. Mean pressure is least affected by the condition of the vascular system and is therefore the best indicator of total body perfusion; however, measurements taken at one location may not reflect the perfusion of a remote organ since each organ has a unique perfusion control system.

2. **Direct pressure measurement** is accomplished by connecting the intravascular space to a transducer.
   a. **External transducers.** An external transducer is connected to the bloodstream using a fluid-filled connecting tube. The intravascular pressure signal displaces the fluid within the connecting tubing, forcing a corresponding displacement of the transducer diaphragm. The displacement is transformed into an electrical signal for amplification and display by the monitor. The entire link between the intravascular cannula and the monitor display defines the measurement system.
   b. **Catheter-tipped transducers.** Indwelling transducers are available on catheters, but current devices have little use in the ICU because of instability, unreliability, and high cost. Catheter-tipped transducers eliminate the fluid coupling link required for external transducers. This feature allows for higher fidelity recordings that may be required for measurements such as dP/dt (change in pressure/unit time).
   c. **Continuous flush device.** Continuous flush devices are employed to prevent clot formation at the tip of the catheter, which would eventually result in signal loss. They consist of a small capillary tube interposed between the monitoring tubing and the pressurized infusion bag. Under an infusion bag pressure of 300 mm

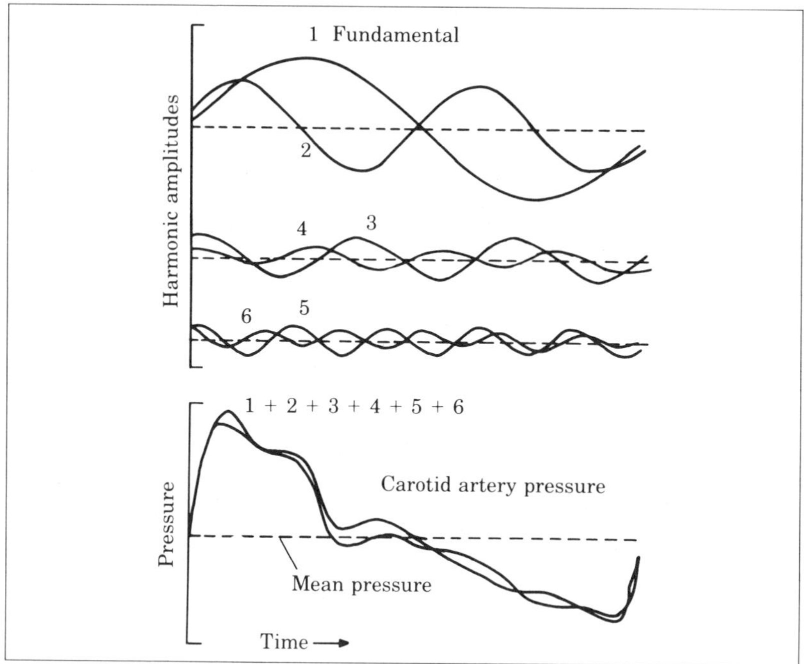

Fig. 5-4. A BP pulse can be minimally estimated by the sum of the mean pressure, the fundamental frequency (heart rate), and the first six harmonics. Higher harmonics are required for greater definition.

Hg, the capillary infuses 3–5 ml per hour of heparinized solution into the arterial catheter. Care should be taken in using continuous flush devices for pediatric monitoring where the constant infusion rate can cause volume overload. A bypass fast-flush valve is also incorporated to facilitate line filling and flushing after drawing blood samples. The complexity of the continuous flush device can contribute to signal distortion because it adds compliance to the system and may trap small air bubbles, further increasing system compliance.

3. The **pressure waveform characteristics** must be well defined in order to establish performance requirements for a direct-pressure monitoring system. The pressure signal can be viewed as a chain of repetitive waveforms of the same shape. This shape can be approximated by adding together a specific mixture of sinusoidal signals (Fig. 5-4).
   a. **Frequency content.** Each sinusoidal signal in the mixture is a multiple (harmonic) of the fundamental frequency (the heart rate). Each harmonic contributes to the overall shape of the contour. The amplitude and timing (phase) relationship between harmonics determines the shape of the displayed waveform. A typical BP pulse can be minimally approximated by the fundamental frequency and six harmonics. Higher harmonics may be required to define unusual pressure pulses. Heart rate and the contour of the pressure pulse determine frequency content.
   b. **Dynamic response** is the quality of the measurement system that

reflects its capability to follow the fastest changing component of the signal. It is usually characterized by the system bandwidth in hertz, or cycles per second (1 hz equals 60 cycles/min). The system bandwidth defines which signal frequencies pass through the system unattenuated. If important information is contained in frequencies outside the range of the system bandwidth, the displayed waveform (and the digital readout that is based on the waveform) will not accurately reflect the actual waveform within the intravascular space. The higher the heart rate, the higher the frequency content, and the greater the need for a system with a good dynamic response. For example, a pulse rate of 90 beats per minute (1.5 hz) has the sixth harmonic at 9 hz and requires a minimum system bandwidth of 0–9 hz. If the patient's heart rate increased to 120 beats per minute (2 hz), both the fifth and sixth harmonics (10 and 12 hz) would be above the bandwidth of the 9-hz system, and the true pressures would not be reported by the instrument.

4. The **minimal performance requirement** of a monitoring system, therefore, is to amplify at least the first six harmonics of the pressure signal equally. Failure to do so will result in signal distortion and false readings. The complete monitoring system consists of a fluid coupling system, a transducer, an amplifier, and a display. The ability of this system to follow fast-changing signals is limited by the component with the most restricted bandwidth. The weakest link is usually the fluid coupling section. Dynamic response can be impaired by any of the following:
   - **a.** Stopcocks and flush devices that tend to trap air and add compliance to the system
   - **b.** Long tubing lengths that add mass to the system (Fig. 5-5)
   - **c.** Small air bubbles that increase system compliance, resulting in ringing waveforms with false-high systolic readings. Small air bubbles are the major cause of poor performance of a given system.
   - **d.** Excessive air or a partially clotted catheter tip that will damp the waveform, causing a loss in signal definition, resulting in false low systolic and false high diastolic readings (Fig. 5-5)

5. The **fluid coupling system** performs in a predictable fashion.
   - **a.** Performance of the fluid coupling system can be described by two parameters: resonant frequency and damping factor.
     - (1) The **resonant frequency** of a system is the frequency at which the system naturally oscillates when disturbed, such as the tone a bell sounds when struck. The resonant frequency of a clinical system is the signal frequency at which maximal amplitude distortion occurs (Fig. 5-6). At resonance, clinical systems have amplitudes roughly twice the undistorted, low-frequency amplitude. Resonant frequency is dependent on the mass of fluid within the tubing and transducer dome, the compliance of the individual parts, the fluid resistance of the tubing, and most important, the care in debubbling the system.
     - (2) **Damping factor** is an indication of how quickly resonant oscillations decay. Damping factor is calculated from the ratio of the low-frequency amplitude to resonant frequency amplitude. If the decay is slow, the system is underdamped, and the damping factor is low (<1). Damping factor is affected by the same system characteristics as resonant frequency (e.g., mass, compliance, viscous resistance) but in a different proportion. Systems used clinically begin to distort well below the resonant frequency because of their low damping factors.
   - **b.** The **bandwidth** of the typical clinical system is determined by both resonant frequency and damping factor. The useful band-

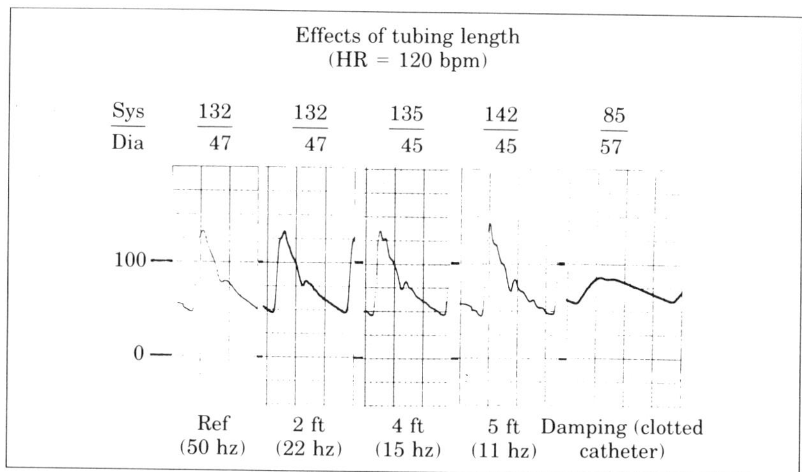

Fig. 5-5. Poor transducer-coupling system performance results in inaccurate systolic measurements. Longer tubing lengths encourage poor performance. Damping produces false-low systolic and false-high diastolic measurements. *bpm* = beats per minute; *Dia* = diastolic; *HR* = heart rate; *Sys* = systolic.

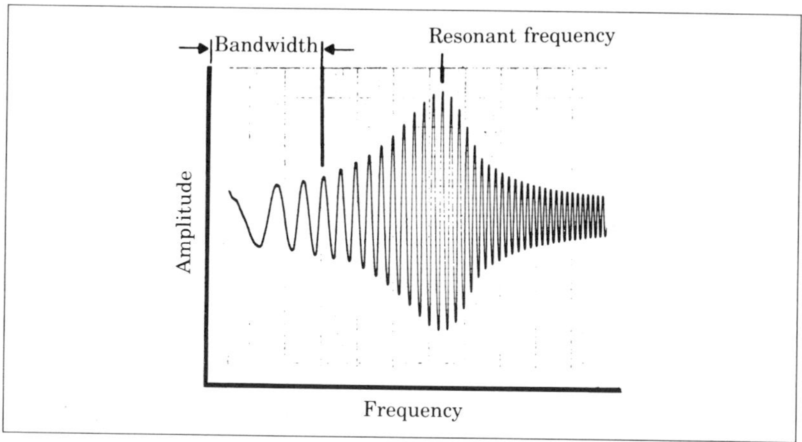

Fig. 5-6. A frequency sweep of an underdamped system demonstrates a useful bandwidth much below the resonant frequency.

width ("flat" response region) is typically six-tenths of the resonant frequency (Fig. 5-6) because of the underdamped behavior of clinical systems. As a result, much higher resonant frequencies are required to ensure the necessary flat bandwidth to recover the six harmonics of interest.

c. The best way to improve performance is to reduce the number of components (e.g., stopcocks) in the fluid coupling system and reduce the tubing length. A carefully filled system consisting of 4 feet of tubing, a continuous flush device, two stopcocks, and a disposable dome will exhibit a resonant frequency of 14 hz with a useful bandwidth of about 8 hz. Reducing this 4-foot tubing to 2 feet will increase the resonant frequency to about 20 hz and the useful bandwidth to 12 hz. Disposable transducers with an integrated flush device and 4 feet of tubing have demonstrated resonant frequencies around 25 hz. Ringing waveforms with as much as 20 mm Hg systolic error can be shown for systems that resonate below 12 hz.

6. **Electronic filters.** All BP amplifiers have filters that restrict bandwidth. Some monitors have electronic filters that restrict the pressure amplifier bandwidth to 12 hz and below. These filters were originally designed to improve agreement between direct and cuff readings. The result has been greater error and more confusion about the measurement. It is important to be aware of the bandwidth of a given monitor. Monitors with 12-hz filters can distort the true signal by limiting the number of signal harmonics displayed by the monitor. Systolic readings may be falsely low if the true waveform has significant harmonic components above 12 hz. Low frequency filters are particularly problematic in pediatric BP monitoring, where heart rates are high, with significant harmonics above 12 hz. Faithful reproduction of pressure pulses at a heart rate of 150 beats per minute requires a monitoring amplifier that does not filter below 25 hz.
7. **Intrathoracic pressure measurements.** Pressure measurements should be taken from a calibrated screen at end expiration. External transducers are referenced against atmospheric pressure when they are "zeroed." However, all intrathoracic pressures (i.e., pulmonary artery, central venous, pulmonary capillary wedge, and left atrial) should be referenced against intrathoracic pressures, which vary with the ventilatory cycle. Thus intrathoracic pressure readings are best taken when pleural pressure comes closest to atmospheric pressure (i.e., end expiration).
   - **a.** During spontaneous inspiration, intrapleural pressure decreases, causing a net increase in transmural pressure and cardiac volumes. However, the displayed signal shows a decrease in pressure because the pressures sensed by the transducer have decreased relative to atmospheric pressure.
   - **b.** Positive end-expiratory pressure (PEEP) raises the end-expiratory pressure reference relative to the atmospheric pressure reference of the transducer, resulting in a systematic error. At low PEEP levels, the displayed signal indicates an increase in end-expired pressure, although the transluminal pressure has decreased. Conversely, high levels of PEEP may compress intrathoracic circulatory structures, resulting in a decrease in left atrial filling and lowering of pulmonary artery wedge measurements.
   - **c.** During controlled ventilation, phenomena opposite to spontaneous inspiration occur. Transmural pressures decrease during inspiration, but the monitor displays an increased pressure signal.
   - **d.** Intermittent mandatory ventilation exhibits either of the previously mentioned inspiratory measurement errors, depending on whether the breath is spontaneous or controlled. The only consistent point in the respiratory cycle to measure intrathoracic pressures regardless of the type of ventilation is at end expiration, when intrapleural pressure approaches atmospheric pressure (see Fig. 5-16).
   - **e.** Catheter whip can also cause erroneous digital display values. However, catheter whip, or fling, is often confused in pulmonary artery recordings with superimposed regurgitant left arterial waves, especially when large A or V waves are present (see Figs. 5-10 and 5-13). Therefore, a calibrated screen and a skilled observer are required for accurate measurements. Digital displays

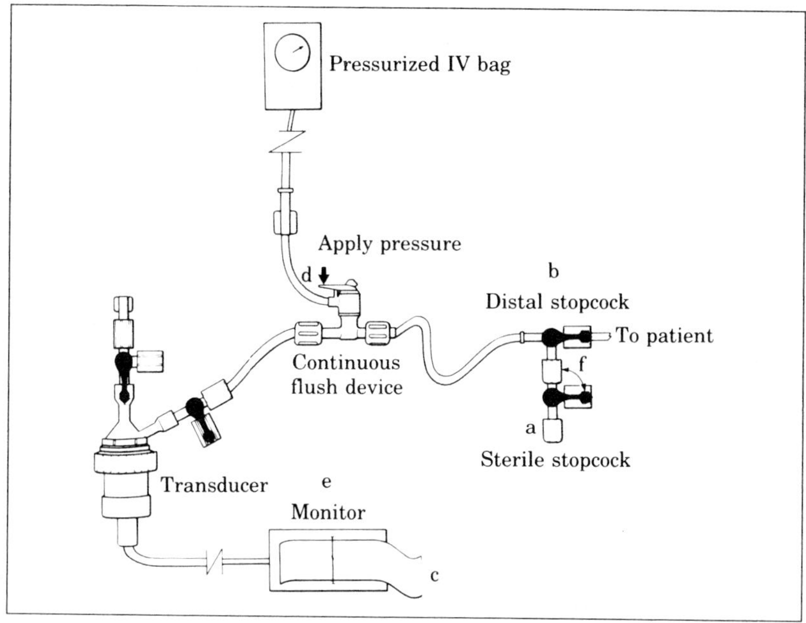

Fig. 5-7. Dynamic performance can be determined in the clinical setting by adding a sterile stopcock at the distal end and recording the response to a step-pressure perturbation.

should not be relied on for critical measurements because they usually depend on algorithms that do not take into account the respiratory cycle.

8. **Transducers drift** during the first half-hour of use and therefore should be rezeroed before critical measurements.
9. **Calibration.** All BP monitors should be statically calibrated against a mercury manometer to ensure accuracy. The "cal" button found on most monitors does not calibrate the transducer. It merely tests the amplifier and display by providing an electronic signal that represents an ideal transducer measuring an exact pressure.
10. **Dynamic testing.** Unexpected waveforms are quite often seen in direct pressure monitoring. These different pulse shapes may be the result of the effects of the cardiovascular system or of poor system dynamics. It is useful to test the monitoring system for dynamic response. A simple test can be performed by exciting the system with a square wave pressure signal and observing the displayed response. Both resonant frequency and damping factor can then be estimated at the bedside. Resonant frequency is the more important of these parameters and is the easiest to determine. This **pop test** (Fig. 5-7) can be performed in a sterile manner as follows:
    a. Mount a separate sterile stopcock at the side port of the distal stopcock (patient end), and close this stopcock off to the system (see *a* in Fig. 5-7).
    b. Isolate the intravascular cannula from the fluid-filled system by turning the distal stopcock (patient end) off to the patient. The system is now completely closed (see *b* in Fig. 5-7).
    c. Set the amplifier to display midscreen on the oscilloscope. The

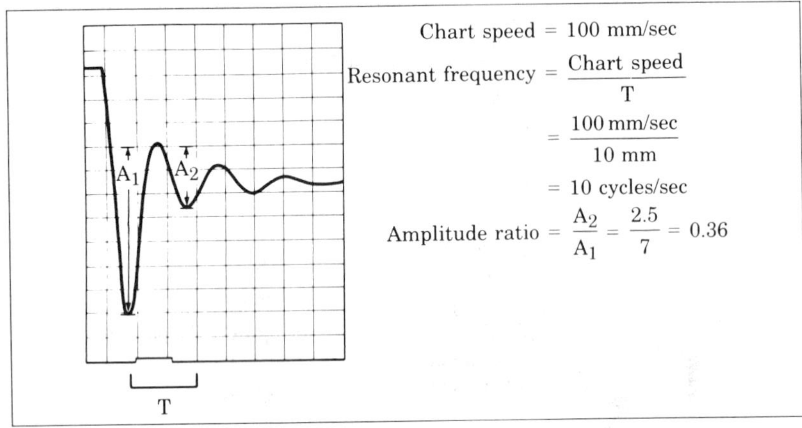

Fig. 5-8. Resonant frequency and amplitude ratio can be measured from the system response to pressure-step change.

screen or monitor does not need to be calibrated for this test (see *c* in Fig. 5-7).

d. Pressurize the entire fluid-filled system to a level beyond the range of the input amplifier (200 mm Hg usually works well). This is easily done by pressurizing the pressure infusion bag to 200 mm Hg and depressing the continuous flush device (fast-flush). Alternatively, a 12-ml syringe can be used to pressurize the system (see *d* in Fig. 5-7).

e. Set the monitor or recorder to the fastest possible sweep speed (see *e* in Fig. 5-7).

f. Suddenly vent the system to room air via the stopcock mounted in **a.** Be sure the patient stopcock is turned off to the intravascular cannula before performing this test (see *f* in Fig. 5-7).

g. Measure the distance of one complete cycle in millimeters, and estimate resonant frequency by dividing sweep speed (mm/sec) by the distance of one cycle (Fig. 5-8). It is easier if a strip chart recorder is used. The measurement is difficult if there are no time calibration marks on the monitor. Using the freeze trace capability on these scopes and a ruler with millimeter markings may help.

h. Resonance less than 12 hz should be considered unsatisfactory for monitoring pulse rates greater than 60 beats per minute, and the cause should be sought.

i. Damping coefficient is determined by calculating the amplitude ratio of the first and second cycles (Fig. 5-8) and looking up the corresponding damping coefficient (Fig. 5-9).

C. Combined invasive and noninvasive techniques

Direct and indirect arterial pressure methods can be combined by placing a properly sized occlusion cuff around the limb proximal to the radial artery catheter. Pressure measurements can be estimated by decreasing the cuff while observing the monitor display for a distal pulse.

1. The systolic measurement is the cuff pressure at which the first distal pulse is observed.

2. This combination technique is an indirect measurement because it relies on the occlusion cuff. As a result, it is subject to all of the measurement problems of cuff occlusion methods (e.g., cuff size, cuff

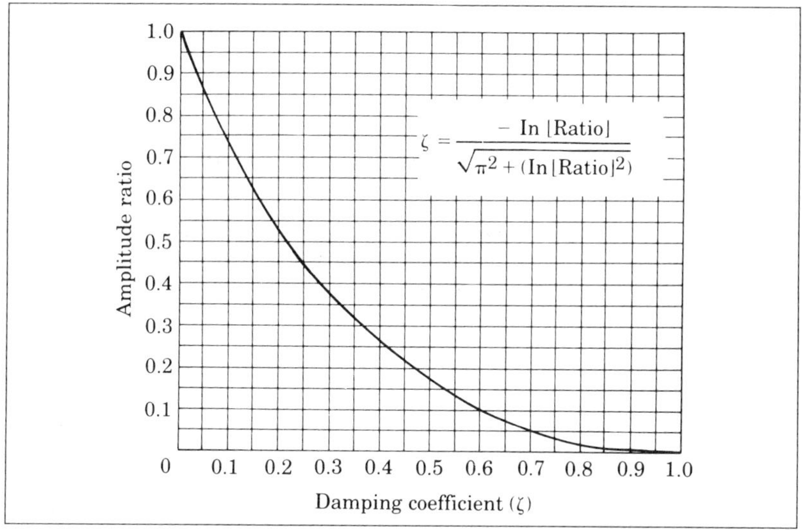

Fig. 5-9. Damping coefficient can be estimated from the amplitude ratio determined from the step response using the graph or directly calculated. (From R. M. Gardner, Direct blood pressure measurement—direct response requirements. *Anesthesiology* 54:227, 1981. With permission.)

deflation rate, cuff application, respiratory variation). The radial artery line acts as the distal sensor, replacing the stethoscope.

3. This method provides a qualitative means to confirm direct pressure measurements but should not be considered more accurate than a properly calibrated direct measurement system. Sharp systolic spikes observed on direct manometer systems may be real, and cuff-based measurements may not have the sensitivity to detect them.

IV. Cardiac output

Physiologic values of primary interest in the management of the critically ill patient are the concentrations of oxygen and other nutrients in the cells of vital tissues. Since concentration measurements at the cellular level are unavailable, a measurement of flow (e.g., CO) gives a general indication of the transport energy available to carry these nutrients to the organs. Indicator dilution methods directly measure CO. They are based on the principles of conservation of mass and energy. The indicator can be continuously added (Fick method) or introduced as a bolus (dye or thermal method). A more rigorous mathematic consideration of the Fick and bolus injection methods is given in the appendix at the end of this chapter.

A. The Fick method

1. The Fick method is based on the principle that for a closed circulation system of constant flow, the flow through the system is proportional to the rate at which the indicator (m) must be added continuously (dm/dt) in order to maintain a constant change in concentration (C2–C1). Oxygen is a natural physiologic indicator that can be used to measure CO.

$$\frac{(dm/dt)}{(C2 - C1)} = \frac{\text{oxygen consumption}}{\text{arterial} - \text{venous } O_2 \text{ gradient}} = CO \qquad (1)$$

2. Oxygen consumption is a complex measurement. The subject breathes from a fixed volume of known oxygen concentration (Doug-

las bag) for a fixed period of time. Exhaled gas is collected in a separate 50-liter bag. Oxygen consumption can be determined by the equation

$$\dot{V}O_2 = (F_IO_2 \times \dot{V}_I) - (F_EO_2 \times \dot{V}_E) \quad (2)$$

where F_IO_2 is the fractional proportion of inspired oxygen and F_EO_2 is the fractional proportion of expired oxygen. $\dot{V}_I$ is the minute volume of inspired gas, and $\dot{V}_E$ is the minute volume of expired gas.
Since patients on mechanical ventilators cannot breathe from the Douglas bag, oxygen consumption can be measured by an alternate method. Inspired tidal volume can be calculated by substituting nitrogen for oxygen in equation 2:

$$\dot{V}N_2 = 0 = (F_IN_2 \times \dot{V}_I) - (F_EN_2 \times \dot{V}_E) \quad (3)$$

Rearranging thus,

$$\dot{V}_I = \dot{V}_E \times \frac{F_EN_2}{F_IN_2} \quad (4)$$

F_IO_2, F_EO_2, and $\dot{V}_E$ can be measured. $\dot{V}_E$ is determined by collecting expired gas with a Douglas bag and measuring the gas volume with a spirometer. F_EN_2, F_IN_2, F_IO_2, and F_EO_2 are measured. $\dot{V}_I$ is calculated, and the numbers are substituted into the (Fick) equation 2. This method for calculating $\dot{V}_I$ is good only at an F_IO_2 where there are measurable differences in F_IN_2 and F_EN_2. If F_IN_2 is low, small measurement errors will have large effects.

3. During gas sampling, blood samples are taken from the pulmonary artery and a systemic artery and analyzed for oxygen content. The venous sample must be taken from the pulmonary artery because blood returning from the upper and lower circulatory loops has different oxygen contents, and the right atrium does not provide adequate mixing.

   The measurement of oxygen content is dependent on multiple variables: hemoglobin concentration and saturation and solubility of oxygen in plasma.

4. The assumptions of the Fick method
   - **a.** Oxygen consumption and CO are at a steady state.
   - **b.** No arteriovenous shunts are present.
   - **c.** Blood samples represent true arterial and mixed venous oxygen contents.
   - **d.** Blood samples are taken simultaneously.
   - **e.** Oxygen consumption measurement error is minimal.

B. Dye dilution

1. The continuous infusion of indicator can be replaced by a sudden infusion to obtain a measurement of flow. The principal assumption of this method is that the same quantity of indicator must pass through the outlet (i.e., aortic valve) as was delivered at the inlet (conservation of mass).
2. The sensors used in bolus indicator dilution techniques do not measure mass but concentration at the outlet. The flow of the system washes out the mass of indicator in the mixing chamber and results in a concentration curve at the outlet sensor. The concentration of indicator present at the outlet C(t) at any given moment in time is equal to the mass of dye in the solution passing by the sensor divided by the increment of the total system volume sampled by the sensor at that instant. Cardiac output can be determined from the equation.

$$CO = \frac{M}{\int_0^\infty C(t)dt} \quad (5)$$

where
M = mass of indicator injected
CO = average cardiac output over the sampled period
C(t) = indicator concentration sensed in the outlet (artery)

3. A variety of indicators can be used to measure CO. The following are requirements for the ideal indicator:
   a. Nontoxic
   b. Rapid mixing with blood
   c. No diffusion into the lungs or vessel walls
   d. Quickly metabolized by the body, but conserved during the course of the measurement
   e. Easy to measure
   f. Measured concentration is a valid sample
   g. No significant recirculation
4. **Dye dilution method:** Indocyanine green dye (5 mg) is diluted in aqueous solvent (1 ml). The indicator solution is bolus-injected into a central vein. An arterial sample is rapidly withdrawn (approximately 50 ml) through an optical densitometer (sensitivity at 8050 Å) and reinfused following the determination. Computation and extrapolation are performed by the instrument.
5. Assumptions of the dye dilution method
   a. The measured concentration is representative of the entire flow of the system. This holds true when the indicator is perfectly mixed.
   b. Flow rate is constant during the measurement. Any arrhythmias occurring during the determination will cause errors. Similarly, respiratory effects can cause periodic changes of 20% in CO. Repeated determinations averaged over the respiratory cycle are required to minimize respiratory effects.
   c. There is no recirculation of the indicator. Some recirculation occurs at the end of the washout curve. To correct for this, the measurement instrument will integrate only part of the curve. The instrument assumes that the washout curve is an exponential decay curve and extrapolates the tail end of the curve where recirculation occurs. If recirculation occurs prior to this point (as is seen in intracardiac right-to-left shunts), the flow measurement will be falsely low. Evaluating the washout curve itself is important for the diagnosis of any shunting.
6. **Sources of error** of the dye dilution method include
   a. Incomplete infusion of the injectate
   b. Use of old dye (unstable in light)
   c. Prolonged injection time
   d. Inadequate mixing
   e. Inaccurate calibration of the densitometer
   f. Nonuniform blood withdrawal rate
   g. Presence of air bubbles during withdrawal
   h. Dye buildup in the patient from sequential measurements
7. Dye dilution measurements should be reproducible within 5%. However, techniques necessary to avoid the sources of error listed in **6** make the method impractical for repeated routine measurements.

C. **Thermal dilution**
   1. Cold (or heat) may be used as an indicator, thereby providing a technique where repeated measurements are possible because the indicator does not accumulate in the circulation.

2. The indicator in thermodilution is thermal energy, as opposed to mass. A known volume of saline at a temperature lower than blood temperature is used as the indicator. In principle, the indicator dilution equation, with some modification, applies:

$$CO = 1.08 \times \frac{(-\text{Tbaseline}) \times V_i}{\int_0^{\infty} \text{Tout}(t)dt} \qquad (6)$$

where
Tbaseline = baseline blood temperature
Tout = temperature measured at the outlet of the system (pulmonary artery catheter)
V_i = injectate volume

3. Equation 6 represents an ideal system with no heat losses. In practice, some of the injectate volume is lost in the dead space of the catheter lumen, and some of the injectate heat is lost through the observer's hand during injection and across the catheter to air or blood before reaching the atrium. Some indicator may also be absorbed by vascular or ventricular walls. A catheter-specific correction factor is used to account for these losses. The correctional constant is entered into the CO measurement instrument. This correctional constant is dependent on injectate volume, catheter design, and injectate fluid characteristics.
4. Cardiac output measurements typically employ a pulmonary artery balloon flotation catheter with a thermal sensor mounted near the distal tip. Saline is drawn into a 10-ml syringe and cooled to 0°C. The saline is bolus-injected into the central venous blood via a proximal catheter port. The thermal sensor detects the washout curve in the pulmonary artery, and the computer integrates the temperature (thermal concentration) curve. As with the dye dilution method, the last part of the curve is extrapolated to correct for recirculation artifact, but recirculation is far less of a problem with the thermodilution method.
5. The **assumptions** made for the dye dilution method hold for the thermal dilution method. The advantages of the thermal method over the dye method are the following:
   a. Less recirculation of the thermal indicator
   b. Less accumulation of the indicator
   c. Signal sensing is more economic.
   d. The indicator is inexpensive and readily available.
   e. The calibration is implicit.
6. The common **sources of error** of the thermal method are
   a. Unstable baseline temperature due to cardiac and respiratory cycling
   b. Indicator (heat) lost in the syringe and catheter body
   c. Incomplete mixing in the right ventricle, especially during low COs
   d. Variability due to flow augmentation during the respiratory cycle
   e. Incorrect syringe volume
   f. Indicator not cooled to expected temperature

V. Waveforms

The usefulness of waveform monitoring is directly related to the methods employed to present and store the data. The ideal monitoring environment includes a large screen display for resolution of traces, plus an easily accessible, simultaneous hard copy of all waveforms. The examples presented in (Figures 5-10 through 5-19) represent such hard copy and demonstrate some of the common waveforms encountered in patient monitoring. The legends point out techniques for integration of information from multiple simultaneous waveforms that are useful to solve common clinical problems such as how to distinguish the wedge trace from the pulmonary artery trace in the presence of large, regurgitant waves in the left atrium.

In these examples, we point out a method of interpreting pressure waveforms that depends on the simultaneous monitoring of arterial and pulmonary artery catheters. The typical method of analyzing pressure tracings is to use the ECG for identifying the components of the waveforms. This method presents some problems for real-time analysis in that there is a variable electromechanical delay between the ECG and the pressure tracings, and the quality of a displayed ECG signal is often difficult to control (P and T waves are not always easy to see). An alternative is to display systemic arterial and pulmonary artery pressures simultaneously. The usefulness of this approach is discussed in the legends.

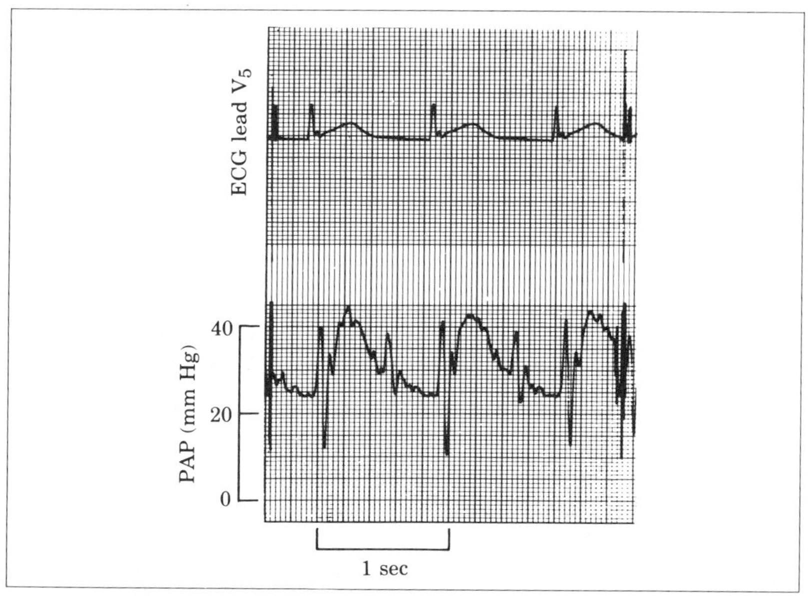

Fig. 5-10. Catheter whip aggravation by system resonance results in "fling." Pulmonary artery line fling is most often seen at the end of diastole. The true diastolic pulmonary artery pressure (*PAP*) in this patient is 24 mm Hg. If one were misled by the distorted trace (or if one were relying on digital readouts), one would be likely to read diastolic PAP as 11–12 mm Hg.

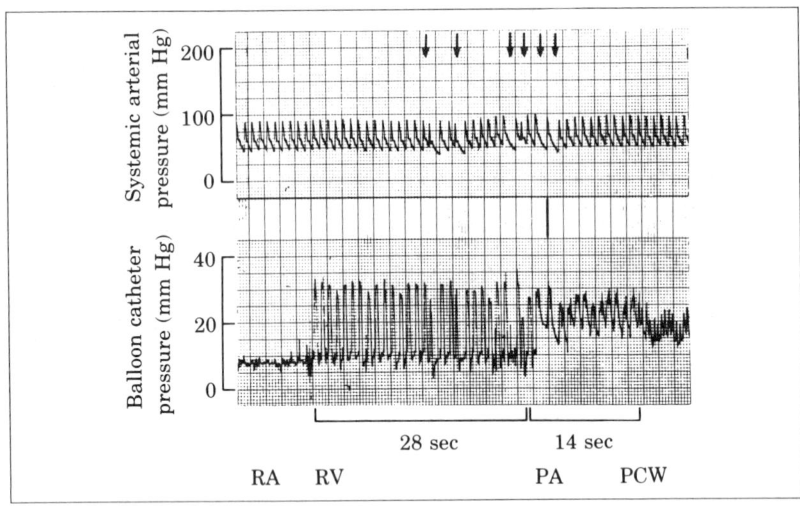

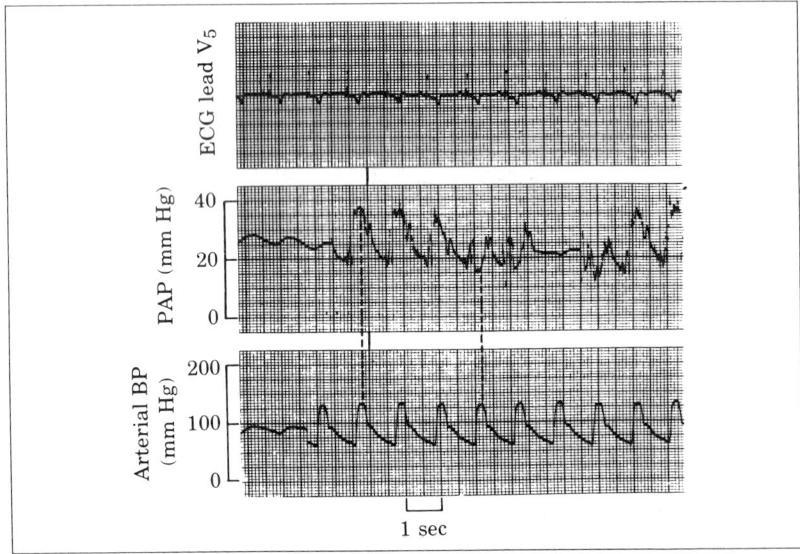

Fig. 5-12. Pulmonary artery and pulmonary capillary wedge pressure tracings with timing lines (*dotted lines*) relating peak radial artery pressure to pulmonary artery pressure (*PAP*). The dotted line on the left relates a normal pulmonary artery trace to the peak radial artery pressure. Note that the onset of PAP rise precedes the onset of arterial pressure rise by approximately 50–100 milliseconds. Right ventricular ejection precedes left ventricular ejection when there is sinus rhythm with a normal conduction system. Also note that peak PAP coincides with the radial artery pressure peak in this setting. When the balloon is inflated, pulmonary capillary wedge waves emerge with a rightward shift, as seen at the dotted line on the right. The left peak on the pulmonary capillary wedge wave is the A wave and that on the right is the V wave.

◄ **Fig. 5-11. Insertion of balloon-tipped pulmonary artery catheter. As the catheter is passed from right atrium (*RA*) to right ventricle (*RV*), note that pressure in the RA equals RV diastolic pressure. As the catheter traverses the ventricle and passes through the RV outflow tract, premature ventricular contractions are often seen (*arrows*). The pulmonary artery (*PA*) is entered, and the waveform changes to reflect the effect of a competent pulmonic valve (i.e., diastolic PA pressure is maintained well above RV diastolic pressure). At the far right of the figure, the catheter has been advanced to the pulmonary capillary wedge (*PCW*) position. Note that the wedge tracing oscillates at about a pressure roughly equivalent to the PA diastolic pressure. The relationship of PA diastolic pressure to mean PCW pressure holds occasionally but cannot be depended on in all cases and may change over time in any given individual. Also note that in this tracing there are abnormal regurgitant waves.**

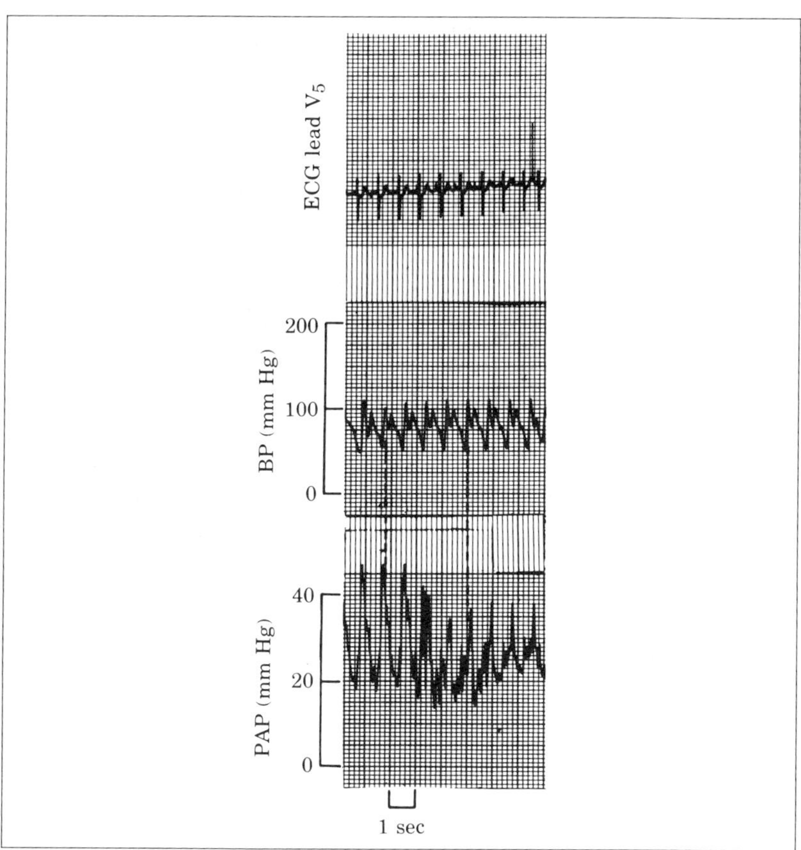

Fig. 5-13. A patient on an intraaortic balloon pump has pulmonary hypertension and large regurgitant waves on his pulmonary capillary wedge pressure tracing. Note that the key to distinguishing pulmonary artery from wedge is timing the wave peaks in relation to the arterial pressure trace. Use the dotted lines to compare timing of the pulmonary artery waveforms on the left with the pulmonary capillary wedge with large V waves on the right. A good way to distinguish these waveforms is to run a strip chart recorder that has visible pens and watch the relative timing of the upstroke of the arterial and pulmonary artery pens. With normal atrioventricular conduction, the pen tracing the pulmonary artery pressure (*PAP*) will stroke upward prior to the upstroke of the systemic arterial pen. As the balloon is inflated and the V waves emerge, this sequence reverses.

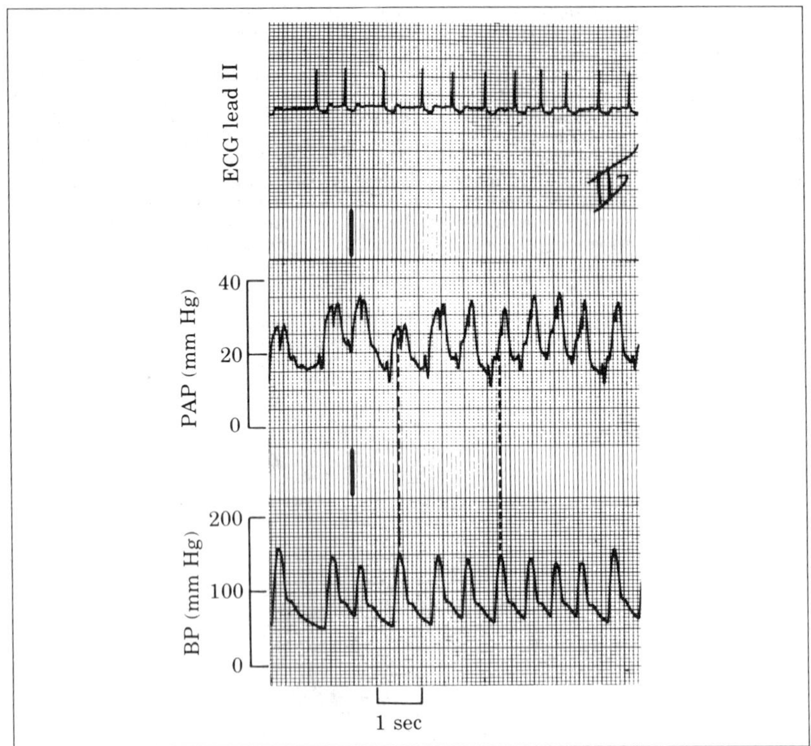

Fig. 5-14. A patient in atrial fibrillation with 3+ mitral regurgitation has V waves that are visible in the pulmonary artery trace and emerge as the balloon is inflated. Using the arterial pressure trace as a basis for timing waves is even more useful in atrial fibrillation where stroke volumes and hence regurgitant pressure waves vary from beat to beat. The importance of recognizing wedge position of the catheter in this setting cannot be overestimated. Although the mean wedge pressure reading has little relationship to left ventricular diastolic filling, diastolic wedge pressure does. More important, mistaking V waves for pulmonary artery waves may lead to the advancement of the catheter well beyond a safe distance into the pulmonary circulation. ***PAP*** **= pulmonary artery pressure.**

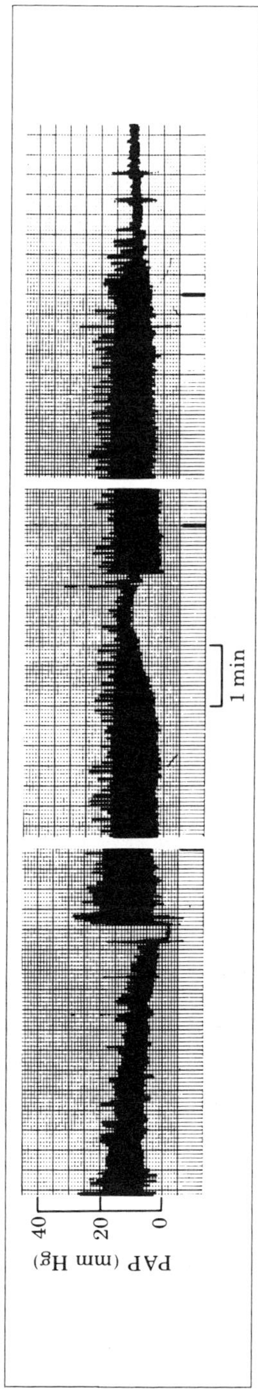

Fig. 5-15. Damping of pulmonary artery waveforms is caused by partial occlusion of the pathway between transducer and bloodstream. This example shows that pulmonary artery traces do not always damp to the mean. Indeed this patient's pulmonary artery pressure (*PAP*) measurement damps sequentially to diastolic, systolic, and finally mean pressures.

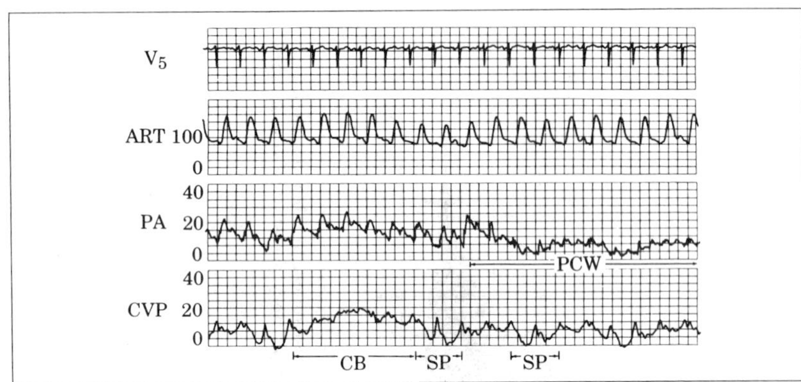

Fig. 5-16. A patient on intermittent mandatory ventilation demonstrates respiratory effects on hemodynamic pressure measurements. Pulmonary artery (*PA*) and central venous (*CVP*) tracings show the complex effects of both controlled and spontaneous breaths. Controlled mechanical breaths (*CB*) elevate the intravascular traces, although actual transmural pressure decreases. Spontaneous breaths (*SP*) depress the recorded pressures due to the decrease in pleural pressure, although transmural pressure and intrathoracic blood volume increase. The correct intrathoracic pressure reading should be taken at end expiration. End expiration after a spontaneous breath is the most consistent measurement point for this particular patient. Arterial (*ART*) pressure fluctuations of 35 mm Hg systolic and 10–15 mm Hg diastolic are evident. These recordings are true pressure signals without the reference artifacts.

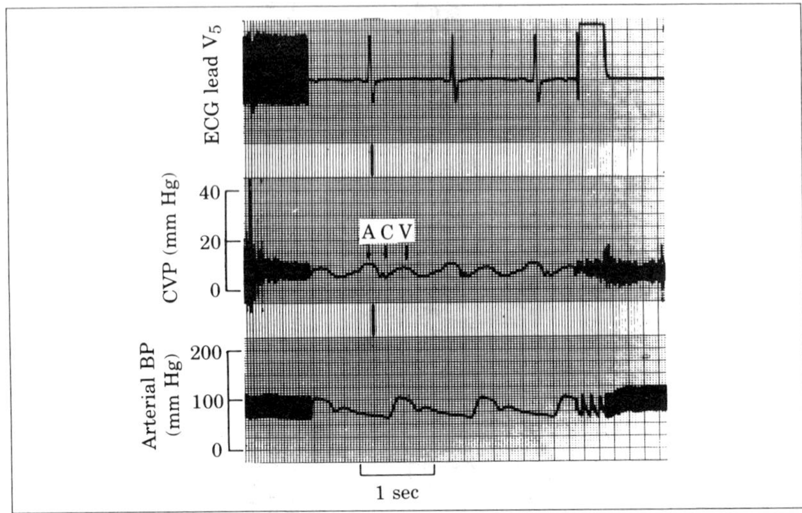

Fig. 5-17. A normal central venous pressure (*CVP*) tracing contains three discrete components. The A wave reflects atrial systole and is aligned in time with the QRS complex of the ECG (a result of the time delay between electrical and mechanical systole). The V wave occurs in concurrence with ventricular mechanical systole (associated with the T wave on the ECG). The C wave is seen here as a notching between the A and V waves.

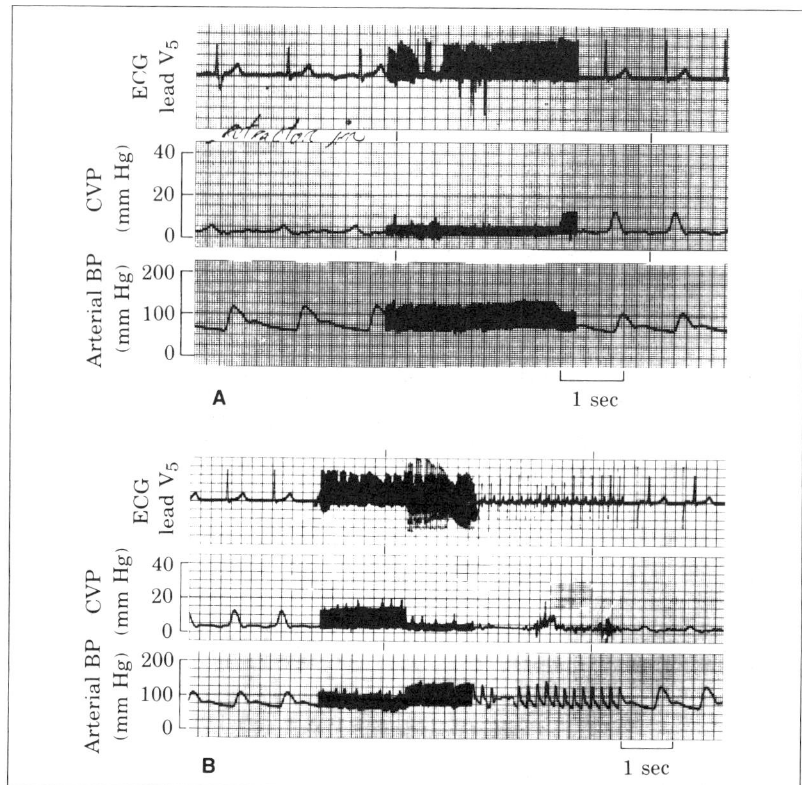

Fig. 5-18. The usefulness of transduced central venous pressure (*CVP*) monitoring to aid in the evaluation of disturbances of the cardiac rhythm. A. Note a sudden drop in the arterial BP. The diagnosis is immediately apparent with a glance at the CVP trace. Note the augmented waves occurring synchronously with the T wave of the ECG (mechanical ventricular systole). These are so-called cannon waves, actually representing a summation of normal V waves and atrial systole that is triggered by retrograde conducted P waves. B. This documents the reversal of the nodal rhythm with atrial pacing.

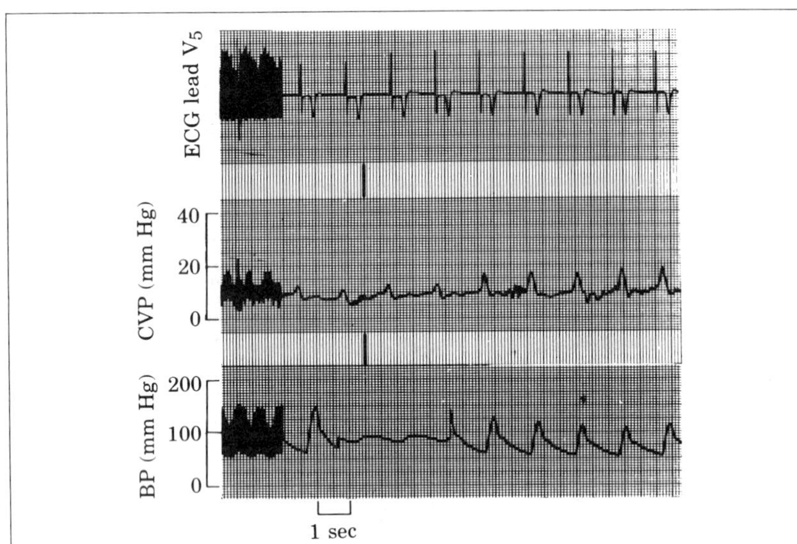

Fig. 5-19. Another example of the usefulness of the central venous pressure (*CVP*) trace to aid in the diagnosis of dysrhythmias. Note the large swings in systemic BP in the left portion of the tracing. In the expanded section, note that when the BP is lowest, the CVP wave is largest. Study of the ECG will disclose that the patient is in a totally dissociated rhythm, with the atrial rate slightly faster than the ventricular rhythm, thus causing atrial systole to "march through" the V waves in the CVP trace.

Appendix

Fick Method

If a known amount of indicator (mass or energy) is added to an unknown volume and the resulting change in concentration is determined, the change in concentration will be directly proportional to the total volume in the system:

$$\text{Concentration} = \frac{\text{indicator mass added (mg)}}{\text{unknown volume (ml)}} = \frac{\text{m}}{\text{V}} = \text{C} \tag{1}$$

Rearranging equation 1, this equation becomes

$$\text{Volume (unknown)} = \text{V} = \frac{\text{m}}{\text{C}} \tag{2}$$

If the fluid volume is moving (dV/dt) as in a cardiovascular system, then flow (F) can be determined if one adds a known indicator mass to the system at a known constant rate (dm/dt). Measuring the indicator concentration gradient (C2–C1) between the inlet and the outlet flowstreams of the system provides the basis for the Fick method.

$$\text{C2–C1} = \frac{\text{(dm/dt)}}{\text{(dV/dt)}} \tag{3}$$

Since dV/dt is flow (F),

$$\text{F} = \frac{\text{(dm/dt)}}{\text{(C2–C1)}} = \frac{\text{rate of indicator delivery}}{\text{concentration gradient}} \tag{4}$$

That is, the flow (F) through the system is proportional to the rate at which indicator must be added continuously (dm/dt) in order to maintain a constant change in concentration (C2–C1).

Oxygen consumption (in cc/min) is measured and substituted in the (dm/dt) term, and arterial and mixed venous blood oxygen content (in cc/L) is substituted for the concentration terms C2 and C1.

$$F = \frac{(dm/dt)}{(C2-C1)} = \frac{\text{oxygen consumption}}{\text{arterial} - \text{venous } O_2 \text{ gradient}} \tag{5}$$

Dye Dilution

The principal assumption of this method is that the same quantity of indicator must pass through the outlet as was delivered at the inlet (conservation of mass).

$$M = \int_0^\infty m(t)dt \tag{6}$$

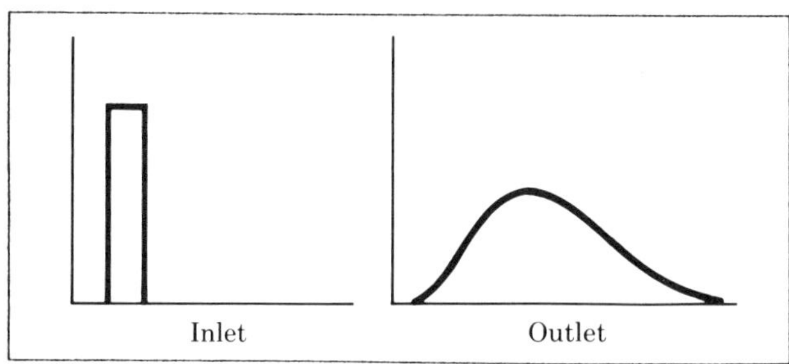

The sensors used in bolus indicator dilution techniques do not measure mass but measure concentration at the outlet. The flow of the system washes out the mass of indicator in the mixing chamber and results in a concentration curve at the outlet sensor. The concentration of indicator present at the outlet C(t) at any given moment in time is equal to the mass of dye in the solution passing by the sensor divided by the increment of the total system volume that is sampled by the sensor at that instant.

$$C(t) = dm(t)/dV \tag{7}$$

Equation 7 can be rearranged to show the instantaneous amount of indicator (dm/dt) seen at the outlet at time t_i by dividing both sides by dt:

$$\frac{dm}{dt} = C(t) \times \frac{dV}{dt} \tag{8}$$

If it is assumed that the flow is constant over the measurement, then

$$\frac{dV}{dt} = F = \text{flow} \tag{9}$$

Then integrating equation 8,

$$M = F \times \int_0^\infty C(t)dt \tag{10}$$

Rearranging this, it becomes

$$F = \frac{M}{\int_0^\infty C(t)dt} \tag{11}$$

Thermal Dilution

The indicator in thermodilution is thermal energy, as opposed to mass. A known volume of saline at a temperature lower than blood temperature is used as the indicator. In principle, the indicator dilution equation 11 applies with some modification:

$$M = (\text{Tadded} - \text{Tbaseline}) \times p_i \times cp_i \times V_i \tag{12}$$

where
p_i = density of the indicator
cp_i = specific heat of the indicator
V_i = volume of indicator (injectate)
Tbaseline = baseline blood temperature
Tadded = injectate temperature

The concentration (C(t)) at the system outlet becomes

$$C(t) = (\text{Tout}(t) - \text{Tbaseline}) \times p_b \times cp_b \tag{13}$$

where
Tout(t) = temperature signal sensed at the outlet
p_b = density of blood
cp_b = specific heat of blood

These relationships can be substituted into equation 11 developed for dye dilution.

$$F = \frac{(\text{Tadded} - \text{Tbaseline}) \times V_i \times p_i \times cp_i}{p_b \times cp_b \times \int_0^\infty (\text{Tadded} - \text{Tout}(t))dt} \tag{14}$$

$$F = \frac{-\text{Tbaseline} \times V_i \times p_i \times cp_i}{p_b \times cp_b \times \int_0^\infty \text{Tout}(t)dt} \tag{15}$$

Since the heat capacities of the indicator (saline) and blood are known, the equation becomes

$$F = \frac{1.08 \times (-\text{Tbaseline}) \times V_i}{\int_0^\infty \text{Tout}(t)dt} \tag{16}$$

Equation 16 represents an ideal system with no heat losses. In practice, some of the injectate volume is lost in the dead space of the catheter lumen, and some of the injectate heat is lost during the measurement through the observer's hand during injection and across the catheter to air or blood before reaching the atrium. Some indicator may also be absorbed by vascular or ventricular walls. A catheter-specific correction factor is used to account for these losses.

For indicator volume of 10 ml (0.01 L), the equation becomes

$$\begin{aligned} F(\text{L/min}) &= 0.836 \times 1.08 \times \frac{60\ (\text{sec})}{1\ (\text{min})} \times \frac{-\text{Tbaseline}}{\int_0^\infty \text{Tout}\ dt} \\ &= 0.542 \times \frac{-\text{Tbaseline}}{\int_0^\infty \text{Tout}\ dt} \end{aligned} \tag{17}$$

where
0.836 = correctional constant for Edwards No. 93A-131-7F catheter

The correctional constant 0.542 is entered into the CO measurement instrument.

Selected References

Bruner, J. M., Krenis, L. J., Kunsman, J. M., and Sherman, A. P. Comparison of direct and indirect methods of measuring arterial blood pressure, part I. *Med. Instrum.* 15:11, 1981.

Bruner, J. M., Krenis, L. J., Kunsman, J. M., and Sherman, A. P. Comparison of direct and indirect methods of measuring arterial blood pressure, part II. *Med. Instrum.* 15:97, 1981.

Bruner, J. M., Krenis, L. J., Kunsman, J. M., and Sherman, A. P. Comparison of direct and indirect methods of measuring arterial blood pressure, part III. *Med. Instrum.* 15:182, 1981.

Gardner, R. M. Direct blood pressure measurement—dynamic response requirements. *Anesthesiology* 54:227, 1981.

Geddes, L. A. *The Direct and Indirect Measurement of Blood Pressure.* Chicago: Year Book, 1970.

Geddes, L. A., Voelz, M., Combs, C., et al. Characterization of the oscillometric method for the measuring of indirect blood pressure. *Ann. Biomed. Eng.* 10:271, 1982.

McDonald, D. F. *Blood Flow in Arteries.* Baltimore: Williams & Wilkins, 1974.

Matthay, M. A. Invasive Hemodynamic Monitoring in Critically Ill Patients. In R. A. Matthay, M. A. Matthay, and D. R. Dantzker (eds.), *Chest Medicine.* Philadelphia: Saunders, 1983.

Posey, J. A., Geddes, L. A., Williams, H., and Moore, A. G. The meaning of maximum oscillations in cuff pressure in the indirect measurement of blood pressure—part I. *Cardiovasc. Res. Cent. Bull.* 8:15, 1969.

Ramsey, M., III. Noninvasive automatic determination of mean arterial pressure. *Med. Biol. Eng. Comput.* 17:11, 1979.

Severinghaus, J. W., and Astrup, P. B. History of blood gas analysis. *J. Clin. Monitor.* 2:270, 1986.

Trautman, E. D., and Newbower, R. S. The development of indicator-dilution techniques. *IEEE Trans. Biomed. Eng.* 12:800, 1984.

Yelderman, M., and Ream, A. K. Indirect measurement of mean blood pressure in the anesthetized patient. *Anesthesiology* 50:253, 1979.

6

Cardiopulmonary Resuscitation in the Acute Care Setting

James K. Alifimoff

Optimal outcome after cardiac arrest depends on several factors. Rapid diagnosis and prompt restoration of spontaneous circulation are probably the most crucial because standard cardiopulmonary resuscitation basic life support (CPR-BLS) usually results in only 6–30% of normal blood flow. Nevertheless, during attempts at restoration of spontaneous circulation with advanced life support (ALS) measures, it is imperative that CPR-BLS be performed efficiently and with only minimal interruption to ensure maximal CNS oxygenation and circulation of resuscitative drugs to their target organs.

The efficient organization of the resuscitative team is of importance. When cardiac arrest occurs in the acute care setting, adequate personnel are usually available; their deployment should be the responsibility of a single experienced individual who makes therapeutic decisions, while considering suggestions from other members of the team.

This chapter focuses on an approach to the management of cardiac arrest as it occurs in the ICU and operating room. Discussion of airway management is not included here; it may be found in Chapter 1. Pharmacologic agents used to support the circulation once restoration of spontaneous circulation has been achieved are discussed separately. Finally, resuscitation of pediatric patients is considered in Chapter 28.

I. **Pathophysiology of cardiac arrest.** With the onset of cardiac arrest, oxygen delivery to tissues ceases, and anaerobic metabolism begins. This results in the production of lactic acid, which produces vasodilatation and failure of catecholamine action.

II. **Causes of cardiac arrest**

A. **Primary cardiac arrest** is due to myocardial ischemia, leading to electrical irritability and ventricular fibrillation (VF) or to asystole secondary to intrinsic heart disease.

B. **Secondary cardiac arrest** may be precipitated by a number of different etiologies.

1. **Decreased preload** may be due to hypovolemia, tension pneumothorax, venal caval obstruction, or cardiac tamponade and leads to poor or inadequate systemic or myocardial perfusion.
2. **Myocardial depression** can result from primary drug effects (antiarrythmics and negative inotropes), electrolyte disturbances (hypokalemia or hypocalcemia), or hypoxemia from inhalation of hypoxic gas mixtures, airway obstruction, pulmonary parenchymal disease, low cardiac output, or apnea/hypoventilation.
3. **Decreased peripheral vascular resistance** may be caused by vasodilating drugs, anaphylaxis, or septic shock.

III. **Diagnosis of cardiac arrest**

A. Two factors are related to optimal neurologic outcome: time from arrest to initiation of CPR-BLS and time to restoration of spontaneous circulation. It is important to make the diagnosis of cardiac arrest quickly and begin treatment expeditiously. However, one must be absolutely certain that technical problems do not lead to an erroneous diagnosis. **Absence of a preexisting pulse in a major blood vessel (carotid or femoral artery) is diagnostic of cardiac arrest and should be employed to confirm the diagnosis prior to initiating CPR.** The following may be highly suggestive as well.

1. VF, ventricular tachycardia (VT), or asystole on EKG
2. Absent blood pressure by direct or indirect monitoring
3. Loss of consciousness
4. Inaudible heart sound
5. Cyanosis or profound desaturation by pulse oximeter

IV. **Treatment of cardiac arrest**

A. The diagnosis of cardiac arrest demands immediate initiation of CPR-BLS.

1. **Basic life support**
   a. Securing and managing the airway
   b. Breathing
   c. Circulation. Artificial circulation is provided by external cardiac compressions. The patient must be placed on a firm, flat surface in order to perform effective compression. Place the heel of one hand two finger breadths above the xiphoid process and the fingers interlocked with those of the opposite hand. Pressure is exerted from the shoulders through locked elbows, depressing the sternum 1.5–2.0 inches. Compression should account for 50% of the compression-relaxation cycle. Compressions are performed at a rate of 80–100 per minute with one breath interposed after every 5 compressions.
   d. **Precordial thump.** A small epicardial potential, which can terminate VF, can be generated by a precordial thump. This maneuver can convert VT or complete heart block into sinus rhythm; it can also precipitate VF. Therefore, whenever a precordial thump is used, a defibrillator should be immediately available.
2. **Advanced life support (ALS)** is the treatment of cardiac arrest with drugs, fluids, DC cardioversion, or pacemaker insertion. Continuation of CPR-BLS is important during this period to provide maximal organ oxygenation and to circulate drugs to their sites of action.
   a. Drugs may be administered through a peripheral or central IV line or by endotracheal tube.
   b. Established venous access should be used initially. If venous access is not present, an antecubital IV should be started. However, drugs administered by this route may take minutes to reach their site of action, depending on the degree of blood flow generated by CPR-BLS.
   c. If restoration of spontaneous circulation is not immediately accomplished, start a central venous line. The internal or external jugular or femoral approaches are preferable to the subclavian because they can be attempted with less interruption of CPR-BLS. The risk of pneumothorax is also lower.
   d. If venous access cannot be readily established, most drugs may be administered through the endotracheal tube (ETT); however, it is preferable to dilute these drugs up to a total volume of 10 ml of sterile saline to ensure a volume sufficient to reach the alveoli. **Never administer sodium bicarbonate and calcium in this manner.**
3. **ALS drugs**
   a. **Oxygen.** 100% oxygen should be used to ventilate all patients during resuscitation. Patients should be ventilated by hand bag so that the interposition of ventilations and compressions may be ensured.
   b. **Epinephrine** has both alpha- and beta-adrenergic effects that result in increased myocardial contractility and perfusion pressure during CPR. In addition, epinephrine coarsens fine VF.
      (1) Initial dose of 0.5–1.0 mg IV (5–10 ml of 1:10,000 solution)
      (2) Repeat q5min
   c. The **routine** use of sodium bicarbonate is no longer recommended since it does not improve defibrillation in experimental animals, may shift the oxyhemoglobin dissociation curve to the right (thereby decreasing oxygen availability), and causes a paradoxical acidosis by enhancing CO_2 production. Sodium bicarbonate may be administered, however, when there is prolonged arrest or documented acidosis by arterial blood gas (ABG) analysis.

(1) Initial dose of 1 mEq per kg IV
(2) Subsequent dose of 0.5 mEq per kg q10min
(3) If ABGs are available, the dose may be calculated as follows:

$$\text{mEq NaHCO}_3 = \text{base deficit (mEq/L)} \times \text{body wt (kg)} \times 0.3$$

d. **Lidocaine** is used to treat refractory or recurrent VF. It should be used cautiously in patients in atrial fibrillation or flutter because it may result in dangerous acceleration of the ventricular rate.
(1) Initial dose of 1 mg per kg IV
(2) Repeat doses of 0.5 mg per kg may be given q8min to a total dose of 3 mg per kg.
(3) Decrease dosage in patients with low cardiac output or hepatic dysfunction.

e. Use **procainamide** to treat ventricular dysrhythmias when lidocaine fails or is contraindicated.
(1) 50 mg IV q5min up to a total dose of 1 g may be given until ventricular ectopy resolves, hypotension occurs, or the QRS complex is widened by 50%.
(2) Emergently, 20 mg per minute may be administered, up to a total dose of 1 g.
(3) Maintenance infusion rate of 2–4 mg per minute.
(4) Decrease the dosage in the presence of renal failure.

f. Use **bretylium** to treat refractory ventricular dysrhythmias and VF. Initially it causes the release of catecholamines; however, hypotension may follow due to its ganglionic blocking properties. Bretylium is indicated when lidocaine and DC cardioversion fail to convert VF or when lidocaine and procainamide have not resolved VT.
(1) For VF, initial dose of 5 mg per kg IV, followed by 10 mg per kg q15min, to a total of 10 mg per kg.
(2) For VT, 5–10 mg per kg in 50 ml of 5% dextrose in water IV over 10 minutes; start an infusion of 1–2 mg per minute.

g. **Atropine** decreases vagal tone, increases AV conduction, and stimulates sinus node discharge. It is used for the treatment of sinus bradycardia associated with either ventricular escape beats or hypotension as well as for asystole.
(1) Initial dose of 0.4–1.0 mg IV for bradycardia
(2) For asystole, 1 mg IV, to a total of 3 mg
(3) Doses less than 0.4 mg may be parasympathomimetic (i.e., may produce bradycardia).

h. **Calcium** is no longer recommended for the treatment of asystole or electromechanical dissociation. However, Ca^{++} is indicated for documented or suspected hypocalcemia, treatment of Ca^{++} antagonist overdose, hyperkalemia, and hypomagnesemia.
(1) 2–4 mg per kg IV of $CaCl_2$ (1.5–3.0 ml of 10% $CaCl_2$ solution)
(2) Alternatively, calcium gluconate (10%) or gluceptate may be used at doses of 5–8 ml and 5–7 ml, respectively.

i. **Isoproterenol** was previously recommended for the treatment of asystole. Now, its only use is for the treatment of atropine-resistant bradycardia. The infusion rate is 2–10 μg per minute.

4. **Specific cardiac arrest scenarios.** All resuscitations, to some extent, must be individualized. The following scenarios are those that are most appropriate to the acute care setting. The steps specified, however, do not preclude alternative or additional therapies as deemed appropriate by the treating physician.

a. **Monitored VF** (i.e., <1 minute in duration)
(1) Precordial thump

(2) Start CPR-BSL until defibrillator is charged.
(3) Confirm rhythm with defibrillator oscilloscope or EKG.
(4) Defibrillate with 200 J.
(5) If VF is not terminated, continue CPR-BLS while recharging defibrillator and defibrillate with 200–300 J.
(6) Repeat Step 5, with a third countershock less than 360 J.
(7) If the third countershock is unsuccessful, administer epinephrine, 1 mg IV or by ETT, during CPR.
(8) Defibrillate with 360 J.
(9) Continue CPR, and administer lidocaine, 1 mg per kg IV or by ETT.
(10) Defibrillate with 360 J.
(11) Administer bretylium, 5 mg per kg IV.

b. VT without hemodynamic compromise or change in mental status
(1) Lidocaine, 1 mg per kg IV.
(2) Repeat lidocaine, 0.5 mg per kg, q5min, up to a total dose of 3 mg per kg, or start infusion at 2 mg per minute after the first bolus and increase rate by 1 mg per minute to a maximum of 4 mg per minute after each additional bolus.
(3) Procainamide 20 mg per minute IV, up to 1 g
(4) **Synchronized** cardioversion starting at 50 J. Consider sedation prior to cardioversion.

c. VT with hemodynamic compromise or change in mental status, indicating inadequate cerebral perfusion
(1) **Unsynchronized** cardioversion at 50 J.
(2) If unsuccessful, repeat cardioversion at 100 J, then 200 J, and, if necessary, at 360 J.
(3) For recurrent VT, administer lidocaine and cardiovert at an energy level that was previously successful.
(4) If unsuccessful, procainamide as directed in **4.b.(3)** or bretylium 5 mg per kg IV

d. Asystole may follow VF or may be due to excessive parasympathetic tone. Very fine VF may mimic asystole. Therefore, an initial countershock at 200 J may be justified. For this reason, two different EKG lead readings are required for the diagnosis.
(1) Immediate CPR-BLS
(2) Epinephrine, 1 mg IV or by ETT
(3) Atropine 1 mg IV or by ETT, repeated q5min to a total dose of 3 mg
(4) Consider $NaHCO_3$ IV.
(5) Consider transvenous or transthoracic pacemaker.

e. Electromechanical dissociation is characterized by organized electrical activity of the heart without effective mechanical pumping and carries a grave prognosis.
(1) Immediate CPR-BLS
(2) Epinephrine, 1 mg IV or by ETT
(3) Consider correctable causes such as tension pneumothorax, profound hypovolemia, cardiac tamponade, profound hypoxemia, or acidosis.

5. Open chest CPR is indicated for:
a. A patient whose chest is already open
b. Penetrating thoracic trauma
c. Tension pneumothorax
d. Cardiac tamponade
e. Profound hypothermia
f. Suspected massive pulmonary embolism

   - **g.** Severe chest deformity, as in advanced chronic obstructive pulmonary disease, which prevents adequate external cardiac compression
   - **h.** Failure of adequately performed external compression and refractory VF
6. **When to terminate CPR.** The decision to terminate a resuscitation is difficult for medical, ethical, and legal reasons.
   - **a.** Unambiguous determination that a patient has suffered irreversible brain damage is the main criterion for terminating CPR. However, this is impossible during CPR. Since there are no sound neurologic criteria for termination of ALS measures, the decision must be based on cardiovascular status. As stated in "Standards and Guidelines for Cardiopulmonary Resuscitation and Emergency Cardiac Care," it must be possible to state that both BLS and ALS were employed in a manner and for a time adequate to test the responsiveness of the victim's cardiovascular system. In this context, cardiovascular unresponsiveness indicates that the heart is no longer viable and thus eliminates the need to establish loss of neurologic function.
   - **b.** It is important to document meticulously that resuscitative efforts were pursued to the appropriate end point.
   - **c.** If doubt exists about when to terminate the resuscitation, continue CPR.
7. **Do not resuscitate (DNR) orders**
   - **a.** A perplexing situation arises when patients with DNR orders are scheduled for a surgical procedure. Under these circumstances, resuscitation should still be performed with the understanding that reversibility is possible when the arrest has been caused by or precipitated by a therapeutic maneuver rather than by the underlying disease process itself. In these circumstances, however, it is essential that this be discussed openly, honestly, and in detail with the patient, the family, the primary physician, and the surgeon and that these discussions are documented in the medical record.

Suggested Readings

Alifimoff, J. K. Open versus closed-chest cardiac massage in nontraumatic cardiac arrest. *Resuscitation* 15:13, 1987.

American Heart Association. Standards and guidelines for cardiopulmonary resuscitation (CPR) and emergency cardiac care (ECC). *J.A.M.A.* 255:2095, 1986.

Geller, S. A., Elliot, P. L., and Rodger, M. C. Update on cardiopulmonary resuscitation. *Adv. Anesth.* 3:323, 1986.

Safar, P., and Birher, N. *Cardio-Pulmonary-Cerebral-Resuscitation.* Philadelphia: W. B. Saunders, 1988.

7

Valvular Heart Disease

Jean Elrick

The management of patients with known or suspected valvular heart disease is dependent on a thorough understanding of the hemodynamic consequences of the anatomic lesion. When more than one structural abnormality is present (often the case), management should be guided by the predominant lesion.

As a general rule, all patients with valve lesions should receive prophylactic antibiotics against endocarditis when invasive procedures or surgery are planned. The current recommendations for such coverage are presented in Table 7-1.

Patients who have undergone prosthetic or reconstructive valve surgery generally do not have significant residual stenosis or regurgitation. However, the structural and functional alterations of the heart as a consequence of valve dysfunction, as discussed in this chapter, may persist after corrective operation. Guidelines for antibiotic prophylaxis apply to these patients as well.

I. Aortic stenosis

A. Etiology. The etiology of aortic stenosis can be classified as congenital, rheumatic, or degenerative. Congenital lesions usually take the form of bicuspid valves that often do not become functionally stenosed until middle or late adult life. The bicuspid structure of the valve is believed to promote degenerative changes from abnormal blood flow patterns. **Rheumatic heart disease** causes commissural fusion. Aortic stenosis is rarely the only manifestation of rheumatic heart disease. Degenerative lesions are characterized by excessive calcification of leaflets, especially in the folds. The elderly are the population affected.

B. Pathophysiology. Aortic stenosis presents fixed obstruction to left ventricular ejection. This obstruction causes a systolic pressure gradient to develop between the ventricle and the aorta. Concentric left ventricular hypertrophy occurs to decrease left ventricular wall stress. This hypertrophy results in increased myocardial oxygen consumption and decreased left ventricular compliance. The normal aortic valve orifice is 2.5–3.5 cm^2. Critical aortic stenosis is defined as an orifice less than 0.5 cm^2 or a systolic gradient more than 50 with normal cardiac output. It is crucial to know the cardiac output at the time of gradient measurement because it is directly related to flow. As the ventricle becomes severely dysfunctional, the systolic gradient and cardiac output fall.

C. Evaluation

1. **History.** A murmur of aortic stenosis (AS) may be present for many years before the classic symptoms of angina, syncope, or exertional dyspnea occur. Once symptoms present, the natural history of AS predicts a life expectancy of 2 to 5 years. The angina may be due to associated coronary artery disease (about 50% of patients) or increased myocardial oxygen consumption secondary to ventricular hypertrophy. Dyspnea results from pulmonary congestion due to increased left ventricular end diastolic and left atrial pressures. The cause of syncope may be hypotension resulting from fixed cardiac output in the presence of vasodilation.
2. **Physical examination.** The crescendo/decrescendo systolic murmur is loudest at the aortic area over the second right intercostal space. Transmission to both carotids is usual. The carotid pulse upstroke is delayed. The BP is normal unless severe left ventricular dysfunction exists.
3. **Other.** The ECG shows left ventricular hypertrophy (LVH) with or without a strain pattern. The degree of LVH does not correlate with severity of AS. Conduction defects may result from calcific infiltration of the conducting tissue located next to the valve annulus. **Chest radiography** shows a normal-sized heart or left ventricular dilation in the late stages. A prominent ascending aorta from poststenotic dilatation may be seen.

Table 7-1. Prophylactic antibiotics for protection from bacterial endocarditis

For dental procedures and upper respiratory tract surgery	
I. For most patients: **Oral penicillin**	*Adults:* 2 g of penicillin V 1 hr before procedure and then 1 g 6 h after initial dose *Children less than 60 pounds:* 1 g penicillin V 1 h before procedure and then 500 mg 6 h after initial dose
II. For those *allergic to penicillin* (may also be selected for those receiving oral penicillin as continuous rheumatic fever prophylaxis): **erythromycin**	*Adults:* 1 g orally 1 h before procedure and then 500 mg 6 h after initial dose *Children:* 20 mg/kg orally 1 h before procedure and then 10 mg/kg 6 h after initial dose
III. For patients *at high risk* of infective endocarditis (especially those with prosthetic heart valves) who are not allergic to penicillin: **ampicillin** plus **gentamicin**	*Adults:* 1–2 g plus gentamicin 1.5 mg/kg IM or IV, both given 30 min before procedure; then penicillin V 1 g orally 6 h after initial dose *Children:* Timing of doses is same for adults; dosages are ampicillin 50 mg/kg and gentamicin 2 mg/kg
IV. For *higher-risk* patients (especially those with prosthetic heart valves who are *allergic to penicillin*): **vancomycin**	*Adults:* vancomycin 1 g IV over 60 min, begun 60 min before procedure; no repeat dose necessary *Children:* vancomycin 20 mg/kg IV over 60 min, begun 60 min before procedure; no repeat dose necessary
For gastrointestinal and genitourinary tract surgery and instrumentation	
I. For most patients: **ampicillin** plus **gentamicin**	*Adults:* 2 g ampicillin IM or IV plus gentamicin 1.5 mg/kg IM or IV given 30 min before procedure; may repeat once 8 h later *Children:* same timing of medications as adult schedule; dosages are ampicillin 50 mg/kg and gentamicin 2 mg/kg
II. For patients *allergic to penicillin*: **vancomycin** plus **gentamicin**	*Adults:* 1 g vancomycin IV given over 60 min plus 1.5 mg/kg gentamicin IM or IV, each given 60 min before procedure; doses may be repeated once 8–12 h later *Children:* timing as for adults; doses are vancomycin 20 mg/kg and gentamicin 2 mg/kg
III. Oral regimen for minor or repetitive procedures in low-risk patients: **amoxicillin**	*Adults:* 30 g amoxicillin 1 h before procedure and 1.5 g 6 h after initial dose *Children:* same timing as for adults: 50 mg/kg initial dose and 25 mg/kg follow-up dose

Adapted from *The Report of the Committee on Rheumatic Fever and Infective Endocarditis,* American Heart Association, 1984.

D. Management

1. Symptomatic patients with aortic stenosis should be referred for surgery or percutaneous valvuloplasty as the progressive nature of the lesion from this point is well known. Although the long-term results from valvuloplasty are not favorable, this technique may provide short-term benefit in critical stenosis when other medical problems are overriding.
2. Left ventricular filling is significantly dependent on atrial contraction. In the normal heart, atrial contraction contributes 25% of stroke volume; this increases to 40% in AS. Thus, the maintenance of normal sinus rhythm is important.
3. Heart rate control is similarly key to ventricular filling. Both bradycardia and tachycardia adversely affect cardiac output. If invasive monitoring of pulmonary vascular pressure is planned, consideration should be given to providing atrial and/or ventricular pacing with selection of an appropriate catheter in order to have further control of rate and rhythm, if necessary.
4. Systemic hypotension is to be avoided assiduously because the heart cannot respond by increasing output. Vasoconstrictors are a good choice to preserve vascular tone. Venodilators must be used judiciously for the same reason.
5. In the presence of severe ventricular dysfunction, inotropic support may be indicated. Dopamine, norepinephrine, and epinephrine are acceptable agents. The need to maintain systemic vascular tone precludes use of dobutamine or amrinone, which are likely to have a vasodilatory effect.

II. Aortic regurgitation

A. Etiology. Acute aortic regurgitation (AR) can result from causes such as endocarditis, trauma, or aortic dissection. Valve incompetence results from damage to the leaflets or supporting supra- or subvalvular structures. **Chronic AR** often is associated with aortic stenosis as a consequence of rheumatic heart disease. Connective tissue disorders such as Marfan's syndrome or cystic medial necrosis cause AR by dilation of the aortic root.

B. Pathophysiology. Acute aortic regurgitation in a patient with normal ventricular compliance results in severe left ventricular dysfunction and dilatation. The dilatation may affect mitral annular size and cause acute mitral regurgitation. Premature closure of the mitral valve is common, interfering with left ventricular filling. **Chronic aortic regurgitation**, a more insidious process, permits compensatory left ventricular dilation and hypertrophy in response to the volume overload. The amount of AR is determined by the pressure gradient between the ventricle and the aorta, and the diastolic time period (inversely proportional to the heart rate). Considering all valvular lesions, cardiomegaly is greatest in AR.

C. Evaluation

1. **History.** A long, asymptomatic interval is usual in chronic AR. Symptoms correlate poorly with the degree of left ventricular dysfunction. When function is severely impaired, symptoms of low cardiac output (chronic weakness, fatigue) predominate. Exercise classically improves symptoms due to enhanced forward flow. Presentation in acute AR depends on the time course of valve incompetence. Low cardiac output with poor systemic perfusion is evident, and the patient may be moribund.
2. **Physical examination.** In **chronic AR**, a high-pitched diastolic murmur is present along the sternal border at the third or fourth interstice. The systolic pressure is elevated and the diastolic pressure quite decreased. Characteristic peripheral vascular signs include wa-

ter hammer pulses, capillary pulsations with nail bed compression and to-and-fro murmurs over the femoral arteries. In **acute AR**, the patient is critically ill with poor peripheral perfusion, tachycardia, and likely pulmonary vascular congestion. Systemic vascular signs are absent in acute AR.

3. **Other.** The ECG in acute AR is often normal. In chronic AR, left ventricular hypertrophy and left axis deviation are present. Chest radiography shows left ventricular enlargement. Ascending aortic dilation may be seen.

D. Management

1. Objectives of medical management include reduction of peripheral resistance, inotropic support, and maintenance of adequate heart rate. In acute AR due to aortic dissection, immediate surgical attention is indicated. Valve replacement is indicated in chronic AR when symptoms develop or echocardiography demonstrates a falling ejection fraction.
2. **Vasodilators** decrease systemic vascular tone and the pressure gradient. In the acute setting, nitroprusside or nitroglycerin directly affects systemic vessels. Inotropic support is often necessary to improve left ventricular function. Dobutamine and amrinone are first-choice drugs for this purpose.
3. The diastolic time interval is inversely proportional to heart rate. Bradycardia promotes increased regurgitant flow and should be avoided.
4. Symptoms are unreliable indicators of the degree of volume overload in AR. Invasive monitoring of systemic arterial and pulmonary vascular pressures is indicated for accurate assessment of effects of therapeutic interventions. In acute AR, however, left ventricular end diastolic pressure will be underestimated by these measures due to premature closure of the mitral valve.

III. Mitral stenosis

A. Etiology. Mitral stenosis (MS) most often results from rheumatic heart disease. The affected population is two-thirds female. Typically, there is a latency of 20 years before symptoms begin. Congenital stenosis occurs rarely and usually presents with symptoms in infancy.

B. Pathophysiology. The normal size of the mitral valve orifice in an adult is 4–6 cm^2. Progressive narrowing of the mitral valve orifice due to commissural fusion results in a transmitral diastolic pressure gradient between the atria and ventricle. In critical MS, where the orifice is 1 cm^2, the left atrial pressure is approximately 25 mm Hg. This elevated pressure leads to elevated pulmonary venous and pulmonary capillary pressures. **Left atrial enlargement** occurs in response to the pressure overload. Blood stasis and thrombus formation develop, especially if the rhythm changes to atrial fibrillation, as is the usual case. Left ventricular function is compromised due to chronic abnormal underloading of the ventricle and likely abnormal architecture secondary to rheumatic carditis. This dysfunction may not be apparent until after mitral valve replacement, when loading conditions are changed. In **long-standing MS**, pulmonary vascular hypertension is marked. A component of this hypertension is fixed and will not normalize even after effective surgical correction of the stenosis. Pulmonary hypertension may result in right ventricular failure and dilatation with tricuspid regurgitation.

C. Evaluation

1. **History.** Dyspnea on exertion and cough secondary to decreased pulmonary compliance are usual complaints. Weakness and fatigue are due to low cardiac output.

2. **Physical examination.** The low-pitched, rumbling diastolic murmur of MS is present at the right lower sternal border. Pulmonary congestive signs are present. If right heart failure occurs, systemic congestion with peripheral edema, hepatomegaly, and pleural effusions are evident.
3. **Other.** The ECG shows left atrial enlargement if in sinus rhythm. Right ventricular hypertrophy and right axis deviation are seen in severe pulmonary hypertension. Chest radiography shows left atrial enlargement. The left mainstem bronchus is elevated above this enlarged chamber.
4. **Management**
   a. Heart rate is the most important determinant of left ventricular filling in MS. Tachycardia decreases the time available for filling and increases the transmitral pressure gradient. Control of heart rate can be achieved by the use of digoxin (if the rhythm is atrial fibrillation) and/or beta-blockers. The underlying cause for tachycardia (fever, anemia, sympathetic stimulation, etc.) should be aggressively treated. Bradycardia is to be avoided since the stroke volume is relatively fixed.
   b. Sinus rhythm should be maintained, if possible, although permanent atrial fibrillation is usual in long-standing MS and heralds exacerbation of symptoms. Electric or pharmacologic conversion of new onset trial fibrillation should be attempted.
   c. Left atrial enlargement and atrial fibrillation permit stasis of blood and potential for thrombus formation. Appropriate anticoagulation should be maintained, especially if the heart rhythm changes from atrial fibrillation to sinus rhythm.
   d. Invasive monitoring of systemic arterial and pulmonary arterial pressures is indicated for patients with severe MS if significant fluid requirements or fluctuations in hemodynamics is anticipated. Passage of a pulmonary artery catheter in patients with severe pulmonary hypertension and tricuspid regurgitation may be difficult and require fluoroscopically guided placement.
   e. Inotropes are indicated to improve cardiac output in the majority of patients. Vasodilators decrease left ventricular filling and stroke volume except in patients with combined MS/MR, where forward fraction may be increased by dilation, or in patients with severe pulmonary hypertension, where vasodilation may increase transpulmonary blood flow and improve cardiac output. Vasoconstrictors may exacerbate pulmonary hypertension and further decrease transpulmonary blood flow. Serial measurements of cardiac output and pulmonary artery vascular pressures are necessary if such therapeutic manipulations are attempted.
   f. Diuretics are indicated to control volume status. Continued administration of these drugs is particularly important for patients on long-standing therapy.

IV. Mitral regurgitation

A. Etiology. Mitral regurgitation (MR) results from dysfunction of one or more components of the mitral apparatus: the valve annulus, leaflets, chordae tendineae, and papillary muscles. Chronic mitral regurgitation is usually associated with MS as a consequence of rheumatic heart disease. Other causes of MR are annular calcification and mitral valve prolapse syndrome. **Acute MR** may occur due to chordae rupture, endocarditis, myxomatous degeneration, or, rarely, trauma. Ischemia of the papillary muscle(s) and annular dilatation secondary to left ventricular dysfunction are other causes of acute regurgitation.

B. Pathophysiology. Chronic MR is generally well tolerated hemodynamically. The left atrium gradually enlarges, accepting the regurgitant volume from the left ventricle without a significant change in left atrial pressure. The left ventricle ejects into the low impedance atrium, an ideal loading situation for the ventricle. The left ventricle responds to the chronic volume condition by dilating and increasing wall thickness. This preserves the ratio of left ventricular mass to end diastolic volume. Left ventricular contractility is not impaired, and the oxygen cost of contraction is normal. Regurgitant flow depends on the size of the mitral orifice, the pressure gradient between the atrium and ventricle, and the heart rate. The pressure gradient, in turn, is dependent on the compliance of the left ventricle and the impedance to left ventricular ejection. When MR is associated with MS, left ventricular filling is highly dependent on appropriately timed left atrial contraction. In isolated MR, maintenance of sinus rhythm is less critical. Severe MR is defined by a forward ejection fraction of less than 0.6. Acute MR is not well tolerated hemodynamically due to the inability of the left atrium to accept the regurgitant volume without markedly increased pressure. Pronounced pulmonary vascular congestion and its sequelae are immediately apparent. As the left ventricle dilates in response to increased volume, regurgitation is further enhanced by annular dilatation.

C. **Evaluation**

1. **History.** Patients with chronic MR are virtually symptom free until ongoing left ventricular dilatation, resulting in left ventricular failure; then weakness, fatigue, and other symptoms of low cardiac output become apparent. In patients with MR secondary to rheumatic heart disease, the symptom-free interval is considerably longer than in patients where mitral stenosis predominates.
2. **Physical examination.** In chronic MR, the systolic murmur is holosystolic in duration, blowing, high pitched, and loudest at the apex. The murmur may radiate to the axilla and back. The precordial impulse is hyperdynamic and displaced to the left. In acute MR, the murmur is lower pitched and softer. Signs of pulmonary vascular congestion are prominent. In severe MR, right-sided failure and venous congestion are present.
3. **Other.** The ECG in chronic MR often shows atrial fibrillation with evidence of left ventricular hypertrophy and left atrial enlargement. In acute MR, the ECG may demonstrate the underlying etiology (ischemia or infarction). In chronic MR, chest radiography shows a moderately enlarged heart with left atrial enlargement, and annular calcification may be seen. In acute MR, the heart is often normal in size with pulmonary vascular congestion evident.
4. **Management**
   a. **Management of acute or chronic MR** should be directed toward decreasing forward impedance to left ventricular ejection, decreasing LV size, and maintaining adequate heart rate to promote forward flow. Invasive monitoring of systemic and pulmonary vascular pressure is necessary in acute or chronic MR when therapeutic maneuvers are attempted to improve cardiac output.
   b. **Vasodilators** that result in arteriolar dilation decrease the pressure gradient across the valve and promote forward flow. Direct-acting agents such as nitroprusside are used acutely. Angiotensin-converting enzyme inhibitors and hydralazine are appropriate drugs for chronic therapy.
   c. **Adequate volume status** should be ensured. Hypervolemia is preferable to hypovolemia.
   d. **Inotropic support** will decrease left ventricular size and annular dilatation, thereby improving forward flow and decreasing the regurgitant volume. Amrinone or dobutamine will improve contractility while decreasing systemic vascular tone; either is the initial agent of choice.

e. **Heart rate** should be maintained at relatively tachycardic levels to decrease regurgitant flow.

V. **Mitral valve prolapse syndrome**

A. **Etiology. Mitral valve prolapse** is reported to affect 5–10% of the population, making it the most common valvular abnormality. It is often associated with connective tissue disorders such as kyphoscoliosis and Marfan's syndrome and has a hereditary component. Women are affected twice as often as men.

B. **Pathophysiology.** Dysfunction of a component of the mitral apparatus, usually a redundant or floppy leaflet, interferes with left ventricular emptying during systole. This obstruction is intensified by underfilling of the left ventricle or increased left ventricular contractility.

C. **Evaluation**

1. **History.** The majority of patients are asymptomatic. Symptomatic patients may report syncope, palpitations, or lightheadedness from hemodynamic effects of arrhythmias or pulmonary congestive symptoms due to mitral regurgitation. Precipitant for the development of symptoms, if any, should be elicited.
2. **Physical examination.** A nonejection click and systolic murmur, heard best at the apex with the patient in the left lateral decubitus position, are characteristic findings. The murmur is intensified by the Valsalva maneuver or standing and attenuated by squatting or isometric exercise.
3. **Other.** The ECG may show premature ventricular contractions, paroxysmal supraventricular tachycardia, or ventricular arrhythmias. T waves may be inverted inferiorly.

D. **Management**

1. Antibiotic prophylaxis against infective endocarditis is a controversial topic in this syndrome. The American Heart Association has no specific guidelines for these patients as of this writing.
2. Ventricular arrhythmias are best treated with Class 1a agents (lidocaine, procainamide). Supraventricular arrythmias can be managed with beta-adrenergic blockers.
3. Prolapse will be accentuated by any factor that promotes more complete emptying of the left ventricle: hypovolemia, increased contractility, tachycardia, impaired venous return, and decreased systemic vascular tone. Adequate volume status and control of sympathetic responses should be maintained.

VI. **Tricuspid stenosis**

A. **Etiology.** Isolated tricuspid stenosis rarely occurs and includes congenital malformations such as Ebstein's anomaly. Rheumatic carditis can result in tricuspid stenosis, most often in conjunction with mitral stenosis.

B. **Pathophysiology.** A diastolic pressure gradient of greater than 5 mm Hg between the right atrium and ventricle will result in systemic venous congestion, evidenced by hepatomegaly, ascites, peripheral edema, and jugular venous distension. The gradient is proportional to transvalvular blood flow, thereby increasing during inspiration or exercise and decreasing during expiration. Significant stenosis may mask underlying mitral stenosis as blood flow through the lungs is progressively impaired.

C. **Evaluation**

1. **History.** Symptoms result from systemic venous congestion and impaired systemic perfusion due to low cardiac output.
2. **Physical examination.** A giant "a" wave is detectable in the jugular venous pulse if sinus rhythm is present. A diastolic, rumbling murmur is present and most prominent at the left lower parasternal border in the fourth intercostal space. Physical findings consistent

with low cardiac output (cool extremities, hypotension, pallor) and systemic venous congestion (edema, hepatomegaly, ascites) are evident.

3. **Other.** The ECG demonstrates right atrial enlargement (tall peaked P in II, upright P in VI). Chest radiography shows a prominent right atrium and superior vena cava. The pulmonary vasculature is not prominent.

D. **Management**

1. Surgical correction of tricuspid stenosis and associated mitral stenosis, if present, may be required to control symptoms. Diuretics and fluid restriction may be helpful. Digoxin is indicated for control of the ventricular response in atrial fibrillation. Systemic venous hypertension and low cardiac output result in fatigue and chronic weakness.
2. **Physical examination.** Distended neck veins, hepatomegaly, ascites, and peripheral edema are prominent secondary to venous congestion.
3. **Other.** Chest radiography shows right ventricular and right atrial enlargement. Pleural effusions may be present. The ECG indicates the underlying disorder. Right ventricular hypertrophy and right bundle branch block are often present.

VII. **Tricuspid regurgitation**

A. **Etiology.** The most common etiology of tricuspid regurgitation is functional, secondary to right ventricular dilatation and failure. The usual cause of right ventricular failure is aortic or mitral valve disease. The tricuspid valve may be directly affected by rheumatic carditis, usually with associated mitral valve disease. Infective endocarditis resulting from intravenous drug abuse, trauma, congenital valve incompetence, and the carcinoid syndrome are less common causes.

B. **Pathophysiology.** The volume overload of TR is generally well tolerated by the right atrium. If the regurgitation is secondary to right ventricular failure, the regurgitation will lead to a decreased left ventricular stroke volume by two mechanisms. First, there is a decrease in transpulmonary blood flow due to the decreased forward stroke volume; second, the dilated right ventricle causes a septal shift that results in decreased ventricular compliance. Left ventricular diastolic function is thus impaired.

C. **Evaluation**

1. **History.** Symptoms of the underlying aortic or mitral valve disease may precede those of tricuspid regurgitation.
2. Interventions that impede venous return (positive pressure ventilation) are poorly tolerated, especially in the presence of hypovolemia. Adequate volume status should be maintained.
3. A right atrial pressure higher than the left atrial pressure favors right-to-left shunting if a patent foramen ovale is present, as is true in approximately 10% of adults. Particular attention should be directed toward the prevention of air emboli by this route.

D. **Management.** Therapy should be directed toward management of the underlying disorder. Right ventricular volume may be decreased with vasodilators (nitroprusside, nitroglycerin) and inotropes (dopamine, dobutamine). Left ventricular function may be improved with these drugs. Since central venous pressure will be a poor reflection of preload in TR, pulmonary artery pressure monitoring is necessary to evaluate volume status accurately. Thermodilution cardiac outputs will be inaccurate in TR due to loss of the indicator in the regurgitant stroke volume.

VIII. **Pulmonic valve disease.** Pulmonic valve disease is rarely a cause of significant hemodynamic compromise. Congenital pulmonic stenosis does occur and presents in infancy or childhood with right heart failure. Acquired pulmonic stenosis is exceedingly rare. Pulmonic incompetence is well tolerated hemodynamically, regardless of etiology, as long as right ventricular function is adequate. Acquired regurgitation can result from infective endocarditis or rheumatic heart disease. Operative intervention in pulmonic regurgitation due to endocarditis usually consists of valve excision rather than replacement with a prosthetic device.

Selected References

Braunwald, E. *Heart Disease: A Textbook of Cardiovascular Medicine* (3d ed.). Philadelphia: W. B. Saunders, 1988.

Harvey, A. et al. *The Principles and Practice of Medicine* (21st ed.). Norwalk, CT: Appleton-Century-Crofts, 1984.

Kaplan, J. A. *Cardiac Anesthesia* (2d ed.). London: Grune & Stratton, 1987.

Petersdorf, R. *Harrison's Principles of Internal Medicine* (10th ed.). New York: McGraw-Hill, 1983.

Stoelting, R. K., and Dierdorf, S. F. *Anesthesia and Co-Existing Disease*. New York: Churchill Livingstone, 1983.

8

Myocardial Ischemia and Infarction

Charles W. Hogue, Jr.

The perioperative period is characterized by multiple stresses that may exacerbate myocardial ischemia in patients with both known and unknown coronary artery disease. The primary goal in the management of susceptible patients is prevention of myocardial ischemia. However, when ischemia occurs, rapid detection and intervention are essential to prevent progression to myocardial infarction.

The complicated pathophysiology of myocardial ischemia and infarction can be simplified to a model of myocardial oxygen supply and oxygen demand. Alterations in the balance of this supply and demand result in ischemia. Myocardial oxygen supply is affected by factors that interfere with coronary blood flow (e.g., obstruction of a coronary artery by a stenosis or vasospasm, hypotension, tachycardia, increased left ventricular pressures) and the oxygen content of the blood. Determinants of myocardial oxygen demand include heart rate, preload, afterload, and myocardial contractility.

Risk factors for coronary artery disease include smoking, hypertension, diabetes mellitus, hypercholesterolemia, and a familial history of atherosclerotic heart disease. The presence of these risk factors in the ICU patient population should make physicians suspicious of the presence of coronary artery disease.

I. Diagnosis

A. History

1. Residual anesthesia, intubation, and sedation may make obtaining a patient history difficult in the perioperative period.
2. The classic symptom of myocardial ischemia, angina pectoris, occurs after predictable levels of exertion and is relieved with rest and sublingual nitroglycerin. Variant angina, secondary to coronary artery vasospasm, in contrast, usually occurs at rest or upon awakening and is not preceded by exertion. Variant angina may also occur in clusters, with intervals between episodes of chest pain ranging from days to weeks.
3. Mixed angina follows exertion but is unpredictable in occurrence. Patients with this form of angina describe chest pain after a certain level of exertion one day but not occurring after the same level of exertion on other days. These patients are believed to have coronary artery stenosis in addition to intermittent vasospasm and are at increased risk of myocardial infarction (MI).
4. Unstable angina occurs when the anginal episodes are increasing in severity, occurring more frequently, lasting longer, and failing to respond to usual therapy. New-onset angina is often included in this category. Unstable angina is a medical emergency requiring prompt intervention to limit the progression to MI. Proposed mechanisms to explain unstable angina include ulceration or hemorrhage into an atherosclerotic plaque, rapid progression of a stenotic plaque, vasospasm, and platelet aggregation with coronary artery thrombus formation.
5. Episodes of silent ischemia, as detected by ECG, occur frequently in patients with known histories of angina. Asymptomatic myocardial ischemia may occur three to four times more frequently than symptomatic ischemia. The significance of silent ischemia in totally asymptomatic patients (those lacking a history of angina or anginal equivalents) is still under investigation. However, in patients with known stable angina, unstable angina, or recent myocardial infarction, the most important factor in predicting an MI or the need for coronary revascularization is ischemia regardless of the presence or absence of symptoms.

B. Electrocardiography

1. Myocardial ischemia (Fig. 8-1)

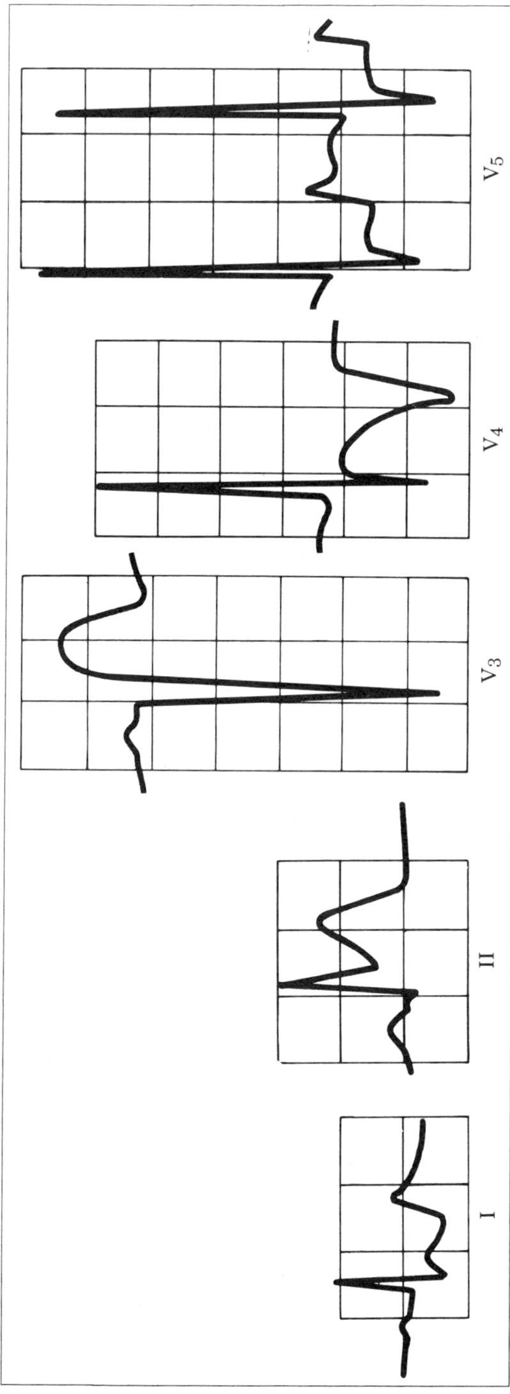

Fig. 8-1. Electrocardiographic changes consistent with acute myocardial ischemia include ST-segment depression or elevation or T-wave inversion.

a. ECG manifestation of myocardial ischemia includes ST-segment depression, peaked T waves, or T-wave inversions. Ischemia secondary to coronary vasospasm may result in ST-segment elevation.
b. ECG findings require correlation to clinical history because ischemia may occur in the absence of ECG changes and not all ECG changes are the result of ischemia. Factors that may alter ST segments and T waves in the absence of ischemia include electrolyte imbalances, left ventricular hypertrophy, conduction abnormalities, drugs (digoxin and quinidine), hiatal hernia, biliary disease, intracranial processes, pericarditis, myocarditis, and body temperature alteration. Isolated elevation of the J-point may occur as a normal variant in young, healthy adults.
c. Reversibility of ECG changes after therapeutic interventions strengthens the diagnosis of myocardial ischemia.
d. Bedside ECG monitors filter interference from patient movement and from electrical equipment. These filters may distort ST segments, limiting the reliability of these monitors in the diagnosis of myocardial ischemia. When available, switching from the "monitor" mode to the "diagnostic" mode lowers the filtering threshold, resulting in less ST-segment distortion and the reliable interpretation of ST-segment changes.

2. Myocardial infarction
   a. The ECG undergoes a series of changes during myocardial infarction beginning with T-wave inversions, followed by ST-segment elevation and the development of Q waves. Isolated Q waves are considered significant when they are at least 0.03 ms or greater than one-third the height of the QRS complex.
   b. Myocardial damage may occur without the "classic" ECG changes noted in **a**, and infarction may be present with only minor ST changes or with a normal ECG.
   c. Enzyme analysis
      (1) Isoenzymes of creatinine phosphokinase (CPK) and lactate dehydrogenase (LDH) are released with myocardial damage. Due to the time lag in obtaining results, enzyme analysis does not alter the initial management of MI. However, elevated isoenzymes in the correct clinical setting document the infarction.
      (2) CPK consists of three isoenzymes, with the MB band being specific for myocardium. CPK-MB increases 4–5 hours after the onset of MI, peaks at 24 hours, and returns to normal by 3 days after an uncomplicated MI. The size of the infarction can be assessed by the peak of CPK-MB elevation. Situations that may also increase CPK-MB include cardioversions with large energy settings, myocardial contusion, pericarditis, Reye's syndrome, prostate and breast cancer, and hypothyroidism. The diagnosis of MI is usually made when the CPK-MB band is greater than 5% of total CPK, except after cardiac surgery, where the diagnosis of MI requires the CPK-MB to be 2 standard deviations above the mean seen in patients with uncomplicated coronary surgery.
      (3) LDH is found in the heart, red blood cells, kidney, brain, stomach, lung, skeletal muscle, liver, and certain tumors. Five isoenzymes of LDH exist, with LDH_2 having the highest level. After an MI, the ratio of LDH_1 to LDH_2 becomes greater than unity. LDH_1 rise occurs 12–24 hours after the onset of the infarction, peaking at 48 hours and returning to normal in 10–14 days.

d. Echocardiography

(1) Both M-mode and 2-D echocardiogram combined with Doppler ultrasound have several applications in the evaluation of myocardial ischemia and MI. Assessment of ventricular function, valvular function, ventricular size, and inspection for the presence of pericardial fluid, ventricular septal perforation, ventricular aneurysm, or ventricular thrombus are all possible with cardiac ultrasound.

(2) Echocardiography can be employed to examine for myocardial wall motion abnormalities. These abnormal myocardial contraction patterns may follow ischemia or infarction. The specificity of regional wall motion abnormalities (RWMA) is not clear; that is, ischemia does cause RWMA, but not all RWMA occur because of ischemia. The appearance of RWMA during ischemia precedes ECG evidence of ischemia and may occur in the absence of ECG changes. Wall motion abnormalities can be localized or generalized and are classified during systole in the following categories:

(a) Hypokinesis: The myocardium thickens and moves inward more slowly than normal.

(b) Akinesis: There is no thickening or inward motion of the myocardium.

(c) Dyskinesis: There is paradoxical outward motion of the ventricle with no thickening.

(3) Transthoracic echocardiography allows rapid, noninvasive evaluation of the heart in the ICU. Thorough examination may not be possible in individuals who are obese, have chronic obstructive pulmonary disease (COPD), or whose chest wall does not allow an adequate examination.

(4) Transesophageal echocardiography (TEE) is gaining acceptance as a sensitive, intraoperative monitor for myocardial ischemia. The advantages of TEE in the ICU result from the position of the ultrasound probe in close proximity to the heart, unobstructed by bony structures or air-containing spaces. TEE should be considered in patients whose examination is inadequate by the transthoracic approach or where the clinical suspicion of pathology is high despite a normal transthoracic examination. Situations where TEE may be superior to transthoracic echocardiography include examination of aortic and mitral valves for vegations and perivalvular abscesses in endocarditis, diagnosing atrial septal defects, evaluating chordae tendineae for suspected rupture, evaluation of the left atrial appendage for thrombus, and examination of the ascending aorta for dissection. Contraindications to TEE include pathology of the esophagus, such as tumors, strictures, varices, or recent surgery. The presence of a coagulopathy or anticoagulation, a left atrial myxoma, or a large, descending thoracic aneurysm should be considered relative contraindications for TEE.

C. Nuclear radiology

1. Thallium 201 is distributed to perfused myocardium, a property useful in the diagnosis of myocardial ischemia.

a. Thallium 201 imaging in conjunction with exercise stress testing (EST) increases the sensitivity of ischemia detection and is especially useful in individuals whose ECG hinders the diagnosis of ischemia (e.g., bundle-branch blocks). Because thallium 201 is distributed only to perfused myocardium, ischemic areas of the myocardium induced by EST appear as perfusion defects. Infarcted myocardium also appears as a perfusion defect; however, if serial thallium 201 scans are obtained, ischemic areas, but not infarcted areas, will show redistribution of the isotope to areas where previous perfusion defects existed.

b. Individuals who are unable to undergo an adequate EST (e.g., those with COPD or peripheral vascular disease) can be evaluated with a dipyridamole-thallium examination. Dipyridamole dilates coronary arterioles and therefore may distribute blood away from ischemic myocardium. Thallium 201 scanning after dipyridamole is given may show reversible perfusion defects that may represent ischemia. Aminophylline can reverse the effects of dipyridamole.

2. Gated blood pool scans (GBPS) involve administering technetium 99–labeled red blood cells to the patient. A GBPS can evaluate ventricular wall motion and ventricular performance by calculation of ejection.
3. Technetium 99 pyrophosphate collects in infarcted myocardium, a property that can be utilized to diagnose an MI. The scans are usually performed 48–72 hours after the MI. Small infarctions, particularly subendocardial infarctions, are usually not diagnosed by this type of imaging. Technetium 99 pyrophosphate scans are useful in diagnosing MI after the period of peak isoenzyme elevation has passed.

II. Treatment of myocardial ischemia and infarction

A. General comments

1. The goal of treatment is to improve the myocardial oxygen supply and demand balance.
2. The initial aim in treating myocardial ischemia is to terminate the ischemic episode and to relieve anginal pain. Nitroglycerin is usually the first line of therapy, but narcotics or other interventions may be indicated for angina not responding to nitroglycerin. Once the ischemic episode abates, therapeutic interventions should be maximized to prevent recurrent ischemia.
3. Adequate oxygenation and ventilation must be assured. Supplemental oxygen or therapy should be initiated.
4. Precipitating causes of the ischemic episode should be sought and controlled. Perioperative events that may precipitate ischemia include pain, agitation, anxiety, tachycardia, hypotension, arrhythmias, and profound hypertension.

B. Nitrates

1. The beneficial effects of nitrates include
   a. Reduction in preload secondary to venodilation
   b. Arteriolar dilation
   c. Dilation of coronary arteries

   These effects result in decreased myocardial oxygen demand and improved oxygen supply.
2. Adverse effects of nitrates include tolerance, headache, reflex tachycardia, hypotension, impairment of hypoxic pulmonary vasoconstriction, and methemoglobinemia.
3. **Administration**

   a. Sublingual nitroglycerin (NTG) is administered as 0.15–0.6-mg tablets. Usually 0.4-mg tablets are given, with onset of action occurring in 1–2 minutes and duration of effect lasting 20–30 minutes. Sublingual NTG is useful to terminate an acute ischemic event, especially if IV preparations are not immediately available. Repeat the drug if the ischemic episode persists after 5–10 minutes. Failure of the ischemia to resolve after 3 doses should prompt aggressive intervention. Store NTG tablets in light-protected, airtight bottles. Because the shelf life is relatively short, a fresh supply of NTG must always be ensured by the ICU staff.

b. Intravenous NTG offers rapid onset, ability to titrate to hemodynamic response, and rapid termination of effect when discontinued. Usually 30–50 mg is added to 250 ml of 5% dextrose in water (NTG adheres to polyvinyl chloride, so it should be mixed in glass bottles and given with nonabsorbing IV tubing). Typically, IV NTG is started at 10 μg per minute, titrating by 5–10 μg per minute until the desired effect is achieved or side effects occur. A usual dose range is 50–300 μg per minute.

c. Topical nitroglycerin can be applied as an ointment (paste) or transdermal patch. Onset of nitro paste occurs in 15 minutes, with a duration of 4 hours. Dosage ranges from 1–2 inches, usually starting with 1/2–1 inch and titrating up as tolerated. Transdermal patches are available in 2.5–15-mg forms, with an onset of 30 minutes and a duration of 24 hours. Tolerance from topical preparations is common.

d. Oral forms of nitroglycerin are available in sustained-release capsules of 2.5–9 mg. Onset is in 60 minutes, with duration lasting 8–12 hours.

e. Isosorbide dinitrate can be given sublingually in 2.5–10-mg tablets or orally in tablet (20–60 mg) or sustained-released capsules (40–80 mg). Onset of effect with sublingual isosorbide dinitrate occurs in 2–5 minutes, while onset after oral administration is 15–30 minutes. Duration of effect is 1–2 hours after sublingual use, 4 hours after oral tablets, and 6–12 hours after sustained-released capsule.

C. Beta-blockers

1. Beta-adrenergic receptors are divided into $beta_1$ and $beta_2$ due to differing pharmacologic responses. $Beta_1$-receptor agonists produce an increase in heart rate, myocardial contractility, and membrane excitability. $Beta_2$ receptor agonists produce bronchodilation, peripheral vasodilation, renin release, uterine relaxation, glycogenolysis, and gluconeogenesis. Exclusive location of one receptor type on any given organ does not occur.
2. Beta-blocking drugs act as beta-receptor antagonists.
3. Beta-blockers are classified as selective or nonselective depending on selective antagonism of the $beta_1$-receptor versus nonselective antagonism of both $beta_1$ and $beta_2$ receptors. Pure $beta_1$ selectivity does not occur because large doses of $beta_1$ antagonist will antagonize both B_1- and B_2-receptors.
4. Beta-blocking drugs are classified by lipid solubility and the ability of certain drugs to be partial agonists. The former characteristic may result in more CNS side effects. The latter effect is termed intrinsic sympathomimetic activity (ISA) and may lead to less peripheral vasoconstriction and less depression of resting heart rate.
5. The anti-ischemic properties of beta-blocking drugs result from lowering of the heart rate, decreasing contractility, and the BP.
6. Beta-blockers rapidly and reliably control tachycardia. They are the first-line therapy for myocardial ischemia related to tachycardia when the precipitating cause of the tachycardia cannot be controlled. Common causes of tachycardia in the perioperative period include pain, anxiety, hypovolemia, fever, sepsis, pulmonary embolism, drug withdrawal (e.g., narcotics, alcohol, clonidine, beta-blockers), hypoxemia, and hypercapnia.
7. Beta-blockers may decrease the frequency of MI in patients with unstable angina.
8. The use of beta-blockers during MI may decrease the infarct size, reduce the incidence of nonfatal reinfarction, and decrease mortality. Intravenous beta-blocking therapy followed by oral treatment should be started, when possible, in this setting.

9. Preparations
   a. Propranolol is a nonselective beta-blocker that can be given orally or parenterally. Oral dosage ranges from 120–400 mg per day divided into intervals of 6–12 hours. Intravenous propranolol is given in 0.25-mg increments while monitoring heart rate and BP.
   b. Metoprolol is a $beta_1$ selective agent in low doses. Oral dosage range is 100–300 mg per day, with intervals of 12–24 hours between doses. Intravenous metoprolol is available but approved only for treatment of MI. If tolerated, 15 mg of metoprolol is given IV in 5-mg increments with at least 2 minutes between doses while ECG, heart rate, and BP are monitored. Patients tolerating the 15-mg IV dosage should be started on 25–50 mg PO q6h for 48 hours. Patients are then converted to a maintenance dosage of 100 mg q12h.
   c. Atenolol is a $beta_1$ selective drug given orally in 50–100-mg doses daily. Atenolol is less lipid soluble than metoprolol or propranolol.
   d. Pindolol is a nonselective beta-blocker with ISA. Usual oral dosage is 10–40 mg q6h.
   e. Acebutol is a $beta_1$ selective agent with low lipid solubility and mild ISA approved for treating hypertension. The initial dose is usually 200–400 mg, either BID or daily with optimal control of blood pressure obtained with 400–800 mg per day.
   f. Labetalol is a nonselective beta-blocking drug that also possesses selective alpha-1 blocking effects. The estimated ratio of alpha to beta-blockade is 1 : 7 IV. Labetalol is indicated primarily for the treatment of hypertension. The effectiveness of labetalol in treating angina has not been fully tested; however, the combined alpha- and beta-blocking properties may be beneficial in some patients. The usual starting dose of intravenous labetalol is 5–20 mg, with additional doses ranging from 20–80 mg given at 10-minute intervals until either the desired blood pressure is achieved or 300 mg is administered. The half-life of IV labetalol is 5½ hours. Oral labetalol is started with 100-mg doses BID, increasing the dose, as tolerated, every 2–3 days to a typical maintenance dose of 200–400 mg BID.
   g. Esmolol is a beta 1 selective drug with an elimination half-life of 9 minutes, allowing rapid onset and termination of action. Although the antianginal effects have not been extensively studied, esmolol has been shown to be effective in the control of tachycardia and hypertension in the perioperative period. Esmolol is also effective for treating supraventricular tachycardia and controlling the ventricular rate during atrial flutter and fibrillation. The ultrashort duration of effect allows titration of beta-blockade during periods of profound stress (e.g., intubation), with withdrawal of effect after the stressful period is completed. Esmolol is given IV by infusion after mixing the drug in a solution that does not contain sodium bicarbonate to yield a concentration of 10 mg per ml. Recommendations for the treatment of supraventricular tachycardia are to give a loading dose of 500 μg/kg/min for 1 minute followed by a maintenance infusion of 50 μg/kg/min. If the tachycardia persists after a 5-minute interval, the loading dose should be repeated and the maintenance infusion increased to 100 μg/kg/min. The bolus and incremental increases in maintenance infusion are continued every 5 minutes until the desired heart rate is achieved or hypotension occurs.

10. Side effects of beta-blocking drugs include congestive heart failure, sinus bradycardia, sinus arrest, AV block, bronchospasm, hypotension, masking the symptoms of hypoglycemia, claudication, headache, fatigue, hallucination, sleep disturbances, and malaise. Abrupt

withdrawal of beta-blockers should be avoided because angina, MI, and ventricular arrhythmias may result. When discontinuing beta-blocking drugs, the dose should be tapered over a period of several days.

11. Relative contraindications to beta-blockers include severe left ventricular dysfunction, history of bronchospasm, and atrioventricular (AV) block. Because of its short termination of effect, esmolol may be useful in several of these conditions to allow a trial to test the tolerance of beta-blockade.

D. Calcium channel blockers

1. The calcium channel blockers interfere with the flux of calcium through the slow calcium channels present in the heart and vascular smooth muscle. The antiischemic effects of this group of drugs result from systemic vasodilation. The coronary artery vasodilating effects of these drugs are particularly useful in treating coronary artery vasospasm seen with variant and mixed angina. Diltiazem and verapamil slow the heart rate, improving myocardial oxygen balance. Diltiazem and verapamil slow AV conduction and are useful in treating supraventricular tachycardias.
2. Calcium channel blockers may decrease the chest pain of unstable angina; however, unlike beta-blockers, they have not been shown to reduce the incidence of MI.
3. Patients with non–Q wave MI given diltiazem may have a reduced incidence of early recurrent MI. However, despite the favorable effects of calcium channel blockers on myocardial oxygen balance, their use does not seem to reduce mortality after MI.
4. **Preparations** (Table 8-1)
   a. Nifedipine is a systemic and coronary arterial vasodilator. The former effect may result in a reflex tachycardia. Negative inotropic effects of nifedipine are offset by a decrease in afterload and an increase in heart rate. Nifedipine is supplied in 10-mg capsules that can be punctured to give the drug sublingually. Treatment is usually started with 10 mg of nifedipine PO q6h. The dose is increased tolerated to a usual range of 120–180 mg per day.
   b. Nicardipine is the newest calcium channel blocker. It is similar to nifedipine and is approved for the treatment of angina and hypertension. The purported advantages of nicardipine are a preferen-

Table 8-1. Comparative effects of calcium channel blockers*

	Nifedipine	Nicardipine	Nimodipine	Diltiazem	Verapamil
Decreased blood pressure	+ + +	+ + +	+ + +	+ + +	+ + +
Coronary vasodilation	+ + +	+ + +	+ + +	+ +	+ +
Increased heart rate	+ +	+ +	+ +	+/−	+/−
Venous capacitance	0	0	0	0	0
Decreased inotropy	+	0	+	+ +	+ + +
Decreased AV conduction	0	0	0	+ + +	+ + +

* 0 denotes negligible effect; + greater effect, − lesser effect

tial decrease in coronary artery resistance compared to systemic vascular resistance. Nicardipine may possess less negative inotropic effects than other calcium channel blockers. The dose of nicardipine is 20 mg q8h, with increases up to 30–40 mg q8h as tolerated.

c. Diltiazem is the most potent negative chronotropic agent of the calcium channel blockers. It causes systemic vasodilation to a lesser degree than nifedipine or verapamil. Diltiazem depresses myocardial contractility. The usual starting dose of diltiazem is 30 mg PO q6h with the dose increased to 240 mg per day or even higher as tolerated.

d. Verapamil slows AV conduction more than the other calcium channel blocker. It is useful in treating supraventricular tachycardia. Heart rate is slowed less than with diltiazem, and systemic vasodilation is less than nifedipine but more than diltiazem. Verapamil depresses myocardial contractility. Oral verapamil is given as 80 mg PO q8h, up to a maximum of 480 mg per day. Intravenous verapamil is useful in treating supraventricular tachycardia and is given in a dose of 0.075–0.15 mg per kilogram. A repeat dose may be given after 30 minutes if required.

5. Side effects of calcium channel blockers include hypotension and congestive heart failure. The peripheral vasodilation after nifedipine can cause a reflex tachycardia that may worsen myocardial ischemia. Other side effects of nifedipine are flushing, headache, dizziness, and peripheral edema. Diltiazem and verapamil can cause bradycardia and AV conduction disturbances. The side effects of nicardipine are similar to those of nifedipine. Diltiazem and verapamil should be used with caution in patients taking other drugs that slow AV conduction, including beta-blockers and digoxin.

E. **Anticoagulation.** Patients with unstable angina may have a lowered risk of MI and death by the use of aspirin and possibly heparin. The use of anticoagulation after MI may be indicated in patients who have had an embolic event and in patients with an MI complicated by a mural thrombus. The presence of anterior akinesis or dyskinesis after an anterior MI indicates the potential for mural thrombosis formation. The use of anticoagulation must be cautiously weighed against the risk of bleeding in postsurgical patients. Relative contraindications to anticoagulation include peptic ulcer disease, severe hypertension, retinopathy, history of cerebrovascular accident (CVA), or invasive procedure.

F. **Intraaortic balloon pumps**

1. Intraaortic balloon pumps (IABPs) reduce afterload and improve diastolic coronary blood flow. Patients with unstable angina refractory to medical treatment, in cardiogenic shock, with refractory post-MI angina, and acute mitral regurgitation or acute ventricular septal defect may benefit from IABP.
2. Contraindications to IABPs include recent aortic surgery, aortic aneurysm, aortic occlusive disease, and aortic valve regurgitation.

G. **Thrombolytic therapy**

1. The majority of patients suffering an MI have a thrombus obstructing the coronary artery. Thrombolytic agents may reestablish blood supply to myocardium in jeopardy of necrosis and limit the infarct size. The early use of thrombolytic therapy during an MI has been shown to improve left ventricular function and reduce mortality.
2. Thrombolytic therapy is most effective when started within 4–6 hours after the onset of an MI. Longer intervals between onset of infarction and initiation of treatment do not necessarily rule out a beneficial effect.

3. Streptokinase and recombinant tissue plasminogen activator (rtPA) are the most frequently used agents; both are effective when given intravenously. Controversy exists as to the superiority of either agent when compared to the other. While more expensive, rtPA may be more efficacious than streptokinase when thrombolytic therapy is begun 3 hours after the start of the MI.
4. Contraindications of thrombolytic therapy include surgery or other invasive procedure within 2 weeks, gastrointestinal or genitourinary bleeding within 4 weeks, history of CVA, CNS trauma or surgery within 4–6 months, pregnancy, intracranial aneurysm, arteriovenous malformation, severe hypertension, or presence of a coagulopathy. Hypersensitivity to streptokinase necessitates the use of rtPA. Relative contraindications are liver or renal disease, diabetic retinopathy, age greater than 75 years, CPR lasting longer than 10 minutes, systolic BP greater than 180 or diastolic greater than 110, and intrathoracic or abdominal trauma within 6 months.
5. Side effects of thrombolytic therapy include systemic fibrinolysis and consumption coagulopathy. Reperfusion ventricular irritability can lead to ventricular tachycardia and fibrillation. Hypotension and allergic reactions may follow the administration of streptokinase.
6. The pathologic abnormality of the infarct-related artery (e.g., critical stenosis, ulcerated plaque) persists after successful thrombolysis, possibly leading the patient to reinfarction. Management strategies are under investigation. Anticoagulation with heparin and aspirin is usually begun after treatment. Early coronary angiography and angioplasty is advocated by some groups. Evidence also exists in support of conservative management after thrombosis, with angiography and angioplasty reserved for patients with post-MI chest pain or for those who demonstrate myocardial ischemia by exercise testing.

H. Treatment of arrhythmias

1. Arrhythmias can both cause and result from myocardial ischemia. In the latter case, management of ischemia may lead to resolution of the arrhythmias.
2. Ventricular fibrillation (VF) and ventricular tachycardia (VT) are major causes of mortality following an MI. VF may or may not be preceded by ventricular premature beats (VPB). Routine use of antiarrhythmias after an MI is not always warranted in the absence of other indicators. While effective in preventing VF, "prophylactic" antiarrhythmics may increase the incidence of asystole.
3. **Ventricular arrhythmias**
   a. Treatment for VPB is considered when they occur with a frequency greater than 5 per minute, when two VPBs are coupled between sinus beats, occur close to the peak of the T wave (vulnerable period), are multiform, or are associated with hemodynamic compromise.
   b. Ventricular tachycardia is treated as VF if the patient is unconscious and without a pulse. Patients who have a pulse should be considered for cardioversion starting with 20–50 J, increasing the energy as required in addition to starting antiarrhythmic therapy. Treatment for patients in VT who are conscious and have a pulse is with antiarrhythmics (see **d**). Further treatment should follow the guidelines in Chapter 6.
   c. The treatment for VF is immediate defibrillation, starting with 200–300 J in the average adult, increasing to 360 J and repeated if necessary (Table 8-2). Further treatment should follow recommendations in Chapter 6.

Table 8-2. Electrical therapy of cardiac arrhythmias

Rhythm	Electrical therapy
Ventricular fibrillation	Countershock 200–360 J (adult) 2 J/kg–4 J/kg (pediatric)
Ventricular tachycardia	Synchronous cardioversion, 50–100 J–360 J
Atrial fibrillation	Synchronous cardioversion
Atrial flutter	25 J
Paroxysmal supraventricular tachycardia	50–300 J
Bradyarrhythmias	Ventricular pacing

Emergency cardioversion for treatment of ventricular and supraventricular tachydysrhythmias in the setting of severe hypotension or myocardial ischemia requires higher energy levels than in nonemergent cases. Initial countershock in these situations should be with 200 J and energy levels increased as per defibrillation if the initial attempt is unsuccessful.

d. Antiarrhythmic drugs

(1) Lidocaine, 1 mg per kg IV bolus, followed by infusion of 20–50 μg/kg/min (approximately 2 mg per minute for the average adult) is usually the first drug used in treating ventricular arrhythmias. This dose should be reduced in the elderly or in the presence of congestive heart failure (CHF) or hepatic dysfunction. Side effects include seizures, mental status change, respiratory arrests, decreased myocardial contractility, and AV conduction disturbances.

(2) Procainamide is considered when lidocaine is ineffective. Intravenous administration at a rate of 20 mg per minute is recommended until a total of 1 g is given, the arrhythmia abates, hypotension occurs, or the QT interval increases greater than 50%. Maintenance infusion is 2–6 mg per minute. Side effects include hypotension, worsening of ventricular arrhythmia, mental status changes, and nausea and vomiting. Serum levels of procainamide and its metabolic *N*-acetyl procainamide should be followed when a continuous infusion is required.

(3) Bretylium is used when ventricular arrhythmias fail to respond to the drugs noted in **(1)** and **(2)**. The initial dose is 5–10 mg per kg IV followed by an infusion at a rate of 1–2 mg per minute. Side effects of bretylium may include hypotension, nausea, and vomiting.

(4) Atrial arrhythmias

(a) Tachyarrhythmias and bradyarrhythmias may be deleterious to patients with myocardial ischemia.

(b) Paroxysmal supraventricular tachycardia (PSVT) that results in hypotension, produces worsening ischemia, aggravates chest pain, or results in CHF should be treated with cardioversion starting with 25–100 J. PSVT in the absence of these complications can sometimes be converted to sinus rhythm by a carotid massage (if no bruits are present). Verapamil, 0.075 mg per kg IV (usually 5 mg), is often effective in terminating PSVT, with the dose repeated in 15–30 minutes if necessary. Other drugs that may be useful to slow the PSVT are beta-blockers and digoxin.

(c) Sinus bradycardia complicated by hypotension or worsening of ischemia on CHF requires treatment, usually with 0.4–1.0 mg atropine.

(d) Atrial flutter and fibrillation with a fast ventricular response is not tolerated in the presence of myocardial ischemia. Rapid control of the ventricular response should be obtained with verapamil, beta-blockers, or digoxin. In the presence of hemodynamic compromise, worsening ischemia, CHF, or a poor response to drug therapy, synchronous cardioversion should be undertaken.

(5) Conduction defects

(a) Mobitz's type I second-degree heart block (Wenckebach's phenomenon) results from an AV block high in the His bundle. It does not typically progress to higher degrees of heart block and usually does not require treatment unless accompanied by bradycardia with associated hypotension, myocardial ischemia, or CHF. Mobitz's type II second-degree heart block results from an AV block below the bundle of His and may progress to complete AV heart block.

(b) Heart blocks associated with inferior MI are often transient. In contrast, AV blocks following anterior MI result from the injury of large portions of myocardium and may swiftly proceed to critical conduction blocks.

(c) Symptomatic bradycardia from a conduction block in the periinfarction period is treated with a temporary pacemaker. Bifascicular blocks, Mobitz's II heart block, and possibly new bundle branch blocks are also treated with temporary pacemaker insertion, even if asymptomatic. Third-degree heart blocks require pacemaker insertion.

Selected References

DeWood, M. A., Spores, J., Notske, R., et al. Prevalence of total coronary occlusion during the early hours of transmural myocardial infarction. *N. Engl. J. Med.* 303:897, 1980.

Egstrup, K. Asymptomatic myocardial ischemia as a predictor of cardiac events after coronary artery bypass grafting for stable angina pectoris. *Am. J. Cardiol.* 61:248, 1988.

Epstein, S. E., Quyyumi, A. A., and Bonow, R. O. Myocardial ischemia—silent or symptomatic. *N. Engl. J. Med.* 318:1038, 1988.

Gibson, R. S., Boden, W. E., Theroux, P., et al. Diltiazem and reinfarction in patients with non-Q-wave myocardial infarction. Results of a double-blind, randomized, multicenter trial. *N. Engl. J. Med.* 315:423, 1986.

Gottlieb, S. O., Gottlieb, S. H., Achuff, S. C., et al. Silent ischemia on Holter monitoring predicts mortality in high-risk post-infarction patients. *J.A.M.A.* 259:1030, 1988.

ISIS-1 (First International Study of Infarct Survival) Collaborative Group. A randomized trial of intravenous atenolol among 16,027 cases of suspected acute myocardial infarction: ISIS-1. *Lancet* 2:57, 1986.

Josephson, M. A., Brown, B. G., Hecht, H. S., et al. Noninvasive detection and localization of coronary stenosis in patients: Comparison of resting dipyridamole and exercise thallium-201 myocardial perfusion imaging. *Am. Heart J.* 103:1008, 1982.

Klein, M. S., Coleman, R. E., Weldon, C. S., et al. Concordance of electrocardiographic and scintigraphic criteria of myocardial injury after cardiac surgery. *J. Thorac. Cardiovasc. Surg.* 71:934, 1976.

Lambert, C. R., Hill, J. A., Nichols, W. W., et al. Coronary and systemic hemodynamic effects of nicardipine. *Am. J. Cardiol.* 55:652, 1985.

Leppo, J., Boucher, C. A., Okada, R. D., et al. Serial thallium-201 myocardial imaging after dipyridamole infusion: Diagnostic utility in detecting coronary stenoses and relationship to regional wall motion. *Circulation* 66:649, 1982.

Marriott, H. J. L. *Practical Electrocardiography* (7th ed.). Baltimore: Williams and Wilkins, 1983.

Maseri, A., and Chierchia, S. A new rationale for the clinical approach to the patient with angina pectoris. *Am. J. Med.* 71:639, 1981.

Multicenter Diltiazem Post Infarction Trial Research Group. The effect of diltiazem on mortality and reinfarction after myocardial infarction. *N. Engl. J. Med.* 319:385, 1988.

Myocardial ischemia and perioperative infarction. *Anesth. Clin. North Am.* 6:3, 1988.

Okada R. D., Boucher, C. A., Strauss, H. W., et al. Exercise radionuclide imaging approaches to coronary artery disease. *Am. J. Cardiol.* 46:1188, 1980.

Packer, M. Combined beta-adrenergic and calcium-entry blockade in angina pectoris. *N. Engl. J. Med.* 320:709, 1989.

Rapaport E. Thrombolytic agents in acute myocardial infarction. *N. Engl. J. Med.* 320:861–864, 1989.

Roberts, A. J. Perioperative myocardial infarction and changes in left ventricular performance related to coronary artery bypass graft surgery. *Ann. Thorac. Surg.* 35:208–225, 1983.

Thadani, U., Hamilton, S. F., Olson, E., et al. Transdermal nitroglycerin patches in angina pectoris. Dose titration, duration of effect, and rapid tolerance. *Ann. Int. Med.* 105:485, 1986.

Thys, D. M., Hillel, Z., Konstadt, S. N., et al. Intraoperative Echocardiography. In J. Kaplan (ed.), *Cardiac Anesthesia* (2d ed.). New York: Grune and Stratton, 1987.

TIMI Study Group. The thrombolysis in myocardial infarction trial. Phase I findings. *N. Engl. J. Med.* 312:932, 1985.

TIMI Study Group. Comparison of invasive and conservative strategies after treatment with intravenous tissue plasminogen activator in acute myocardial infarction. Results of the thrombolysis in myocardial infarction (TIMI) Phase II trial. *N. Engl. J. Med.* 320:618, 1989.

Visser, C. A., Koolen, J. J., et al. Transesophageal echocardiography: Technique and clinical applications. *J. Cardiothorac. Anesth.* 2:74, 1988.

White, H. D., Rivers, J. T., Maslowski, A. H., et al. Effect of intravenous streptokinase as compared with that of tissue plasminogen activator on left ventricular function after first myocardial infarction. *N. Engl. J. Med.* 320:817, 1989.

Yusuf, S. Interventions that potentially limit myocardial infarct size: Overview of clinical trials. *Am. J. Cardiol.* 60:11A, 1987.

Yusuf, S., Collins, R., MacMahon, S., et al. Effect of intravenous nitrates on mortality in acute myocardial infarction: An overview of the randomized trials. *Lancet* 1:1088, 1988.

Yusuf, S., and Furberg, C. D. Effects of calcium channel blockers on survival after myocardial infarction. *Cardiovasc. Drug Ther.* 1:343, 1987.

Yusuf, S., Sleight, P., Rossi, P. R. F., et al. Reduction in infarct size, arrhythmias, chest pain and morbidity by early intravenous beta-blockade in suspected acute myocardial infarction. *Circulation* 67 (pt. 2):32, 1983.

Yusuf, S., Wittes, J., and Friedman, L. Overview of results of randomized clinical trials in heart disease. I. Treatments following myocardial infarction. *J.A.M.A.* 260:2088, 1988.

Yusuf, S., Wittes, J., and Friedman, L. Overview of results of randomized clinical trials in heart disease. II. Unstable angina, heart failure, primary prevention with aspirin, and risk factor modification. *J.A.M.A.* 260:2259, 1988.

9

Congestive Heart Failure

David Y. Williams, Phillipa J. Hore, and Terry W. Latson

    d. **Nitroprusside**
    e. **Hydralazine**
    f. **Angiotensin-converting enzyme (ACE) inhibitors**
2. **Inotropic support**
    a. **Dopamine**
    b. **Dobutamine**
    c. **Epinephrine**
    d. **Norepinephrine**
    e. **Isoproterenol**
3. **Phosphodiesterase inhibitors**
    a. **Amrinone and milrinone**
    b. **Digitalis**

I. Background. Congestive heart failure (CHF) is a syndrome characterized by the inability of the heart to pump an adequate flow of blood to meet the metabolic needs of the body.

A. Determinants of cardiac function. The therapeutic goal in the treatment of CHF is to increase oxygen delivery to vital organs and peripheral tissues. Assuming adequate hemoglobin concentration and arterial oxygen saturation, oxygen delivery is dependent on the cardiac output. Cardiac output is the product of heart rate and stroke volume (SV). SV, which relates directly to the extent of myocardial fiber shortening, is determined by preload, contractility, and afterload.

1. Preload is the degree of stretch of the myocardium prior to the onset of contraction. The degree of myocardial stretch or end-diastolic fiber length is represented by left ventricular end-diastolic volume (LVEDV). Three factors influence preload: blood volume, the distribution of blood volume (related to venous tone and intrathoracic pressure), and atrial contraction. In the normal heart, following the Frank-Starling relation, an increase in the end-diastolic volume results in an increase in the SV and cardiac output. Eventually a plateau is reached on the ventricular performance curve such that augmentation of the end-diastolic volume results in little or no increase in SV. Because LVEDV is not readily measured, left ventricular end-diastolic pressure (LVEDP) is used as an index of preload. The in vivo clinical correlate that is most often used to approximate the LVEDP is the pulmonary capillary wedge pressure (PCWP). Measurement of the PCWP as an index of LVEDV, relies on two important assumptions:

a. LVEDP correlates with LVEDV. The relationship between end-diastolic volume and pressure is not linear (Fig. 9-1). In the heart with normal compliance at low volumes, change in the end-diastolic volume causes a relatively small change in LVEDP. Thus, administration of fluid to increase the end-diastolic volume may significantly increase SV with little change in the LVEDP. At higher volumes, augmentation of end-diastolic volumes may cause a disproportional increase in LVEDP. The compliance of the ventricle may be reduced by ischemia, fibrosis, and hypertrophy. Distortion of normal ventricular geometry may also reduce compliance

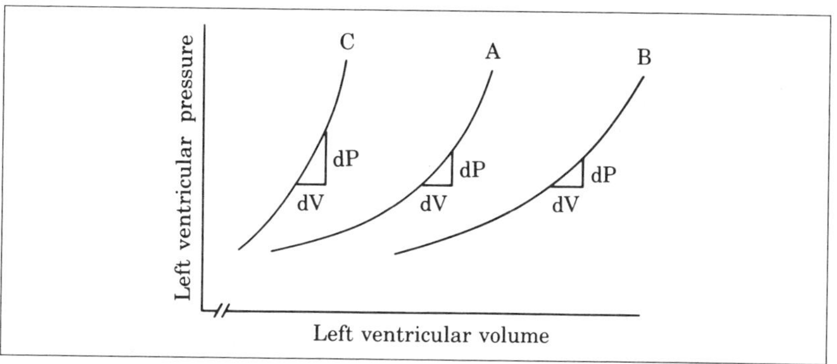

Fig. 9-1. Left ventricular diastolic pressure-volume relationships: normal (*A*), increased volumes and compliance (e.g., effect of chronic volume overload) (*B*), and decreased volumes and compliance (e.g., effect of chronic pressure overload or pericardial tamponade with pressures measured relative to atmosphere) (*C*). For a given change in volume (*dV*), the change in pressure (*dP*) varies inversely with compliance.

by leftward shift of the interventricular septum from high right ventricular (RV) diastolic pressures or by external restrictions to ventricular filling (e.g., constrictive pericarditis, pericardial tamponade).

b. PCWP correlates with LVEDP

(1) In patients with left ventricular dysfunction, LVEDPs may be significantly augmented by left atrial contraction without a proportionate increase in left atrial pressure or PCWP. The pulmonary capillary "a" wave pressure correlates best with the LVEDP, but the tracing of the waveform may be poorly reproduced.

(2) The position of the tip of the pulmonary artery catheter may be important in determining the accuracy of the measurement. A minimal pressure gradient is required between the catheter tip and the left atrium for an optimal reading. This occurs in West's zone 3, where the pulmonary artery and venous pressures are greater than alveolar pressure. Alveolar pressure may exceed pulmonary venous pressure under conditions of high alveolar pressure, low pulmonary venous pressure (hypovolemia), or catheter tip position high in the vertical gradient of the lung (above the left atrium). Under these conditions, the PCWP may overestimate the LVEDP.

(3) Mitral valve disease. The PCWP overestimates the LVEDP at end-diastole. PCWP may exceed LVEDP in patients with mitral incompetence because of the influence of systolic ventricular pressure. The contribution of ventricular pressure to the PCWP in mitral incompetence can be detected by identifying "v" waves on the wedge tracing.

(4) Chronic pulmonary disease may result in PCWPs that overestimate LVEDPs. This may be due to increased collateral pulmonary venous flow and elevated intrathoracic pressures. Pulmonary artery diastolic pressures have also been used to reflect PCWPs. Pulmonary artery diastolic pressures are usually 1–2 mm Hg higher than PCWPs and correlate well with PCWPs and left atrial pressures unless the pulmonary vascular resistance is elevated. In the face of pulmonary hypertension, there is a marked discrepancy between the diastolic and wedge pressures. The difference between the pulmonary artery diastolic pressure and the PCWP may help to determine the degree of pulmonary hypertension; a difference of 4–5 mm Hg can be used as an index to differentiate a normal and an increased pulmonary vascular resistance.

2. Contractility refers to the force or vigor of contraction that can be generated by a given level of diastolic stretch. Enhanced contractility refers to an increase in velocity or extent of muscle fiber shortening that occurs under constant load conditions. At any level of contractility, the extent of contraction varies directly with preload and inversely with afterload. Contractility is the most difficult determinant of SV to measure accurately; every known index of contractility has been found to be dependent to varying degrees on ventricular preload and afterload. The end-systolic pressure volume line (ESPVL) offers a correlate that does not depend on loading conditions (Fig. 9-2). An increase in contractility increases the slope of the ESPVL, which, for a given preload and end-systolic pressure (ESP), will produce an increased stroke volume. Conversely, the slope of the ESPVL becomes flatter as contractility is depressed (Fig. 9-3). ESP is an index of afterload; a change in ESP alters the intersect with the same ESPVL, resulting in a change in SV. Hence, SV for a given preload is deter-

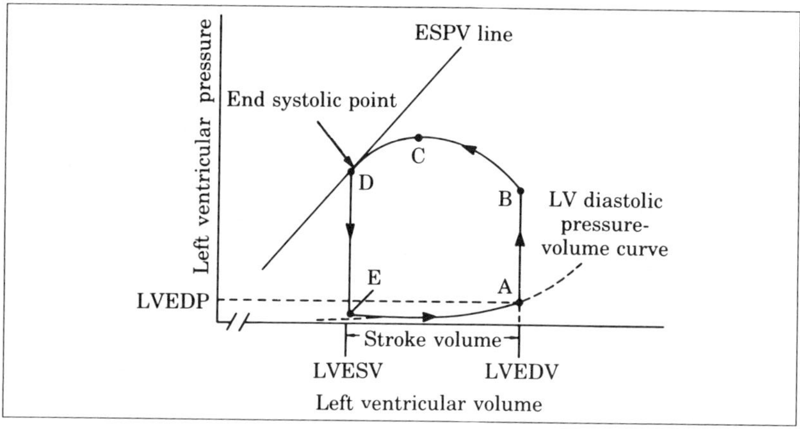

Fig. 9-2. Pressure-volume loops and the ESPV line. The labeled points correspond to the cardiac cycle as follows: End of diastole and start of ventricular contraction (*A*), start of ejection (*B*), peak systolic pressure (*C*), end of ejection (*D*), and start of diastolic filling (*E*). The "end-systolic point," corresponding to the time of maximal ventricular elastance, occurs near end ejection and lies on the ESPV line. *LV* = left ventricular; *LVESV* = left ventricular end-systolic volume.

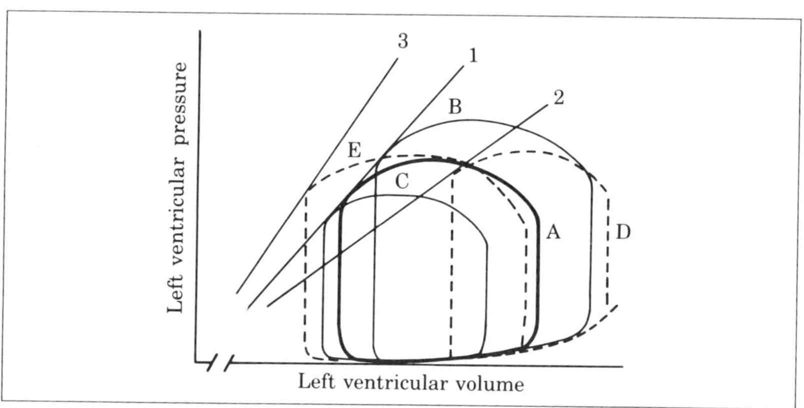

Fig. 9-3. Utility of the ESPV line (*1, 2, 3*). For a given contractile state, the end-systolic points of all PVLs will lie on the same line despite changes in preload and afterload (e.g., control ESPV line *1* and PVLs *A, B, C*). A decrease in contractility will result in a decreased slope of the ESPV line (line *2* and PVL *D*) and an increase in contractility just the opposite (line *3* and PVL *E*).

mined by the pressure at end-systole and the ESPVL. The SV, calculated by dividing cardiac output by heart rate, is essential for assessing ventricular performance. The normal adult SV is 70–80 ml. The information obtained from the cardiac or SV measurement is not increased in indexing for body surface area. Large patients have higher cardiac outputs and SV, but the relationship is not linear and does not have a zero intercept. It is also important to note that cardiac output and SV decrease with age. Thus, it may be impossible to achieve an SV of 70 ml in a patient age 80 years and weighing 50 kg. The utility of SV compared to cardiac output measurements in assessing ventricular performance becomes apparent when the heart rate is taken into account. For example, a cardiac output of 4.0 L per minute at a heart rate of 50 beats per minute (SV–80 ml), which increases to 6.0 L per minute with a concomitant rise in heart rate to 100 beats per minute, actually reflects a decrease in myocardial performance (SV = 60 ml).

3. **Afterload** can be defined as the systolic wall tension or stress that develops during ventricular contraction. Wall stress reflects an integration of two major loads: a vascular load and the load imposed by the ventricle itself. The vascular load is determined by the cross-sectional area of the vascular bed, the elasticity of the vascular wall, and the viscosity of the blood. The ventricular load represents the effects of the physiologic properties of cardiac muscle cells, as well as ventricular shape and size. These factors can be summarized by the Laplace equation, which states that wall stress (S) relates directly to the product or intraventricular pressure (P) and ventricular radius (R) and inversely to ventricular wall thickness (H):

$$S = \frac{PR}{H}$$

Ventricular afterload cannot easily be measured using this physiologic definition. As determined by pressure-volume loops for a given contractility or slope of the ESPVL, an alteration in afterload affects the ESP, resulting in a different intercept on the ESPVL. In theory, for a given contractility, a reduction in afterload resulting in an increase in SV must lead to a fall in BP. In clinical practice, SV may occasionally improve without a fall in systemic blood pressure. Possible explanations include concommitant effects of vasodilator therapy on myocardial ischemia and/or beneficial effects on ventricular mechanics.

B. **Graphic analysis of cardiac function.** Analysis of **pressure-volume loops** gives added insight into the physiologic determinants of SV. These give a graphic representation of the pressure-volume changes throughout the cardiac cycle (see Fig. 9-2).

II. **Pathophysiology.** CHF is caused primarily by failure of the systolic function of the heart and less commonly by failure of diastolic function. Systolic dysfunction represents an inability of the heart to empty normally; the latter represents an abnormality of diastolic myocardial relaxation and results in an inability of the heart to fill properly. Both systolic and diastolic dysfunction depress the clinical ventricular function similarly and lead to a low cardiac output and high ventricular filling pressures.

The causes of systolic dysfunction fall into two broad categories: (1) an excessive cardiac work and (2) destruction or depression of the myocardium. Conditions that most commonly result in systolic dysfunction are hypertensive heart disease, ischemic heart disease, and congestive cardiomyopathy. Diastolic dysfunction results from such conditions as hypertrophic cardiomyopathy and constrictive pericarditis. Systolic dysfunction and diastolic dysfunction may coexist, but usually the importance of one or the other predominates and may evolve at various times in the natural history of the disease.

Biochemical and ultrastructural abnormalities have been identified in myocardial tissue from patients with CHF, including a decreased rate of catecholamine synthesis and norepinephrine levels, a lower level of high-energy phosphate production, disordered mitochondrial structure and function, and abnormalities of cell-cell connections. The role of these abnormalities in the development of CHF remains to be determined. The failing heart depends on cardiac and systemic compensatory mechanisms for the maintenance of cardiac output. The primary cardiac mechanism is through myocardial hypertrophy. Systemic compensatory mechanisms include (1) activation of the sympathetic nervous system, leading to an increase in contractility and heart rate, and (2) renal salt and water retention, mediated by the renin-angiotensin-aldosterone system and by antidiuretic hormone release. Activation of the latter two hormones and the sympathetic nervous system results in intense vasoconstriction. **Vasorelaxant natriuretic substances** are also released during heart failure in an attempt to offset peripheral vasoconstriction and sodium retention. Atrial natriuretic factor (ANF), released by the stimulation of atrial stretch receptors, modulates vasorelaxation of constricted vessels, natriuresis, and fluid extravasation. In addition, ANF suppresses renin, and aldosterone releases and inhibits antidiuretic hormone action. Prostaglandin E2, released by vascular smooth muscle in response to reduced tissue perfusion, may subserve vasodilation and be important in maintaining adequate renal function during reduced cardiac output. Dopamine levels are also higher in patients with heart failure. Dopamine acting on receptors situated on presynaptic sympathetic neurons and renal tubules may modulate norepinephrine release and enhance a natriuresis. The result of this complex interaction of neuroendocrine responses is that peripheral vasoconstriction and sodium retention appear to be dominant, particularly in the advanced stages of heart failure.

III. **Etiology.** The most common cause of decompensation in stable CHF is an inappropriate reduction in therapy or noncompliance by the patient. In the perioperative setting, CHF usually occurs as a result of the additional stresses imposed by an acute illness, major operation, or as a result of the underlying cardiac disease.

A. **Precipitating causes**

1. **Increased preload**

a. Inappropriate intraoperative/perioperative fluid administration

b. Termination of anesthesia is often accompanied by the cessation of positive pressure ventilation, excretion or metabolism of anesthetic vasodilating drugs, and increased sympathetic stimulation. These factors tend to increase venous tone and venous blood return independent of changes in intravascular volume. Hence, even with optimal intraoperative fluid management, a patient may become relatively volume overloaded at the cessation of anesthesia.

c. Epidural analgesia. Postoperative pain management may utilize epidural catheters with the instillation of narcotics, local anesthetic solutions, or both, into the epidural space. The use of local anesthetic solutions may require volume supplementation for BP control in order to compensate for the initial vasodilatory effect and the effective reduction in preload. However, cessation of the epidural and the return of vasoconstrictor tone may augment the intravascular volume, contributing to the development of CHF.

d. **Postoperative fluid "mobilization."** Excess extravascular body fluid accumulates in the intraoperative and early postoperative periods following major surgery due to such factors as "third spacing" with surgical tissue trauma and stress-induced changes in aldosterone and antidiuretic hormone (ADH) levels. Clinically, this fluid appears to mobilize back into the central circulation starting at about 12–36 hours postoperatively. This is usually manifested by a decrease in exogenous fluid requirements or an increase in urine output, or both, the magnitude and time course of which are dependent on numerous factors, including ventricular and renal function and the entire history of fluid management. Resulting increases in intravascular volume may contribute to the development of congestive cardiac failure (CCF).

2. **Hypothermia.** Deleterious effects of hypothermia postoperatively include vasoconstriction (leading to increased afterload) and significantly increased metabolic demands secondary to shivering. Following a major operation with significant hypothermia, muscle relaxants are usually allowed to wear off spontaneously with passive rewarming (with controlled ventilation and adequate sedation) to avoid this stress of shivering.
3. **Decreased blood oxygen content.** Anemia and hypoxemia produce decreased blood oxygen content. The physiologic responses to each are multiple, complex, and sometimes significantly different (e.g., the carotid chemoreceptor is responsive to decreased PaO_2 but not to decreased oxygen content with normal PaO_2). Both lead to graded increases in demands on cardiac function, with simultaneous decreases in cardiac metabolic reserve.
4. **Postoperative respiratory changes.** Following major abdominal and thoracic surgery, multiple respiratory alterations consequent upon the effects of general anesthesia, postoperative pain, decreased activity, abdominal distension, and the effects of sedative-analgesic drugs are commonly seen and may lead to hypoxemia and hypercapnia, which increase demands on cardiac performance. Patients with minimal cardiac reserve who are mechanically ventilated may have stable cardiovascular hemodynamics while being ventilated. During weaning from ventilation, however, the increased work of breathing and an increase in sympathetic tone resulting in an augmented preload may add a further stress to the myocardium, leading to CHF.
5. **Increased sympathetic tone.** Mild to moderate hypertension and tachycardia are frequently seen early postoperatively following major surgery. Part of this phenomenon may represent increased sympathetic tone in response to pain, anxiety, increased work of breathing, hypoxemia, hypercapnia, fluid shifts, and multiple other factors. The net result on cardiac performance is determined by the interplay of multiple factors, including effects on contractility, preload, afterload, heart rate, and myocardial oxygen supply-demand balance.
6. **Sepsis.** Endotoxin causes vasodilation and peripheral shunting, requiring increased cardiac output for maintenance of BP and equivalent tissue perfusion. Accompanying hyperthermia increases metabolic demands and carbon dioxide production. Concomitant metabolic acidosis and myocardial depressant factors of sepsis may decrease cardiac reserve further.
7. **Increased RV afterload.** Pulmonary embolism, respiratory failure, hypoxemia, hypercapnia, the effects of positive end-expiratory pressure (PEEP), or a combination, may elevate pulmonary vascular resistance and increase pumping demands on the right ventricle.

B. Cardiac reserve may be decreased.

1. Depression of myocardial contractility may occur in the perioperative period secondary to a number of factors.
   - **a. Drug-induced depression**
     - (1) Residual anesthetic drugs
     - (2) Narcotic-sedative drugs
     - (3) Beta-adrenergic blockade
     - (4) Calcium channel antagonists
     - (5) Antiarrhythmic agents

b. Acid-base and electrolyte disturbances (e.g., severe alkalosis, acidosis, hypocalcemia, hypophosphatemia)
c. Myocardial ischemia
d. Myocardial depressant factor of sepsis and humoral mediators following pulmonary embolus

2. Mechanical factors may decrease cardiac output despite normal contractility.
   a. **Arrhythmias**
      (1) **Supraventricular tachyarrhythmias** may lead to decreased cardiac output secondary to limitation of ventricular diastolic filling. They also increase myocardial oxygen consumption and shorten the time for diastolic coronary perfusion, which can further depress cardiac function if obstructive coronary disease is present.
      (2) **Nodal rhythms or atrial fibrillation** can cause loss of atrial contraction, which may be particularly important in patients with decreased ventricular compliance where the atrial contribution is essential for adequate ventricular filling.
      (3) **Bradycardia** may significantly decrease output in patients who cannot compensate for decreased heart rate with appropriate increases in SV.
   b. **Valvular regurgitation** secondary to any of the following:
      (1) Ventricular overdistension
      (2) Papillary muscle dysfunction
      (3) Endocarditis
      (4) Preexisting valvular disease
   c. **Cardiac tamponade,** especially following cardiac surgery
   d. **Cardiac herniation** out of a partially opened pericardium (after cardiac or thoracic surgery)
   e. **Mediastinal shift** secondary to pneumothorax or following pneumonectomy
   f. **Severe abdominal distension** (including pregnancy) with inferior vena cava compression, mechanical restriction to cardiac filling from diaphragmatic displacement, or both
   g. **RV distension** (from ischemia or elevated pulmonary vascular resistance). Changes in left ventricular (LV) function, notably a decrease in SV, are due to decreased LV filling secondary to decreased RV output or alterations of LV geometry and diastolic compliance, or both. The latter changes are due to increases in RV diastolic volumes and pressures that produce relative displacement of the interventricular septum into the LV cavity. LV compliance may be restricted by pericardial constraint if the right ventricle is excessively dilated.
   h. **PEEP**
      (1) **Right and left ventricular preload** is reduced. RV preload is reduced secondary to increased intrathoracic pressers. Although CVP, PA, and PAOP measured relative to atmospheric pressure may be increased following application of PEEP, the net transmural pressure (CVP or PCWP-intrathoracic pressure) can be decreased. LV filling may be decreased by a reduction in RV output, decreased LV diastolic compliance, or a combination of both factors. High levels of PEEP—20 cm H_2O or greater—may be associated with a shift of the interventricular septum toward the left ventricle, reducing diastolic compliance.
      (2) RV afterload is increased when the elevated alveolar pressure exceeds pulmonary microvascular pressure, resulting in a raised pulmonary vascular resistance. The effect of PEEP on RV function depends on the preexisting RV function. Patients

with a right ventricular ejection fraction (RVEF) of greater than 30% beforehand show no change in RVEF or RV volume even with high levels of PEEP. In patients with a decreased RVEF, application of PEEP is associated with an elevated RV volume and underlying coronary disease.

(3) **LV contractility** is unchanged despite changes in PEEP.

(4) The adverse effects of PEEP on cardiac output tend to be diminished as the compliance of the lungs decreases. In this setting, a given level of PEEP produces less lung expansion and a consequent reduction in intrathoracic expansion. Hence, the effects on preload and afterload are reduced.

IV. Therapy

A. Philosophy

1. **Principles of management**
   a. Removing the underlying or precipitating cause
   b. Controlling the heart failure state
2. **Therapy direction**
   a. Attaining an optimal cardiac output and systemic pressure sufficient to achieve normal mentation, an adequate renal output, peripheral perfusion (without a metabolic acidosis), and general organ viability
   b. Resolving pulmonary edema to ensure adequate oxygenation
   c. Reducing cardiac work to resolve myocardial ischemia
3. **Management goals** may involve conflicting therapeutic strategies. For example, the goal of attaining an optimal cardiac output may conflict with the resolution of other problems:
   a. **Systemic pressure.** Treatment of hypotension may require the use of a vasoconstrictor, which may limit the cardiac output.
   b. **Pulmonary edema.** This may require the reduction of extracellular fluid volume, which may conflict with the need to maintain ventricular filling pressures.
   c. **Oxygenation.** PEEP may be required to ensure adequate oxygenation but may have an adverse effect on cardiac output.
   d. **Cardiac work.** Inotropic support may be required to maintain cardiac output, but the associated increase in heart rate may aggravate myocardial ischemia.

B. Therapeutic strategies in managing CHF, aside from specific therapy directed at precipitating causes, are aimed at optimizing preload, contractility, and afterload.

1. **Preload reduction**
   a. Patients with CHF have an elevated peripheral venous tone and an expanded extracellular volume to augment their end-diastolic volume and improve their SV. However, elevated filling pressures cause progressive cardiac dilation, myocardial ischemia, worsening congestive symptoms, increased mitral insufficiency, and a reduced cardiac output.
   b. Preload is reduced in CHF to relieve pulmonary edema and improve contractility by lessening myocardial ischemia and improving ventricular compliance.
   c. Reduction of preload may have a variable effect on cardiac output (Fig. 9-4).
      (1) A reduction in end-diastolic volume, and particularly pressures using vasodilators, can reduce LV wall stress and, in turn, decrease myocardial oxygen consumption. This may result in relief of coronary ischemia and an increase in SV. Vasodilators can increase blood flow to an ischemic area by improving collateral flow. This is controversial. SV can also increase from an improvement in ventricular compliance (see Figs. 9-1 and

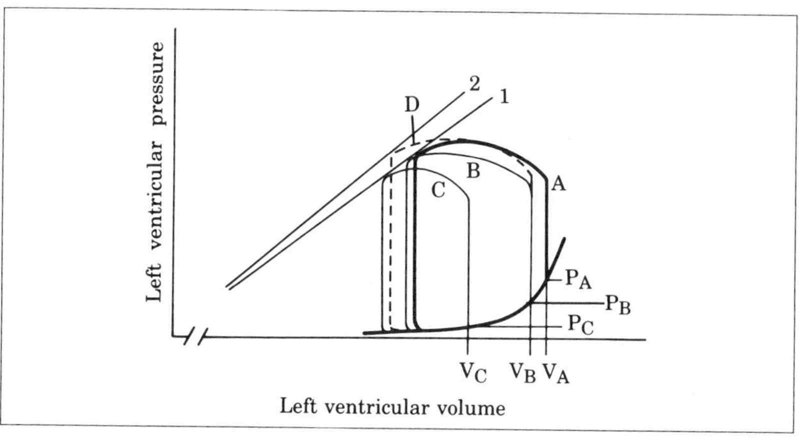

Fig. 9-4. Effects of preload reduction. Reduction in LVEDP from P_A to P_B causes little change in ventricular end-diastolic volume (because of the steepness of the ventricular diastolic pressure-volume curve in this region) with little resultant change in stroke volume. Equal reduction in LVEDP from P_B to P_C, however, causes a much greater change in end-diastolic volume and resultant decrease in stroke volume (compare to points A, B, and C in Fig. 9-5). The PVL *D* depicts one possible response if the decrease in LVEDP from P_A and P_B were to result in decreased myocardial ischemia leading to an effective increase in contractility and a shift in the ventricular ESPV line from *1* to *2*.

9-4). Some evidence suggests that vasodilation shifts the pressure-volume curve to the right, allowing a greater increase in end-diastolic volume without attaining a pressure that induces pulmonary edema. The increase in volume at a lower pressure produces better ventricular performance. Mechanisms for the increase in compliance are uncertain but include a reduction in ischemia, an intrinsic increase in diastolic relaxation, and RV relaxation, causing increased LV compliance within a confined pericardium. In some patients with CHF, LV distension may result in mitral regurgitation. A decrease in end-diastolic volume may reduce the regurgitant load and improve cardiac output.

(2) The failing heart usually operates on the plateau portion of the depressed Starling curve. Thus, a reduction in preload does not reduce SV. However, at lower levels of end-diastolic volume (operating on the slope rather than the plateau of the ventricular function curve), vasodilators may cause a decrease in SV and systemic pressure (Fig. 9-5).

(3) The optimal preload usually occurs at a PCWP of approximately 15 mm Hg. Reduction in the preload beyond this may result in a fall in cardiac output, while an elevation may result in pulmonary edema. However, situations may occur in which a PCWP greater than 15 mm Hg may be required:

(a) **Abnormal ventricular compliance.** A stiff ventricle (e.g., patients with aortic stenosis or hypertension) may require higher filling pressures to achieve an optimum end-diastolic volume.

(b) **Atrioventricular valvular disease.** Mitral or tricuspid stenosis impedes ventricular filling such that higher atrial pressures (and therefore measured PCWPs) are needed to

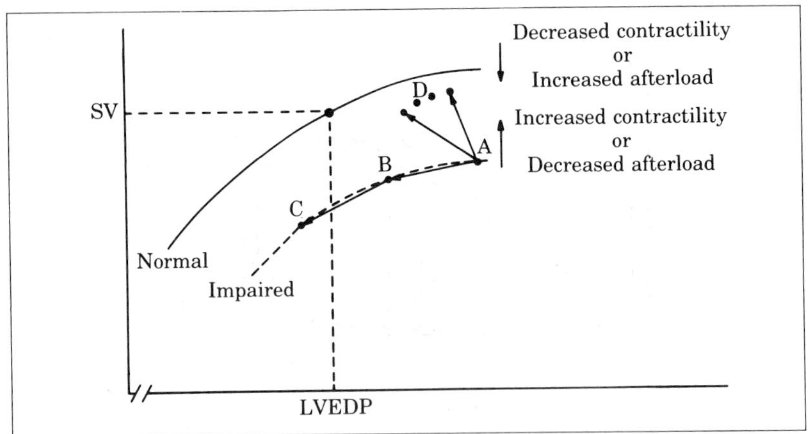

Fig. 9-5. Frank-Starling ventricular function curves. Each curve describes the relationship between ventricular end-diastolic pressure (a correlate of end-diastolic volume or preload) and stroke volume (*SV*) for a given contractile state and afterload. Changes in contractility, afterload, or both will shift the curve as shown. Point *A* corresponds to a failing ventricle with high LVEDP and low SV. Reduction in LVEDP from *A* and *B* along the flat portion of the Frank-Starling curve results in little change in SV; further reduction in LVEDP as from *B* and *C* along a steeper portion of the curve causes a much greater decrease in SV (compare to *A*, *B*, and *C* in Fig. 9-4). Points labeled *D* indicate possible responses to enhanced contractility, afterload reduction, or both; the resultant increase in SV is often associated with a concomitant decrease in LVEDP (LVEDV) (see text for further explanation).

provide adequate ventricular filling. It is important to remember that the PCWP may not accurately reflect the LVEDP; that is, a high wedge pressure may reflect a normal end-diastolic pressure.

(c) **Pericardial tamponade.** Increased filling pressures may be required to overcome the external restriction to ventricular filling.

(d) **RV distension.** Elevation in RV diastolic volumes and pressures may produce relative displacement of the interventricular septum into the LV cavity. Higher LVEDV may be needed to compensate.

(e) **Positive end-expiratory pressure** may reduce right and left ventricular preload, requiring higher filling pressures to improve SV.

(4) The beneficial effect of preload reduction must be balanced against the effects on cardiac output. In assessing the results of preload reduction, monitoring of the PCWP, the cardiac output, and the ECG if ischemia is involved is important. Maintenance of the PCWP at or below 15 mm Hg in the presence of normal pulmonary capillary permeability usually results in the resolution of pulmonary edema. In optimizing preload for the best cardiac output in a situation other than **3.(a)–(e),** it is uncommon to derive much benefit from increasing the PCWP beyond 15–18 mm Hg. Patients who require higher PCWPs to ensure an adequate LVEDP have usually developed physiologic mechanisms to ensure that these higher pressures do not lead to pulmonary edema, such as pulmonary vascular changes in patients with long-standing mitral stenosis. Increased alveolar

pressure in patients receiving PEEP may also offer a degree of protection.

2. Inotropic support

a. The primary effect of inotropic support in the treatment of CHF is to increase cardiac output.

(1) An increase in contractility increases the slope of the ESPVL, which for a given preload and end-systolic pressure/afterload will produce an increased SV (see Fig. 9-3). Hence, SV is determined only by the pressure at end-systole and the slope of the ESPVL.

(2) An increase in contractility effects displacement of the ventricular curve back toward "normal," resulting in an increase in SV for the same LVEDP.

(3) The result of an increased contractility is a reduction in the LVEDV and an increase in the systemic pressure. The latter effect assumes the use of a pure inotrope without vasodilator effects, which may cause a decrease in BP.

b. The net effect on myocardial oxygen supply-demand balance is less predictable than with preload reduction. Thus, careful titration of inotropes is required, particularly in the setting of myocardial ischemia.

(1) In the failing dilated heart, the increased myocardial oxygen demand from increased contractility may be offset by a decreased oxygen requirement due to a reduced ventricular volume and the increased myocardial perfusion from increased systemic pressures, decreased ventricular diastolic pressures, or both.

(2) In the nonfailing or normal-sized heart, the increased oxygen demand from increased contractility may not be offset by the above factors, thus worsening ischemia. This occurs particularly with an excessive increase in heart rate.

(3) Rate-related ischemia may be the important limitation in the use of inotropic agents. In patients with ventricular hypertrophy or coronary stenoses, increases in heart rate may exceed the limits of coronary blood flow to supply oxygen to the myocardium, resulting in ischemia.

3. Afterload reduction

a. In patients with CHF, arterial impedance, systemic arteriolar resistance, and peripheral venous tone are elevated. Circulating vasoconstrictors such as catecholamines, angiotensin II, and ADH serve initially to maintain BP. However, the failing heart responds to arteriolar constriction with a further reduction in SV, contributing to deteriorating ventricular function.

b. Increased peripheral venous tone helps to maintain intracardiac volumes and adequate ventricular preload. Excessive increase in intracardiac volumes may result in increased wall stress (i.e., an increase in the true ventricular afterload). "Afterload reduction," a term clinicians use, refers to a reduction in arterial impedance induced by pharmacologic agents. The term will be used in this manner.

c. The effects of afterload reduction may be illustrated graphically (Fig. 9-6). This results in a lowering of the pressure at which aortic ejection commences and results in the conversion of pressure work to volume work; an increase in stroke volume results. In patients with decreased contractility (reduced slope of the ESPVL), a small amount of afterload reduction results in a larger increment in SV than in the heart with normal contractility. The ESP/systemic pressure will fall with the fall in afterload. For the same increase

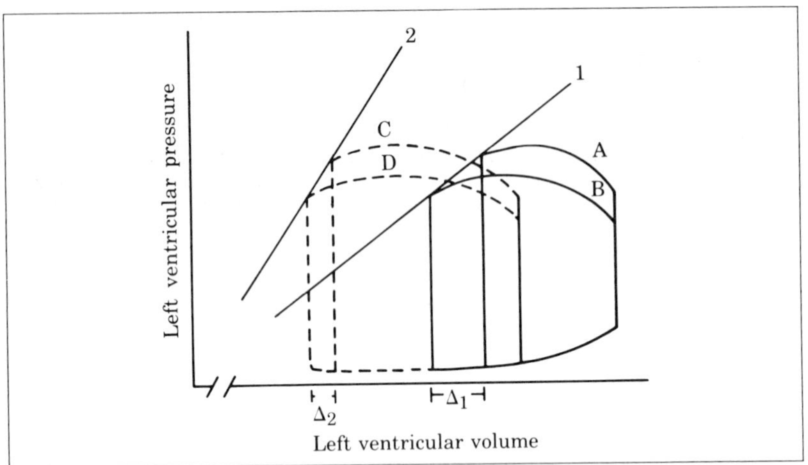

Fig. 9-6. Effects of afterload reduction. Reduced afterload results in lower end-systolic pressures and hence greater ejected volume (shown for constant preload). The change in stroke volume for a given change in end-systolic pressure will be greater in a ventricle with depressed contractility (ESPV line *1,* PVLs *A* and *B,* Δ_1) than in one with a normal or enhanced contractility (ESPV line *2,* PVLs *C* and *D,* Δ_2).

in SV, however, the fall in BP is less in the depressed heart than in the normal heart due to the slope of the ESPVL.

d. Some evidence suggests that afterload reduction may increase SV as a result of a reduction in vascular impedance and an improvement in ventricular compliance due to a downward shift of the pressure-volume curve. An increase in compliance implies a decrease in end-diastolic pressure for the same end-diastolic volume.

e. The decrease in end-diastolic volume and pressure with an improved LV function favorably alters the myocardial oxygen supply-demand balance. This may be important in patients with ischemia. Vasodilators may also increase blood flow to an ischemic area by improving collateral flow. This is controversial.

f. The major hazard and limitation associated with afterload reduction is hypotension, with a concomitant fall in perfusion pressure to vital organs.

g. The resultant effect of a reduction in afterload depends on the summative effect of several factors, including preexisting myocardial ischemia, contractility, intravascular volume status, and baseline arterial impedance. The net effect, assuming perfusion pressure can be maintained, is an increase in cardiac output with no change or an improvement in the myocardial oxygen supply-demand balance.

h. Survival of patients with moderate to severe heart failure has improved with vasodilator therapy. A combination therapy of hydralazine and isosorbide dinitrate, compared to prazosin or placebo, has been shown to improve mortality in patients with heart failure already receiving digitalis and diuretics. Another study demonstrated that the addition of enalapril to conventional therapy in patients with severe heart failure can reduce mortality and improve symptoms. These studies were performed on patients with chronic severe heart failure. It is unknown whether vasodilator therapy will improve survival in patients with acute heart failure in a critical care setting.

C. **RV dysfunction**

1. **Isolated RV failure** without concomitant LV failure is less common than isolated LV failure or biventricular failure.
2. **RV dysfunction** is most commonly seen when the impedance to RV ejection is acutely increased. This can occur during acute pulmonary artery hypertension secondary to severe acute respiratory failure or embolism, positive pressure ventilation, especially with PEEP applied, or when pulmonary vasoconstriction follows severe hypoxemia.
3. **Pulmonary hypertension** may have several effects on RV and LV performance. The RV ejection fraction is inversely correlated with the mean pulmonary artery pressure. RV end-diastolic volume increases with increasing pulmonary artery pressure but the increase in RV and diastolic volume may not correlate with the central venous pressure because of the high compliance of the RV. Pulmonary hypertension may reduce the gradient for tissue perfusion at the rigt ventricle during systole. The right ventricle is normally perfused during both systole and diastole. Reduction of systolic flow may contribute to RV ischemia. A reduction in left ventricular SV may occur as a result of decreased LV filling secondary to decreased RV output and/or alterations of LV geometry and diastolic compliance. The latter changes occur due to shifts in the position of the septum as the right ventricle dilates.
4. The effects of positive pressure ventilation and PEEP on RV function have been described (**IV.C.4**).
5. **Acute inferior or right ventricular infarction** may cause RV dysfunction, resulting in a decreased RV ejection fraction and enlargement of the RV.
6. **Assessment of RV function.** Apart from the standard techniques of two-dimensional echocardiography and radionuclide angiocardiography, a pulmonary artery catheter can measure RV ejection fraction. Derived variables include RV end-diastolic and end-systolic volumes. The current technique is to inject a bolus of iced saline into the right atrium, followed by mixing in the right ventricle. The reduction in temperature is measured in the pulmonary artery blood by a rapid-response thermistor. The accuracy of the technique compares favorably with 2-D echocardiography and gated angiography. The clinical importance of RV volume and ejection fraction estimations remains to be determined; however, the information gained from the RV end-diastolic volume and ejection fraction as an index of RV preload greatly exceeds that of the CVP.
7. The therapeutic approach of preload manipulation, afterload reduction, and inotropic support remains valid in the treatment of right ventricular failure. An approach includes:
   a. **Assess ventricular volumes.** Methods are described **IV.B**.
   b. **Maintain normal volume status.** Preload augmentation may be relatively ineffectual, with minimal response in SV and RV ejection fraction.
   c. **Treat hypotension.** The failing ischemic RV may respond to increases in blood pressure. Despite a potential increase in RV afterload, the increase in right coronary perfusion may relieve ischemia and increase contractability. This is achieved by augmentation of aortic BP with inotropes or mechanical assist devices such as an intraaortic balloon pump.
   d. **Consider an inotrope.** Inotropes such as dopamine and norepinephrine may increase the RV ejection fraction via a direct

inotropic effect on the RV. This is independent of the effect an increase in aortic BP has on decreasing RV ischemia.

e. **Consider a selective pulmonary vasodilator.** Prostaglandin E1 (PGE1) has been used in the therapy of acute and chronic pulmonary hypertension. It is a potent vasodilator of pulmonary veins and has been shown to decrease markedly pulmonary artery pressure and pulmonary and systemic vascular resistances and increase cardiac output, arterial PO_2, oxygen delivery, and oxygen consumption. It has shown promise in patients with RV failure and with severe pulmonary hypertension who are undergoing mitral valve replacement. However, large trials have been unable to demonstrate an enhanced survival in patients with adult respiratory distress syndrome, a condition in which acute pulmonary hypertension is a consistent feature.

D. Specific therapeutic agents

1. Preload and afterload reduction

a. **Fluid restriction.** Maximal restriction of fluid intake and concentration of all IV medications is an important measure for contributing to preload reduction.

b. **Diuretics**

(1) Diuretics have few acute side effects and promote removal of excess body fluid (in contrast to vasodilators). Commonly used diuretics are hydrochlorothiazide, chlorothiazide, furosemide, and ethacrynic acid. The first two act mainly at the distal tubule but also have some action at the proximal tubule by inhibiting carbonic anhydrase. The last two are more potent loop diuretics that primarily affect chloride transport in the loop of Henle.

(2) Diuretics are useful as the primary therapeutic agent in mild to moderate CHF and as adjunctive therapy in more severe CHF. The speed and onset of their actions are limited by the renal response to their pharmacologic actions. When rapid lowering of PCWP is necessary or when CHF is accompanied by renal dysfunction, supplemental or alternate modes of therapy may be needed.

(a) **Synergistic effects** may sometimes be obtained by the simultaneous administration of a potassium-sparing diuretic (e.g., spironolactone) to one of the loop diuretics, which will reduce the hypokalemic alkalosis that accompanies the use of loop diuretics, or by the simultaneous administration of metolazone or a thiazide diuretic (both distal tubule diuretics) to a loop diuretic. Another option is an infusion of furosemide combined with mannitol, an osmotic diuretic.

(b) **Furosemide,** in addition to its diuretic action, is a weak venodilator and may effect a mild to moderate decrease in PCWP prior to diuresis.

(3) **Common side effects of diuretics** are hypokalemia, hyponatremia, hypochloremic alkalosis, hyperglycemia, hyperuricemia, and hearing impairment (especially ethacrynic acid and furosemide).

c. **Nitroglycerin**

(1) The primary systemic effect of nitroglycerin and other organic nitrates is venodilation, although it mildly decreases arterial resistance as well.

(2) Nitrates also dilate epicardial coronary vessels and coronary collateral vessels, thereby reducing myocardial ischemia (in addition to its beneficial effect on preload).

(3) Because of its rapid onset, short half-life, easy controllability, beneficial effects on myocardial ischemia, and relative lack of serious hemodynamic side effects or metabolic toxicity, nitroglycerin is frequently employed for rapid preload reduction and relief of ischemia.

(4) Nitrate tolerance may occur with chronic dosing, resulting in partial or complete attenuation of hemodynamic benefits, such as increases in SV and decreases in LV filling pressures and systemic vascular resistance. This may occur within 24 hours of transdermal nitrate use or after 48 hours of IV administration of nitroglycerin. Chronic use requires the use of shorter-acting nitrates with a nitrate-free interval to avoid this problem.

(5) Mortality over the long term has been shown to be reduced in patients with CHF when the combination of hydralazine and isosorbide dinitrate is added to routine therapy of digoxin and a diuretic.

(6) **Side effects**

(a) **Hypotension,** due to over-vigorous preload reduction, usually can be easily managed with reduction or cessation of therapy, leg elevation, temporary fluid administration, or the use of a vasopressor such as phenylephrine.

(b) **Reflex tachycardia** can occur but is much less common than with nitroprusside.

(7) Intravenous infusions provide the optimal titration of effects. Sublingual, transcutaneous, or oral routes of administration may be used when close titration is not necessary.

d. **Nitroprusside**

(1) Nitroprusside significantly dilates the venous and arterial vasculature.

(2) It is, thus, very effective for both preload and afterload reduction. Because of the greater effect on afterload, a larger increase in SV and cardiac output can be expected compared to nitroglycerin.

(3) **Side effects**

(a) **Hypotension.** Nitroprusside is a potent but short-acting agent, allowing rapid titration of effects. It is not recommended for use in patients who have a systolic BP less than 100 mm Hg because of its greater tendency to cause hypotension. A precipitous fall in BP should raise the possibility that the filling pressures are lower than expected, leading to a reduction rather than an increase in the cardiac output.

(b) Coronary steal. This is the preferential shunting of blood flow away from ischemic to normal myocardium. Conflicting reports on the efficacy of nitroprusside in the setting of acute myocardial infarction (MI) have been published; however, it appears safe and effective in the setting of coronary ischemia and CHF.

(c) Thiocyanate/cyanide toxicity. Thiocyanate toxicity is manifest by confusion, hyperreflexia, and convulsions. Cyanide toxicity is first manifest by a metabolic acidosis due to cyanide's combining with cytochromes and inhibiting aerobic cellular metabolism. Thiocyanate or cyanide toxicity usually occurs in the setting of high doses for a prolonged period (greater than 3 μg/kg/min for more than 72 hours).

(d) **Hypoxemia.** Mild reductions in arterial oxygen tension may occur due to nitroprusside-induced inhibition of the pulmonary vasoconstrictor response.

(e) **Reflex tachycardia.** This may occur if the systemic BP drops severely.

(4) Continuous IV infusion is the only mode of administration of nitroprusside. In patients with severe heart failure, a nitroprusside infusion is started at 10 μg per minute; most patients show a positive response by 1–2 μg/kg/min, although there is great variability in the individual response.

e. **Hydralazine**

(1) **Hydralazine** is almost a pure arterial vasodilator.

(2) It may have a reflex or direct cardiac inotropic effect.

(3) It may be used for afterload reduction by itself or in combination with other shorter-acting drugs (e.g., to reduce required dosages of nitroprusside).

(4) **Side effects**

(a) Hypotension

(b) Reflex tachycardia

(c) Systemic lupus erythematosus syndrome/Coomb's positive hemolytic anemia

(5) It may be administered intermittently IV, IM, or PO. It is not highly suitable for administration as an IV infusion because of its long life (2–4 hours). Interval dosing is recommended.

f. **Angiotensin-converting enzyme (ACE) inhibitors**

(1) **ACE inhibitors** are balanced vasodilators reducing both systemic and pulmonary vascular resistances. Vasodilation is mediated by a decline in angiotensin II, catecholamine, and ADH levels and by increasing levels of bradykinin and prostaglandins.

(2) Right atrial, pulmonary artery, and capillary wedge pressures decrease, while cardiac output and SV increase with ACE inhibition. Heart rate remains unchanged or decreases.

(3) The CONSENSUS trial recently demonstrated a 31% reduction in mortality in patients with severe chronic CHF who had enalapril added to their standard regime of digitalis and diuretics. The clinical efficacy of captopril has also been confirmed.

(4) **Side effects**

(a) **Hypotension** can be minimized by starting with low doses.

(b) **Renal function** may deteriorate after ACE inhibition in patients dependent on angiotensin II-mediated efferent arteriolar vasoconstriction to maintain glomerular filtration. ACE inhibitors are contraindicated in bilateral renal artery stenosis.

(c) **Hyperpotassemia.** ACE inhibitors cause a reduction in aldosterone, resulting in potassium retention.

(5) Therapy is begun with captopril at a dose of 6.25 mg PO or enalapril at a dose of 2.5 mg PO. Maintenance doses are approximately 75 mg per day for captopril and 20 mg per day for enalapril. Enalapril has a slower onset (2 hours) and longer duration of action (12 hours) than captopril. IV enalapril is given at doses of 0.625–1.25 mg IV q6h.

2. **Inotropic support**

a. **Dopamine**

(1) **Effects of dopamine** are dose related.

(a) At 0.5–2.0 μg/kg/min, renal blood flow and urine output increase secondary to selective dopaminergic receptor activation. Sodium excretion is enhanced by the increase in renal blood flow, dopamine-mediated inhibition of proximal tubule sodium reabsorption, and a reduction in aldosterone secretion.

(b) Doses of 2–5 μg/kg/min can cause an increase in cardiac contractility and cardiac output with little change in heart rate, BP, or systemic vascular resistance. Alpha adrenergic effects usually begin to appear in doses of 5–10 μg/kg/min. Doses up to 10 μg/kg/min further increase cardiac output but may be accompanied by tachycardia, hypertension and/or elevated filling pressures in some patients. Infusions in excess of 10 μg/kg/min result in an increasing alpha-adrenergic effect, with increases in systemic vascular resistance. This may override the salutary effect of dopamine on renal blood flow.

(2) Dopamine is used for inotropic support in moderate to severe CHF and pump failure after cardiopulmonary bypass.

(3) **Side effects**

(a) **Elevation of the PCWP** may result from constriction of pulmonary capacitance veins.

(b) **Increases in myocardial oxygen demands and afterload** at high infusion rates may worsen myocardial ischemia and impair cardiac output. Hence, addition of a vasodilator may improve SVs.

(c) **Dopamine does not influence infarct size,** whereas dobutamine decreases it.

(d) **Tachycardia and dysrhythmia** are variable, dose-related side effects.

b. Dobutamine

(1) Dobutamine, at infusion rates of 5–15 μg/kg/min, results in an increase in contractility with less tachycardia than dopamine. Systemic and pulmonary vascular resistances are unaltered or decreased. Although dobutamine does not have a selective renal vascular effect, it often increases urine output by improving cardiac output and renal perfusion. Dobutamine generally improves the balance between myocardial oxygen supply and demand.

(2) Dobutamine is currently the inotrope of choice in low cardiac output states if an acceptable BP can be maintained. Compared with dopamine, dobutamine is more appropriate in patients with a low cardiac output and high PCWP who are normotensive or with borderline hypotension, especially if cardiogenic pulmonary edema is present. In contrast, dopamine is a better choice in patients with a low cardiac output, low or normal PCWP, and hypotension in which positive inotropic and pressor responses are needed.

(3) **Side effects**

(a) Tachycardia and dysrhythmia occur less frequently compared to dopamine.

(b) Hypotension may occur, especially if the PCWP is below 15 mm Hg.

c. Epinephrine

(1) Effects of epinephrine are dose related.

(a) At rates of 0.005–0.02 μg/kg/min epinephrine stimulates beta-adrenergic receptors, resulting in an increase in cardiac output and heart rate and a decrease in systemic and pulmonary vascular resistances.

(b) Higher infusion rates result in more alpha-adrenergic effects, leading to an increased systemic vascular resistance, elevation of BP, and variable effects on the cardiac output (the last action depending on the heart's ability to maintain SV as afterload is increased).

(2) **Epinephrine** remains the mainstay of cardiac resuscitation. Its potency and greater maximal inotropic effect compared to dopamine and dobutamine ensure its place in the treatment of severe CHF.

(3) **Side effects**

(a) **Tachycardia and dysrhythmia**

(b) **Extreme hypertension** may occur with high doses.

(c) **Myocardial oxygen demand** often exceeds supply, in spite of an increase in coronary perfusion, aggravating ischemia.

d. Norepinephrine

(1) **Norepinephrine** has potent beta- and alpha-adrenergic receptor activity. The resultant alpha-adrenergic-mediated vasoconstriction raises BP, but heart rate remains unchanged because of reflex baroreceptor mechanisms. SV increases if the augmentation in afterload is tolerated by the ventricle. Initial infusion rates are 1–2 μg per minute.

(2) The major role of norepinephrine is in the treatment of septic shock, where inotropy and restoration of arteriolar tone are required. Norepinephrine is less useful in CHF unless the benefits of an increase in BP and coronary perfusion outweigh the detrimental increases in afterload and myocardial work. The main indication for norepinephrine is shock resulting from myocardial infarction. The goal is to increase mean arterial pressure to 70–80 mm Hg, at which time coronary blood flow improves. This is balanced against the increase in afterload and myocardial oxygen demand.

(3) **Side effects**

(a) **Renal vasoconstriction** may compromise renal function. Low-dose dopamine may ameliorate the vasoconstrictive action of norepinephrine.

(b) **Tachycardia and dysrhythmia** are less common compared to other potent inotropes.

e. Isoproterenol

(1) **Isoproterenol** has potent beta-adrenergic activity but no alpha activity. Cardiac output increases when filling pressures are adequate. The rise in cardiac output is often related to the rise in heart rate rather than an increase in SV. Due to the potential for marked tachycardia, it has little therapeutic role in the treatment of CHF in adults.

(2) Isoproterenol is useful for marked bradycardia and high-degree atrioventricular block unresponsive to atropine.

(3) **Side effects**

(a) **Tachycardia and dysrhythmia** are more common with isoproterenol.

(b) **Myocardial ischemia.** An increase in heart rate and contractility in association with a reduction in diastolic coronary perfusion pressure worsens myocardial oxygen supply-demand mismatch.

(c) **Vasodilation**

3. Phosphodiesterase inhibitors

a. Amrinone and milrinone

(1) **Amrinone and milrinone** are nonadrenergic, nonglycosidic agents that effect their inotropic and vasodilator action through phosphodiesterase inhibition, thereby indirectly elevating cyclic adenosine monophosphate and increasing calcium availability. Both agents cause dose-dependent increases in SV and heart rate with independent reductions in systemic

and pulmonary vascular resistances. Systemic BP is often unchanged because the increase in SV compensates for the fall in resistance. However, in anesthetized patients, some decrease in blood pressure is not uncommon. Myocardial oxygen consumption is unchanged or reduced. Amrinone and milrinone have hemodynamic effects similar to a combination of dobutamine and nitroprusside.

(2) These drugs have been shown to improve ventricular relaxation, and their use has been suggested in diastolic cardiac failure. To date, they have been used in patients with severe heart failure, primarily in combination with other inotropic agents. Their long half-life and individual variation in the peripheral vascular and myocardial response make them less easily titratable compared with catecholamines and intravenous vasodilators.

(3) **Side effects**

(a) **Hypotension** may occur as a result of their vasodilator action, which may compromise diastolic coronary filling.

(b) **Amrinone** may produce thrombocytopenia and liver dysfunction, which precludes it from long-term oral administration. It is infused intravenously at a dose of 5–10 μg/kg/min after an initial bolus of 0.75 mg per kilogram. Milrinone is not currently available as an IV preparation.

(c) **Both agents** have much less potential to cause arrhythmia than other inotropes.

b. **Digitalis**

(1) **Digoxin** has a diminished role in patients with acute heart failure. Its use is limited by a slow onset of action (40–60 min) and by mild hemodynamic effects in comparison to catecholamines and phosphodiesterase inhibitors. In the acute setting, the role of digoxin should probably be limited to the therapy of arrhythmia, such as atrial fibrillation, atrial flutter, or supraventricular tachycardia. Digoxin therapy may benefit some patients with chronic CHF, particularly if atrial fibrillation is present and is used as an adjunct with diuretics and vasodilators in the long-term management of severe heart failure.

(2) **Side effects**

(a) Arrhythmia. Virtually every known ECG abnormality may be produced by digoxin toxicity.

(b) **Gastrointestinal and necrologic symptoms** may be a manifestation of digoxin toxicity.

(c) Digoxin administration **may potentially exacerbate myocardial ischemia** by causing both increased oxygen demand and coronary vasoconstriction.

Selected References

General Background and Therapy

Braunwald, E. *Heart Disease: A Textbook of Cardiovascular Medicine.* Philadelphia: W. B. Saunders, 1988.

Chernow, B. *The Pharmacologic Approach to the Critically Ill Patient.* Baltimore: Williams & Wilkins, 1988.

The CONSENSUS Trial Study Group. Effects of enalapril on mortality in severe congestive heart failure. Results of the cooperative North Scandinavian Enalapril Survival Study (CONSENSUS). *N. Engl. J. Med.* 316:1429, 1987.

Left Ventricular Pressure-Volume Relationships

Sagawa, K., Maughan, L., Suga, H., and Sunagawa, K. *Cardiac Contraction and the Pressure-Volume Relationship*. New York: Oxford, 1988.

Right Ventricular Failure and Ventricular Interactions

Hurford, W. E., and Zapol, W. M. The right ventricle and critical illness: A review of anatomy, physiology, and clinical evaluation of its function. *Int. Care Med.* 14:448, 1988.

Pulmonary Capillary Wedge Pressure

O'Quin, R., and Marini, J. J. Pulmonary artery occlusion pressure: Clinical physiology, measurement and interpretation. *Am. Rev. Respir. Dis.* 128:319, 1983.

10

Shock

Albert T. Cheung

I. Classification
- **A. Hypovolemic shock**
- **B. Cardiogenic shock**
- **C. Distributive shock**
- **D. Obstructive shock**
- **E. Mixed states**

II. General approach
- **A. Initial diagnosis and therapy**
  - **1. Diagnosis**
    - **a. Hypotension**
    - **b. Organ dysfunction**
    - **c. Inadequate tissue perfusion**
  - **2. Immediate therapy**
    - **a. Airway**
    - **b. Breathing**
    - **c. Circulation**
    - **d. Arrhythmias**
    - **e. Tension pneumothorax**
    - **f. Pericardial tamponade**
    - **g. Disconnected vasoactive drug**
    - **h. Anaphylactic shock**
- **B. Subsequent diagnosis and therapy**
  - **1. History**
  - **2. Associated metabolic disorders**
  - **3. Physical and laboratory examination**
    - **a. Central nervous system**
    - **b. Cardiovascular system**
    - **c. Respiratory system**
    - **d. Renal blood flow and function**
    - **e. Hematologic**
    - **f. Gastrointestinal**
    - **g. Muscle fatigue**
  - **4. Monitoring**
    - **a. ECG**
    - **b. Foley bladder catheter**
    - **c. Arterial line**
    - **d. Central venous pressure (CVP)**
    - **e. Pulmonary artery catheters**
      - **(1) Pulmonary artery pressure (PAP)**
      - **(2) Pulmonary artery occlusion pressure (PAOP)**
    - **f. Cardiac output (CO)**

III. Hypovolemic shock
- **A. Diagnosis**
- **B. Causes**
- **C. Management**
  - **1. Crystalloid solutions**
  - **2. Colloid solutions**
    - **a. Human albumin**
    - **b. Dextran**
    - **c. Blood and blood products**
  - **3. Pneumatic antishock garment (PASG)**
  - **4. Vasopressors and inotropes**

- **IV. Septic shock**
  - **A. Pathophysiology**
  - **B. Diagnosis**
  - **C. Management**
    - **1. Circulatory support**
      - **a. Volume expansion**
      - **b. Vasopressors**
    - **2. Treatment of infection**
    - **3. Experimental approaches**
      - **a. Immunotherapy**
      - **b. Nonsteroidal antiinflammatory drugs**
      - **c. Glucocorticoids**
- **V. Anaphylactic shock**
  - **A. Pathophysiology**
  - **B. Management**
    - **1. Identification of the allergen**
    - **2. Airway management**
    - **3. Intravenous volume expansion**
    - **4. Epinephrine**
    - **5. Antihistamines**
    - **6. Glucocorticoids**
- **VI. Cardiogenic shock**
  - **A. Pathophysiology**
  - **B. Etiology**
  - **C. Management**
    - **1. Volume expansion**
    - **2. Inotropic agents**
    - **3. Afterload reduction**
    - **4. Intraaortic balloon pump (IABP)**

Shock is a general term applied to pathological states characterized by a failure of the circulation to supply essential metabolic substrates necessary to maintain the function and the cellular integrity of vital organ systems. Irreversible cellular injury and multisystem organ failure ensues if the condition is not promptly remedied.

I. Classification

A. **Hypovolemic shock** (Table 10-1) is caused by intravascular volume depletion leading to a reduction in cardiac output. Normally 70–80% of the total blood volume is contained within the venous capacitance bed. With progressive loss of intravascular volume, venous return to the heart is reduced, and cardiac stroke volume decreases. Shock occurs when adrenergically mediated venoconstriction and augmentation of heart rate can no longer compensate for the reduced cardiac filling pressure and reduced cardiac output. Arteriolar vasoconstriction occurs in an attempt to maintain perfusion pressures. The renin-angiotensin-aldosterone system is activated to conserve sodium and water.

B. **Cardiogenic shock** is caused by failure of the heart to function as a pump in order to deliver adequate systemic blood flow. Myocardial dysfunction can result from acute myocardial infarction, cardiomyopathies, arrhythmias, or valvular heart disease.

C. **Distributive shock** is caused primarily by vasomotor dysfunction, resulting in excessive venous pooling, loss of arteriolar tone, and redistribution of blood flow. This pathological condition can occur during sepsis, with the loss of neurogenic control of the vasculature (neurogenic shock) and through the vasoactive actions of certain drugs. Cardiac output and intravascular volume may be low, normal, or increased in the presence of hypotension in distributive shock.

D. **Obstructive shock** is caused by mechanical obstruction of channels of blood flow—for example, aortocaval obstruction by a gravid uterus or increased intraabdominal pressure, pericardial tamponade, herniation of the myocardium through the pericardial sac following chest surgery, pulmonary embolism, obstruction of the inferior vena cava by tumor or thrombus, intramyocardial tumors, tension pneumothorax, and aortic dissection.

E. **Mixed states.** In practice, the various subtypes of shock already mentioned usually occur in combination. In anaphylactic shock, for example, hypovolemia caused by capillary leakage coexists with abnormalities in distribution due to the release of endogenous vasoactive substances. Hypovolemia caused by capillary leak, inflammation, and insensible losses from fever often complicates the distribution defect in septic shock. Inadequate perfusion in the advanced stages of hypovolemic shock results in myocardial dysfunction. Drug therapy and preexisting disease states add to the complexity of the condition. A comprehensive

Table 10-1. Hemodynamic parameters in shock

Type of shock	BP	CO	PCWP/CVP
Hypovolemic	↓	↓	↓
Septic	↓	↑	± ↓
Cardiogenic	↓	↓	↑
Anaphylactic	↓	↑	↓
Neurogenic	↓	±	↓

↑ = increase; ↓ = decrease; ± = variable.

approach to diagnosis and therapy must address each individual problem and underlying pathological condition.

II. General approach

A. Initial diagnosis and therapy. The critical nature of the condition requires that diagnosis and therapy begin concurrently. Diagnosis is based on evidence of hypotension, inadequate tissue perfusion, and organ dysfunction. The history usually suggests a precipitating event, such as exposure to an allergen, trauma, infection, or localized pain. Therapy begins with the "ABCs" of resuscitation: airway, breathing, and circulation.

1. Diagnosis

a. Hypotension is generally defined as a systolic BP of less than 80 mm Hg or mean arterial pressure (MAP) of less than 50 mm Hg. These parameters are chosen because autoregulation of regional blood flow is impaired and becomes pressure dependent below these levels in the normal individual.

b. Organ dysfunction can present as altered mentation, oliguria, respiratory distress, myocardial ischemia, or coagulopathy.

c. Inadequate tissue perfusion can be demonstrated by detecting the presence of lactic acidosis. Signs of poor perfusion are cool, clammy skin, slow capillary refill, tachycardia, thready pulses, acrocyanosis, and mottled skin. An exception occurs with distributive shock, in which inadequate tissue perfusion is accompanied by warm skin and a hyperdynamic cardiovascular state.

2. Immediate therapy begins with cardiopulmonary life support followed by the diagnosis and treatment of immediately reversible life-threatening causes contributing to the condition of shock.

a. Airway. Endotracheal intubation is necessary in the presence of altered mentation as a prophylactic measure against aspiration, to provide mechanical ventilation, and to deliver high inspired concentrations of oxygen.

b. Breathing. Respiratory distress or failure is a common feature of shock. Mechanical ventilation is often necessary to reduce the metabolic cost of breathing and to ensure maximum oxygen availability for delivery to tissues.

c. Circulation. Immediate establishment of IV access is essential for drug administration and volume expansion.

d. Arrhythmias can be detected with ECG monitoring.

e. Tension pneumothorax should be suspected with precipitous hypotension during mechanical ventilation. Jugular venous distention, contralateral tracheal deviation, ipsilateral hyperresonance to chest percussion, diminished breath sounds, shift in position of the point of maximum cardiac impulse, a sudden increase in central venous pressure, or a sudden increase in peak inspiratory pressure can support the diagnosis of a tension pneumothorax. A chest radiograph is not necessary to confirm the diagnosis in the presence of life-threatening hemodynamic instability. Decompression can be accomplished with the insertion of a 14-gauge needle or catheter into the second intercostal space at the midclavicular line, followed by insertion of a chest tube.

f. Pericardial tamponade can occur as a consequence of penetrating injury, thoracic surgery, transmural myocardial infarction, dissecting aortic aneurysm, malignant disease, uremia, or pericarditis. Clinical signs in order of frequency are jugular venous distension, tachypnea, tachycardia, and pulsus paradoxus. The ECG may show electrical alternans. Right heart catheterization typically demonstrates the equalization of central venous, right atrial, right ventricular diastolic, pulmonary artery diastolic, and pulmonary artery occlusion pressures with intrapericardial pressure. Echocardiography is extremely useful to confirm the diagnosis. Volume expansion and beta-adrenergic agonists, such as epinephrine, can be used for support prior to pericardiocentesis.

g. **Disconnected vasoactive drug** or the unintentional interruption of an intravenous carrier infusion can result in precipitous hypotension in patients dependent on those medications.

h. **In anaphylactic shock**, all suspect drugs and ongoing transfusions of blood products should be discontinued immediately.

B. **Subsequent diagnosis and therapy** is directed toward a full evaluation of the possible etiologies contributing to the condition of shock.

1. **History.** Obtain a full history from all individuals involved in the care of the patient prior to admission.

2. **Associated metabolic disorders** can contribute to hypotension. Adrenal insufficiency, hypothyroidism, hypopituitarism, hypoglycemia, hypocalcemia, and acid-base disorders can be excluded by laboratory testing. Patients on chronic glucocorticoid therapy, who are at risk of acute stress-induced adrenal insufficiency, can be given hydrocortisone 100 mg IV while awaiting the results of laboratory tests.

3. **The physical and laboratory examination** is directed at determining the presence and extent of multisystem involvement.

a. **Central nervous system.** In the absence of cerebrovascular disease, autoregulation of the cerebral circulation is independent of the systemic circulation. Cerebral blood flow is maintained until MAP falls to less than 50 mm Hg. Confusion, obtundation, and the appearance of focal neurologic deficits are possible indications of inadequate cerebral perfusion. Metabolic encephalopathy from sepsis can also produce delirium. Metabolic disorders, infection, trauma, or mass lesions of the CNS need to be excluded before attributing neurologic disturbances to shock.

b. **Cardiovascular system.** Autoregulation of blood flow in the coronary circulation is a function of myocardial oxygen demand. In shock, tachycardia and increased circulating concentrations of catecholamines can increase myocardial oxygen demand while hypotension decreases coronary perfusion pressure. This condition predisposes the myocardium to ischemia, myocyte necrosis, decreased contractility, and arrhythmias, even in the absence of underlying heart disease. Left ventricular depression has been attributed to the presence of circulating myocardial depressants.

c. **Respiratory system.** The early effects of shock on pulmonary function include ventilation and perfusion mismatching, increased physiologic dead space, and increased oxygen demand of the respiratory muscles to compensate for metabolic acidosis. Increased capillary membrane permeability can lead to the accumulation of extravascular lung water, hypoxemia, and decreased diffusing capacity. The presence of tachypnea, labored breathing, stridor, wheezing, rales, or cyanosis is a sign of impending respiratory failure.

d. **Renal blood flow and function** are often diminished in the attempt at preserving intravascular volume by normal physiologic mechanisms during shock. Renal blood flow may be reduced further by exogenously administered vasopressors. Aminoglycoside antibiotics and other nephrotoxic drugs can add to the renal injury. As a consequence, acute tubular necrosis is a frequent complication during shock.

e. **Hematologic.** In addition to the loss of intravascular volume, hemorrhage decreases the total red cell mass and can impair oxygen-carrying capacity. Dilution, loss, and consumption of platelets and coagulation factors can lead to impaired clot formation. Hypothermia from rapid infusions of cold solutions will impair clotting. Endothelial injury, the liberation of procoagulants, and slowing of blood flow as a consequence of shock can lead to disseminated intravascular coagulation. Intravascular microthrombosis and aggregation of erythrocytes, leukocytes, and platelets exacerbate the perfusion defect in shock. Hematocrit, platelet count, prothrombin time, and partial thromboplastin time should be followed closely to detect these problems.

f. **Gastrointestinal.** Activation of the sympathetic nervous system and the reduction of splanchnic blood flow lead to gastric and intestinal hypomotility. Absorption of food is delayed, and gastric dilation can occur. Gastrointestinal bleeding from stress-induced gastritis and ulceration can complicate shock. Liver dysfunction and abnormal liver function tests in a nonspecific pattern occur commonly during shock. Hypoperfusion can predispose to pancreatitis.

g. **Muscle fatigue** occurs quickly during shock when metabolic substrate availability is diminished. Muscle weakness and atrophy can result from enhanced proteolysis of skeletal muscle during critical illness.

4. **Monitoring** the cardiovascular and respiratory status of patients in shock is one of the primary purposes of an ICU. Monitoring is used to diagnose problems rapidly and serves as an immediate guide to determine the effectiveness of therapy.

a. **ECG.** Continuous monitoring of the ECG is useful for detecting arrhythmias. A properly calibrated ECG monitor in the diagnostic mode is also useful for detecting ischemia and metabolic disturbances.

b. **Foley bladder catheter** is used for the hourly quantitation of urine output. Urine output can provide an indirect indicator of intravascular volume and renal function in the absence of diuretic therapy.

c. **Arterial line.** The direct, continuous measurement of blood pressure with an intraarterial cannula is helpful in shock. An arterial line provides a convenient site of access for obtaining blood for laboratory analysis.

d. **Central venous pressure (CVP)** can be monitored from an intravascular catheter with a port in the superior vena cava or right atrium. Since the CVP does not reflect left ventricular filling pressure, a normal or high CVP (>10–12 mm Hg) does not necessarily indicate that the patient will respond to volume expansion. A high CVP and inadequate left ventricular preload can occur with cardiac tamponade, tension pneumothorax, mitral stenosis, pulmonary embolus, pulmonary hypertension, and high levels of PEEP. Analysis of the CVP waveform can aid in the diagnosis of arrhythmias. For example, A waves are not present during atrial fibrillation, and cannon A waves become prominent with atrial-ventricular dissociation and junctional rhythms.

e. **Pulmonary artery catheters** enable the direct measurement of CVP, pulmonary artery pressures, cardiac output, and the indirect measurement of left atrial pressure. Monitoring these parameters provides a means of rapidly determining the effects of therapeutic interventions on the cardiovascular system.

(1) **Pulmonary artery pressure (PAP)** can increase in conditions of hypoxia, hypercarbia, acidosis, chronic lung disease, adult respiratory distress syndrome (ARDS), mitral valve disease, and pulmonary embolism. The PAP also provides an indication of right ventricular afterload.

(2) **Pulmonary artery occlusion pressure (PAOP)**, often referred to as pulmonary capillary wedge pressure (PCWP), correlates accurately with left ventricular end-diastolic pressure (LVEDP) in the absence of mitral valve disease. LVEDP is one of the determinants of preload to the left ventricle and therefore a major factor affecting cardiac output. The effectiveness of volume expansion for hypovolemia can be determined by serial measurement of the PAOP and stroke volume (cardiac output divided by heart rate) following IV fluid boluses. An increase in stroke volume in response to an increase in the PAOP with volume expansion indicates a therapeutic response. The absolute value of the PAOP should not be used alone to guide volume expansion. Patients with a noncompliant left ventricle as in hypertensive cardiomyopathy or aortic stenosis may require a relatively higher PAOP to achieve the desired increase in stroke volume. The PAOP can also be used to monitor changes in left ventricular performance. An acute increase in the PAOP that is not accompanied by a change in intravascular volume can indicate global left ventricular dysfunction caused by ischemia, dysrhythmias, hypertension, or valvular heart disease. The presence of large V waves on the PAOP waveform is a nonspecific indication of mitral regurgitation or decreased left ventricular compliance. A decrease in the PAOP with maintenance or improvement in stroke volume can indicate the therapeutic effectiveness of inotropes or afterload reduction in patients with heart failure.

f. **Cardiac output (CO)** is easily measured using the thermodilution technique. CO is reduced in hypovolemic, cardiogenic, and obstructive shock. A normal or increased CO can be present in septic shock. Stroke volume calculated from the CO gives an indication of myocardial performance independent of the heart rate. Pulmonary vascular resistance and systemic vascular resistance can also be calculated from the CO.

III. Hypovolemic shock

A. **Diagnosis.** Early signs of hypovolemic shock occur with an acute 15–25% loss of intravascular volume. The clinical signs of hypovolemia may be modified or masked among patients who are elderly, under anesthesia, on beta-adrenergic antagonists, on calcium channel blockers, or on antihypertensive therapy. Hypovolemia is less well tolerated when sympathetic reflexes are impaired. Hypovolemia often coexists with other forms of shock.

B. **Causes** of hypovolemia are multiple. External fluid losses can be caused by hemorrhage, vomiting, diarrhea, gastric suctioning, uncontrolled diabetes mellitus or insipidus, excessive diuretic use, postdialysis hypovolemia, excessive drainage from wounds, chest tubes, surgically placed drains, acute drainage and reaccumulation of ascites or pleural effusions, or plasma loss from burns. Hypovolemia caused by internal displacement of intravascular volume includes hemoperitoneum, hemothorax, hematoma from long bone fractures, intestinal obstruction, intraabdominal surgery, and acute pancreatitis. Hypovolemia can be caused by inadequate fluid intake or volume replacement.

C. **The management** of hypovolemic shock is based on rapid restoration of intravascular volume and control of ongoing volume loss. Attention should be directed at maintaining normal body temperature during the resuscitation since hypothermia can predispose to arrhythmias, coagulopathies, and immune suppression. Vasopressors and inotropes are sometimes useful to maintain the perfusion pressure to vital organs while the volume deficit is being restored. The advantages and disadvantages of various solutions for intravascular volume expansion are discussed below.

1. **Crystalloid solutions** such as lactated Ringer's solution (LR) and normal saline (NS) contain sodium as the major osmotically active solute. These solutions are isotonic with human plasma and distribute uniformly throughout the extracellular space. Approximately one-fifth to one-fourth of the intravenous volume administered will remain in the intravascular space after 1 hour. Advantages of crystalloid solutions are their low cost, easy storage, and ready availability. Crystalloid solutions are especially useful when the volume deficit is predominantly an ultrafiltrate of plasma, as in the conditions of renal fluid losses, gastrointestinal fluid losses, and dehydration. Hemodilution with crystalloid solutions decreases blood viscosity and theoretically can improve tissue perfusion. The concern that crystalloid solutions contribute to pulmonary injury by increasing extracellular lung water has not been substantiated. LR should be used cautiously in patients with renal failure or the potential to develop hyperkalemia since it contains 4 mEq per liter of KCl. Dextrose-containing solutions should be avoided since hyperglycemia may exacerbate ischemic cerebral injury.
2. **Colloid solutions** contain high-molecular-weight substances as the osmotically active agents. Intravascular infusion of colloids can increase intravascular volume by increasing plasma oncotic pressure, leading to the displacement of water from the extracellular and intracellular spaces into the intravascular space. Advantages of colloids include their ability to expand intravascular volume quickly at smaller infused volumes as compared to crystalloids and their ability to remain in the intravascular space. Disadvantages include their high cost compared to crystalloids and their specific side effects.
   a. **Human albumin**, the major osmotically active plasma protein, is available as a 5% or 25% solution in normal saline. Ninety percent of the albumin remains in the intravascular space 2 hours after intravenous administration and has a plasma half-life of 20 days. Heat treatment of human albumin eliminates the risk of transfusion-associated infections.
   b. **Dextran** is a solution of synthetic glucose polymers of either 40 KDaltons (D-40) or 70 KDaltons (D-70). D-40 is available as a 10% solution and D-70 as a 6% solution in either normal saline or 5% dextrose in water. It has a variable plasma half-life and is cleared predominantly by the kidneys, although uptake by the reticuloendothelial system (RES) and subsequent metabolism does occur. Potential problems with its use include a 1–5% chance of anaphylactic reactions, impairment of coagulation, the inability to crossmatch blood as a result of coating of cellular elements, osmotic diuresis (greater with D-40), renal failure from precipitation in renal tubules, and impairment of RES function. Its use in patients should be restricted to less than 1.5–2.0 g/kg/day.
   c. **Blood and blood products** are administered to maintain a hematocrit to ensure adequate oxygen delivery and to replete factors necessary to enable clot formation. In an emergency, the use of type O or type-specific, uncrossmatched blood carries a less than 0.1% chance of a transfusion reaction. Autotransfusion systems are also an effective source of volume replacement.
3. **Pneumatic antishock garment (PASG)** or military antishock trousers (MAST) were designed for emergency use in the field to temporize the effects of acute blood loss and assist in the insertion of venous catheters prior to definitive therapy. The device applies external pressure to the lower extremities, pelvis, and abdomen. It increases

blood pressure by increasing preload, increasing systemic vascular resistance, mobilizing 500–1,000 ml of blood into the upper body compartment, and decreasing blood loss by tamponading sites of active bleeding within the suit. Optimal inflation pressure of the suit is between 60 and 80 mm Hg. Few complications are associated with the use of the PASG when inflation time is less than 90 minutes. Deflation of the suit should be performed gradually, starting first with the abdominal portion. The team should be prepared to monitor the patient's blood pressure closely and rapidly administer IV fluids and control the sites of active bleeding upon deflation of the suit.

4. **Vasopressors and inotropes** are used to support the blood pressure initially until intravascular volume can be restored. The pharmacologic support of blood pressure in the setting of hypovolemic shock may be particularly important in patients with underlying coronary or cerebral vascular disease.

IV. **Septic shock**

A. **Pathophysiology.** Hypotension and impaired tissue perfusion as caused by the systemic response to infection is termed "septic shock." In addition to gram-negative bacterial infections, septic shock can be caused by viral, fungal, or gram-positive bacterial infections. Septic shock is a common problem among debilitated patients in the ICU and has a mortality ranging between 25% and 60%. Patients receiving immunosuppressive therapy, or multiple antibiotics, in addition to those who are malnourished or who have been chronically instrumented, are at risk of developing this syndrome. Although the pathogenesis of septic shock is not fully understood, evidence suggests that cellular products such as endotoxin produced by bacteria triggers the production of endogenous mediators. These mediators may have deleterious effects and produce a condition of distributive shock. Endogenous mediators that have been implicated include: cytokines, such as tumor necrosis factor and interleukin-1; eicosanoids such as the prostaglandins, prostacyclins, thromboxanes, and leukotrienes; endogenous opioid peptides; histamine-activated complement components; kinins; lysosomal enzymes; and oxygen-free radicals.

B. **Diagnosis** of septic shock is based on clinical criteria. A positive blood culture, although helpful, is not essential to make the diagnosis. Accepted criteria for septic shock are hypotension (systolic blood pressure of less than 90 mm Hg or a decrease in systolic blood pressure of more than 40 mm Hg from baseline), hypothermia (<98°F) or hyperthermia (>101°F), tachycardia (>90 beats per minute), tachypnea (>20 beats per minute), clinical evidence of a site of infection, and at least one end organ demonstrating inadequate perfusion (e.g., oliguria, lactic acidosis, hypoxemia, or altered mentation). When these are present in the absence of hypotension, the condition is often referred to as the sepsis syndrome. The presence of warm skin, bounding pulses, and a low systemic vascular resistance is helpful in establishing the diagnosis of sepsis. In the late stages of septic shock, progressive end-organ injury produces hypotension with diminished cardiac output, a narrowed pulse pressure, and increased systemic vascular resistance.

C. **Management** of patients in septic shock is based on supporting the circulation and optimizing organ perfusion until the infection can be controlled with appropriate antibiotic therapy. The only proved definitive therapy is to eliminate the source of infection. Experimental approaches using specific agents to neutralize bacterial toxins or to modify the systemic response to the infection are under study, but their clinical efficacy has yet to be determined.

1. **Circulatory support** is directed at improving oxygen delivery. Oxygen requirements are often increased during sepsis because of fever and hypermetabolism. Maldistribution of blood flow, hypotension,

and impaired oxygen utilization at the cellular level can limit oxygen availability to metabolically active tissue.

a. **Volume expansion** should be tried first. Patients with septic shock are often volume depleted because of poor fluid intake during the course of the illness, insensible fluid losses from fever, and extravasation of intravascular fluid through leaking capillaries. Observing a marked improvement in cardiac output and stroke volume upon increasing cardiac filling pressures indicates a therapeutic response.

b. **Vasopressors** are used to maintain perfusion pressure in the settings of a normal-to-high cardiac output and normal-to-high cardiac stroke volume in the presence of hypotension. Dopamine is often used initially since it has dose-dependent inotropic and vasoconstrictive effects. If additional vasopressors are necessary, norepinephrine, phenylephrine, or epinephrine can be added.

2. **Treatment of infection.** The early recognition and treatment of the infection is probably the most important factor influencing survival. Broad-spectrum antibiotic therapy is instituted after obtaining specimens of blood, urine, sputum, wound exudates, or cerebrospinal fluid for culture. An exhaustive search for a source of the systemic infection should be performed, although a discrete source of infection cannot be identified in 10–20% of patients with septic shock. Indwelling vascular catheters should be removed or changed since they are a common source of infection in the ICU. Radiographic studies such as chest radiographs, computerized axial tomography (CAT) scans, or sinus films of the head are sometimes useful to locate the site of infection. Prompt surgical therapy for drainage of abscesses, debridement of devitalized tissue, cholecystitis, or intestinal perforation can be lifesaving.

3. **Experimental approaches** directed at modifying or interrupting specific steps in the pathogenesis of septic shock are of interest since they may become important therapeutic options in the future. At present, their clinical efficacy remains unproved.

a. **Immunotherapy** in the form of specific antibodies against endotoxin and tumor necrosis factor–alpha are being investigated since these two compounds are thought to be mediators of the sepsis syndrome. Antiserum with specificity for endotoxin core antigen have been demonstrated in a clinical trial to decrease mortality in patients with gram-negative bacteremia and shock. Monoclonal antibodies against tumor necrosis factor–alpha are protective against lethal bacteremia in animal models.

b. **Nonsteroidal antiinflammatory drugs** such as ibuprofen and specific antagonists of arachidonic acid metabolites may attenuate fever and cardiovascular and metabolic changes produced by increased circulating concentrations of eicosanoids during sepsis. Ibuprofen pretreatment attenuates the fever, tachycardia, and stress hormone response to experimental administration of endotoxin to normal human volunteers.

c. **Glucocorticoids** in pharmacologic doses have been investigated for the treatment of septic shock and ARDS. Several recent prospective multicenter randomized studies have failed to demonstrate clinical effectiveness of glucocorticoids therapy in sepsis.

V. Anaphylactic shock

A. **Pathophysiology.** Anaphylactoid reactions are caused by the endogenous release of chemical mediators in response to exposure to substances such as food, drugs, blood products, insect venoms, or pollen in susceptible individuals. When these reactions are antigen induced and IgE mediated in a previously sensitized individual, they are specifically referred to as anaphylactic reactions. For practical purposes, the treatment of anaphylactic and anaphylactoid reactions are identical, and the terms will be used interchangeably. The endogenous mediators released during anaphylactic and anaphylactoid reactions include histamine, slow-reacting substance of anaphylaxis (leukotrienes: LTC4, LTD4, and LTE4), prostaglandins, thromboxanes, platelet activating factor, bradykinin, serotonin, complement components (C3a and C5a), and various chemotactic factors. These substances produce flushing, urticaria, angioedema, increased capillary permeability, bronchoconstriction, increased pulmonary secretions, and vasodilation. The clinical manifestations of anaphylactoid reactions can occur immediately following an antigenic challenge or occur as a delayed reaction 15–60 minutes after antigenic challenge. Late reactions are usually less severe. Cardiovascular collapse and shock as a consequence of anaphylactoid reactions are caused primarily by the loss of plasma volume through extravasation of plasma water and vasodilation.

B. **Management.** The successful management of anaphylactic and anaphylactoid reactions requires prompt diagnosis and early intervention. The assessment and therapeutic interventions outlined below should be carried out simultaneously when possible.

1. **Identification of the allergen.** An effort to identify and prevent the continued systemic absorption of the offending allergen may decrease the severity of the reaction.
2. **Airway management** can range from the administration of supplemental oxygen by facemask to emergent intubation or tracheostomy for angioneurotic edema of the airway. Severe, life-threatening bronchospasm may require mechanical ventilatory support.
3. **Intravenous volume expansion** is the initial therapy for hypotension since hypovolemia is a cause of the cardiovascular collapse seen in anaphylactic shock.
4. **Epinephrine** is considered the drug of choice for the initial emergency treatment of anaphylaxis. Epinephrine has multiple actions that counter the detrimental systemic effects of anaphylaxis. Its $alpha_1$ adrenergic agonist activity causes vasoconstriction and decreases angioedema and urticaria. Its beta-adrenergic agonist actions promote bronchodilation and increase cardiac output. Epinephrine causes an increase in intracellular cyclic adenosine monophosphate (cAMP) concentration through adrenergically mediated activation of adenylate cyclase. Increased concentrations of cAMP have been demonstrated to inhibit both mast cell degranulation and the intracellular synthesis and release of leukotrienes and histamine. The dose and route of administration of epinephrine for the initial treatment of anaphylaxis are controversial. A generally accepted regimen consists of 0.1–0.5 mg of a 1:1,000 dilution (0.1–0.5 ml) of epinephrine subcutaneously. If the initial reaction is localized, part of this dose can be administered near the site of the reaction. In the presence of cardiovascular collapse, the IV route of administration is recommended. An initial dose of 5–10 μg (0.05–0.10 ml of a 1:10,000 dilution) of epinephrine IV can be given in incremental fashion followed by a continuous infusion of 1.0–4.0 μg per minute in adults. Epinephrine can be administered through an endotracheal tube if an IV access is not immediately available. IV epinephrine should be used cautiously in patients with ischemic heart disease.
5. **Antihistamines.** Histamine-1 (H-1) antagonists administered together with histamine-2 (H-2) antagonists will attenuate the cardiovascular effects of drug-induced histamine release H-1 together with H-2 antagonists can be administered as adjuvant therapy in anaphylaxis but should not be considered as the sole therapy since

histamine is not the only endogenous mediator responsible for the systemic effects in anaphylaxis. The dosages for these drugs are: diphenhydramine 50 mg or chlorpheniramine 10 mg IV and cimetidine 300 mg or ranitidine 150 mg IV.

6. **Glucocorticoids,** though unproved, may be effective for the treatment of anaphylaxis since they have been demonstrated to increase cellular responsiveness to adrenergic agents, inhibit mast cell and basophil degranulation, prevent leukocyte and platelet aggregation, and inhibit phospholipase A2, which is the rate-limiting step for prostaglandin and leukotriene synthesis. If the decision to administer glucocorticoids is made, they should be given early since their actions are often not observed until 4–6 hours after administration.

VI. Cardiogenic shock

A. Pathophysiology. Cardiogenic shock occurs when the myocardium is unable to generate a sufficient cardiac output to meet systemic demand. The hemodynamic state is characterized by hypotension with a decreased cardiac output. Left ventricular filling pressure, as measured by PAOP, is usually increased except in the setting of isolated right ventricular infarction, cor pulmonale, or massive pulmonary embolism.

B. Etiology. Acute myocardial infarction affecting greater than 40% of the left ventricle is the most common cause of cardiogenic shock. The mortality of this condition ranges from 85% to 100%. An isolated right ventricular infarction producing cardiogenic shock is relatively rare. Patients with left main coronary artery disease and reversible ischemia can present in cardiogenic shock. Ischemia-induced atrial and ventricular dysrhythmias, atrioventricular block, papillary muscle dysfunction, interventricular septal perforation, and myocardial rupture with cardiac tamponade can impair cardiac output further. Nonischemic causes of cardiogenic shock include valvular heart disease, proximal aortic dissection with acute aortic insufficiency (ischemia can occur in this condition if the dissection extents into the coronary ostia), extreme tachycardia or bradycardia, cardiomyopathies, hypertrophic obstructive cardiomyopathy (e.g., idiopathic hypertrophic subaortic stenosis), intracardiac masses or tumors, pericardial disease causing cardiac tamponade, congenital heart disease, or cardiac dysfunction following cardiopulmonary bypass.

C. Management of cardiogenic shock is based on medical or surgical correction of reversible etiologies contributing to the low cardiac output state, optimizing the hemodynamic state through the use of inotropic and vasoactive agents, the use of temporary ventricular assist devices, or cardiac transplantation. Intubation and mechanical ventilatory support are often necessary for patients in pulmonary edema. Invasive monitoring with arterial and pulmonary artery catheters is essential to guide diagnosis and therapy.

1. **Volume expansion** sometimes improves cardiac output. Maintaining intravascular volume and preload is especially important for patients with hypertrophic obstructive cardiomyopathy, cardiac tamponade, or an isolated right ventricular infarction.
2. **Inotropic agents** such as dopamine, dobutamine, amrinone, and epinephrine can be used in patients with increased left ventricular filling pressures and decreased cardiac stroke volume not responding to volume expansion. Inotropic therapy used together with vasodilating agents is an effective combination for patients with valvular insufficiency or dilated cardiomyopathies. Digoxin is generally not useful for acute management because of the risk of precipitating arrhythmias.
3. **Afterload reduction** is accomplished with vasodilators such as nitroprusside, nitroglycerin, captopril, or enalapril. Vasodilator therapy can be initiated alone when BP is adequate or in combination

with inotropic agents. This mode of therapy is particularly useful for increasing forward ejection in patients with aortic insufficiency or mitral regurgitation. Morphine in incremental doses alone or in combination with benzodiazepines to ameliorate pain and anxiety may be effective agents to reduce preload and systemic vascular resistance.

4. **The intraaortic balloon pump (IABP)** is useful for temporarily supporting the circulation while awaiting definitive therapy or the resolution of ischemia. The IABP is inserted percutaneously through the femoral artery or transthoracically into the ascending aorta through a surgical approach. It is inflated immediately after closure of the aortic valve to augment diastolic perfusion pressure and deflated just before the onset of systole to decrease afterload in synchrony with the ECG or arterial waveform. It is effective in separating from cardiopulmonary bypass in patients with poor left ventricular function, in the treatment of postoperative ischemia after myocardial revascularization, and in patients with ischemia-induced ventricular dysfunction awaiting surgery or balloon angioplasty. The IABP is sometimes used prophylactically in the perioperative management of patients with critical ischemic coronary artery disease undergoing noncardiac surgery. Complications of the IABP are frequent and include aortic perforation or dissection, lower extremity ischemia, arterial embolization, renal failure, hemolysis, and thrombocytopenia. The IABP is contraindicated in patients with aortic insufficiency or aortic aneurysms.

Selected References

Altura, B. M., and Schumer, W. (eds.). *Handbook of Shock and Trauma.* New York: Raven Press, 1983.

Barach, E. M., Nowak, R. M., Lee, T. G., et al. Epinephrine for treatment of anaphylactic shock. *J.A.M.A.* 251:2118, 1984.

Cheung, A. T., and Chernow, B. The Stress Responses to Critical Illness. In B. Chernow and I. D. Todres (eds.), *Critical Care Medicine: Cutting Edge Issues. Problems in Anesthesia* (Vol. 3), April/June, 1989.

Chernow, B. (ed.). *The Pharmacological Approach to the Critically Ill Patient.* Baltimore: Williams and Wilkins, 1988.

Harris, R. L., Musher, D. M., Bloom, K., et al. Manifestations of sepsis. *Arch. Intern. Med.* 147:1895, 1987.

Higgins, T. L., and Chernow, B. Pharmacotherapy of circulatory shock. *Disease-a-Month* 33:1987 (June).

Hoellerich, V. L., and Chernow, B. Shock: Vasoactive mediators and pharmacologic manipulation. *Probl. Crit. Care* 1:538, 1987.

Levy, J. H. Allergic reactions during anesthesia. *J. Clin Anesth.* 1:39, 1988.

Macciolo, G. A., Lucas, W. J., and Norfleet, E. A. The intraaortic balloon pump: A review. *J. Cardiothorac. Anesth.* 2:365, 1988.

Michie, H. R., Manogue, K. R., Spriggs, D. R., et al. Detection of circulating tumor necrosis factor after endotoxin administration. *N. Engl. J. Med.* 318:1481, 1988.

Rackow, E. C., Astiz, M. E., and Weil, M. H. Cellular oxygen metabolism during sepsis and shock. The relationship of oxygen consumption to oxygen delivery. *J.A.M.A.* 259:1989, 1988.

Sibbald, W. J., and Sprung, C. L. (eds.). *Perspectives on Sepsis and Septic Shock.* Fullerton, CA: Society of Critical Care Medicine, 1986.

Soreide, E., Buxrud, T., and Harboe, S. Severe anaphylactic reactions outside hospital: Etiology, symptoms and treatment. *Acta Anesthesiol. Scand.* 32:339, 1988.

Sprung, C. L., Caralis, P. V., Marcial, E. H., et al. The effects of high-dose cortiocosteroids in patients with septic shock. A prospective, controlled study. *N. Engl. J. Med.* 211:1137, 1984.

Weiz, M. H., Von Planta, M., and Rackow, E. C. Acute Circulatory Failure (Shock). In E. W. Braunwald (ed.), *Heart Disease*. Philadelphia: W. B. Saunders, 1988.

Zeigler, E. J., McCutchan, J. A., Fierer, J., et al. Treatment of gram-negative bacteremia and shock with human antiserum to a mutant *Escherichia coli*. *N. Engl. J. Med.* 307:1225, 1982.

11

Hypertension

William J. Hoffman and Lee Ann McGinnis

I. Hypertension defined
  A. Measurement of BP
    1. Riva-Rocci method
    2. Automated oscillotonometers
    3. An indwelling arterial cannula
  B. Determinants of BP
II. Etiology of hypertension
  A. Essential hypertension
  B. Secondary hypertension
    1. Pheochromocytoma
    2. Renal parenchymal disease
    3. Endocrine causes of hypertension
      a. Primary aldosteronism
      b. Oral contraceptives
      c. Cushing's syndrome
    4. Catecholamine excess states
      a. Pain and anxiety
      b. Hypoxemia and hypercapnia
    5. Other causes of hypertension
III. Hypertensive emergencies
  A. Hypertensive encephalopathy
  B. Intracerebral hemorrhage
  C. Aortic dissection
IV. Pharmacology of antihypertensive medications
  A. Central sympatholytic drugs
    1. Methyldopa
    2. Clonidine
  B. Adrenergic antagonists
    1. Beta-blockers
      a. Propranolol
      b. Labetalol
      c. Esmolol
      d. Other common beta-adrenergic blockers
    2. Phenoxybenzamine and phentolamine
  C. Vasodilators
    1. Hydralazine
    2. Sodium nitroprusside
    3. Minoxidil
    4. Diazoxide
  D. Calcium channel blockers
  E. Angiotensin-converting enzyme inhibitors
  F. Ganglionic blockers

Blood pressure is related to morbidity and mortality; however, there is no agreed-upon dividing line between normal and elevated BP. Adequate treatment of diastolic BPs above 105 mm Hg to less than 90 mm Hg significantly decreases morbidity and mortality. An increased systolic pressure with a normal diastolic pressure is also related to increased cardiovascular morbidity; however, the benefit from treatment of systolic hypertension has not yet been demonstrated.

I. Hypertension is generally defined as follows:

Females of all ages: Over 160/90 mm Hg
Males over 45: Over 140/95 mm Hg
Males under 45: Over 130/90 mm Hg

Systolic hypertension is defined as systole pressures greater than 150 mm Hg with diastolic pressures below 90 mm Hg.

A. Measurement of BP (see also Chap. 6)

1. **Riva-Rocci method.** Auscultation of Korotkoff's sounds is done with cuff deflation. This is the method on which epidemiologic data are based. This method of BP determination is based on the detection of **flow**, whereas a transduced arterial catheter reflects actual pressure, not flow. Small cuffs give falsely elevated readings.
2. **Automated oscillotonometers** are programmed to derive systolic, diastolic, and mean BPs. Some brands can determine BP at every minute. In conscious patients, such frequent measurement can be uncomfortable, and IV infusions in that extremity can become discontinuous.
3. **An indwelling arterial cannula** gives beat-to-beat pressure, which can be useful when hypertension is being treated with potent drugs.

B. Determinants of BP. The mean arterial pressure (MAP) reflects the pressure gradient caused by blood being moved through a vessel with a given resistance at a given flow. The flow is the cardiac output (CO), and the resistance is the systemic vascular resistance (SVR). The relationship to BP is:

$$BP = CO \times SVR$$

Thus, an increase in either CO or SVR will increase BP. Cardiac output and SVR are affected by the autonomic nervous system and the renin-angiotensin-aldosterone system. Increased sympathetic stimulation increases CO and SVR, decreases venous capacitance, and can induce renin release. Renin release resulting from beta-adrenergic stimulation, hypernatremia, or decreased renal perfusion leads to production of angiotensin II, a potent vasoconstrictor and stimulus for aldosterone production. Aldosterone then increases sodium and water resorption, increasing intravascular volume and thus CO.

II. Etiology of hypertension

A. Essential hypertension is the most common form of hypertension. Several studies point to genetic factors, stress, and diet as contributing to the development of essential hypertension.

B. Secondary hypertension

1. **Pheochromocytoma** is rare and accounts for less than 1% of patients with hypertension. Pheochromocytoma arises from the enterochromaffin cells of the sympathetic nervous system. The majority of tumors are located within one of the adrenal glands. Typical symptoms are palpitations, sweating, headache, and hypermetabolism. One of the most common signs during the examination is orthostatic hypotension, which results from depletion of volume. Other associated findings are polycythemia, glucose intolerance, cholelithiasis, constipation, and enhanced pressor responses. During attacks of the

disease, the patient's systolic pressure can exceed 300 mm Hg. The primary cause of death, if untreated, is cerebral hemorrhage.

2. **Renal parenchymal disease.** Chronic glomerulonephritis occurs in approximately 3% of hypertensive individuals. In children, acute infection from polynephritis is the leading cause of hypertension. Hypertension results from volume excess and renin-mediated vasoconstriction. Renovascular hypertension secondary to renal artery stenosis can be detected by measurements of renin levels. Treatment for patients with renovascular hypertension and unilateral disease is nephrectomy.
3. **Endocrine causes of hypertension**
   a. **Primary aldosteronism** is caused by adrenal adenoma or hyperplasia. Patients present with hypertension and hypokalemia. The diagnosis is difficult because most patients do not show both elevated sodium and decreased potassium, as well as muscle weakness and polyuria. Thus, these patients are difficult to differentiate from those with essential hypertension. The mechanism of hypertension is an expanded volume with reduced renin activity. Surgical treatment is indicated for patients with adrenal adenomas, and spironolactone and diuretic therapy is used for patients with adrenal hyperplasia.
   b. **Oral contraceptives.** These drugs are among those most commonly prescribed in the United States. About 5% of women using oral contraceptives develop hypertension. Incidence of hypertension increases with usage over time. Elevation of systolic and diastolic pressure is minimal, but it may become significant.
   c. **Cushing's syndrome.** The majority of patients with Cushing's syndrome have hypertension. The mechanism is cortisol excess leading to volume expansion due to salt retention and stimulation of renin secretion.
4. **Catecholamine excess states**
   a. **Pain and anxiety.** Endotracheal tubes, nasogastric tubes, chest tubes, bright lighting, sleep deprivation, and noisy monitors can cause considerable patient discomfort. In addition, surgical patients have obvious requirements for pain relief. The treatment of postoperative pain is covered in Chapter 12.
   b. **Hypoxemia and hypercapnia** should always be suspected in evaluating postoperative hypertension. Residual effects of narcotics, inhalation anesthetics, or muscle relaxants commonly contribute to postsurgical hypoxemia and hypercapnia. In addition, thoracic and upper abdominal incision decrease functional residual capacity (FRC), thereby inducing airway closure and hypoxemia.
5. **Other causes of hypertension** are preeclampsia, pregnancy-induced hypertension, coarctation of the aorta, severe burns, thyroid storm, and carcinoid syndrome.

III. **Hypertensive emergencies.** Hypertensive emergencies exist where severe hypertension is present and is aggravating an end organ system. These emergencies, which are rather uncommon, need to be treated immediately. Identification of hypertensive emergency is critical, and BP reduction takes precedence over time-consuming diagnostic evaluations. Common causes of hypertensive emergencies are acute myocardial ischemia, acute pulmonary edema, acute aortic dissection, acute renal insufficiency, cerebral vascular accidents, subarachnoid hemorrhage, thrombic cerebral vascular accidents, hypertensive encephalopathy, and eclampsia. Diastolic pressures may be fairly low—95–110 mm Hg—or quite high—above 130 mm Hg. Regardless of the absolute diastolic number, treatment is indicated. There are three common types of hypertensive emergencies.

A. **Hypertensive encephalopathy.** Patients with hypertensive encephalopathy commonly have essential hypertension. Cerebral edema occurs in these patients because of their lack of cerebral autoregulation. The signs and symptoms are variable and include severe headache, visual changes, paresthesias, hemiparesis, positive Babinski reflex, and seizures. Acute lowering of BP can result in cerebral cardiac or renal ischemia. Thus, BP must be reduced carefully over time.

B. **Intracerebral hemorrhage** is one of the most devastating aspects of hypertensive emergencies; the mortality rate is usually in excess of 75%. Normal cerebral vascular autoregulation usually occurs over an MAP range of 50–150 mm Hg. Cerebral blood flow is maintained as a constant over this pressure range by constriction and vasodilation of cerebral arterioles. This mechanism is lost in areas of hemorrhage, complicating the optimal level of BP reduction. Most authorities state that intracerebral hemorrhage is benefited by lowering the BP to prevent further bleeding. The choice of drugs in this situation is usually sodium nitroprusside or trimethaphan. Other drugs, such as labetalol, have been tried.

C. **Aortic dissection.** Usually patients present to the emergency room with severe pain in the chest, neck, or midback and/or with a host of other symptoms depending on which aortic branch has become obstructed. Acute aortic dissection can be stabilized by reducing the diastolic pressure to halt the extension of dissection. The treatment of choice is sodium nitroprusside or trimethaphan. Beta-blockers may be used to decrease myocardial contractility.

IV. Pharmacology of antihypertensive medications

A. Central sympatholytic drugs

1. **Methyldopa** has been a common agent and has been used for many years to treat hypertension. Methyldopa is converted to alphamethyl norepinephrine, and this molecule stimulates central alpha-adrenergic receptors, blocking the further release of norepinephrine. Thus, methyldopa lowers BP predominantly by reducing peripheral vascular resistance, causing little change in heart rate or cardiac output. The usual dose is 1–2 g per day, divided into 3 or 4 doses. Maximal hypertensive effects usually occur in 4–6 hours and persist for up to 24 hours. Common side effects are orthostatic hypertension in volume-depleted patients and sedation. Another adverse effect of methyldopa may be the development of a positive Coombs test. This usually occurs in patients who have been undergoing therapy for longer than 12 months.
2. **Clonidine.** Clonidine is an alpha$_2$-adrenergic agonist with pre- and postsynaptic action. The main antihypertensive action of clonidine occurs by presynaptic activation of alpha$_2$-adrenergic receptors, causing decreased release of norepinephrine and increased vagal stimulation. Patients also demonstrate lower levels of renin. The primary mode of action occurs in the CNS. Clonidine also activates postsynaptic alpha$_2$-receptors, and this most likely mediates the analgesic effects of clonidine. Clonidine becomes an appropriate drug in the postoperative ICU setting due to its antihypertensive and analgesic actions. Clonidine can be administered orally or as a transdermal patch. After oral administration of clonidine, peak plasma levels usually occur within 60–120 minutes, and the half-life of the drug is 8–12 hours. Therapeutic doses are commonly 0.2–1.2 mg per day. Common side effects are orthostatic hypotension with initial doses and sedation. Another problem with clonidine arises with acute withdrawal of the drug, which may preface life-threatening hypertensive crises due to a sudden increase in sympathetic nervous system activity. If the drug has to be stopped, it should be stopped gradually while other agents are being instituted.

B. Adrenergic antagonists

1. **Beta-blockers** antagonize the effect of catecholamines at beta-adrenergic receptors. The exact mechanism of how beta-blockers lower the blood pressure is not known. Beta-blockers inhibit the stimulation of renin release by catecholamines. There are other mechanisms for lowering BP besides decreased renin release, as demonstrated by patients with low renin activity. BP decreases primarily as a result of decreased cardiac output associated with bradycardia. With further therapy, cardiac output returns to normal as peripheral vascular resistance decreases.
   a. **Propranolol.** Propranolol is one of the most commonly used beta-blockers because of its low cost. Initial treatment usually starts with 60–100 mg per day in divided doses. Daily dosage can be increased up to 500 mg per day. Some of the side effects are constriction in patients with bronchial asthma and hypoglycemia in patients on insulin or oral hypoglycemic agents: $beta_2$ receptor stimulation causes bronchial smooth muscle constriction and prevents glycogenolysis during hypoglycemia. Propranolol may be administered intravenously starting with 1 mg and titrating dose to desired effect.
   b. **Labetalol** is an excellent choice for patients with hypertension because of its combined effect at both alpha and beta receptors. Labetalol blocks beta receptors to a greater extent than alpha receptors. BP is lowered by decreased systemic vascular resistance and a mild reduction in heart rate. Labetalol may be administered IV or orally. The initial IV dose is 5 mg and can be given in increasing incremental doses. Oral dosage of labetalol for control of hypertension ranges from 200 to 1,800 mg per day. The most common side effect is orthostatic hypotension. Nausea, vomiting, and fluid retention may occur with administration of labetalol.
   c. **Esmolol** is an ultra-short-acting beta-blocker. Its half-life is 9 minutes because esmolol is hydrolyzed by red cell esterases. An IV loading dose for esmolol is 500 μg per kilogram, followed by an infusion of 100–300 μg/kg/min. This drug is useful in the postoperative setting for states of increased sympathetic activity that may occur commonly after coronary bypass surgery or vascular surgery. Side effects are nausea, vomiting, headache, and dizziness.
   d. **Other common beta-adrenergic blockers** are atenolol, metoprolol, nadolol, pindolol, sotalol, and timolol. Atenolol and metoprolol have relative beta-receptor selectivity. All of these medications are given orally, except for metoprolol, which also is available as an IV preparation. The usual starting dose is indicated in Table 11-1. Common side effects are nausea, vomiting, diarrhea, sexual dysfunction, and insomnia.

Table 11-1. Starting doses for various beta-adrenergic blockers

Drug	Oral dose (mg)	Intravenous dose (mg)	Half-life (hr)
Atenolol	50–100	—	6–9
Metoprolol	100–400	5–15	3–4
Nadolol	80–320	—	14–24
Pindolol	15–60	—	3–5
Sotalol	80–320	—	8–10
Timolol	20–60	—	3–5

2. **Phenoxybenzamine and phentolamine** are nonspecific for the alpha$_1$-adrenergic receptor. These drugs are commonly used for patients with pheochromocytoma. The dosage for phenoxybenzamine usually begins at 10 mg PO, increasing to 160 mg per day in divided dosages. Phentolamine comes in an IV form of 5-mg ampules. A 5-mg IV bolus results in a dramatic decrease in BP; therefore, a continuous infusion is generally preferred. The usual dosage of phentolamine as an infusion is 30–70 μg per kg, which produces a prompt reduction in BP. Phentolamine is used as an IV infusion during resections of pheochromocytomas.

C. **Vasodilators**. Most vasodilators work by affecting the smooth muscle of the arterioles. Vasodilators should be used with other antihypertensive drugs to counteract the compensatory reflexes that occur with activation of baroreceptors.

1. **Hydralazine**, an arterial dilator, acts primarily on the coronary, cerebral, and renal vasculatures. The reflex tachycardia that often occurs with hydralazine can be countered by starting patients on beta-blockers. Hydralazine can be used in IV form in an initial dose of 5–40 mg. Therapeutic effects can usually be seen in 10–20 minutes after IV administration. Hydralazine comes in oral tablet form, with a usual dose of 100–200 mg per day, starting with 10–20 mg 2–4 times daily. Headache, nausea, dizziness, sweating, and palpitation are common side effects. In patients receiving in excess of 400 mg per day of the drug, a lupus-like syndrome may occur.
2. **Sodium nitroprusside** produces vasodilation of the arterial and venous system by its direct action on vascular smooth muscle. In normal patients, cardiac output and systemic vascular resistance decrease. In patients with congestive heart failure and an increased afterload, the cardiac output increases. Sodium nitroprusside is an effective medication for hypertensive emergencies where rapid control of BP is needed. The infusion rate of sodium nitroprusside starts at 0.1–0.2 μg/kg/min and should not exceed 10 μg/kg/min. An arterial line is needed on all patients to monitor beat-to-beat pressure with infusion of sodium nitroprusside. Infusion is prepared by placing 50 mg of the drug into 250 ml of a 5% dextrose solution. Because the drug decomposes with light exposure, the infusion bag must be covered with an opaque cover. Metabolism of sodium nitroprusside is by uptake into red cells and release of cyanide ions. The liver enzyme, rhodanase, converts cyanide ions into thiocyanate in the presence of sulfur donor groups. Finally, thiocyanate is eliminated by the kidney. With prolonged administration of sodium nitroprusside or renal disease, thiocyanate toxicity may develop. The symptoms of thiocyanate toxicity are nausea, vomiting, muscle spasm, tenderness, and psychosis. Maximum recommended level of thiocyanate is 100 μg per milliliter. Cyanide toxicity is an uncommon complication. Signs of cyanide toxicity are tachyphylaxis with an accompanying metabolic acidosis. Administration of thiosulfate (150 mg/kg over 15 min) is the recommended therapy for cyanide toxicity. With any signs of toxicity, sodium nitroprusside should be discontinued.
3. **Minoxidil** works as a vasodilator for prevention of hypertension. The primary mode of action of minoxidil is via decreasing systemic vascular resistance. Retention of fluid and salt occurs with the use of minoxidil; therefore, a diuretic should be used in combination with the drug. Initial dose is 1 mg given orally three times a day. Orthostatic hypotension or syncope can occur with the initial doses if more than 1 mg is given. Over the next several days, dosages can be increased to 20–40 mg per day, given in divided doses. The side effects of minoxidil are relatively infrequent—dizziness, palpitations, hirsutism, and headaches.

4. **Diazoxide**, a long-acting arteriolar dilator, causes a drop in MAP, which is accompanied by an increase in cardiac output and heart rate. The side effects are sodium and water retention and hyperglycemia. The administration of diuretics and beta-blockers reduces the undesirable hemodynamic side effects. The initial dosage of diazoxide is 75–100 mg IV. The drug can be administered every 5 minutes until the MAP is lowered. The effects of diazoxide last from 4–12 hours. The drug is excreted unchanged by the kidney.

D. **Calcium channel blockers.** By inhibiting calcium uptake in arterial smooth muscle vasculature, smooth muscle relaxation occurs and peripheral arterioles dilate. The major clinical use of calcium channel blockers is for treatment of coronary artery vasospasm, antianginal effects, cerebral artery vasospasm, and superventricular tachycardia. These drugs can be effective in the treatment of essential hypertension but offer no advantage over other antihypertensives. **Nifedipine** is probably the most commonly used antihypertensive medication. This drug can be used effectively in the ICU because it can be administered sublingually as well as orally. A sublingual dose of 10 mg can be repeated every 5 minutes to desired effect. Heart rate may increase from reflex sympathetic activation.

Nicardipine is a new calcium channel blocker that can be administered IV in an initial dose of 2 mg per minute over a 5-minute span, followed by an infusion of 200 μg per minute. Besides producing arteriolar vasodilation, nicardipine causes a small natriuretic effect. Diltiazem and verapamil are not usually used in the acute setting in the ICU for control of hypertension.

E. **Angiotensin-converting enzyme (ACE) inhibitors.** Captopril inhibits peptidyldipeptidase, the enzyme that hydrolyzes inactive angiotensin I to angiotensin II. Angiotensin II is an arterial vasoconstrictor and also stimulates the release of aldosterone. Captopril decreases systemic vascular resistance and has minimal effects on cardiac output and heart rate. ACE inhibitors not only are effective for patients with renovascular hypertension or patients with elevated renin activity but also have been found to be beneficial in patients with normal renin activity. Dosage should start at 12.5 mg orally, given in 3 doses per day, and increasing to a total of 50–150 mg per day. Severe hypotension can occur with the initial dose of ACE inhibitors. Side effects are acute renal failure, hypokalemia, nausea, and vomiting. Other ACE inhibitors available are enalapril and lisinopril. The effective dosage of enalapril is 5–10 mg once or twice daily. Enalapril may also be administered IV, with the initial dosage of 1.25 mg increasing to a total dose of 5 mg. Lisinopril is given in a daily oral dosage ranging from 10–80 mg.

F. **Ganglionic blockers.** Trimethaphan blocks ganglionic transmission in the sympathetic and parasympathetic system. By occupying postsynaptic receptors, trimethaphan prevents the release of acetylcholine by presynaptic nerve endings. Ganglionic blockade causes vasodilation, decreased venous return, and decreased cardiac output. Trimethaphan can be used in hypertensive emergencies because of easy titration and a short half-life of the drug. The initial dosage of trimethaphan is usually 1–4 mg per minute via infusion pump. An indwelling arterial line should be in place before starting the infusion. The drug may also be advantageous in situations where increased intracranial pressure is a concern since it is not a pure vasodilator. Side effects of trimethaphan occur secondary to effects on the sympathetic and parasympathetic system and include orthostatic hypotension, visual disturbances, precipitation of glaucoma, dry mouth, constipation, and visual disturbances.

Selected References

Blaschke, T. E., and Melmon, K. L. Antihypertensive Agents and Drug Therapy of Hypertension. In A. G. Gilman, L. S. Goodman, and A. Gilman (eds.), *Goodman and Gilman's The Pharmacological Basis of Therapeutics (6th ed.)*. New York: Macmillan, 1980.

Gilman, A. G., Rall, T. W., Nies, A. S., and Taylor, P. (eds.) *The Pharmacological Basis of Therapeutics* (8th ed.). New York: Pergamon Press, 1990.

Grossman, S. H., and Grinells, J. C. Recognition and Treatment of Hypertensive Emergencies. In C. Rackley (ed.), *Critical Care Cardiology*. Philadelphia: Davis, 1981. Vol. 11, No. 3.

Haber, E., and Slater, E. E. High Blood Pressure. In E. Rubenstein and D. D. Federman (eds.), *Scientific American Medicine*. New York: Scientific American, 1983. Vol. 1.

Husserl, F. E., and Messerli, F. H. Adverse effects of antihypertensive drugs. *Drugs* 22:188, 1981.

12

Pain Management in Critically Ill Patients

Alvin Morales

I. Physiology of acute pain
II. Chronic pain in patients in the intensive care unit
III. Modalities for pain control
    A. Pharmacologic intervention
        1. Parenteral narcotics
        2. Patient-controlled analgesia
        3. Nonparenteral intervention
    B. "Single-shot" techniques
        1. Intercostal nerve blocks
        2. Epidural and intrathecal techniques
        3. Other nerve blocks
    C. Catheter technology
        1. Intercostal catheters
        2. Epidural catheters
    D. Transcutaneous electrical nerve stimulation
IV. Benefits and risks of pain control
V. Conclusion

Patients in the intensive care environment sustain pain that may be considerable yet unrecognized or undertreated. Many have undergone major surgical procedures or have intrinsic medical states that significantly endanger their lives. Thus, many intensivists focus on stabilizing organ systems and relegate pain management to a secondary role in this setting. Pain management in the intensive care environment is complicated by the frequent inability of patients to characterize their pain. The experience of pain is highly variable and subjective. Moreover, patients who are intubated, under the influence of sedatives or muscle relaxants, or whose coexisting illnesses impair cognitive function are hardly able to voice their feeling of pain as a primary concern. Physicians must rely on indirect evidence of altered autonomic activity: increases in heart rate, systolic blood pressure, muscle tension, or perspiration. This chapter presents an overview of pain physiology in an intensive care setting. It reviews the common modalities of pain therapy in the ICU and some problems of under- and overtreatment of pain.

I. Physiology of acute pain

A. Acute pain begins with the noxious stimulation of somatic or visceral tissue. Tissue damage results in the release of algesic substances such as bradykinin, prostaglandins, histamine, or 5-hydroxytryptamine that bind to nerve endings known as nociceptors.

B. Two major types of nociceptors are the high threshold mechanoreceptors (HTM) and polymodal nociceptors (PN). HTMs respond to pressure and stimulate small-diameter, fast-conducting, delta-afferent fibers. Stimulation of HTMs results in an initial sharp pain that is highly localized and of short duration. PNs respond to pressure, heat, and algesic substances, and their afferents are predominantly slow-conducting, unmyelinated C fibers. This second and much slower dull pain mediated by PNs is poorly localized. Thus, noxious stimuli activate pathways that yield an initial sharp pain followed by a dull, aching pain. Primary afferent fibers originating from nociceptors eventually terminate in the various laminae of the dorsal horn in the spinal cord. The substantia gelatinosa, found within laminae I–III, is an important processing center of transmitted noxious signals. Some primary afferent nerve cells synapse on somatic motor neurons, sympathetic fibers, or both. Other afferent cells synapse on ascending secondary neurons responsible for central transmission of noxious stimuli. The spinothalamic tract contains secondary neurons that transmit noxious stimuli to the contralateral side and ascend to the thalamus. Tertiary neurons subsequently transmit these stimuli to somatosensory areas of the cerebral cortex. The spinoreticular tract contains the other major group of ascending secondary neurons that transmit noxious stimuli. It travels on both sides of the anterolateral spinal cord and sends fibers to the medulla, pons, periaqueductal gray area of the midbrain, the thalamus, and hypothalamus. The spinoreticular neurons mediate poorly localized, burning pain. The modulation of noxious stimuli utilizes a complex series of neurotransmitters. The most important are the endogenous opioid neurotransmitters, including beta-endorphin, enkephalin, and dynorphin. These neuromodulators are morphinelike in their analgesic quality; they bind to opioid receptors located throughout the limbic system, respiratory centers, substantia gelatinosa, and periaqueductal gray area. Their analgesic effect is supported by the Tamsen research (1982) that studied patients who had undergone major abdominal procedures and were allowed to self-administer small doses of meperidine. These patients demonstrated an inverse relationship between their preoperative cerebrospinal fluid (CSF) endorphin level and the mean plasma meperidine concentration required for them to achieve analgesia. That is, the lower the endorphin level found preoperatively, the higher was the required mean plasma meperidine level. Tamsen also found that substance P, which is thought to be an algesic mediator of pain, was elevated in a number of patients who required large doses of meperidine. Other mediators of pain were the neurotransmitters serotonin and gamma-aminobutyric acid (GABA). The acute postoperative pain of most patients in ICUs arises from direct somatic or visceral stimulation or from inflammatory changes in peripheral neural tissue that lower the excitation threshold of nociceptors. Somatic pain comes from activation of the mechanical, thermal, or chemical nociceptors already noted. This pain tends to be localized if it arises from superficial tissues. Localization is less clear if deep somatic nociceptors are stimulated in the muscles, ligaments, tendons, periosteum, or joints. Deep somatic nociceptors are activated by muscle contraction, stretching, ischemia, heat, or algesic substances. Visceral pain is much more diffuse and is provoked by spasm of smooth musculature, distention of a hollow viscus, traction or twisting of mesenteric tissue, chemical irritants, or inflammatory changes. Unlike somatic pain, visceral pain may be referred to cutaneous dermatomes corresponding to the spinal cord projections of the viscus. Mechanistically, branches of visceral fibers synapse in the spinal cord with afferent pain fibers from the skin. For example, a perforated duodenal ulcer causes diaphragmatic irritation and referred shoulder pain.

II. **Chronic pain in patients in the intensive care unit.** Although this chapter focuses on the management of acute pain in patients in the ICU, chronic pain, defined as a painful condition existing longer than 6 months, also appears in such patients. Many sick patients have preexisting pain overshadowed by nociceptive stimulation in the postsurgical period. A major group of chronic pain conditions is neurogenic pain, which includes neuralgias of peripheral or cranial nerves, neuropathies, radiculopathies, plexopathies, nerve compression or entrapment, and neuromas. Patients with cancer, for example, may exhibit neuropathic pain from compression of axons or other neural structures that produce an abnormal discharge pattern of these nerves. Neuropathic pain may arise as a secondary effect of chemotherapy, radiation fibrosis, or bone fractures at sites adjacent to a nerve root or from tumor compression of a spinal nerve root. Pain may come from nociception that has evoked abnormal motor and sympathetic reflexes. In such cases, patients develop painful skeletal muscle spasms or pain secondary to sensitization of nociceptors supplied by a compromised microcirculation. Other patients have deafferentation pain, which is characterized as an aberrant central interpretation of peripheral nerve impulses—for example, phantom limb pain. A few unfortunate patients, classically those who have suffered thalamic infarcts, exhibit central pain. Treatment response is poor, and neurosurgical intervention offers only modest benefit to such patients. Referral to a comprehensive or multidisciplinary pain service may help delineate the specific problems and offer suggestions on pain control for all of these conditions.

III. **Modalities for pain control**

A. **Pharmacologic intervention**

1. **Parenteral narcotics.** Narcotics in the ICU are most commonly given intravenously. Intramuscular injections have the disadvantage of slower onset, increased sedation, and intermittent gaps in analgesia. The advantage of immediate onset, complete absorption, and ease of administration makes the IV route ideal. Morphine sulfate is the prototype narcotic and has a peak onset time of 20 minutes, duration of 4 hours, and IV bolus dosing range of 0.05–0.2 mg per kilogram. It promotes cardiovascular stability in normovolemic patients but may cause histamine release with cutaneous changes when given in bolus

form. Other common narcotic choices used in the ICU are fentanyl, meperidine, hydromorphone, and methadone. Fentanyl has an onset time of 30 seconds, duration of less than 1.5 hours, but an elimination half-time almost twice that of morphine. Fentanyl's IV bolus dosing range is 0.5–2 μg per kilogram. Meperidine has a duration of action of 3 hours and a bolus dosing range of 0.5–2 mg per kilogram. Unlike most other narcotics that tend to lower heart rate, meperidine has an atropinelike effect. Meperidine may cause cardiovascular depression and CNS excitability. It may cause cardiovascular collapse if given concurrently with monoamine oxidase (MAO) inhibitors. Hydromorphone has a duration of 4–5 hours and an IV bolus dosing range of 10–30 μg per kilogram; it tends to produce more sedation and less euphoria compared to morphine. Methadone doses are the same as those of morphine, but it has a plasma half-life of 15–30 hours; it is an alternative drug when a true allergy to morphine exists. Of these narcotics, morphine and fentanyl are the ones most commonly given as continuous infusions for analgesia. Agonist/antagonist drugs are not used often in the ICU because they run the risk of precipitating withdrawal in patients with narcotic tolerance. In selected circumstances, agonist/antagonist drugs can provide analgesia while limiting the risk of respiratory depression and smooth muscle spasm, but this theoretical advantage is easy to overstate.

2. **Patient-controlled analgesia.** Patient-controlled analgesia (PCA) has gained increasing popularity in the intensive care setting. This system utilizes a computerized pump that allows the patient to self-administer incremental doses of narcotics over a specified period of time. The physician sets the dose volume (the dose the patient may self-administer), the lock-out time (the interval of time before the machine will allow another self-administration of narcotic), the basal rate (a continuous infusion), and the 1-hour or 4-hour limit of narcotic (a long-term protective mechanism). Patients must have intact cognitive and emotional function to allow proper use of the pump. Indications for its use include nearly any surgical procedure and a select number of medical conditions (e.g., sickle cell disease or an acute exacerbation of pancreatitis). Contraindications include an allergy to the available narcotics (morphine sulfate, meperidine, or hydromorphone), hemodynamic or pulmonary instability, psychosis, confusion, major depression or poor comprehension, violent or volatile behavior, active drug-seeking behavior, severe hepatic or renal dysfunction, or mechanical inabilities to push a button, such as bandaged hands, severe hand arthritis, or quadriplegia due to spinal cord injury at C4 or higher. The benefits include increased patient comfort secondary to a steadier narcotic blood level, more immediate pain relief, less patient anxiety awaiting the next analgesic dose, greater nursing flexibility, decreased sedation, and decreased incidence of atelectasis. Typical orders for PCA morphine sulfate include a demand dose of 1 mg, lock-out of 10 minutes, basal rate of 0.5 mg per hour, and a 1-hour limit of 7 mg. A loading dose of 2 mg of morphine q5min, titrated to effect, is sufficient for most patients. In some cases, PCA may be continued upon patient transfer to a medical or surgical floor.

3. **Nonparenteral intervention.** In some circumstances, nonparenteral administration of medicines may play a role in the management of ICU patients with pain. One may choose oral administration of maintenance narcotics when gut absorption is likely. This has the advantage of increasing the patient's sense of well-being and perhaps accelerating recovery. The disadvantage is an unpredictable absorption secondary to decreased gastrointestinal motility and first-pass

metabolism. Moreover, most oral maintenance narcotics—MS Contin (controlled-release morphine sulfate) (30 mg PO bid), methadone (5 mg PO tid), levorphanol (2 mg PO qid)—may require up to 24 hours for full effects. One may choose rectal administration of indomethacin (50 mg PRN tid) in select circumstances. Indocin, a prostaglandin inhibitor, decreases the inflammatory changes seen in postsurgical patients. On rare occasions, it may cause platelet, hepatic, and renal dysfunction.

B. "Single-shot" techniques

1. **Intercostal nerve blocks.** Intercostal nerve blocks are exceedingly useful in managing the pain of postthoracotomy incisions, rib fractures, neuritis, or acute herpes zoster and improving the impairment in pulmonary function caused by these conditions. The technique uses 0.5% bupivacaine with epinephrine (1 : 200,000) and, less commonly, 2% lidocaine with epinephrine. The toxic doses of these local anesthetics are 3 mg per kilogram versus 4 mg per kilogram for bupivacaine, without and with epinephrine respectively, and 4.3 mg per kilogram versus 7 mg per kilogram for lidocaine, without and with epinephrine respectively. One must pay close attention to signs of toxicity since even in the absence of intravascular injection, intercostal nerve blocks yield the highest blood levels of local anesthetics compared to caudal, epidural, or peripheral nerve blocks. Signs of progressive toxicity from local anesthetics include numbness of the tongue, lightheadedness, visual and auditory disturbances, muscular twitching, unconsciousness, and convulsions. Intercostal nerve blocks serve to anesthetize the lateral cutaneous division of the intercostal nerve that arises from the intercostal nerve in the midaxillary line. This block anesthetizes somatic but not sympathetic nerves.

   The patient is placed in the lateral decubitus or sitting position. The anesthetist makes indentations on the skin posteriorly using the hub of a needle at 7 cm from the spinous process at the most caudad palpated portion of the rib. The appropriate ribs are prepared and draped in sterile fashion, and the skin is infiltrated with 1% lidocaine using a 25-gauge short needle. This infiltration is continued in perpendicular manner, always heading for the lowermost border of the rib, using no more than 1–2 cc of local anesthetic per rib. A 1½-inch, 22-gauge needle is inserted similarly. Once rib is contacted, the needle is slightly withdrawn with the right hand, and the left hand is used to pull skin tissue and the needle caudad, always maintaining the direction of the needle perpendicular to the skin. The physician walks the needle tip off the rib, advances 2 mm, aspirates checking for air, fluid or blood, and, if clear, injects 2–4 ml of local anesthetic per rib. Bupivacaine 0.5% with epinephrine has an onset time of 6 minutes and duration of 7 hours or more. Occasionally the presence of edema or adiposity may prevent easy palpation of the ribs and require the use of a 1½-inch, 25-gauge needle to localize the rib. Intercostal nerve blocks have multiple risks. Hemorrhage can occur in patients with a prothrombin time greater than 15, platelet count less than 100,000, or bleeding time greater than 8 minutes. The risk of infection is minimized by not injecting through cutaneous lesions. Pneumothoraxes have an incidence of less than 0.5%; a negative aspiration test does not rule them out. Dural puncture can occur in some patients since the dural root sleeve extends laterally a variable distance. Systemic neurotoxicity typically occurs with intravascular injection; tachycardia or hypertension developing after injection of local anesthetic containing epinephrine may be the first sign of intravascular injection. Maximum recommended doses of local anesthetics can be seen in Table 12-1.

Table 12-1. Maximum recommended dosages of local anesthetics*

Agent	Plain solution (mg)	Solution with epinephrine (1:200,000) (mg)
Lidocaine	300	500
Bupivacaine	175	225
Tetracaine	100	200
Etidocaine	300	400

* In a given patient, the toxic dosage may vary from this table with variations in habitus and overall physical status. Dosages are based on injections for neural blockade in a healthy 70-kg patient and presuppose slow absorption consistent with such extravascular injection.

Table 12-2. Onset and duration of sensory blockade

Type of blockade	Approximate onset (min)	Approximate duration (min)
Brachial plexus		
Lidocaine 1% with epinephrine (1:200,000)	15	195
Bupivacaine 0.25% with epinephrine	25	610
Epidural		
Lidocaine 2% with epinephrine	5	150
Bupivacaine 0.5% with epinephrine	10	225
Intercostal (4 ml/nerve)		
Lidocaine 1%	5	160
Bupivacaine 0.5%	6	450

2. **Epidural and intrathecal techniques** (Table 12-2). The placement of local anesthetic and/or opiates in the epidural or intrathecal space may be utilized for pain control in the ICU. This technique is useful in postthoracotomy, abdominal, pelvic, aortic, major vascular, or orthopedic procedures. Epidural techniques are preferred over intrathecal because of a theoretically lower risk and severity of infection, lower risk of postdural puncture headaches, and less acute hypotension after using local anesthetics. Opiates act on intra- and supraspinal opiate receptors, and local anesthetics block axonal sodium channels and thus decrease nerve conduction. Local anesthetics when applied epidurally initially produce sympathetic blockade followed by sensory and motor blockade. The block is segmental and migrates in a rostral manner. Of the local anesthetics used in "single-shot" epidural techniques for pain control, 0.5% bupivacaine with epinephrine (6–9 ml) is preferred over 2% lidocaine with epinephrine (6–9 ml) because of a longer duration (6 hours versus 2 hours) and a more gradual onset with less hypotension. In either case, be prepared to treat hypotension with fluids and vasoconstrictive agents (ephedrine in 5–10 mg increments or phenylephrine by standard IV drip). Preservative-free morphine sulfate is the narcotic most commonly administered into the epidural space. Because of its hydrophilicity, it produces a nonsegmental effect and has a significant risk of rostral spread. Epidural morphine has a peak analgesic effect at 20–30 minutes and a duration of 8 to 18 hours depending on the bolus

range. As a rough approximation, an IV dose of morphine is equivalent to one-tenth the dose given epidurally and one–one hundredth the dose given intrathecally. Common side effects of epidural or intrathecal morphine are nausea and vomiting, pruritus, urinary retention, constipation, early respiratory depression (seen 2–3 hours after an epidural morphine bolus), and late respiratory depression seen 10–18 hours after an epidural bolus. Respiratory depression tends to develop gradually along with somnolence. The respiratory rate may not reflect the true minute ventilation, or more important, carbon dioxide retention. Nevertheless, impedance apnea monitors are the most common devices utilized for these patients. Pulse oximeters are also used but offer no warning of carbon dioxide retention. Nausea and vomiting may respond to droperidol or hydroxyzine and pruritus to Benadryl, although all side effects, including respiratory depression, generally respond to titrated doses of naloxone. Interestingly, reversal of side effects by low doses of naloxone may not decrease the analgesic benefit. An infusion of 5 μg/kg/hour of naloxone is a good starting point. One can mix 5 ampules of naloxone (0.4 mg/ml) in 195 cc of 5% dextrose in water to yield a concentration of 10 μg/ml. For a 70-kg patient, one may infuse this mixture at 35 ml per hour or higher, according to effect. As an intermittent treatment, patients without coronary artery disease may be treated safely with 0.1 mg of naloxone boluses q15min. Risk factors for late respiratory depression include an age of 70 years or older, intrinsic pulmonary disease, high lumbar or thoracic epidural placement, the supine position, a large epidural narcotic dose, or concomitant doses of parenteral narcotics or sedative medicines. Fentanyl and sufentanil are other commonly used epidural narcotics. They produce segmental analgesia as a result of their avid opiate receptor binding (i.e., their lipophilicity). Fentanyl and sufentanil sometimes produce truncal rigidity, with a higher incidence seen after sufentanil. Respiratory depression may occur, but there are no reported cases of late respiratory depression with either fentanyl or sufentanil. Either can cause nausea or vomiting, pruritus, urinary retention, and constipation. The epidural bolus dose of fentanyl is 50–100 μg in preservative-free normal saline to a total volume of 10 ml. For sufentanil, it is 12.5–25 μg in a total volume of 10 ml. The intrathecal bolus dose of fentanyl is 10–15 μg. The peak onset of analgesia for fentanyl is 10–15 minutes, and duration is 1–2 hours. Epidural blocks provide anesthesia and analgesia that spreads rostrally and caudally. Placing the needle at the middle dermatome where analgesia is desired reduces the local anesthetic and opiate requirement.

One begins by placing the patient in a lateral decubitus or sitting position. Using the iliac crest as approximating the body of L4 and the subscapular border as approximating the body of T7, the appropriate intervertebral space is identified. Using spinous processes as landmarks, an indentation is made into the lowermost border of the space. After a wide preparation and draping, the skin is infiltrated with 1% lidocaine using a 25-gauge needle and then a 22-gauge, 1½-inch needle, infiltrating slightly cephalad to a depth of 1 inch into subcutaneous fat and tissue. This infiltration allows the localization of the supraspinous and intraspinous ligaments and bony protrusions. A 17-gauge epidural needle (Weiss, Crawford, or Touhy) is advanced midline, angled cephalad at 15 degrees when approaching the lumbar epidural space and 5 degrees when approaching a thoracic space. The epidural space is identified by loss of resistance to air (in a well-lubricated glass syringe) or preservative-free normal saline. One carefully aspirates for cerebrospinal fluid or blood and notes paresthesias. A paramedian approach is used in the case of bony spurs that prevent midline entry or for structural reasons, as in the narrow intervertebral spaces above T7–8. With the epidural space identified, a test dose of 2 cc (2% lidocaine or 0.5% bupivacaine) will produce sensory anesthesia but not motor blockade; the latter would strongly suggest a dural puncture. One proceeds with either a one-shot epidural or continuous infusion via a biologically inert catheter.

Multiple complications can develop from epidural blocks. Clinical or subclinical dural puncture can occur and cause headaches. Post-dural puncture headaches are uncommon in patients older than age 50 years. The most feared complication is an epidural hematoma, which can occur in patients who are anticoagulated, have thrombocytopenia or platelet dysfunction, or have had an epidural catheter placed after an initial positive aspiration test for blood. Placement of catheters in the upper lumbar or thoracic interspaces also poses a risk of epidural hematoma. Although the incidence is small, vigilance with a diagnostic computerized tomography (CT) scan may help avoid irreversible paralysis; neurosurgical decompressive laminectomy is the definitive treatment. Epidural hematoma classically presents as severe central back pain with new and rapid onset of paralysis and bowel or bladder dysfunction. Cutaneous infections can occur in the face of poor aseptic technique or cutaneous lesions. Epidural abscesses, on the other hand, are extremely rare and most often occur in the presence of septicemia secondary to staphylococcus.

3. **Other nerve blocks.** Many prefer general endotracheal anesthesia for patients destined for an ICU. In some cases, however, regional techniques using long-acting local anesthetics may provide better ongoing pain control. Patients who have undergone knee surgery and receive femoral nerve blocks can move their affected limb and tolerate traction better. Patients who have undergone shoulder surgery may have significant pain on respiration relieved by brachial plexus blocks. Renal stones produce intense stimulation that may be relieved by epidural analgesia or lumbar sympathetic blocks. Acute herpes zoster may develop in immunocompromised patients. Sympathetic blocks, such as blocks of the stellate ganglion (intermittent or continuous), can relieve the pain and decrease the incidence of chronic postherpetic neuralgia.

   Patients with pain due to lower extremity reflex sympathetic dystrophy respond best to lumbar sympathetic blockade performed earlier than 6 weeks from the injury. The techniques for these blocks are not presented here but merit consideration and referral to a comprehensive pain service.

C. Catheter technology

1. **Intercostal catheter** placement allows continuous analgesia and improved respiratory function for postthoracotomy patients. In contrast to intercostal nerve blocks, fewer ribs are involved, and more local anesthetic is applied per rib. The technique requires identification of the seventh, eighth, and ninth ribs with planned placement of catheter under one of these, depending on the analgesic requirement.

   With the patient in the lateral decubitus or sitting position, an indentation is made at 7 cm from the midline in the upper portion of the rib. After sterile preparation, draping, and skin infiltration, a 17-gauge needle is advanced perpendicular to the rib so as to touch it with the bevel angled medially. While securing the skin and needle with the left hand and maintaining the 17-gauge needle perpendicular to the rib, the needle is alternately advanced and withdrawn slightly, bouncing off the rib until the needle slips off the lower border of the rib. The needle is advanced 2–3 mm, and it is checked for aspiration of blood, fluid, or air. If negative for these, an epidural catheter is advanced 4 cm through the needle, and the needle is withdrawn. A dry, sterile dressing is applied. After a test dose, a total dose of 20 ml of 0.5% bupivacaine without epinephrine is infused through the catheter. Analgesia lasts approximately 7 hours. This procedure is ideal for patients with existing chest tubes on the side of the catheter placement. The risks of intercostal blockade have been noted in **III.B.1.**

2. **Epidural catheters** allow continuous analgesia and differ from "single-shot" techniques that require careful management and labeling. The catheter is typically advanced 3–4 cm into the epidural space, with a rostral direction being most common in lumbar-placed catheters, even if the bevel direction is caudad. A large, nonocclusive skin dressing is typically placed over the entry site to permit inspection of the catheter for skin irritation, inflammation, blood, or fluid accumulation. Irritation may occur at 3–5 days and may necessitate discontinuation of the catheter. Surface-dried blood is common in patients who have been heparinized for an intraoperative procedure such as an aortic aneurysm resection. It is generally harmless unless it continues. Fluid accumulation most often represents leakage of the catheter secondary to the burrowing effects of the catheter on the skin and subcutaneous tissue or from microscopic catheter tears. Fluid leakage is rarely due to a CSF drainage, which would reveal itself by a dramatic response to the local anesthetic and opiate. Continuous epidural infusions require watching for side effects, catheter migration, and tachyphylaxis. The rapid onset of side effects, along with sensory and motor blockade, may suggest catheter entry into the intrathecal space. Some catheters migrate into epidural veins and others into foraminal structures, producing a unilateral block. In either case, the catheter may become nonfunctional. Over days, the local anesthetic effects will accumulate, and a sensory blockade may develop. If these problems are not recognized, a motor block may ensue. Thus, the infusion rate should be tapered. Interestingly, decubiti are rarely seen. Tachyphylaxis (resistance) to local anesthetics may develop in patients—typically those whose anesthesia is allowed to wear off. Tachyphylaxis can be confirmed by initiating a sensory or motor blockade via a short-acting local anesthetic given through the epidural catheter. This should be done while anticipating a possible sympathetic blockade and ensuing hypotension. Bolus treatment with local anesthetic may serve to resensitize nerves. Typical mixtures for epidural infusion utilize a total volume of 200 ml and are composed of preservative-free morphine sulfate 20 cc of a 1 mg per milliliter concentration, or fentanyl 40 cc of a 50 μg per milliliter concentration, or sufentanil 10 cc of a 50 μg per milliliter concentration. This is added to 100 cc of 0.25% bupivacaine; the difference of any of these three mixtures is completed with preservative-free, normal saline. For lumbar catheters the infusion rate starts at 5 cc per hour, and thoracic catheters start at 3 cc per hour. Morphine is not recommended through thoracic catheters. In some cases, epidural analgesia may be continued upon patient transfer to a surgical or medical floor. There are some additional advantages to epidural analgesia. Bromage (1980) found that thoracic epidurals are helpful in minimizing the decrease in forced expiratory volume in 1 second and vital capacity seen postoperatively. The benefits have been demonstrated in effort-related pulmonary function tests though their benefit is less clear in improving volume, such as functional residual capacity (FRC). The main advantages of thoracic epidurals, when compared to lumbar epidurals, are a more localized analgesia, decreased drug require-

ment, and improved tolerance of chest physiotherapy. In orthopedic procedures, epidurals have been shown to decrease blood loss and subsequently decrease the need for transfusions. There also appears to be a decreased incidence of thrombosis and thrombophlebitis, which may mean a lower risk for pulmonary emboli. Epidural analgesia decreases the risk for myocardial ischemia in susceptible individuals.

D. **Transcutaneous electrical nerve stimulation** (TENS) has been used effectively as an adjunct to pain management in the intensive care setting. TENS reportedly works by stimulating large myelinated A fibers that subsequently serve to suppress the activity and pain transmission of small unmyelinated C fibers. Melzack and Wall (1965) proposed the gate control theory, which claimed that a "gate" for pain transmission could be closed in response to electrical stimulation. TENS utilizes low-voltage, high-frequency (20–100 Hz) stimulation of involved nerves to achieve this goal. Indications for its use are not absolute, but patients who have significant sensitivity to narcotics from intrinsic pulmonary or cardiovascular dysfunction and those with chronic pain who have previously used it successfully seem to benefit most. The advantages relate to the negligible respiratory depression it causes, the ease in placement, and the overall decrease in narcotic requirement. The disadvantages are that pain relief may be only slight, lead placement may require some experimentation, skin irritation can occur, and patients with cardiac pacemakers may render the units dysfunctional, or vice versa. Placement of the leads over the carotid can produce significant bradycardia, and leads over the larynx can cause laryngeal occlusion. Consultation for a TENS unit is usually sought through a physical therapy department.

IV. **Benefits and risks of pain control.** Systemic narcotic administration is the most common mode of treating pain in the ICU and in the postoperative period. The vigilance required for the safe administration of these medicines has often led to their overcautious underuse. The general consensus is that physicians tend to undermedicate patients for pain. There is evidence that maintaining adequate analgesia in ICU patients accelerates recovery and decreases the incidence of postoperative complications. From a pulmonary standpoint, adequate analgesia serves to minimize the reflex contraction of expiratory muscles and splinting and reduces the incidence of atelectasis. Patients clear their secretions better and have a decreased incidence of postoperative pneumonias. Patients who have significant coronary artery disease or are otherwise at risk for myocardial ischemia benefit from adequate analgesia on at least two levels. Adequate analgesia helps to minimize anxiety and subsequently decreases myocardial stress, and it helps to break the cycle of catecholamine release during angina so as to decrease myocardial oxygen demand. Pain retards gastrointestinal motility, decreasing clearance of gastric contents, and leads to an unpredictable absorption rate of orally administered medicines. Pain and overnarcotization reduce patient activity and indirectly increase the incidence of thrombophlebitis. There is also some evidence that pain may impair immunologic function.

The benefits of providing adequate analgesia are often overshadowed by a fear of overdosing. Narcotization poses an acute risk from a pulmonary, cardiovascular, and neurologic point of view. Narcotization of gravid patients, those with obstructive or restrictive pulmonary disease, or those who have undergone thoracic or upper abdominal procedures will significantly increase their carbon dioxide retention and hypoxemia beyond an existing compromised state. Narcotization can inhibit cough and frequency of sigh so as to increase the incidence of alveolar collapse and poor clearance of secretions. Patients who are taking sedatives or other respiratory depressants, the elderly, and infants, particularly infants with a history of prematurity, are at increased risk. Significant hepatic or renal dysfunction may delay clearance of narcotics and pose another hazard: potential respiratory arrest. Patients with intracranial pressure are at risk from narcotization since an increase in PCO_2 leads to cerebral vasodilation. Narcotics can produce significant neonatal depression and must be used sparingly in the gravid patient.

Some concerns raised over the use of narcotics in the intensive care setting are more theoretical than practical. Some surgeons argue that narcotization may blunt the benefit of pain as a sensitive diagnostic barometer in certain medical or surgical states. For example, pain is useful in evaluating the patient with an acute abdomen, yet pain in isolation is rarely used diagnostically in this scenario. Narcotics are well known to increase the incidence of biliary smooth muscle spasm. At equianalgesic doses, fentanyl is the worst offender, with meperidine, morphine and pentazocine following. In general, the mixed agonist-antagonists appear to cause the least biliary spasm. Small, titrated doses of narcotics rarely lead to biliary spasm. Some physicians avoid analgesic doses of narcotics because of a theoretical risk of producing physical dependence. In fact, it is exceedingly rare for narcotic dependence to occur in the immediate postoperative period, the very time when the narcotic requirement is greatest. Physical dependence to morphine may require as much as 25 days of analgesic dosing, much beyond the perioperative course for most surgeries. Tolerance, on the other hand, can occur with increasing doses. Some patients have a high baseline narcotic requirement that increases in their postoperative course. Common examples are patients with extensive burns and those with cancer pain. These patients often fail to receive adequate analgesia. To the uninitiated, their doses may seem frighteningly high, and, thus, narcotic dosing may not be adequate. These patients may have their pain controlled, albeit with some predictable narcotic side effects. Nausea, vomiting, constipation, pruritus, urinary retention, sedation, euphoria or dysphoria, and respiratory depression are common; the last is less pronounced than expected. Other patients develop delirium, hyperalgesia, and seizures. Normeperidine, a metabolite of meperidine, has been implicated in inducing seizures. Fentanyl can produce truncal rigidity and muscular activity resembling seizures. Glucoronidation products of morphine are increased with high morphine dosing, and some of these metabolites are hyperalgesic (they increase the analgesic requirement).

V. **Conclusion.** Pain management in the intensive care setting presumes that postoperative pain is, to some degree, predictable and is expected to decrease as patients recover. Deviation from this natural progression should always alert the physician of a possible evolving surgical or medical condition. In this art and science, a differential diagnosis is evaluated while attempting to provide pain relief. Pain control can be achieved through basic pharmacology and simple procedures without destabilizing the patient's medical condition. Treating the pain of patients in the immediate postoperative period, as well as those with coexisting chronic pain, can be a challenge. In the long run, however, the effort is repaid by a faster and stronger psychological and physical recovery. In some patients who are terminally ill and not expected to leave an ICU, pain may be the overriding concern. Absence of movement or apparent consciousness does not exclude the presence of pain. Maintenance narcotic and sedating regimens are generally appropriate and humane. One must also treat the family, which may be concerned about the patient's pain and will seek comfort measures for their family member. Often the additional supportive and sympathetic tone of the medical staff provides the best medicine.

Selected References

Alexander, J. I., and Hill, R. G. *Postoperative Pain Control*. London: Blackwell Scientific Publications, 1987.

Bromage, P. R., Camporesi, E., Chestnut, D. Epidural narcotics for postoperative analgesia. *Anesth. Analg*. 59:473, 1980.

Chapman, C. R. Pain related to cancer treatment. *J. Pain Symptom Manag*. 3:188, 1988.

Cousins, M. J., and Bridenbaugh, P. O. (eds.). *Neural Blockade in Clinical Anesthesia and Management of Pain*. Philadelphia: Lippincott, 1988.

Dodson, M. E. *The Management of Post-Operative Pain*. London: Edward Arnold Ltd., 1985.

Fields, H. L. *Pain*. New York: McGraw-Hill, 1987.

Melzack, W., and Wall, P. D. *Pain Mechanisms: A new theory*. Science 150:971, 1965.

Raj, P. P. *Practical Management of Pain*. Chicago: Year Book Medical Publishers, 1986.

Stoelting, R. K. *Pharmacology of Pain*. Chicago: Year Book Medical Publishers, 1986.

Tamsen, A., Hartvig, P., Fagerlund, C., et al. Patient-controlled analgesic therapy, part II. Individual analgesic demand and analgesic plasma concentrations of pethidine in postoperative pain. *Clin. Pharmacokinet*. 7:164, 1982.

Wall, P. D., and Melzack, R. (eds.). *Textbook of Pain*. New York: Churchill-Livingstone, 1984.

13

Postoperative Care of Neurosurgical Patients

John D. Wasnick

- **I. General considerations**
  - **A. Ventilation**
  - **B. Hemodynamic stability**
    - **1. Hypertension**
    - **2. Hypotension**
  - **C. Fluid and electrolyte abnormalities**
    - **1. Hypovolemia**
    - **2. Hypokalemia**
    - **3. Hypernatremia**
  - **D. Neurologic examination**
  - **E. Other critical care issues**
- **II. Specific considerations**
  - **A. Intracranial aneurysm**
    - **1. Why?**
    - **2. When?**
      - **a. Vasospasm**
      - **b. Early versus late surgery**
    - **3. Where?**
    - **4. What?**
      - **a. Electrocardiogram changes**
      - **b. Hydrocephalus**
  - **B. Arteriovenous malformations**
  - **C. Intracranial mass resection**
  - **D. Carotid endarterectomy**
    - **1. Hypotension**
    - **2. Hypertension**
    - **3. Nerve damage**
    - **4. Regulation of breathing**
    - **5. Neck hematoma**
    - **6. Myocardial ischemia**
    - **7. Cerebral ischemia**
  - **E. Neurosurgical trauma**
    - **1. Managing intracranial hypertension**
    - **2. Coagulopathy**
    - **3. Associated injuries**

The perioperative care of neurosurgical patients reflects the principles and the practices of many medical disciplines. Elements of internal medicine, neurology, neurosurgery, neuroanesthesiology, and critical care medicine blend together in sharing postoperative patient management.

I. General considerations

A. Ventilation. Adequacy of ventilation is essential to the recovery of all postoperative patients. Following emergence from anesthesia the patient is evaluated by the anesthetist in regard to the patient's ability to protect his or her airway. An awake and ventilating patient may be safely extubated. A patient who remains somnolent, due to either residual anesthetic effects or neurologic injury, should be transferred from the operating room to the ICU intubated. Mechanical ventilation may be necessary in the postoperative period. Ventilatory settings should be made as described in Chap. 3. Frequently, patients are at increased risk for cerebral edema and increased intracranial pressure in the perioperative period. Elective hyperventilation may be instituted in this setting in an effort to decrease cerebral edema and intracranial pressure. Increased partial pressure of carbon dioxide can lead to cerebrospinal fluid acidosis. This change in cerebrospinal fluid (CSF) pH results in an increase in cerebral blood flow and potentially in an increase in intracranial pressure. Elective hyperventilation decreases CSF pH and results in decreased cerebral blood flow. In the immediate recovery period, the ventilatory pattern of the extubated patient must be carefully monitored. Changes in the pattern of breathing may reflect airway obstruction, narcotic effects, or postoperative intracranial mass effects. Any change in ventilatory pattern must be evaluated in the context of the neurologic examination.

B. Hemodynamic stability. Rigorous blood pressure control is essential in the perioperative management of neurosurgical patients.

1. **Hypertension.** Uncontrolled hypertension presents numerous risks to patients immediately following craniotomy. The blood-brain barrier is interrupted in areas of recent neurosurgical manipulation. Hypertension can produce potentially dangerous cerebral edema due to the lack of blood-brain barrier integrity. Hypertension may also aggravate postoperative bleeding in the event of inadequate surgical hemostasis.
2. **Hypotension.** Hypotension must also be avoided in postoperative neurosurgical patients. Hypotension can lead to inadequate cerebral perfusion in the setting of altered autoregulation of cerebral blood flow. Due to autoregulation cerebral blood flow (CBF) is relatively constant over a wide range of systemic blood pressures. Postoperative craniotomy patients may have areas in which cerebral autoregulation is impaired. Consequently, lower systemic pressures may lead to a decrease in cerebral perfusion pressure (cerebral profusion pressure = mean arterial pressure − intracranial pressure). Cerebral ischemia and infarction may result from impaired cerebral perfusion. Like other postoperative patients, neurosurgical patients are at risk for all of the systemic problems associated with uncorrected hypotension.

C. Fluid and electrolyte abnormalities. Neurosurgical patients are given furosemide and mannitol intraoperatively to facilitate surgical exposure. Mannitol creates an osmotic gradient across the blood-brain barrier, which results in the transudation of fluid from the brain into the intravascular space. Furosemide is given to augment the mannitol-induced osmotic diuresis. These fluid shifts, accompanied by surgical blood loss, may produce a number of postoperative fluid and electrolyte disturbances.

1. **Hypovolemia.** The goal of intraoperative fluid therapy is to achieve a

state of hyperosmolality and euvolemia. Profound hypovolemia should be avoided. Nevertheless, postoperative neurosurgical patients frequently present to the ICU with some degree of hypovolemia. Hypotension, tachycardia, and mild metabolic acidemia are signs of inadequate volume replacement. Should hypovolemia occur, the judicious administration of volume should be undertaken.

2. **Hypokalemia.** The osmotic diuresis results in the loss of potassium. Potassium supplements should be given postoperatively to correct hypokalemia and its associated metabolic alkalemia.
3. **Hypernatremia.** Osmotic diuresis results in a loss of free-water-producing hypernatremia. Postoperative diabetes insipidus can occur following pituitary surgery and severe neurologic injury. Diabetes insipidus occurs because of a lack of antidiuretic hormone. Hyperosmolality and hypernatremia may be treated by the administration of free water (D_5W). Guides for the specific treatment of diabetes insipidus can be found in Chap. 30.

D. **Neurologic examination.** The serial neurologic examination remains the cornerstone of monitoring in the neurosurgical ICU.

1. **Tests.** The examination should be easily reproducible and include tests of:
   a. **Motor.** The patient should be asked to show two fingers on each hand. Upper and lower extremity strength is assessed. Cranial nerves must be carefully tested.
   b. **Mental status:** orientation to person, place, and time
   c. **Recall**
   d. **Identification of objects**
   e. **Vision/pupil size**
2. **Assessment.** After examining the patient in the five areas listed, a rough assessment of neurologic status can be made. Deterioration in any particular area of examination could herald intracranial catastrophe. The serial examination may be altered to address specific concerns as warranted by the type of surgery performed. For example, following pituitary surgery, the visual fields are carefully followed due to the proximity of the optic chasm to the sella turcica. In neurovascular surgery, specific attention may be given to tests that reflect neural tissue at risk for cerebral ischemia. Thus, the patient having a left carotid endarterectomy who is left hemispheric dominant may develop right-sided hemiplegia and aphasia. This same patient having right-sided surgery could develop a left-sided hemiplegia and the signs of nondominant hemisphere impairment. Should any deterioration be noted by ICU personnel these changes must be communicated with the neurosurgical staff. Follow-up radiologic studies may then be ordered.

E. **Other critical care issues.** Much of postoperative neurosurgical intensive care focuses on the diagnosis and treatment of cardiopulmonary disease as with other patients.

III. **Specific considerations**

A. **Intracranial aneurysm.** The postoperative care of intracranial aneurysm patients reflects many of the medical issues seen in the preoperative care of subarachnoid hemorrhage. In approaching the specific concerns of intracranial aneurysm patients, four questions must be asked.

1. **Why?** Why has this patient been taken to surgery? Intracranial aneurysms present to the operating room in a number of ways. Most frequently, subarachnoid hemorrhage (SAH) leads the patient to angiography, at which time the aneurysm is discovered. Thus, the perioperative concerns in treating aneurysm patients who present in this manner center on managing the complications of subarachnoid hemorrhage. SAH is not the only occurrence that leads to the discovery of an intracranial aneurysm. Seizures or other neurologic symptoms

may uncover the aneurysm before subarachnoid hemorrhage has occurred. The presentation of the intracranial aneurysm patient is important because the morbidity and the mortality from elective surgical clipping is less than 2% in patients operated on before SAH.

2. **When?** When did the SAH occur? The relationship between the timing of intracranial aneurysm surgery and SAH remains controversial. In the past, aneurysm clipping was delayed for upwards of 14 days following the ictus because early efforts at clipping immediately following SAH were complicated by cerebral edema and vasospasm. New anesthetic and surgical techniques have permitted a renewed interest in aneurysm clipping within the first 24 hours following SAH. The time course of surgery is important in managing the postoperative complications of aneurysm clipping. Much of the morbidity and the mortality of SAH occur between days 3 and 14 postictus. Patients are at risk for cerebral artery vasospasm at this time.
   a. **Vasospasm.** Vasospasm is the narrowing in the lumen of major cerebral arteries that occurs for unknown reasons following SAH. Significant morbidity and mortality result from the cerebral ischemia produced as a consequence of the vasospasm-induced reduction in cerebral blood flow. Up to 40% of patients who survive the initial bleed suffer some form of vasospasm. Because of the time course of vasospasm, the patient taken to surgery within 24 hours of the ictus may present with vasospasm during the postoperative recovery period.
      (1) **Diagnosis.** The diagnosis of vasospasm is made angiographically by demonstrating lumenal narrowing of the major cerebral arteries. The diagnosis is often empirically made when SAH patients show a deterioration in neurologic function during the third to fourteenth day postictus and there is no computed tomography (CT) evidence of rebleed or hydrocephalus.
      (2) **Therapy.** Treatments of vasospasm are controversial. Two approaches are taken to improve cerebral blood flow: Vasodilators are employed to dilate spastic vessels, and induced hypertension is designed to augment cerebral blood flow in areas of impaired autoregulation.
         (a) **Vasodilators.** Nimodipine is a calcium channel antagonist that crosses the blood-brain barrier. It is employed to dilate cerebral arteries and improve cerebral blood flow. Nimodipine may act by preventing calcium from entering ischemic cells. This protects against vasospasm induced neuronal ischemia. Nimodipine therapy in the perioperative period is associated with increased volume requirements, decreased hemodynamic responses to noxious stimuli, and decreased requirements for hypotensive agents. Intravenous nitroglycerin has been used as vasodilator therapy for vasospasm. In vasospasm unresponsive to medical therapy, cerebral artery angioplasty may be attempted.
         (b) **Volume augmentation and induced hypertension.** Following SAH, autoregulation of cerebral blood flow is impaired. Under these conditions, increasing the systemic BP produces an increase in cerebral blood flow. Elevation of BP with vasopressors and volume is now used as a therapy for vasospasm. In patients with coronary artery disease and congestive heart failure, close hemodynamic monitoring with a pulmonary artery catheter is warranted when treating vasospasm by induced hypertension.
   b. **Early versus late surgery.** Induced hypertension improves cerebral perfusion in the setting of vasospasm. Of course, the elevation

of BP in the patient with an unclipped aneurysm places the patient at an increased risk from aneurysmal rupture. By undergoing early surgery, within 24 hours of the ictus, the patient may have the aneurysm clipped before the onset of vasospasm. Vasospasm that does develop may be maximally treated with vasodilators and induced hypertension without concern for rebleed.

3. **Where?** Where is the aneurysm? The location and the size of the aneurysm are important because this information gives some indication of what area of the brain is at risk for cerebral ischemia following placement of the occlusive clip. Ideally the aneurysm is isolated from the parent artery by placement of an occlusive clip about the neck of the aneurysm. Infrequently, these clips may cut off flow to areas of the brain supplied by branches of the parent artery. Should blood flow be occluded, cerebral ischemia/infarction may occur.
4. **What?** What other systems are altered by SAH?
   a. **Electrocardiogram changes.** Following intracranial catastrophes, varying changes in the ECG may appear. Changes include ST-T segment abnormalities, alterations in the T wave, appearance of U waves, varying forms of ectopy, and heart block. Studies have failed to demonstrate any increase in cardiac enzymes associated with these changes. However, patients at risk for SAH are also in the same population at risk for coronary artery disease. If hemodynamic instability develops in the SAH patient with ECG changes, close hemodynamic monitoring should be instituted. Echocardiography may be helpful to identify areas of ventricular dyskinesis in the setting of a questionable ECG.
   b. **Hydrocephalus.** Postoperatively patients may become increasingly somnolent. A CT scan aids in the diagnosis of the patient with decreased neurologic function. Bleeding and hydrocephalus will be detected by CT scan. In the event of intracranial bleeding, the patient will most likely require decompression and reexploration. Should signs of hydrocephalus be noted, a ventriculostomy may be placed to remove cerebrospinal fluid. The therapy for vasospasm was described in **2.a.(2)**.

B. **Arteriovenous malformations (AVM).** AVMs are intertwining collections of vessels with numerous arteriovenous connections found in varying locations in the CNS. Like intracranial aneurysm patients, AVM patients often present with SAH. Seizure may be the first symptom in up to 30 percent of AVM patients. The perioperative care of these patients is similar to that of aneurysm patients.

C. **Intracranial mass resection.** The postoperative care of patients following the resection of an intracranial mass reflects the general principles outlined at the beginning of this chapter. Special attention must be given following posterior fossa surgery because patients may develop altered patterns of breathing. This results from the close proximity of the surgery to the respiratory control centers in the brainstem.

D. **Carotid endarterectomy (CEA).** The principal concern in approaching the postoperative management of carotid endarterectomy patients is the realization that carotid occlusive disease is but one aspect of widespread atherosclerosis. Patients frequently have significant coronary artery disease and are at high risk for postoperative myocardial ischemia. Additionally, these patients often have long smoking histories and some element of chronic obstructive pulmonary disease. Sundt et al. (1975) have shown that a patient's risk of significant postoperative morbidity and mortality is related to his or her preoperative neurologic and medical condition. The goal in caring for post-CEA patients is to treat the preexisting medical conditions so as to minimize morbidity. Common problems seen following CEA include:

1. **Hypotension.** Hypotension occurs as a consequence of the carotid

baroreceptors' "seeing" a relatively higher BP than that which they sensed before removal of the carotid artery plaque. Therapy for postoperative hypotension should center on pressor support of the BP until the baroreceptors reset themselves. Patients following CEA are rarely hypovolemic, and volume is not recommended as a therapy for post-CEA hypotension. Indeed, excessive volume administration may place these patients at risk for congestive heart failure. Other causes of hypotension must be ruled out before attributing post-CEA hypotension to baroreceptor dysfunction.

2. **Hypertension.** Often CEA patients have a history of preexisting hypertension. Immediate control of the BP can be achieved with a number of drugs. It is imperative that the patient's baseline medical regimen be resumed at the earliest opportunity in the postoperative period.
3. **Nerve damage.** Surgical retraction can lead to damage of the cervical nerves, producing annoying paresthesias. Damage to the recurrent laryngeal nerve may also occur, leading to a vocal cord palsy. This is especially of concern in patients undergoing a second carotid endarterectomy. The potential exists for bilateral recurrent laryngeal nerve damage and postoperative airway obstruction.
4. **Regulation of breathing.** Oxygen sensors are located in the carotid bodies. Patients who have had bilateral carotid endarterectomies may be at risk for the loss of hypoxic ventilatory drive.
5. **Neck hematoma.** Postoperative bleeding into the neck can cause hematoma formation with airway obstruction and respiratory embarrassment. Stridor and complaints of dyspnea by a patient with a neck hematoma require emergent surgical attention. It may not be possible to intubate patients whose trachea is being compressed by a hematoma. Release of the hematoma may be necessary in order to secure the airway. The incision may be opened, allowing for release of the compressing hematoma. Beware in undertaking this action because the source of bleeding may be under arterial pressure, leading to exsanguinating hemorrhage. If time permits, such maneuvers should be undertaken in the operating room by the attending surgeon.
6. **Myocardial ischemia.** Myocardial ischemia is discussed in Chapter 8. It is important that the patient's baseline antiischemic regimen be started early in the postoperative period. Postoperative myocardial infarction is the leading cause of perioperative death.
7. **Cerebral ischemia.** Postoperative stroke may occur following CEA. The number of patients who suffer postoperative stroke varies from study to study and from center to center. Figures from 2–10% are usually cited.

E. **Neurosurgical trauma.** Head injury patients may range from closed head injury to decompression of subdural hematoma to widespread cerebral debridement. Postoperative care centers on:

1. **Managing intracranial hypertension.** The majority of patients will have intracranial pressure (ICP) monitors in place (see Chap. 14). ICP monitors are employed to guide medical therapy in lowering ICP and in watching for sudden increases in intracranial volume. Sudden increases in ICP may represent increased cerebral edema or intracranial hemorrhage. Therapeutic interventions designed to lower ICP are centered on decreasing the volume of the three components of the content of the intracranial vault.
   a. Cerebral blood volume
   b. Cerebrospinal fluid (CSF)
   c. Brain tissue. Therapy at decreasing ICP is aimed at reducing the volume of each of the component parts.
      (1) Cerebral blood volume by decreasing cerebral blood flow agents: hyperventilation and cerebrovasostrictors—barbiturates

(2) CSF: ventriculostomy

(3) Brain tissue edema: mannitol or furosemide

2. **Coagulopathy.** CNS injury can lead to the development of disseminated intravascular coagulation.
3. All patients with severe head trauma must be viewed as having other associated injuries. Abrupt changes in patient condition may be attributed to previously undetected associated injuries:
   - **a.** Cervical neck injury
   - **b.** Pulmonary/myocardial contusion
   - **c.** Aortic dissection
   - **d.** Abdominal trauma
   - **e.** Hip fracture
   - **f.** Long bone injuries

Selected References

Cafferata, H. T., Merchant, R. F., Jr., and DePalma, R. G. Avoidance of postcarotid endarterectomy hypertension. *Ann. Surg.* 196:465, 1982.

Fisher, C. M., Kistler, J. P., and Davis, J. M. Relation of cerebral vasospasm to subarachnoid hemorrhage visualized by computerized tomographic scanning. *Neurosurgery* 6:1, 1980.

Heros, R. C., and Kistler, J. P. Intracranial arterial aneurysm—an update. *Stroke* 14:628, 1983.

Hertzer, N. R., and Lees, C. D. Fatal myocardial infarction following carotid endarterectomy. *Ann. Surg.* 194:212, 1981.

Kassell, N. F., Boarini, D. J., Adams, H. P., et al. Overall management of ruptured aneurysm: Comparison of early and late operation. *Neurosurgery* 9:120, 1981.

Pine, R., Avellone, J. C., Hoffman, M., et al. Control of postcarotid endarterectomy hypotension with baroreceptor blockade. *Am. J. Surg.* 147:763, 1984.

Ropper, A. H., and Kennedy, S. K. Postoperative Neurosurgical Care. In A. H. Ropper and S. K. Kennedy (eds.), *Neurologic and Neurosurgical Intensive Care.* Rockville, MD: Aspen Publications.

Sundt, T. M., Jr., Sandok, B. A., and Whisnant, J. P. Carotid edarterectomy. Complications and preoperative assessment of risk. *Mayo Clin. Proc.* 50:301, 1975.

Wasnick, J. D., and Kennedy, S. K. Anesthesia for Cerebrovascular Surgery. In M. P. Yeager and D. P. Glass (eds.), *Anesthetic Management of the Vascular Surgery Patient.* Norwalk, CT: Appleton and Lange, 1990.

14

Intracranial Hypertension

W. Andrew Kofke, Krishna N. Nirmel, and Allan H. Ropper

Intracranial hypertension frequently is the final pathway leading to cerebral death. This chapter reviews clinical situations where it tends to occur and options in management. In addition, intracranial pressure (ICP) concerns during management of nonneurologic conditions are discussed.

I. Background

A. **Anatomy.** The craniospinal space consists of the rigid cranial vault and the somewhat less rigid vertebral canal. The volume of the intracranial space is virtually constant and is divided by the tentorium into the supratentorial space and the posterior fossa. The intracranial space communicates with the vertebral canal via the foramen magnum. The spinal dura mater, not being closely adherent to the vertebral canal, can distend slightly at the expense of spinal epidural veins. Thus, the volume of the craniospinal space is nearly incompressible and nearly constant.

B. **Definitions**

1. **Cerebral perfusion pressure** (CPP) is the effective pressure of blood perfusing the brain. It is defined as mean arterial pressure (MAP) minus intracranial pressure (or central venous pressure [CVP] if higher). Normal CPP is 60–90 mm Hg.
2. **Intracranial pressure** is the pressure exerted by cerebrospinal fluid (CSF) inside the skull and can be measured by a variety of methods (subarachnoid bolt, ventriculostomy). Normal supine ICP is less than 10 mm Hg.
3. **Intracranial hypertension** can be defined as an ICP greater than 10 mm Hg, although 20 mm Hg is usually the pressure above which ICP-reducing therapy is escalated.

C. **Intracranial compliance.** Minor fluctuations in the volume of intracranial blood, tissue, or CSF are normally well tolerated, producing minimal changes in ICP. However, there is a critical volume at which minimal increases in intracranial volume will abruptly produce intracranial hypertension (Fig. 14-1). This critical volume will vary depending on the rapidity of the process. Experimental data suggest that a gradual increase in intracranial volume will shift the curve to the right, presumably due to egress of CSF, while in an acute increase in intracranial volume, there is not time for such diminution of CSF volume.

D. ICP is normally determined by the volume in the craniospinal space of CSF, brain tissue, and interstitial fluid and blood. In pathologic states, other masses also contribute to the ICP.

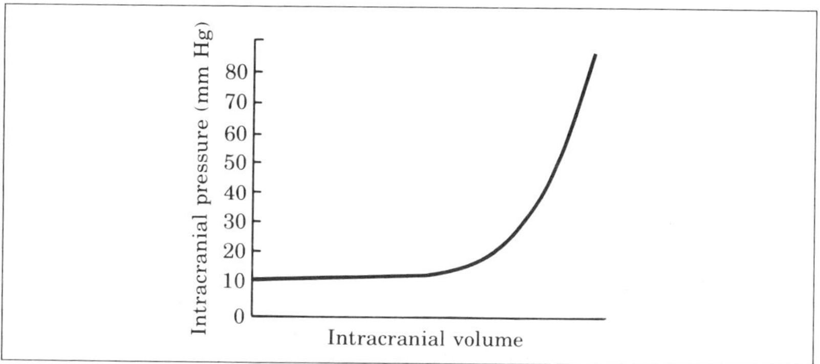

Fig. 14-1. Intracranial compliance curve. In the normal ICP range, increases in intracranial volume produce minimal changes in ICP initially. Further small increases in intracranial volume at the "elbow" of the curve, however, can produce an abrupt increase in ICP.

1. **Cerebrospinal fluid.** Under normal conditions, the balance between production and absorption of CSF determines the intracranial CSF pressure. Cerebrospinal fluid is produced predominantly in the choroid plexus at about 20 ml per hour and is absorbed via unidirectional valves in the arachnoid villi. The amount of CSF in the normal adult is 140–170 ml and normally occupies 10% of the intracranial volume. The entire CSF volume is exchanged 5 times a day. Cerebrospinal fluid production decreases with hypothermia and respiratory and metabolic alkalosis and decreases acutely with administration of acetazolamide, furosemide, ouabain, amphotericin, and vasopressin. Fluctuations in ICP do not affect CSF production, although increased ICP increases CSF absorption. Cerebrospinal fluid absorption can be impaired in several pathologic conditions, which include intracranial hemorrhage, central nervous system infection, and congenital malformations.
2. **Brain tissue volume** can vary with tissue-blood osmolar or hydrostatic gradients, leading to fluid shifts into or out of the brain. The volume of brain tissue and interstitial fluid increases, for example, with infections, tumors, or ischemia. Brain tissue normally occupies 80% of the intracranial volume.
3. **Cerebral blood volume** (CBV) changes reflect alterations in cerebrovascular resistance, which normally occur secondary to pressure or metabolic autoregulation of cerebral blood flow (CBF). In addition, cerebrovascular resistance can be altered by pathologic conditions or drug administration. Blood normally occupies 10% of the intracranial volume.
   a. **Pressure autoregulation** is the mechanism by which CBF is maintained constant over a range of perfusion pressures. With variations in BP, the autoregulatory range normally varies from a CPP of approximately 50–150 mm Hg. Thus, decreases in MAP or increases in ICP in addition to decreasing CPP per se may contribute to an increase in ICP secondary to vasodilation in brain areas with intact autoregulation (increasing CBV).
   For reasons that are unclear, the lowest CPP producing normal CBF may be lower with an increase in ICP than with a decrease in MAP.
   b. **Metabolic autoregulation** is the mechanism by which CBF is adjusted locally in response to focal variations in cerebral metabolic rate. Seizures wherein very high metabolic demands substantially increase CBF and CBV, can exacerbate intracranial hypertension.
   c. **Pathologic conditions** may blunt pressure autoregulation, decreasing cerebrovascular resistance and consequently increasing CBV. Such conditions include hypoxemia, hypercapnia, malignant hypertension, ischemia, trauma, extensive neurosurgery, and prolonged seizures. Increases in BP with such vasoparalysis can further increase CBV and exacerbate intracranial hypertension.
   d. **Drugs.** Cerebrovascular resistance is increased with barbiturates and decreased with vasodilators such as nitroprusside and nitroglycerin.
4. **Masses** such as a tumor or hemorrhage tend to increase ICP. Masses that arise gradually tend to be larger when intracranial hypertension develops than those that arise acutely.

E. **Interpretation** of ICP measurements
   1. Elevation of ICP should prompt consideration of the **cause.** There are four general causes of (or contributors to) intracranial hypertension:
      a. Mass lesions
      b. Hydrocephalus

c. Brain edema
d. Cerebrovascular dilatation

2. Intracranial hypertension reflects the brain's inability to compensate further for an intracranial space-occupying lesion. Ultimately, brain dysfunction arises because of decreased CBF secondary to decreased CPP or transtentorial, subfalcial, or foramen magnum herniation with focal brain compression.
3. The ICP waveform usually shows pressure variations with breathing and with each cardiac pulsation. The amplitude of the cardiac pulsation normally is approximately 1 mm Hg and increases with elevations in ICP.
4. Heterogeneities in pressure can exist within the craniospinal space. During expansion of mass lesions, CSF pressure transmission may be obstructed at the incisura and the foramen magnum, thereby dissociating supratentorial from lumbar spinal pressures. Whether supratentorial pressure heterogeneities exist is unclear as experimental data are conflicting. It is likely, however, that pressure within or immediately adjacent to a rapidly expanding supratentorial mass is higher than pressures in other supratentorial areas.
5. **Pressure waves** are rhythmic variations in ICP described as A, B, and C waves (Lundberg, 1960). Only the A waves are clinically significant.
   a. A waves are 50–100 mm Hg waves, lasting 5–20 minutes and occurring at variable intervals. When they are sustained and very high (e.g., 100 mm Hg), they are called **plateau waves** and are often associated with clinical deterioration. Plateau waves can arise spontaneously or may be precipitated by minor events such as increased mentation, muscular activity, pain, anxiety, and nursing procedures.
   b. B waves are sharper 50 mm Hg waves occurring at about 1-minute intervals. They can be associated with normal sleep or pathologically decreased levels of consciousness occurring at both high and normal ICP.
   c. C waves are up to 20 mm Hg waves, occurring about 6 times per minute and may indicate a decreased intracranial compliance. They usually occur in the presence of elevated ICP.

II. **Diagnosis.** The definitive diagnosis of intracranial hypertension can be made only by direct measurement of ICP (see Chap. 13). There are a variety of clinical situations and presentations in which it should be suspected.

A. **History**

1. **Symptoms.** Increased ICP should be suspected in a patient with a history of headache, nausea, vomiting, progressive drowsiness, or episodic blindness, especially when associated with a predisposing clinical situation.
2. **Clinical situations** where intracranial hypertension should be suspected include head trauma, intracranial hemorrhage, massive stroke, post–ischemic-anoxic encephalopathy, hydrocephalus, encephalitis, and intracranial neoplasia.

B. **Physical findings**

1. The **physical examination** can be variable. Serial physical examinations may reveal progression of the following abnormalities:
   a. Decreased level of consciousness
   b. Third nerve palsy (pupillary dilatation or asymmetry, decreased light reactivity)
   c. Alterations in the spontaneous breathing pattern
   d. Abnormal motor responses to noxious stimulation
   e. Papilledema (may lag temporally after the onset of high ICP)
   f. Sixth nerve palsy (mechial eye movement)

g. Abnormal oculocephalic or oculovestibular responses
h. Cerebellar fits (i.e., sudden opisthotonos, pupillary dilatation, and clonus—usually due to posterior fossa tumors)

2. The **Glasgow coma score** can facilitate recording and communication of trends in neurologic function (Table 14-1).
3. **Systemic effects** of intracranial hypertension may be present, including the following:
   a. **Systemic hypertension** occurs as part of the overall vasopressor response to intracranial hypertension.
   b. **Cardiac dysrhythmias.** Classically, bradycardia has been described. However, atrial tachyarrhythmias and ventricular ectopy can occur, especially when intracranial hemorrhage is present.
   c. **Electrocardiographic repolarization abnormalities.** Ischemic heart disease can be closely simulated with a variety of S–T-segment and T-wave abnormalities. Histologic examination has revealed subendocardial damage in some (but not all) patients (Weintraub, 1974). Such ECG abnormalities are associated primarily with subarachnoid hemorrhage.
   d. **Pulmonary edema** is an occasional concomitant of intracranial hypertension and probably reflects the intense sympathetic response that can occur.
   e. **Respiratory irregularities.** A variety of respiratory dysrhythmias can arise, including bradypnea, apneustic breathing, Cheyne-Stokes breathing, hyperventilation, and apnea.

C. **Computed tomography** can elucidate the cause of intracranial hypertension.

III. Monitoring

A. **Intracranial pressure.** The decision to institute ICP monitoring is a clinical judgment based on several considerations.
   1. **Clinical condition.** Decreasing level of consciousness, unconsciousness, or Glasgow coma score of less than 8 suggests intracranial

Table 14-1. The Glasgow coma scale*

Category	Score
I. Best motor response	
Obeys	6
Localizes	5
Withdraws (flexion)	4
Abnormal flexion	3
Extensor response	2
Nil	1
II. Verbal response	
Oriented	5
Confused conversation	4
Inappropriate words	3
Incomprehensible sounds	2
Nil	1
III. Eye opening	
Spontaneous	4
To speech	3
To pain	2
Nil	1

*Coma score = I + II + III.

hypertension. Intracranial pressure monitoring will confirm the diagnosis and allow safe, rational use of modalities that have the potential to raise ICP (e.g., positive end-expiratory pressure [PEEP], chest physical therapy, vasodilators) and prevent unnecessary use of some ICP-reducing therapies.

2. **Therapeutic modalities.** If aggressive pharmacologic or physiologic interventions are contemplated (e.g., barbiturates, high PEEP), ICP monitoring is essential.
3. **Risks of monitoring.** Risks of ICP monitoring are minimal and are related mostly to infection and technical problems with insertion and maintenance.

B. An **intraarterial cannula** facilitates frequent arterial blood gas measurements and maintenance of hemodynamic stability.

C. **Laboratory data** that should be followed include arterial blood gases, hematocrit, serum osmolality, electrolytes, blood urea nitrogen (BUN), urine specific gravity, weight, and blood glucose.

D. A **CVP or Swan-Ganz catheter** may help assess intravascular volume status as urine output in these patients may be unreliable due to diuretic administration or abnormalities in antidiuretic hormone secretion.

IV. **Therapy**

A. **General goals** in treating intracranial hypertension
1. Promote adequate cerebral oxygen and nutrient supply by the following:
   a. Maintaining adequate CPP
   b. Maintaining adequate arterial oxygenation
   c. Avoiding hypoglycemia and hyperglycemia
2. Prevent excessive increases in cerebral metabolic rate (e.g., fever, seizures) that can exacerbate intracranial hypertension.

B. **Clinical strategy**
1. **Exacerbating factors are avoided,** including the following:
   a. Fever
   b. Seizures
   c. Agitation, pain
   d. Use of central nervous system stimulants (e.g., ketamine)
   e. Hypercapnia, hypoxemia
   f. Coughing, vomiting, "fighting" the ventilator
   g. Hypotension, hypertension
   h. Hypoglycemia, hyperglycemia
   i. Hyponatremia
2. **The underlying cause is treated.**
   a. **For a mass:** early surgical resection or evacuation, if indicated
   b. **For hydrocephalus:** CSF drainage
   c. **For cerebral edema,** decrease brain fluid content with the following:
      (1) Hyperosmolar therapy
      (2) Fluid restriction
      (3) Diuretics
      (4) Avoidance of hypertension
      (5) Glucocorticoids
   d. **For cerebrovascular dilation,** decrease CBF (or prevent further increases) with the following:
      (1) Hypocapnia
      (2) Barbiturates
      (3) Avoidance of fever, hypertension, or central nervous system stimulation
      (4) Hypothermia

3. **Intracranial pressure is reduced.** Therapy aimed at decreasing volume of CSF and unaffected brain may be instituted. Hyperventilation and osmotherapy are the mainstays of such therapy, to which the following may be added:
   a. Glucocorticoids
   b. Loop diuretics and fluid restriction
   c. Best head position
   d. Barbiturates
   e. Lidocaine
   f. Cerebrospinal fluid removal
   g. Surgical decompression
   h. Hypothermia (rare)

C. **Therapeutic modalities** used primarily to decrease ICP

1. **Mannitol**
   a. Mannitol creates an osmotic gradient across the blood-brain barrier, effecting a decrease in overall brain size. Clinical effects can be expected within 15 minutes, lasting from less than 1 hour to several hours.
   b. Mannitol is useful as a temporizing measure when a rapid decrease in ICP is desirable pending definitive therapy (e.g., rapidly rising ICP or an acute herniation syndrome). Repeat dosages are frequently required to maintain serum hyperosmolality.
   c. Adverse effects of mannitol
      (1) Immediate transient systemic and cerebral vasodilation when given rapidly in high dosages
      (2) Transient intravascular hypervolemia followed by diuresis and hypovolemia
      (3) Electrolyte abnormalities
      (4) Hyperosmolar state
      (5) Possibly a rebound increase in ICP on discontinuation
      (6) Exacerbation of active intracranial bleeding
      (7) An increased risk of hypovolemia, hemoconcentration, hyperglycemia, metabolic acidosis, and renal failure with very high dosages (at osmolality >330–350 mOsm).
   d. For urgent treatment of intracranial hypertension, mannitol can be given 0.25–1.50 g per kilogram IV, followed by 0.25–0.50 g per kilogram every 4–6 hours as needed to maintain ICP within reasonable limits without exceeding a serum osmolality of 320 mOsm. Lower dosages require more frequent administration, although fluid and electrolyte abnormalities may be less problematic.
   e. The therapeutic end point for mannitol administration is a decrease in ICP to normal or unacceptable side effects (usually at osmolality >330 mOsm).
2. **Hyperventilation**
   a. Hyperventilation can acutely decrease CBF and CBV, thereby decreasing ICP. However, CBF ultimately returns to its original levels, possibly within 1–2 hours. It also decreases CSF production.
   b. Hyperventilation is useful in intubated patients when a very rapid ICP reduction is required. Manual hyperventilation can be used to treat plateau waves or can be used prophylactically prior to endotracheal suctioning.
   c. Adverse effects of mechanical hyperventilation
      (1) Complications of endotracheal intubation (see Chap. 1)
      (2) Hypotension
      (3) Paradoxically increased ICP due to increased cerebral venous pressure, although this is less pronounced with noncompliant lungs

(4) Alkalemia
(5) Decreased CBF
(6) Increased affinity of hemoglobin for oxygen
(7) Paradoxic CSF acidosis with increased CBF on resumption of normal ventilation
(8) Decreased seizure threshold

d. Hyperventilation may be initiated with manual ventilation, subsequently adjusting the ventilator to obtain a $PaCO_2$ of 25–35 mm Hg. The end point is a decrease in ICP or unacceptable side effects. Hyperventilation should be weaned over 12–24 hours, preferably with ICP monitoring.

3. Corticosteroids

a. Corticosteroids have a controversial role in the treatment of intracranial hypertension. They probably decrease brain swelling with vasogenic edema (e.g., with mass-occupying lesions).
b. Their use in head trauma is controversial.
c. Adverse effects associated with prolonged steroid use include immunocompromise, adrenal suppression, hyperglycemia, hypokalemia, metabolic alkalosis, fluid retention, impaired wound healing, psychosis, myopathy, gastric ulceration, and hypertension.
d. Dexamethasone (or another corticosteroid in an equivalent dosage) can be administered 4–20 mg IV q6h.

4. Furosemide

a. Furosemide and other loop diuretics may be useful for intracranial hypertension, possibly by decreasing edema and CSF production.
b. Furosemide is useful in the more prolonged therapy of high ICP. Its role is controversial, however, when acute ICP reduction is required.
c. Potential adverse effects include hypovolemia, azotemia, metabolic alkalosis, electrolyte abnormalities, nephrotoxicity, and ototoxicity.
d. Furosemide can be given IV, 10–20 mg, titrating additional doses q4–6h (or more frequently as needed).

5. Head position

a. Head elevation 30–45 degrees facilitates cerebral venous drainage, thereby minimizing the contribution of cerebral venous BP to ICP. Avoiding extreme turning of the head or extrinsic neck vein compression also facilitates cerebral venous drainage.
b. Head elevation is more likely to be useful with supratentorial lesions, although this is difficult to predict in an individual patient prior to diagnostic studies. Additionally, it may be useful with subarachnoid hemorrhage to facilitate blood drainage.
c. Adverse effects include postural hypotension and, with posterior fossa lesions, a paradoxic ICP increase.
d. Head position changes should be done slowly, with the transducer position adjusted to reflect the ICP accurately.

6. Fluid restriction

a. Fluid restriction maintains a high serum osmolality and decreases total body water, presumably decreasing intracranial water.
b. Adverse effects include hypovolemia with hypotension, oliguria, or azotemia.
c. Fluid restriction can be achieved by administering IV fluids at one-half to two-thirds of the usual maintenance requirements while maximally concentrating drug infusions.

7. Barbiturates

a. Barbiturates decrease ICP by decreasing CBF, cerebral metabolic rate, and seizure activity. Barbiturate coma will usually decrease ICP, although it will not necessarily be sustained.

b. Ultra-short-acting barbiturates such as thiopental or methohexital administered as IV boluses can be useful in the intubated patient to treat **acute** ICP increases, especially if associated with arterial hypertension. Boluses, however, will result in only brief ICP reductions. **Prolonged therapy** of intracranial hypertension refractory to conventional treatment requires a thiopental infusion or pentobarbital.
Barbiturates have the added advantage of decreasing the amount of mannitol needed and, because they blunt shivering, are useful adjuncts with hypothermia. They also can be used to blunt ICP rises due to suctioning and other nursing procedures.

c. Adverse effects of prolonged barbiturate use
   (1) **Unconsciousness.** The neurologic examination is lost. Pupillary light responses and brainstem reflexes may be obliterated, although unilateral pupillary dilation remains a dependable sign of brainstem compression. The electroencephalogram (EEG) may become isoelectric.
   (2) **Hypotension and respiratory depression.** Extensive nursing and ICU support is required, including CVP, ICP, and intraarterial pressure monitoring; endotracheal intubation and mechanical ventilation; and possibly circulatory support with fluids, catecholamines, or both.
   (3) **Alimentary tract dysfunction.** Parenteral nutrition may be required.
   (4) **Depressed thermoregulation.** Hypothermia can occur inadvertently.
   (5) **Physical addiction and acute tolerance** are theoretic possibilities.

d. Thiopental can be given IV, 1–4 mg per kg, repeated as needed to control ICP, subsequently infused (4 mg/ml infusion mix) and titrated to desired effects on ICP and BP.

e. Pentobarbital is administered for prolonged barbiturate coma. It can be given as a loading dose of 3–5 mg per kg over 30–60 minutes, followed by 1 mg/kg/hour as an infusion or in hourly boluses. Dosage requirements vary according to patient condition.

f. After the initial dosages of barbiturates have been administered, titration can be difficult. The EEG can be monitored, aiming for a burst suppression pattern, or serum levels can be measured, aiming for pentobarbital levels of about 30–50 μg per milliliter.

g. Discontinuance of barbiturate therapy is an individual decision that may be considered in the following circumstances:
   (1) There is no ICP decrease after the loading dosage and two consecutive hourly dosages.
   (2) Intracranial hypertension recurs at the maximal tolerated barbiturate dosage after an initial favorable response (escape phenomenon).
   (3) Intracranial pressure has remained less than 15 mm Hg for 48 hours.

8. **Lidocaine**

a. Lidocaine can decrease ICP by decreasing CBF and cerebral metabolic rate.

b. Lidocaine can be useful acutely to control intracranial hypertension when there is hemodynamic instability and barbiturate use is too risky. It is also useful prior to airway manipulations.

c. Lidocaine in high dosages can cause seizures or psychotic reactions.

d. Lidocaine can be given IV, 0.5–1.5 mg per kilogram, producing an effective serum concentration for several minutes.

9. **Cerebrospinal fluid removal**
   a. Patients with indwelling intraventricular catheters or lumbar drains can have CSF volume decreased by drainage through these devices.
   b. Cerebrospinal fluid drainage can be particularly useful with hydrocephalus, with acutely increased ICP unresponsive to other modalities, when side effects of other modalities are unacceptable, or with intraventricular or subarachnoid hemorrhage. With hydrocephalus, CSF can be continuously drained externally or into another body cavity.
   c. Cerebrospinal fluid cannot be reliably removed from a lumbar drain. In addition, this can produce a downward craniospinal pressure gradient with a herniation syndrome. Ventricular CSF removal, on the other hand, can produce an upward craniospinal pressure gradient with herniation (e.g., in some posterior fossa lesions).
   d. In the patient with acutely increased ICP, external CSF drainage can be performed by aseptically withdrawing 5–10-ml increments of CSF until ICP decreases or CSF drainage stops.
10. **Hypothermia**
   a. Hypothermia can decrease ICP by decreasing CBF, cerebral metabolic rate, and arterial BP. It is controversial and rarely used.
   b. A multitude of side effects is associated with hypothermia. These include hyperglycemia, increased peripheral vascular resistance, decreased cardiac output, ventricular fibrillation if too low a temperature is obtained (<92°F), increased blood viscosity, blunting of the febrile response to infection, depressed sensorium, the need for concomitant neuromuscular blockade or barbiturate coma to prevent shivering, increased affinity of hemoglobin for oxygen, acid-base abnormalities, EEG abnormalities, decreased gastric motility, and a rebound ICP increase on rewarming.
   c. Hypothermia is instituted by first paralyzing the patient or administering barbiturates to prevent shivering. Temperature is gradually reduced with an external cooling blanket. Hypothermia to 92–94°F can usually be safely achieved in the otherwise hemodynamically stable patient.
11. **Surgical decompression**
   a. A decompressing craniectomy involves opening the dura mater to convert the cranium from a closed to an open vault, allowing decompression and cerebral perfusion. Alternatively, internal decompression (i.e., resection of edematous brain tissue) may be done followed by skull closure. If a mass is the primary cause of the intracranial hypertension, craniotomy with resection of the mass may be the therapy of choice.
   b. Surgical decompression (in the absence of a resectable mass) is reserved for the patient refractory to other therapies.
   c. Adverse effects include those associated with the neurosurgical procedure and its anesthesia. Postoperative ICP monitoring may be unreliable and should be done from the contralateral side. The potential exists for herniation through a craniectomy.

V. Extracranial problems

A. **Systemic hypertension.** Intracranial hypertension may impair cerebral autoregulation such that MAP elevations can further increase ICP. The optimal BP with intracranial hypertension is difficult to ascertain; however, keeping the MAP at the premorbid level may be a reasonable goal. If a low CPP results, then whether to allow a higher MAP is controversial and must be decided on an individual basis. Neurologic considerations in utilizing antihypertensive agents (see Chap. 11) follow:

1. **Nitroprusside and nitroglycerin** can induce cerebral vasodilation, increasing ICP.
2. **Trimethaphan camsylate** has less potential than the vasodilators to increase ICP. It can induce **pupillary dilatation,** abdominal cramps, and prolonged ganglionic blockade.
3. **Hydralazine** can increase ICP. It has a slow onset time and relatively prolonged action (2–3 h), making it difficult to titrate and reverse.
4. **Methyldopa** may have less potential to increase ICP. It is difficult to titrate due to a slow onset time and prolonged effects and can further depress the level of consciousness.
5. **Propranolol** has minimal direct effect on CBF or ICP. It is moderately difficult to titrate IV due to its several-minute onset time and 1–6-hour duration. At very high dosages, it may further depress the level of consciousness. Labefolol similarly has minimal effects on ICP.
6. **Thiopental,** although not typically classified as an antihypertensive agent, can have its depressant hemodynamic effects plus its ICP-decreasing effects advantageously combined. Dosage and side effects are discussed above (see **IV.C.7**).

B. **Hypotension** may be defined as a MAP providing a CPP below 50–60 mm Hg or inducing signs of cerebral hypoperfusion. Patients with chronic systemic hypertension may show neurologic dysfunction at higher BPs because of altered CBF pressure autoregulation. Neurologic considerations in utilizing modalities used for hypotension follow:
1. **Catecholamines** have an unpredictable potential to increase cerebral metabolic rate and CBF. These effects are likely to be more pronounced as BP is increased above normal and in the presence of blood-brain barrier disruption.
2. **Excessive volume infusion** can potentially increase CSF production. Hypoosmolar solutions may exacerbate brain edema. Glucose-containing solutions may produce hyperglycemia, which may lead to a worse neurologic deficit after brain ischemia.
3. **Trendelenburg position** has the potential to increase ICP.
4. **If central venous access is required,** subclavian puncture-induced pneumothorax or carotid puncture can be catastrophic. Internal jugular puncture can cause an ICP rise when the head is turned to gain exposure.

C. **Pain** can increase CBF, and cerebral metabolic rate, and should be an important consideration with intracranial hypertension after trauma or postoperatively. Neurologic considerations in utilizing narcotics are the following:
1. Consciousness can be further depressed. If narcotic overdose occurs or if neurologic changes follow narcotic administration, naloxone can be carefully titrated IV to effect reversal.
2. Mean arterial pressure may decrease.
3. Respiratory depression can produce hypercapnia or hypoxemia.
4. If cardiorespiratory parameters do not change, narcotics may decrease cerebral metabolic rate and CBF.

D. **Hypoxemia and hypercapnia.** Minor degrees of hypoxemia or hypercapnia can have profound neurologic consequences with neurologic injury. Preventing or treating hypoxemia and hypercapnia is essential (although by no means straightforward) in these patients (see Chaps. 1, 2, and 3).
1. **Mechanical ventilation and PEEP**
   a. In general, higher mean airway pressures can have direct intracranial effects. Any maneuver increasing airway pressure such as larger tidal volume or higher PEEP may decrease CPP by increasing ICP or decreasing MAP.

b. As pulmonary compliance decreases, intracranial effects tend to be less pronounced.
c. In addition to direct mechanical effects, PEEP occasionally may increase physiologic dead space, thereby increasing $PaCO_2$.
d. "Fighting" the ventilator, agitation, and coughing can further increase ICP. After excluding new systemic abnormalities, these problems can be treated with one of the following:
(1) A trial of manual ventilation for 3–4 minutes. If successful, this can be followed by institution of intermittent mandatory ventilation (if not already in use) or a higher respiratory rate or tidal volume.
(2) Sedation or paralysis with mechanical ventilation, preferably in the intermittent mandatory ventilation mode.
(3) Allowing spontaneous ventilation if a rise in $PaCO_2$ is acceptable and ventilatory mechanics suggest that weaning from mechanical ventilation is feasible (vital capacity >16 cc/kg, negative inspiratory force $>30–35$ cm H_2O).
(4) Extubation, if the patient has a good gag and cough. This presupposes that the patient is stable and is otherwise ready for extubation (see **3.b.**).

2. **Chest physical therapy, turning, tracheal suctioning**
a. All of these essential maneuvers can increase MAP, ICP, or both.
b. Several interventions can minimize the ICP increase
(1) Timing pulmonary care to follow osmotherapy or other scheduled ICP-reducing therapies
(2) Pretreatment with 50–100 mg IV of thiopental or lidocaine (not more frequently than q1h)
(3) Small dosages of morphine (or other narcotic) prior to suctioning
(4) Neuromuscular blockade if ICP increases appear to be cough-induced (and the patient is being mechanically ventilated)

3. **Airway management** (see Chap. 1)
a. **Intubation** of the trachea can increase ICP.
(1) An indwelling arterial cannula is most useful to facilitate maintenance of hemodynamic stability with laryngoscopy.
(2) An "awake" intubation, with sedation, topical anesthesia, or both has the advantages of no residual CNS depression from IV drugs and no need for neuromuscular blockade. However, gastric fluid aspiration can still occur, and hypertension or coughing may occur.
(3) Endotracheal intubation under deep anesthesia offers the potential advantages of inducing minimal hemodynamic change and avoiding coughing. Disadvantages include CNS depression and the potential for severe hemodynamic instability, gastric fluid aspiration, hypoxemia, and hypercapnia.
(4) An experienced anesthesiologist should be present when intubating a patient with intracranial hypertension or hemorrhage.
b. **Extubation.** Prior to extubation, the following should be present:
(1) Adequate gag
(2) Adequate cough
(3) Level of consciousness consistent with airway maintenance and secretion clearance
(4) Maintenance of adequate gas exchange with spontaneous ventilation
(5) Resolution of the initial indication for endotracheal intubation.
c. Special caution with respect to extubation is required in some situations, which include the following:

(1) **Marginal level of consciousness.** The neurologic status should be stable. If improvement or deterioration is ongoing, extubation should be postponed. If the patient stabilizes neurologically at an intermediate level of consciousness with adequate gas exchange, gag, and cough, then a trial of extubation may be warranted with very close postextubation observation for inadequate gas exchange, aspiration, or inability to clear secretions.

(2) **Cervical spine fracture.** If cervical immobilization, traction, or both are still required to maintain vertebral alignment, extubation should be performed in the presence of an experienced anesthesiologist with a flexible fiberoptic bronchoscope at the bedside.

(3) **Abnormal intracranial compliance.** If there is still evidence of abnormal intracranial compliance (e.g., ICP > 10 mm Hg or altered level of consciousness), hypercapnia related to postextubation airway obstruction may produce an unacceptable increase in ICP. Close observation is thus required after extubation of such patients.

(4) **Airway trauma.** If the integrity of the airway is not certain (e.g., edema from burns or trauma), extubation should be performed in the operating room.

4. **Neuromuscular blockade** is occasionally needed to decrease oxygen consumption, facilitate endotracheal intubation, or prevent fighting the ventilator (which has not responded to narcotics). There are several agents available, all of which interfere with the neurologic examination.
5. **Hypothermia,** if used for hypoxemia, can supplement ICP-reducing efforts but can also result in ICP increases on rewarming.

E. **Fever** will increase cerebral metabolic rate, carbon dioxide production, and CBF, further increasing ICP. Normothermia should be maintained with acetaminophen or surface cooling with a fan or cooling blanket.

F. **Gastric hyperacidity.** These patients are under great stress and are often on steroids, which may increase the risk of upper gastrointestinal bleeding. Cimetidine may alter the neurologic examination and increase blood levels of drugs that rely on hepatic degradation to be eliminated.

Selected References

Aidinis, S. J., Lafferty, J., and Shapiro, H. M. Intracranial responses to PEEP. *Anesthesiology* 45:275, 1976.

Jafar, J. J., Johns, L. M., and Mullan, S. F. The effect of mannitol on cerebral blood flow. *J. Neurosurg.* 65:754, 1986.

Langfitt, T. W. Increased Intracranial Pressure and the Cerebral Circulation. In J. R. Youmans (ed.), *Neurological Surgery.* Philadelphia: Saunders, 1982. Vol. 2.

Lavyne, M., Wurtman, R. J., Moskowitz, M., and Zervas, N. Brain catecholamines and cerebral blood flow. *Life Sci.* 16:475, 1975.

Lundberg, N. Continuous recording and control of ventricular fluid pressure in neurosurgical practice. *Acta Psychiatr. Neurol. Scand.* 36: [Suppl. 149] 1, 1960.

Miller, J. D., Ecker, D. P., Ward, J. D., Sullivan, H. G., Adams, W. E., and Rosner, M. J. Significance of intracranial hypertension in severe head injury. *J. Neurosurg.* 47:503, 1977.

Muizelaar, J. P., Lutz, H. A., III, and Becker, D. P. Effect of mannitol on ICP and CBF and correlation with pressure autoregulation in severely head-injured patients. *J. Neurosurg.* 61:700, 1984.

Perloff, J. K. Neurological Disorders and Heart Disease. In E. Braunwold (ed.), *Heart Disease, A Textbook of Cardiovascular Medicine*. Philadelphia: Saunders, 1980. P. 1801.

Piatt, J. H., Jr., and Schiff, S. J. High dose barbiturate therapy in neurosurgery and intensive care. *Neurosurgery* 15:427, 1984.

Poungvarin, N., Bhoopat W., Viriyavejakul, A., et al. Effects of dexamethasone in primary supratentorial intracerebral hemorrhage. *New Engl. J. Med.* 316:1229, 1987.

Raichle, M. D., and Plum, F. Hyperventilation and cerebral blood flow. *Stroke* 3:566, 1972.

Rockoff, M. A., Marshall, L. F., and Shapiro, H. M. High-dose barbiturate therapy in humans: A clinical review of 60 patients. *Ann. Neurol.* 6:194, 1979.

Ropper, A. H., Kennedy, S. K., and Zervas, N. T. (eds.). *Neurological and Neurosurgical Intensive Care*. Baltimore: University Park, 1983.

Ropper, A. H., O'Rourke, D., and Kennedy, S. K. Head position, intracranial pressure, and compliance. *Neurology* 32:1288, 1982.

Ropper, A. H., and Rockoff, M. A. Treatment of Intracranial Hypertension. In A. H. Ropper and S. K. Kennedy (eds.), *Neurological and Neurosurgical Intensive Care*. Rockville, MD: Aspen, 1988.

Ropper, A. H., and Shafran, B. Brain edema after stroke. Clinical syndrome and intracranial pressure. *Arch. Neurol.* 41:26, 1984.

Rosner, M. J., and Coley, I. B. Cerebral perfusion pressure, intracranial pressure, and head elevation. *J. Neurosurg.* 65:636, 1986.

Shapiro, H. M. Intracranial hypertension: Therapeutic and anesthetic considerations. *Anesthesiology* 43:445, 1975.

Shenkin, H. A., and Bouzarth, W. F. Clinical methods of reducing intracranial pressure. *N. Engl. J. Med.* 282:1456, 1976.

Teasdale, G., and Jennett, B. Assessment of coma and impaired consciousness. *Lancet* 2:81, 1974.

Ward, J. D., et al. Cerebral Homeostasis and Protection. In F. P. Wirth and R. A. Ratcheson (eds.), *Neurosurgical Critical Care*. Baltimore: Williams and Wilkins, 1987.

Weintraub, B. M., and McHenry, L. K., Jr. Cardiac abnormalities in subarachnoid hemorrhage: A resumé. *Stroke* 5:384, 1974.

Woodcock, J., Ropper, A. H., and Kennedy, S. K. High dose barbiturates in nontraumatic brain swelling: ICP reduction and effect on outcome. *Stroke* 13:785, 1982.

Youmans, J. R. Cerebral Blood Flow in Clinical Problems. In J. R. Youmans (ed.), *Neurological Surgery*. Philadelphia: Saunders, 1982. Vol. 2.

15

Status Epilepticus

Debra Petrucci

I. Classification of seizures and of status epilepticus
   A. Grand mal status epilepticus
   B. Simple partial or focal motor status epilepticus
   C. Complex partial (psychomotor, temporal lobe) status epilepticus
   D. Absence (petit mal) status epilepticus
   E. Myoclonic status epilepticus
   F. Nonconvulsive status epilepticus
II. Etiology of status epilepticus
   A. Noncompliance or withdrawal from anticonvulsant medications
   B. Head trauma
   C. Neoplasms
   D. Cerebrovascular disease
   E. Central nervous system infections
   F. Drugs and toxins
   G. Metabolic and systemic derangements
III. Management of status epilepticus
   A. General measures
   B. Drug therapy of status epilepticus
      1. Phenytoin (diphenylhydantoin, Dilantin)
      2. Diazepam (Valium)
      3. Phenobarbital
      4. Paraldehyde
      5. General anesthetic agents
         a. Thiopental (Pentothal)
         b. Pentobarbital (Nembutal)
         c. Inhalation agents
      6. Other anticonvulsants
         a. Carbamazepine and clonazepam
         b. Lorazepam
         c. Valproic acid

Seizures represent abnormal neurologic function resulting from intermittent, excessive neuronal discharges that cause abnormal cerebral electrical activity and behavior. There are several etiologies of seizures. Epilepsy is a disorder in which there are recurrent seizures over months to years; if an underlying cause of seizures is known, then it is symptomatic epilepsy; if no etiology is evident, it is termed idiopathic. Status epilepticus refers to continuous seizure activity lasting greater than 30 minutes or the presence of repeated seizures in which the onset of the next seizure occurs before the patient recovers from the postictal phase of the previous seizure. There is no interictal return to consciousness. Status epilepticus can result in irreversible cerebral neuronal damage. Some animal models demonstrate that neuronal changes can result following only 30 minutes of prolonged seizure activity. The mortality of tonic-clonic status epilepticus is 3–20%. Therefore, status epilepticus is a medical emergency.

I. **Classification of seizures and of status epilepticus.** Table 15-1 gives the current classification of seizures. Status epilepticus can be classified as tonic-clonic (grand mal), simple partial (focal motor), complex partial (psychomotor or temporal lobe), absence (petit mal), myoclonic, and unilateral.

A. **Grand mal status epilepticus** is the most common and most life-

Table 15-1. Classification of seizures

Traditional terminology	New nomenclature
	I. Partial seizures (seizures beginning locally)
	A. Simple (without impairment of consciousness)
Focal motor; Jacksonian seizures (occasionally become secondarily generalized)	1. With motor symptoms
	2. With special sensory or somatosensory symptoms
	3. With autonomic symptoms
	4. With psychic symptoms
	B. Complex (with impairment of consciousness)
	1. Simple partial onset followed by impairment of consciousness, with or without automatisms
Temporal lobe or psychomotor seizures	2. Impaired consciousness at onset, with or without automatisms
	C. Secondarily generalized (partial onset evolving to generalized tonic-clonic seizures)
	II. Generalized seizures (bilaterally symmetrical and without local onset)
Petit mal	1. Absences
Minor motor	2. Myoclonic
Limited grand mal	3. Clonic
	4. Tonic
Grand mal	5. Tonic-clonic
Drop attacks	6. Atonic
	7. Infantile spasms
	III. Unclassified seizures (because of incomplete data)
	IV. Status epilepticus (prolonged partial or generalized seizures without recovery between attacks)

Rothner, A. D. *Recent Developments in the Treatment of Epilepsy.* Philadelphia: Borland-Coogan Associates, 1987.

threatening form of status epilepticus, responsible for one-third of all epilepsy-related deaths. These seizures are not preceded by an aura. The patient loses consciousness, and the body becomes tonically rigid in extension. There is often clonic jerking of the limbs, trunk, or face, and the patient may be incontinent of urine and feces. This tonic-clonic activity persists for longer than 30 minutes, or there may be repeated seizures occurring so frequently that a new attack begins before the postictal period of the preceding one ends.

Most cases of tonic-clonic status occur in patients with a known seizure disorder that is symptomatic rather than idiopathic epilepsy. Usually it is due to a structural or metabolic lesion such as tumors, posttraumatic injuries, CNS infections, strokes, and pre- or perinatal injuries. There is usually a definable precipitant to status in such cases. Noncompliance or withdrawal from anticonvulsant medications and fever are frequently causes in developing grand mal status epilepticus. Other causes are alcohol or drug withdrawal; metabolic disorders such as hyponatremia, hypoglycemia, hypocalcemia, or hepatic or renal failure; drug intoxication (e.g., cocaine, tricyclic antidepressants); or an acute CNS event such as trauma, stroke, or infection. The underlying cause of status must be investigated and treated in order to facilitate treatment.

B. **Simple partial or focal motor status epilepticus** is the second most common type of status epilepticus, usually the result of focal cortical pathology (such as an acute vascular or traumatic event) or metabolic disturbance. It involves rapid, focal, clonic movements of one part or one side of the body, often localized to the face and eyes or face and upper limbs. Consciousness is usually retained; however, impairment of consciousness and autonomic disturbances can occur. These seizures can become generalized. An aura generally precedes focal seizures. **Epilepsia partialis continua** is a type of focal motor seizure that involves myoclonic jerking of a discrete part of the body. Treatment is difficult since this type of status is often refractory to anticonvulsant medications.

C. **Complex partial (psychomotor, temporal lobe) status epilepticus** is rare. It is characterized by confusion and partial responsiveness, speech arrest or impairment, stereotyped automisms, and hallucinations.

D. **Absence (petit mal) status epilepticus** is characterized by altered consciousness, mild clonic movements of the eyelids and hands, and automatisms. These attacks can last 12 hours or longer. These seizures are more common in pediatric rather than adult patients. The typical electroencephalographic (EEG) pattern associated with this type of seizure is the 3 Hz spike-wave activity.

E. **Myoclonic status epilepticus** consists of bilateral rapid, irregular jerking movements of the body. Consciousness is variably affected. It is often the result of degenerative, hypoxic, toxic, or metabolic insults to the CNS.

F. **Nonconvulsive status epilepticus** involves behavioral disturbances ranging from mild confusion with stereotyped movements to near-complete unresponsiveness and mutism. It can result from continuous, partial, or absence seizures. An EEG is helpful in making the diagnosis.

II. **Etiology of status epilepticus.** It is important to identify and treat the underlying cause of seizures to facilitate their control. Head computed tomography (CT) and examination of the spinal fluid are helpful in trying to determine the etiological factor producing seizures. Table 15-2 summarizes causes of status epilepticus.

A. **Noncompliance or withdrawal from anticonvulsant medications** can result in status in a patient with chronic seizure history. It is essential to obtain such information.

Table 15-2. Causes of status epilepticus

Trauma
Fluid and electrolyte disturbances
Water intoxication, including syndrome of inappropriate antidiuretic hormone
Hypocalcemia and hypomagnesemia
Miscellaneous
ECT (bilateral or unilateral)
Pyridoxine deficiency or dependency
Multiple sclerosis
Eclampsia
Hypoxia
Hypoglycemia
CNS infections
Meningitis
Encephalitis
Brain abscess
Subdural empyema
Cerebrovascular disease
Venous thrombosis
Thromboembolic arterial occlusion

Aminoff, M. J., and Simon, R. P. Status epilepticus. Causes, clinical features and consequences in 98 patients. *Amer. J. Med.* 69:657, 1980; Pilke, A., Partinen, M., and Kovanen, J. Status epilepticus and alcohol abuse: an analysis of 82 status epilepticus admissions. *Acta Neurol. Scand.* 70:443, 1984.

B. **Head trauma** can result in immediate or delayed seizures. The more severe the head injury is, the more likely is the possibility of seizure, such as injuries resulting in brain contusion, intracerebral hemorrhage, prolonged unconsciousness, and skull fracture.

C. **Neoplasms,** especially tumors near or involving cerebral cortex, are epileptogenic.

D. **Cerebrovascular disease.** Cerebral emboli or thrombi resulting in ischemia can cause status epilepticus. Acute hemorrhages can also produce seizures. Vascular lesions such as arteriovenous malformations, especially if they involve cerebral cortex, often cause seizures.

E. **Central nervous system infections** such as meningitis, encephalitis, and brain abscess may cause status epilepticus. This is especially true in infants.

F. **Drugs and toxins.** Alcohol and drug withdrawal or drug overdose may present as myoclonic or grand mal status epilepticus.

G. **Metabolic and systemic derangements.** These seizures are often refractory to anticonvulsant medications until the underlying abnormality is corrected. Several such abnormalities producing seizures are hypo- and hypernatremia, hypocalcemia, hypomagnesemia, hypoglycemia, hypoxia, renal and hepatic failure, sepsis, shock, and drug toxicity.

III. **Management of status epilepticus.** Status epilepticus is an emergency requiring prompt, aggressive therapy (Table 15-3). The goals of acute management are intensive support of vital signs, identification and treatment of underlying cause of status, and correction of medical complications. Administration of a loading dose of a long-acting anticonvulsant medication is essential in the long-term control of seizures.

A. **General measures.** Assess and maintain adequate airway and vital signs. Endotracheal intubation may be necessary, particularly if respi-

Table 15-3. General therapy in treating status epilepticus

Airway oxygenation
Obtain baseline blood samples, including drug levels
Dextrostix estimation of blood glucose
Administer glucose intravenously
Pediatric dose: 1–2 ml/kg of 25% glucose
Adult dose: 50 ml of 50% glucose
Infusion of 10% glucose solution
Consider thiamine, 100 mg IV
Administer antiepileptic drugs
Administer bicarbonate if pH <7.2
Correct fluid and electrolyte disturbances
Consider corticosteroids
ECG and EEG
Specific treatment of etiology

Bleck, T. Therapy for status epilepticus. *Clin. Neuropharmacol.* 6:255, 1983; Bruni, J. Treatment of status epilepticus in adults. *Can. Med. Assoc. J.* 128:531, 1983.

ratory depressant drugs are administered for seizure control. Blood pressure should be monitored and supported as needed. An ECG should be checked. A large IV catheter should be placed for administration of fluids and drugs. Blood should be drawn for determination of electrolytes (especially sodium), glucose, urea, calcium, magnesium, anticonvulsant levels, and toxic screen. Rapid determination of serum glucose with Dextrostix is advisable and 50% dextrose IV quickly administered if hypoglycemia is found (1–2 ml/kg in children or 50 cc of 50% dextrose in adults). In adult patients who appear malnourished or are alcoholic, thiamine 100 mg IV or IM should be given prior to infusion of glucose to avoid the possible development of Wernicke's encephalopathy. An arterial blood gas (ABG) should be performed early for determination of oxygenation, acid-base status, and metabolic abnormalities. Sodium bicarbonate (100 mEq IV) is given if pH is less than 7.2 or if status has persisted for longer than 15 minutes and ABG results are not readily available. This is important since metabolic acidosis may prevent seizure control with anticonvulsant drugs. Hyperthermia is treated, especially in children. A Foley catheter may be inserted to relieve bladder distension (often these patients are incontinent). The patient should carefully be restrained, if necessary, to prevent physical harm. Bed rails should be padded and constricting clothing removed from around patient's neck.

The underlying factors precipitating status epilepticus must be diligently identified and corrected to facilitate seizure control and avoid the possibility of irreversible cerebral injury.

B. Drug therapy of status epilepticus. The principal goal of drug therapy for status epilepticus is cessation of seizures. It is unnecessary to achieve therapeutic drug concentrations with acute treatment. Careful monitoring of vital signs is necessary during administration of anticonvulsants, which can cause cardiac and respiratory effects. Endotracheal intubation may be necessary, particularly if Diazepam and phenobarbital are used, both of which can cause respiratory depression.

1. **Phenytoin (diphenylhydantoin, Dilantin),** considered the anticonvulsant drug of choice for treating status epilepticus, can be given IV and is rapidly effective. It does not cause respiratory depression or decrease the level of alertness.

a. Dosage and administration. The loading dose of phenytoin is 15–18 mg per kilogram over 20–30 minutes IV. It should not be given at a rate faster than 50 mg per minute (1 mg/kg/minute in children), or it can cause cardiorespiratory depression. If seizure activity persists despite administration of an adequate loading dose of phenytoin, a second drug should then be given rather than additional phenytoin, since excessively high levels of phenytoin can cause toxic seizures. The phenytoin level should be checked. A maintenance dosage of 300 mg per day is usually adequate for maintaining a therapeutic drug level.

b. Adverse effects. Intravenous phenytoin can cause hypotension, heart block, ventricular fibrillation, and cardiac and respiratory arrest. These serious complications can occur if the drug is given too rapidly. At toxic drug levels, drowsiness, nystagmus, gait ataxia, vertigo, nausea, and vomiting can occur. Allergic reactions are often manifested as a maculopapular dermatitis with fever and eosinophilia. If this occurs, the drug must be stopped. Rarely, phenytoin can cause blood dyscrasia with leukopenia and/or thrombocytopenia. Chronic effects include gingival hyperplasia and hirsutism. Phenytoin can interfere with vitamin B_{12} and folate metabolism and can accelerate vitamin D metabolism, resulting in hypocalcemia and elevation of alkaline phosphatase.

c. Drug interactions. Phenytoin serum level is increased with concomitant administration of Coumadin, isoniazid, disulfiram, chloramphenicol, benzodiazepines, phenothiazines, methylphenidate, ethosuximide, estrogens, phenylbutazone, and alcohol.

2. **Diazepam (Valium).** Diazepam is used as an adjunct in the treatment of tonic-clonic seizures. It has a rapid onset of action but a brief therapeutic effect, lasting 20–30 minutes. Initial administration of a long-acting anticonvulsant such as phenytoin is preferable. Diazepam is given when tonic-clonic seizure activity persists for several minutes while the loading dose of a long-acting anticonvulsant is being given, or if seizure activity recurs in a postictal patient's receiving a loading dose of a long-acting anticonvulsant. It must be given cautiously since it can cause respiratory depression.

a. Dosage and administration. Diazepam in 2.5–5-mg boluses is given IV every minute in adults. Children over 5 years of age may be given 1 mg every 2–5 minutes, to a maximum of 10 mg. A higher dose may be necessary initially for refractory seizures. Respiratory status must be monitored closely. A long-acting anticonvulsant medication is started. Intramuscular diazepam is absorbed slowly, and the drug should not be given IM to treat status. Rectally administered diazepam may be effective in treating status in children.

b. Adverse effects. The most serious side effects from diazepam administration are respiratory depression and hypotension. Repetitive dosing can affect level of alertness and even produce prolonged unconsciousness.

3. **Phenobarbital** is the second-choice drug in treatment of status epilepticus. It is the first-choice drug in patients with known allergy to phenytoin and patients with cardiac conduction defects. It may be the drug of choice in infants, children, and adolescents to avoid the adverse effects of phenytoin. Phenobarbital is used after a full loading dose of phenytoin in treatment of status should seizure activity continue. Respiratory status must be carefully monitored, and intubation may be necessary, especially if phenobarbital is used in combination with diazepam.

a. Dosage and administration. Adequate brain concentrations of phenobarbital are not achieved until about 30 minutes after IV injection. The anticonvulsant effect lasts several hours. The drug is given IV as a bolus of 90–120 mg in adults (5–10 mg/kg in children) and may be repeated every 10–15 minutes, to a maximum dose of 500 mg. A maintenance dose of 30 mg tid is usually required. The drug can be given IM, but this is not recommended for treatment of status because of the slower therapeutic effect.

b. Adverse effects. Intravenous phenobarbital can cause sedation, hypotension, and respiratory depression, especially when used with diazepam.

4. **Paraldehyde** is a potent but uncommonly used anticonvulsant. It can be given IV with rapid onset of action, but the safety of IV administration is controversial. Given IM, it has a therapeutic effect in 20–30 minutes. It can also be given rectally. It is felt that paraldehyde may be the drug of choice for treatment of alcohol withdrawal seizures.

a. Dosage and administration. Paraldehyde should be diluted prior to IV or rectal administration to a 5% solution in normal saline. A maximum dose of 0.1–0.15 ml per kilogram is given. Rectal paraldehyde is used mostly in children. It is diluted 2:1 in olive or cottonseed oil or in 200 ml of normal saline. It can be given IM up to 5 ml per injection site.

b. Adverse effects. Paraldehyde can potentiate metabolic acidosis that occurs during status epilepticus. It has been associated with acute pulmonary edema. It is a noxious drug that reacts with and dissolves plastic tubing and syringes; therefore, glass syringes need to be used. It can sclerose veins and when given IM can cause sterile abscesses. Gastric and rectal bleeding can result from oral or rectal administration, respectively.

5. **General anesthetic agents.** If tonic-clonic seizures are refractory to a full loading dose of phenytoin and phenobarbital and identified precipitating factors have been corrected, general anesthesia can then be induced. General anesthesia will prevent tonic-clonic activity and allow control of respiratory function. It decreases cerebral seizure activity and reduces cerebral metabolic demands. Short-acting barbiturates, such as thiopental and pentobarbital, are used in these cases. As a last resort, inhalational agents have been recommended for treatment of refractory status epilepticus.

a. **Thiopental (Pentothal)** is a potent, short-acting anticonvulsant with rapid central nervous system penetration. It has a half-life of 3–8 hours.

(1) Dosage and administration. Initial dose for treatment of status epilepticus is 25–100 mg IV. The usual dose for induction of general anesthesia is 2–5 mg per kilogram. Higher doses can be given until seizures are controlled or adverse side effects occur and cannot be controlled (e.g., hypotension, apnea). A continuous IV infusion (4 mg/ml mix) is used to maintain a therapeutic level, with the rate adjusted according to clinical and EEG results.

(2) Adverse effects. Thiopental causes respiratory and hemodynamic depression. Endotracheal intubation with mechanical ventilation and hemodynamic support with fluids and/or pressor agents may be required. It causes unconsciousness and suppresses the EEG.

b. **Pentobarbital (Nembutal)** is a potent anticonvulsant similar to thiopental but has a slower CNS penetration and a longer duration of action. It has a half-life of 21–42 hours.

(1) Dosage and administration. An initial dose of 50–100 mg IV is given. The dose is increased until seizure activity ceases or risk of adverse side effects is unacceptable. A continuous IV infusion of 2–3 mg/kg/hour is used to maintain a therapeutic effect. The drip is titrated to effect.

(2) Adverse effects. These are similar to thiopental (see **a.(2)**).

c. **Inhalation agents** are used as a last resort for controlling status epilepticus. An anesthesiologist must be involved in such treatment.

(1) **Isoflurane** has a rapid onset of action and can be stopped to allow neurologic examination.

(a) Dosage and administration. Isoflurane vapor is given via endotracheal tube with controlled ventilation, with incremental 0.25% increases in inhaled concentration until seizure activity stops or hemodynamic effects preclude further increases in concentration.

(b) Adverse effects. Hemodynamic effects include vasodilatation, hypotension, and variable heart rate.

(2) Other inhalation agents: **Halothane** can be used for treatment of status epilepticus but is not recommended. Higher doses than isoflurane are necessary for seizure control, and with such doses, it produces hemodynamic instability. Furthermore, halothane may increase cerebral blood flow and potentially increases intracranial pressure.

6. **Other anticonvulsants.** Several other drugs have been used in the treatment of status epilepticus.

a. **Carbamazepine and clonazepam** are useful for the long-term management of seizures. They cannot be given parenterally.

b. **Lorazepam** can be used instead of diazepam; it is a benzodiazepine with a longer duration of action but slower onset of action than diazepam. It is not approved by the Food and Drug Administration for treatment of status epilepticus; therefore, diazepam is the benzodiazepine of choice.

c. **Valproic acid** is used for chronic management of seizures. It can be given rectally with a loading dose of 17 mg per kilogram in a diluted solution as a last-resort treatment of refractory status epilepticus.

Selected References

Aircardi, J., and Chevrie, J. J. Convulsive status in infants and children. A study of 239 cases. *Epilepsia* 11:187, 1970.

Celesia, G. G. Modern concepts of status epilepticus. *J.A.M.A.* 235:1571, 1976.

Celesia, G. G., Messert, B., and Murphy, M. J. Status epilepticus of adult onset. *Neurology* 22:1047, 1972.

Delgado-Escueta, A. V., et al. *Status Epilepticus. Mechanisms of Brain Damage and Treatment.* New York: Raven, 1983. Vol. 34.

Ginsberg, P. L., Fischer, K. C., and Richey, E. T. Status epilepticus: clinical, electrical and therapeutic considerations in a general hospital population. *Neurology* 26:342, 1976.

Hantman, D., Rossier, B., Zohlman, R., and Schrier, R. Rapid correction of hyponatremia in the syndrome of inappropriate secretion of antidiuretic hormone. *Ann. Intern. Med.* 78:870, 1973.

Janz, D. Conditions and causes of status epilepticus. *Epilepsia* 2:170, 1961.

Kofke, W. A., Snider, M. T., Young, R. S. K., and Ramer, J. C. Prolonged low flow isoflurane anesthesia for status epilepticus. *Anesthesiology* 62:653, 1985.

Schwartz, W. B. Disorders of Fluid, Electrolyte, and Acid-base Balance. In P. B. Beeson and W. McDermott (eds.), *Textbook of Medicine* (14th ed.). Philadelphia: Saunders, 1975. Chap. 805.

Solomon, G., and Plum, F. *Clinical Management of Seizures, A Guide for the Physician.* Philadelphia: Saunders, 1976.

Wolpow, F. R. Neurologic Emergencies. In E. W. Wilkins (ed.), *Massachusetts General Hospital Textbook of Emergency Medicine.* Baltimore: Williams & Wilkins, 1978.

16

Acute Quadriplegia

Krishna N. Nirmel, W. Andrew Kofke, and Allan H. Ropper

Injuries to the spinal cord produce approximately 10,000 new para- or quadriplegic patients per year. Cervical spinal cord trauma produces significant physiologic alterations in many organ systems. Life-threatening problems can arise that include ascension of the lesion, respiratory failure, shock, hypothermia, and large decubiti. This chapter discusses management techniques that are important to circumvent or treat these and other problems related to acute quadriplegia.

I. Stabilization

A. Further injury to the traumatized spinal cord is avoided by maintaining normal body anatomy as closely as possible. The neck-cervical spine must be stabilized in some manner (e.g., Halo thoracic vest, Gardner-Wells tongs, or Crutchfield tongs) with 10–20 lb of traction. Surgery with anterior or posterior fusion of the spine with an external fixation device (e.g., Philadelphia collar, Halo thoracic vest) may be indicated.

B. Stabilization of the spine is continually observed in the ICU. Alignment is assessed with radiologic studies that include cross-table lateral cervical spine radiographs, usually taken with portable equipment.

C. The traction force is often reduced when neck muscle spasm secondary to the injury decreases and alignment is satisfactory. On rare occasions, quadriparesis resolves with adequate realignment.

D. Movement. While the patient is in traction, the head-neck-thorax is moved as a unit. This **log-rolling** requires two to three people. The Roto-Rest kinetic bed can be used to keep the patient in a stable position while automatically turning the patient at regular intervals.

II. Respiratory management. Adequate airway care and ventilation are essential.

A. Respiratory muscle weakness. With a complete cervical cord lesion, there is total paralysis of the intercostal muscles. With the lesion at or below C6, diaphragmatic innervation is intact; at C4 or above, diaphragmatic function is impaired because the phrenic nerve, from roots C3–C5, is damaged. Inadequate ventilation can then occur with decreased vital capacity, retention of secretions, poor cough, and decreased pulmonary compliance. In addition, diaphragmatic efficacy may be further compromised by paralytic ileus. This combination of problems may produce a requirement for endotracheal intubation and mechanical ventilation.

B. Chest physical therapy should be instituted early to prevent respiratory complications. A Roto-Rest kinetic bed can be quite useful, safely providing postural drainage. If a Stryker frame is used, a nurse should be at the bedside to observe for respiratory insufficiency while the patient is prone. In this position, the upper chest and pubis should be on pads to minimize abdominal pressure, thereby allowing diaphragmatic excursion. If conservative chest physical therapy methods are ineffective or if there is radiographic evidence of airway obstruction, therapeutic fiberoptic bronchoscopy should be performed.

C. The spinal cord lesion can ascend. A "low" quadriplegic can become a "high" quadriplegic with severe ventilatory dysfunction, requiring mechanical ventilatory assistance. Thus, the **unintubated acute quadriplegic requires close monitoring.** Ventilatory rate, forced vital capacity (normal 65–75 cc/kg), maximum negative inspiratory force (normal 75–100 cm H_2O), chest auscultation, and arterial blood gases are followed serially to assess trends. Vital capacity is initially checked hourly. If vital capacity is less than 15 cc per kilogram or there is difficulty clearing secretions, especially if trends suggest gradual ongoing deterioration, intubation should carefully be performed prior to frank respiratory failure. This can be done with the patient awake with adequate sedation and topical anesthesia while closely monitoring vital signs.

Nasotracheal or orotracheal intubation is performed, preferably utilizing a fiberoptic bronchoscope without extending or flexing the neck. Cricothyrotomy or tracheotomy is not usually necessary. The subsequent initiation of positive pressure ventilation in the presence of interrupted sympathetic reflexes may produce hypotension. This usually responds to IV fluid infusion.

D. **Pulmonary embolism** is a significant risk. Prophylactic heparin treatment (5,000 units sq q12h) is controversial because there is some suggestion that it, with steroid therapy, increases the risk of gastrointestinal hemorrhage. Regular examinations should be performed to detect signs of lower extremity phlebitis or deep vein thrombosis. Changes in vital signs, respiratory function, and general appearance should be noted. Diagnostic evaluation (e.g., ventilation-perfusion lung scan, lower extremity venogram, or pulmonary angiogram) should be initiated at the earliest sign of pulmonary embolism.

E. **Infection** (see Chap. 19). Surveillance must be ongoing for signs of infection. Unfortunately, the signs can be rather subtle in this patient population, as temperature may not rise as much as normal in response to infection and the white blood cell (WBC) count may be increased by concomitant steroid administration. Surveillance sputum Gram's stains and cultures obtained 2–3 times a week and chest radiographs obtained daily to weekly may provide the only clues of early infection. The trends in WBC counts can also be followed, a new rise suggesting a new infectious process.

III. **Cardiovascular management**

A. **Compromise of sympathetic outflow** from T1 to L2 spinal segments results from complete cervical cord lesions leading to a state of spinal shock, typically presenting with mild to moderate hypotension, bradycardia, and warm, well-perfused skin. Orthostatic hypotension occurs, which usually diminishes with time. Compensatory reflexes will be attenuated. If there is a concomitant hemorrhage or ventricular dysfunction, the patient may not develop the usual cool, clammy appearance and will not become tachycardiac.

B. **Hypotension.** The patient should be kept supine. Blood pressure should be supported with infusions of fluids, vasopressors, or both.

1. **Monitoring** is needed to assess and guide therapy. Usual monitors include a bladder catheter, arterial cannula, ECG, and central venous pressure (CVP) catheter. A pulmonary artery catheter is needed when pulmonary edema is present or the patient is felt to be at risk of pulmonary edema with fluid resuscitation (e.g., continued hypotension or oliguria despite a high CVP, rales, concomitant myocardial contusion, sepsis).
2. **Fluids** should be infused, usually titrated to maintain mean arterial pressure greater than 60 mm Hg and urine output greater than 0.5 ml/kg/hour. Central venous pressures can be followed to prevent overhydration, aiming usually for a CVP less than 15 mm Hg that produces normotension and acceptable urine output.
3. **Catecholamines** are commonly used to treat spinal shock.
   a. **Phenylephrine** to treat low systemic vascular resistance. It may exacerbate bradycardia.
   b. **Norepinephrine** to treat low systemic vascular resistance and absent cardiac sympathetic innervation.
   c. **Dopamine** to treat low systemic vascular resistance and absent sympathetic innervation. It is also useful if oliguria is present despite infusion of an adequate volume of fluid.

C. **Severe bradycardia** and even asystole can occur, particularly with tracheal suctioning, and may be exacerbated by hypoxemia. Thus, preoxygenation is mandatory before tracheal suctioning. If bradycardia is persistent, 0.4 mg of atropine IV is indicated, repeated as needed up to 2 mg (this may exacerbate gastrointestinal-bladder atonia). With bradycardia refractory to atropine, an infusion of isoproterenol or dopamine or insertion of a cardiac pacemaker wire should be considered.

D. **Autonomic dysreflexia** is a syndrome manifesting with paroxysmal hypertension, sweating, facial flushing, nasal congestion, and headache. In severe cases, retinal or cerebral hemorrhage and seizures may occur. It is precipitated by stimuli such as defecation, bladder distention, rectal distention, or muscle spasms. During the spinal shock phase, the first 1–3 weeks postinjury, autonomic dysreflexia seldom occurs. Thereafter, however, with return of spinal reflexes, precautions must be taken to prevent it. The precipitating causes should be prevented and alleviated: empty the bladder continuously or regularly (i.e., temporary indwelling catheter, intermittent catheterization), prevent fecal impaction with regular bowel care (including laxatives and suppositories), and treat severe muscle spasms with diazepam. Medical therapy is rarely indicated for hypertension if these precipitating causes are prevented.

IV. Temperature regulation

A. Disordered temperature regulation results from sympathetic denervation. This is most prominent with lesions at T8 or above.

B. **Hypothermia** to less than 35°C core body temperature can occur initially after cervical spinal cord injury due to cutaneous vasodilation with subsequent heat loss. However, **hyperthermia** may occur with high ambient temperature or humidity, or it may indicate the presence of an infection. It is due to inability to dissipate heat through the normal mechanisms of vasodilation and sweating.

C. Passive warming measures are usually employed for **hypothermia** when it is mild. Such measures include covering the patient with a blanket and warming the room. If hypothermia is severe (e.g., <35°C) and the patient is unstable, additional active measures such as heating and humidifying inspired gas or gastric lavage with warm fluids may be necessary. Similarly, mild **hyperthermia** is managed by keeping the patient uncovered with a fan, sponge bath, or both, and severe hyperthermia (>40.5°C) is managed with ice water, gastric lavage, packing in ice, or a combination.

V. Gastrointestinal management

A. **Gastrointestinal ileus** is frequently present with cervical or thoracic spine lesions. Furthermore, assessment of abdominal injury is difficult, as the lack of appropriate sensation or mental status may prevent development of the usual signs of peritonitis. The stomach becomes atonic and may become quite distended, interfering with spontaneous breathing. A nasogastric tube is used to empty the stomach, reducing the risk of aspiration and preventing gastric distention from aerophagia (common with this lesion). With resolution of the ileus, the nasogastric tube can then be used for nutrition for the duration of skull-cervical traction, which often is required for 1–2 weeks.

B. **Intraabdominal pathology** may be signaled by persistent nausea and vomiting, tachycardia or bradycardia with a pulse that has been normal, or (referred) diaphragmatic pain in the shoulders or cervical region.

C. **Fecal impaction** is a major cause of autonomic dysreflexia. It should be prevented with regular use of stool softeners and judicious use of rectal suppositories and enemas. The aim of bowel care is to obtain patient-controlled reflex evacuation.

D. The **stress ulcer** syndrome with gastrointestinal hemorrhage is a major complication in quadriplegic patients, typically occurring 10–14 days postinjury. It seems to be more common in patients who receive steroids. Antacids and cimetidine are frequently used, with the aim of keeping gastric pH above 3.0.

VI. **Bladder care.** Urinary retention occurs after spinal injury and can cause autonomic dysreflexia. In addition, urine output should be followed closely. Thus, an indwelling bladder catheter (as small a size as feasible) should be inserted for up to the first 48 hours postinjury. After 48 hours, intermittent bladder catheterization, initially every 4–6 hours, is preferred. Immaculate catheter care and catheterization techniques are essential. The catheter should be introduced with scrupulous aseptic technique by an experienced individual.

VII. **Neurologic assessment**

A. Serial **neurologic reassessment with accurate charting of the motor and sensory levels** of function is essential to distinguish between cord and root damage. Neurologic checks should be performed hourly for the first 24 hours. If the level is stable, they can decrease to every 2–4 hours for 2–3 days, then every 4 hours for the next 3 days, after which they can be done every 8 hours. Any change in level at any time mandates an increase in frequency of the checks. If the deficit below a cord lesion remains complete for 24 hours, then the cord is irreparably damaged and recovery does not occur. If there is some return of sensation, however distorted, or some return of motor power in areas innervated by segments below the level of the lesion within 24 hours, then at least part of the cord is intact and recovery may occur.

B. As part of accurate serial neurologic evaluation, the following points should be kept in mind:

1. By comparing the level of vertebral bony injury with the level of paraplegia or quadriplegia, that part of the deficit due to nerve root damage can be separated from that due to cord damage. For example, a patient with a fracture of the first thoracic vertebra with unilateral paralysis up to C6 (biceps weakness) probably has a component of nerve root damage that can be expected to resolve.
2. Deficits due to root injury may persist for many weeks and still recover.
3. Return of reflex activity below the level of the cord lesion in the absence of motor power or sensation is **not** a good prognostic sign.
4. If any motor power or sensation is present below the level of the cord lesion on initial examination, then the cord is only partially damaged, and considerable recovery may be expected.
5. If there is any progressive loss of neurologic function, the patient's neurosurgeon should be notified immediately as urgent surgical intervention must be considered.

C. **Other injuries** are commonly associated with spinal cord trauma, with an incidence ranging from 25–65% (Albin, 1980). Head injuries are the most common, followed by chest injury (especially with thoracic spine trauma).

VIII. **Skin care.** Meticulous attention must be given to the skin. The position of paralyzed or anesthetic body parts should be changed at least every 2 hours and should be washed and massaged with alcohol and powdered daily, especially skin in the perineal and sacral areas. The Roto-Rest kinetic bed can be used to turn a patient automatically. Heels and elbows should be padded. The skin there as well as that under the edge of a cast or brace and the presacral and perineal area must be checked daily. Specialized foam mattresses, horizontally rotating frames, or sheepskin (clean and dry) should be used.

IX. **Rehabilitation.** Physical and psychologic rehabilitation involving the patient, family and, where appropriate, friends, is started in the acute phase. Range-of-motion extremity exercises are begun soon after admission, and after sufficient spinal stability has been achieved, upper extremity resistance exercises are begun. Splinting should be instituted early to prevent development of contractures.

Selected References

Albin, M. S., Hung, T. K., and Babinski, M. Spinal cord injury—epidemiology, emergency care and acute care: Advances in physiopathology and treatment. *Curr. Probl. Surg.* 17:190, 1980.

Bergofsky, E. H. Mechanism for respiratory insufficiency after cervical cord injury. *Ann. Intern. Med.* 61:435, 1964.

Carter, R. E. Medical management of pulmonary complications of spinal cord injury. *Adv. Neurol.* 22:261, 1979.

Chan, R. C., Schweigel, J. F., and Thompson, G. B. Halo-thoracic brace immobilization in 188 patients with acute cervical spine injuries. *J. Neurosurg.* 58:508, 1983.

Eidelberg, E. E. Cardiovascular response to experimental spinal cord compression. *J. Neurosurg.* 38:326, 1973.

Frankel, H., and Mathias, C. Cardiovascular Systems in Tetraplegia and Paraplegia. In P. J. Vinken and G. W. Bruyn (eds.), *Handbook of Clinical Neurology.* Amsterdam: North Holland, 1976. Vol. 26.

Frost, E. R. The physiopathology of respiration in neurosurgical patients. *J. Neurosurg.* 50:699, 1979.

Head, H., and Riddoch, G. The autonomic bladder, excessive sweating and some other reflex conditions in gross injuries of the spinal cord. *Brain* 40:188, 1971.

Hinchey, J., Hreno, A., Benoji, P. R., et al. The Stress Ulcer Syndrome. In C. Welch (ed.), *Advances in Surgery.* Chicago: Yearbook Medical, 1970. Vol. 4.

Holdsworth, F. Fractures, dislocations and fracture-dislocations of the spine. *J. Bone Joint Surg. (Am)* 52A:1534, 1970.

Johnson, R. H. Temperature Regulation and Spinal Cord Injuries. In P. J. Vinken and G. W. Bruyn (eds.), *Handbook of Clinical Neurology.* Amsterdam: North Holland, 1976. Vol. 26.

Mathias, C. J. Bradycardia and cardiac arrest during tracheal suction-mechanisms in tetraplegia patients. *Intensive Care Med.* 2:147, 1976.

Pierce, D. S., and Nickel, V. H. (eds.). *The Total Care of Spinal Cord Injuries.* Boston: Little, Brown, 1977.

Silver, J. R., and Moulton, A. The physiological and pathological sequelae of paralysis of the intercostal and abdominal muscles in tetraplegic patients. *Paraplegia* 7:131, 1969.

Tator, C. H., and Rowed, D. W. Current concepts in the immediate management of acute spinal cord injuries. *Can. Med. Assoc. J.* 121:1453, 1979.

Webb, S. B., Berzin, S. E., Wengardiner, T. S., and Lorenzi, M. E. First year hospitalization costs for the spinal cord patient. *Paraplegia* 15:311, 1978.

Yashon, D. *Spinal Injury.* New York: Appleton-Century-Crofts, 1978.

17

Brain Death

Krishna N. Nirmel and Allan H. Ropper

The pronouncement of brain death should be performed at an appropriate time with adequate documentation. Certain guidelines have been established, but all considerations necessitate the use of clinical judgment in applying objective tests of cerebral function. The pronouncement of death is based on physiologic reasoning and not on total cellular death of the organism. The concept of brain death is based on the inference that without brain function, as carefully defined, other organs will certainly fail with no chance of recovery. Brain death is widely accepted as a criterion of death in the medical and legal communities and in the public opinion. Thus, all patients who fulfill the particular criteria of brain death may have artificial support systems discontinued. In order to define irreversible loss of all brain function, the following should be demonstrated:

1. There is no evidence of brainstem or cortical activity.
2. No patients with the given criteria survive despite intensive therapy.
3. A certain set of clinical criteria predict widespread brain necrosis at autopsy.

The criteria detailed subsequently are consistent with these conditions.

I. Brain death guidelines. The following are locally accepted guidelines, as used at the Massachusetts General Hospital, for the diagnosis of brain death. It is not necessary to use these procedures when the cause of death involves fatal systemic diseases. These guidelines do not replace the physician's judgment in individual cases as brain death is a clinical diagnosis.

A. Clinical

1. **Cerebral unresponsiveness.** Deep coma should be present with no evidence of withdrawal or posturing to painful stimuli. Spinal level movements do not preclude the diagnosis of brain death. Decerebrate or decorticate posturing, however, does.
2. **Brainstem-cephalic unresponsiveness**
   a. **Pupils.** Previously healthy pupils should be larger than 3 mm in diameter and unreactive to bright diffuse light. They should not be oval in shape since this demonstrates residual midbrain function. It is generally agreed that pupillary dilatation is not a necessary criterion for brain death; **fixed pupils,** indicating loss of brainstem pathways, may be satisfactory if other requirements are met.
   b. **Eye movements.** There should be no spontaneous eye movement. Oculovestibular testing with 100 ml of ice water irrigation of each ear separately should produce no eye movement. The patient's head should be elevated 30 degrees during testing and the external auditory canals cleared beforehand.
   c. **Other cranial nerves.** There should be no corneal reflex, facial movement, or bulbar function such as gagging or coughing with tracheal stimulation.
   d. **Spinal reflexes.** The presence of deep tendon reflexes, flexor toe response, isolated triple flexion of the legs, or other spinally mediated reflexes does not preclude the diagnosis of brain death.
   e. **Apnea test.** The patient must be apneic in the presence of hypercapnia: **The proper determination of severe medullary damage requires an apnea test.** The patient should be removed from the respirator and $PaCO_2$ allowed to rise while the thorax is carefully observed and palpated for spontaneous respiration. During this test, vital functions are supported by the use of diffusion oxygenation. This is accomplished by preoxygenation for 5 minutes with 100% oxygen and, during apnea, the use of an oxygen catheter inserted into the trachea (not a T piece), supplying 8–12 liters of oxygen per minute. At the end of a period of time estimated to bring the arterial $PaCO_2$ to above 50 mm Hg, or after 5 minutes

if the initial $PaCO_2$ is unknown, an arterial blood gas sample is obtained, and the patient is reconnected to the ventilator. A $PaCO_2$ rise of approximately 2.5 mm Hg per minute can be expected in most patients. If $PaCO_2$ at the end of the test exceeds 50 mm Hg and the blood pH is below 7.35 without respiratory movement, apnea has been adequately demonstrated. A change of 10% in pulse or BP or the appearance of cyanosis requires termination of apnea testing. This test must be performed in the absence of neuromuscular blockade or serum levels of pharmacologic agents that would depress spontaneous respiration.

B. Laboratory testing

1. **Electroencephalogram** (EEG). An EEG recording of at least a 30-minute duration should show no electrocerebral activity, termed **electrocerebral silence (ECS).** There should be a minimum of eight scalp electrodes and ear lobe reference electrodes with sensitivity increased from 7 μV per mm to 2 μV per mm during most of the recording with inclusion of appropriate calibrations. ECS refers to the absence of nonartifactual activity greater than 2 μV in amplitude, with electrode impedances between 100 and 10,000 ohms and interelectrode distances of at least 10 cm. There should be no change with auditory (loud sound), visual (stroboscopic bright light), or painful (pinch) stimulation. Electrocardiograph artifact should be visible. The recording should be made by EEG technologists with the EEG record interpreted by a staff electroencephalographer as showing ECS prior to the determination of brain death and should be in the patient record. There is no need for the patient to be normothermic. Recordings with a core body temperature above 90°F (32.3°C) are acceptable. A second EEG is not necessary unless CNS depressant drugs may have contributed to coma or doubt exists about ECS. Telephone transmission of the EEG is not to be used for determination of ECS. Intoxication (especially barbiturates with a serum level > 1 mg/dl) and metabolic causes for coma should be excluded.
2. **Ancillary testing.** Radionuclide or contrast angiographic demonstration of absent cerebral blood flows is not necessary but can be used in special cases. Evoked potentials may be helpful in the diagnosis of brain death but are not diagnostic alone.

II. Period of observation and underlying illness. A period of observation of at least 24 hours without clinical neurologic change is recommended and necessary if brain hypoxia-ischemia has occurred. Toxicologic screening for CNS depressant drugs is recommended in all cases where such agents may play a role. If the cause of coma is known with certainty and drug-metabolic causes have been excluded, then in extraordinary circumstances, a period of observation of 6 hours with no change in clinical state is adequate.

III. Special cases

A. Children and neonates. The aforementioned criteria in general form can be applied to children and neonates, but in questionable circumstances, ancillary testing to demonstrate the absence of cerebral blood flow is recommended. A period of observation of 24 hours is necessary.

B. Previous therapeutic use of high-dose barbiturates for raised intracranial pressure or seizures does not preclude the diagnosis of brain death if serum levels at the time of examination are very low (i.e., <1 mg/dl, an arbitrarily selected level). Brain bloodflow examination may be useful in circumstances where barbiturates are present.

C. Inability to examine the brainstem. When circumstances do not permit the examination of the eyes for pupillary reaction and eye movements, the diagnosis of brain death may generally be made by demonstrating ECS and apnea. In questionable cases, cerebral bloodflow studies are recommended.

D. **Hypothermia.** Except when extreme (below 90°F or 32.3°C), hypothermia does not produce the clinical or EEG phenomena associated with brain death.

E. **Hypotension.** The diagnosis of brain death should not be made if the systolic BP is below 90 mm Hg.

IV. **Consultation and recording.** If the patient is under the care of a nonneurologic physician, a staff neurologist or neurosurgeon should concur in the diagnosis of brain death. A note indicating that the patient is declared dead and the explicit criteria used for this determination should be written, dated, and signed, with the time of such determination in the patient chart. Physicians associated with transplantation or a potential organ recipient should not be involved in the determination of brain death.

V. **Commentary on brain death criteria**

A. The **EEG** is valuable in diagnosing brain death but has to be used in the context of the entire clinical situation and must not be used as a single test. Furthermore, to make the clinical diagnosis of brain death, it is not **necessary** to have corroboration by EEG or arteriography except when findings on neurologic examination are equivocal. However, survival after ECS on EEG does not occur if hypothermia, intoxication, and metabolic causes have been excluded.

B. The role of **cerebral angiography** is based on the understanding that demonstrating absence of intracranial circulation is an accurate way of demonstrating irreversible cerebral damage. The special importance of the angiogram is that it allows the distinction of comatose states from brain death. Unlike the EEG, it is not falsely positive in certain overdose states. If there is absence of intracranial circulation for 10–30 minutes, the brain is irreversibly damaged, regardless of the cause. An obvious advantage of cerebral angiography is its speed in making the diagnosis of brain death, for transplantation purposes. It requires only one occasion in which an absence of flow is demonstrated. Isotope angiography, alternatively, has been advocated by some.

C. Once the findings indicate brain death and are recorded, only then are the respiratory and other support systems withdrawn. Medicolegally, this is very important.

D. It is also important to **distinguish between brain death and a persistent vegetative state** (or apallic syndrome), with respect to withdrawal of support systems. According to a 1977 collaborative study (*J.A.M.A.* 237:982, 1977), "cerebral death implies total destruction of the brain such that both volitional and reflex evidence of responsivity are absent." This requires the absence of both cortical and brainstem activity. Persistent vegetative state, on the other hand, is one "in which all functions attributed to the cerebrum are lost but certain vital functions such as respiration, temperature and blood pressure regulation may be retained." Thus, brain death is a condition of impending bodily or somatic death with massive brain destruction, whereas the persistent vegetative state is one with a kind of permanent unresponsiveness with independent respiratory effort, spontaneous movement, and an EEG that shows some activity.

E. **The concept of brain death should be explained to the surviving family and friends.** This requires patience and an understanding of their emotional distress and anger and often needs to be repeated. Nurses and social workers can help.

F. **Organ transplantation** may be suggested by the family, although often it has to come from the physician attending the patient. The physician should assume a positive role, when appropriate, and inform the family of the opportunity to donate healthy organs from the patient with brain death. After effective communication is established in this manner with the grieving family and the criteria for brain death have been met, the declaration of death and transfer of the patient to the operating room for organ removal surgery should cause no difficulty. Furthermore, in arranging this sequence of events, the physician, by his or her compassion, often helps the family in assuaging their grief by helping them to know that the death of their loved one, through organ donation and subsequent transplantation, has given another person the gift of life.

VI. Brain death and transplantation

A. If a patient is brain-dead or is likely to be pronounced brain-dead, and after discussion with the family regarding organ donation, the transplantation or organ procurement service is contacted. In these circumstances, the attending physician should direct efforts toward the continued resuscitation of the brain-dead patient and maintain vital functions (e.g., adequate perfusion, BP, and renal function). The treatment in general should be as unencumbered as possible from the consideration of transplantation, until a diagnosis of brain death is made with adequate documentation.

B. It is the responsibility of the transplantation team to decide whether the brain-dead patient is an appropriate organ donor and to obtain procurement permission from the next of kin. Once consent for organ donation is obtained and the donor has been pronounced brain-dead, the transplantation team manages the donor and coordinates harvest of all potential transplantable tissue and organs. **In no case may the same person certify brain death and perform the transplantation.** The American Medical Association Judicial Council requires that the donor's death be determined by someone other than the recipient's physician. The Committee on Morals and Ethics of the Transplantation Society of the United States has stated that "acceptation of death should be made and declared by at least two physicians whose primary responsibility is care of the potential donor and who are independent of the transplantation team."

C. Legal considerations. If the brain-dead person is liable to be submitted to a legal enquiry (e.g., crime, suicide, accidents at work, occupational disease), the case should be carefully reviewed with the medical examiner prior to consideration for organ donation.

Selected References

A definition of irreversible coma: Report of the Ad Hoc Committee of the Harvard Medical School to examine the definition of brain death. *J.A.M.A.* 205:337, 1968.

American Medical Association Judicial Council Opinions and Reports. Chicago: AMA Press, 1977, P. 23.

An appraisal of the criteria of cerebral death: A summary statement: A collaborative study. *J.A.M.A.* 237:982, 1977.

Black, P. M. Brain death. *N. Engl. J. Med.* 299:338, 1978.

Ivan, L. P. Spinal reflexes in cerebral death. *Neurology* 23:650, 1973.

Merrill, J. P. Statement of the Committee on Morals and Ethics of the Transplantation Society. *Ann. Intern. Med.* 75:631, 1971.

Ovaknine, G., Kosary, I. Z., Braham, J., et al. Laboratory criteria of brain death. *J. Neurosurg.* 39:429, 1973.

Silverman, D., Saunders, M. G., Schwab, R. S., et al. Cerebral death and the electroencephalogram: Report of the Ad Hoc Committee of the American Electroencephalographic Society on EEG criteria for determination of cerebral death. *J.A.M.A.* 209:1505, 1969.

18

Nutritional Support in the Intensive Care Unit

Regina K. Stuart and Bruce R. Bistrian

Modern advances in medical therapy, surgical procedures, and intensive care support have created a new ICU population. Patients who survive for extended periods of time on mechanical ventilation and pharmacologic support may not receive oral nutrition. This combination of starvation and stress leads to the rapid development of malnutrition, with concomitant dysfunction in the immunologic and reparative processes of the body. Except in cases of pure malnutrition, nutritional therapy is not itself the cure for any critical illness. Survival is optimized by the addition of nutritional support to the therapeutic regimen.

I. Assessment

A. Candidates. The first goal in effective nutritional support is to identify those patients who will benefit from this therapy. "Malnutrition" in the ICU setting is a result of the combined effects of starvation and metabolic stress.

1. The patient with a preexisting nutritional deficit is predisposed to the rapid development of severe malnutrition under conditions of stress. Prompt nutritional repletion is indicated, even with mild to moderate stress. Preoperative nutritional deficiency may exist in two forms:
   - **a.** Marasmus results from uncomplicated semistarvation and consists of weight loss from both skeletal muscle and body fat stores with preservation of visceral protein status. It is manifested by a history of weight loss with normal albumin levels and immune function.
   - **b.** Hypoalbuminemic malnutrition or adult kwashiorkor results from conditions that cause an increase in the levels of catabolic hormones (catecholamines, corticosteroids, glucagon) and is characterized by the net catabolism of secretory proteins, extravasation of albumin, and net fat and skeletal muscle loss. Clinically this is manifested by net weight loss, hypoalbuminemia, and energy.
2. The previously well-nourished patient who experiences a severe illness, causing an elevation in the levels of catabolic hormones and the mobilization of nitrogen stores, may also require nutritional therapy. Elective postsurgical patients undergo nitrogen losses of 7–9 g per day, septic patients 11–14 g per day, and severely burned patients 12–18 g per day. With normal total body-expendable nitrogen of 100 g, fasting can be tolerated for only 5–10 days, depending on the degree of stress, before clinically significant depletion of protein stores occurs. If a prolonged course is anticipated, early nutritional support should be started. Nutritional repletion is inefficient in the presence of ongoing stress where protein depletion has already occurred.

B. Methods of assessment. A battery of diagnostic tools can be utilized to define the degree of nutritional depletion.

1. **Physical examination** can give reliable information on subcutaneous fat and skeletal muscle stores; however, weight loss may be masked by edema. Deficits in lean body mass may exist in the setting of obesity.
2. **History.** Significant nutritional depletion is defined by:
   - **a.** Involuntary weight loss exceeding 5% in 1 month or 10% over 6 months
   - **b.** Weight adjusted for height of less than 85% of the standard value
3. **Upper arm anthropometry** involves the measurement of the triceps skinfold (TSF) using skinfold calipers. Utilizing this value together with the total arm circumference, the arm muscle circumference (AMC) can be derived. A value of less than the fifth percentile compared with normal for either TSF or AMC indicates severe depletion of fat or muscle stores, respectively.

4. **The secretory proteins** such as albumin, transferrin and prealbumin are affected by multiple variables in a stressed ICU patient. Preoperative, unstressed values are indicative of baseline nutritional status, but poststress levels are not specific.
5. **Immune function**
   a. Although useful in the assessment of uncomplicated malnutrition, the total lymphocyte count is affected by multiple variables, including any ongoing infections. Thus, the total lymphocyte count is an unreliable index of malnutrition in ICU patients.
   b. The absence of a delayed hypersensitivity response in the setting of ongoing stress is a nonspecific finding.
6. **The creatinine-height index** compares the patient's creatinine excretion, which is a function of lean body mass, with that of a normal individual of the same height. In patients with normal renal function, this yields a reliable index of actual lean body mass regardless of fluid overload or obesity. Values of less than 75% of the standard for height and age are indicative of significant malnutrition.
7. **In summary,** nutritional assessment in postoperative or postinjury ICU patients can be difficult. In general, any patient with evidence of preexisting malnutrition should begin nutritional therapy as soon as possible. Previously well-nourished patients with mild to moderate stress may remain in a fasting state for 5–10 days. In patients whose recovery can be projected to be prolonged or who experience severe stress such as multiple trauma or burns, nutritional support should be instituted immediately.

II. Requirements

A. Estimating requirements

1. The most commonly used method of estimating calorie requirements is the **Harris Benedict formula.** Basal energy expenditure (BEE) is calculated by the equation:

$$\text{BEE (males)} = 66.4 + 13.7\ W + 5\ H - 6.7\ A$$
$$\text{BEE (females)} = 65.5 + 9.6\ W + 1.8\ H - 4.6\ A$$

   where
   A = age in years
   W = weight (in kilograms)
   H = height (in centimeters)

   The total caloric expenditure is then estimated as a multiple of the BEE depending on the degree of stress. An ambulatory person utilizes 1.2(BEE); an infected postoperative patient would metabolize 1.5–1.7(BEE). The upper limit of stress is manifested by the severely burned patient at approximately 2.0(BEE).
2. A more rapid and fairly reliable method of estimating energy expenditure is 25 kcal per kilogram for the typical ICU patient, 30 kcal per kilogram for the more hypermetabolic ICU patient (i.e., persistently febrile, multiple fistulae), and 35–40 kcal per kilogram for the previously well-nourished patient with severe stress (head injury, burns, multiple trauma) or the less ill but fully ambulatory patient.
3. The metabolic cart that calculates energy expenditure via measurements of O_2 consumption and O_2 production is a valuable tool in the ICU setting. Current methods of estimating energy expenditure can be inaccurate in complex ICU patients where multiple variables affect net expenditure. Actual measurements can be invaluable, especially in the setting of ventilator dependence, severe catabolism, or prolonged illness.

B. Protein

1. The recommended daily allowance (RDA) of protein to maintain ni-

trogen balance in healthy adults is 0.8 gm/kg/day; 1.2 gm/kg/day will permit anabolism.

2. Additional protein is required in patients to meet the demands of wound healing, infection, fistula losses, and so forth. Protein intakes of 1.5 gm/kg/day (based on ideal body weight for those with significant weight loss or obesity) have been shown to maximize net protein synthesis in severely catabolic patients.

C. **Nonprotein calories.** Once protein needs have been supplied, the remainder of the energy requirements is provided through glucose and lipids.

1. **Glucose**
   a. Glucose is an essential substrate for the renal medulla, erythrocytes, bone marrow, peripheral nerves, and the ischemic heart. The daily requirement is met first by glycogenolysis, until the glycogen stores are depleted, and then by gluconeogenesis from amino acids at the rate of 200 g glucose per day.
   b. Exogenous glucose infusions suppress endogenous glucose production (and thus conserve protein) at rates up to 4–5 mg/kg/minute (400–500 g/day for a 70-kg person). Increasing the rate above 5 mg/kg/minute leads to glycogenesis and lipogenesis, with the associated problems of additional carbon-dioxide production, O_2 consumption, and hepatic steatosis. Thus, infusion rates above 5 mg/kg/minute are not recommended.
2. **Lipids**
   a. Provision of 2–4% of total calories in the form of long-chain triglyceride (LCT) infusions prevent essential fatty acid deficiency.
   b. Advantages of lipid infusions include decreased carbohydrate requirement, decreased insulin requirement, lower carbon dioxide production and reduced minute ventilation, serum isoosmolarity, and less volume for the same protein-sparing effect.
   c. Depression of reticuloendothelial system function with high-dose lipid infusions has been reported in both animals and humans. For this reason, infusion of LCT lipid emulsions should be kept to less than 100 g per day and preferably infused over 24 hours.
3. Using these basic guidelines and considering the individual characteristics of the patient (e.g., diabetes, fluid overload, obesity), the optimal mixture of nonprotein calories can be determined. The breakdown of total calories typically consists of 25% total calories as protein (1.5 g/kg), 45–65% as glucose, and 10–30% as lipid.

D. **Fluid and electrolytes**

1. Fluid-overloaded patients may not tolerate the volume of fluid necessary to deliver a complete nutritional regimen. The first priority is protein sparing. A "fluid overload formula" of 70 g of protein and 200 g of glucose delivered in 1,000 cc will decrease hepatic gluconeogenesis and result in decreased net catabolism until full nutritional support can be provided.
2. Sodium (Na^+) losses via drains and nasogastric suction can be calculated and replaced by the nutritional mixture. Thus, separate crystalloid infusions are seldom necessary. Most ICU patients are both Na^+ and fluid overloaded, and a low Na^+ or Na^+-free solution will facilitate diuresis.
3. Potassium (K^+) losses may be substantial due to urine and drain outputs. Replacement of K^+ via nutritional mixture will allow for the smooth control of serum levels and minimize the need for frequent K^+ determinations and bolus administration.
4. Ca^{++}, PO_4^-, and Mg^{++} requirements can be estimated by using the RDA. However, unusual losses secondary to disease or therapy are common in the ICU setting. Serum determinations usually suffice as a guide to further supplementation. (See **IV.B.**)

E. Acid-base balance

1. **Metabolic acidosis** in the ICU setting is commonly due to chronic renal failure, acute renal failure, or renal tubular acidosis (often secondary to amphotericin or aminoglycosides). This imbalance should be corrected by acetate administration in the nutritional mixture.
2. **Metabolic alkalosis** can be secondary to diuretics, corticosteroids, nasogastric suctioning, or the administration of large amounts of citrated blood products. Mild degrees of alkalosis can be corrected by the administration of KCl or NaCl. In severe alkalosis, however, or when Na^+ and K^+ must be restricted, HCl is the treatment of choice. HCl may be administered by nonlipid-containing central parenteral formulas. The HCl concentration should not exceed 100 mEq HCl per liter of total parenteral nutrition (TPN), and the rate of administration should be limited to 0.2 mEq/kg/hour. $CaCl_2$ can be used to treat alkalosis via the enteral route.
3. **Calculation of the acid or base deficit**

$$\text{Desired } TCO_2 - \text{measured } TCO_2 \times TBW = \text{base excess/deficit (mEq)}$$

where

TCO_2 = total CO_2 (mEq/L) obtained from blood gas analysis

TBW = total body water(L) = 0.5 × body weight(kg)

Unless a life-threatening abnormality exists, one-half of the calculated excess or deficit should be replaced over 24 hours.

F. Micronutrients. Evidence for the nutritional and metabolic role of most of the **trace elements** is lacking or incomplete. However, several are known to be required.

1. **Iron (Fe).** Since acute and chronic blood loss are common in the ICU setting, many patients are iron deficient. Free iron is necessary for the metabolism of many bacteria. The liver sequesters iron in septic states. Elevated levels of free iron have been reported to make patients more susceptible to bacterial and fungal pathogens. Therefore, care must be taken when administering large amounts of IV iron to septic patients. The small replacement amounts of Fe (2 mg/day) routinely infused in the TPN are not likely to be a problem. Patients who receive blood transfusions acquire 250 mg of iron per unit of packed red blood cells and therefore rarely require additional supplementation. Since the iron is bound to protein, red blood cell transfusion is a safe way to administer IV iron.
2. **Zinc** is a component of numerous metallic enzymes and plays an essential role in metabolism. Excessive gastrointestinal fluid losses via fistula or diarrhea deplete zinc stores. In this setting 5–10 mg per day of zinc replacement, in addition to the RDA of 3 mg per day that all patients receive, is advisable.
3. **Other trace elements** that have known metabolic roles and should be provided by means of commercially available supplements include copper 1.2 mg per day, manganese 0.3 mg per day, selenium 60 μg per day, and chromium 12 μg per day.
4. **Vitamins.** Serum vitamin levels are dependent on the adequate synthesis and release of plasma transport proteins; thus, low levels may not reflect true deficiency. The RDA of each vitamin is supplied daily by means of enteral or parenteral commercial preparations. Weekly subcutaneous injections of vitamin K (10 mg) are necessary for patients on parenteral nutrition.

III. Route of administration

A. Enteral

1. **Malnutrition** is not an automatic indication for parenteral therapy.

Many critically ill, malnourished patients tolerate enteral formulas, especially when administered by nasoduodenal, nasojejunal, or percutaneous jejunal routes. Advantages to enteral nutrition include:

- **a.** Higher rates of secretory protein synthesis
- **b.** Release of gastrointestinal hormones with trophic effects on the gut mucosa
- **c.** Direct trophic effects by the components of the nutritional formula on gut mucosa
- **d.** Possible decreased translocation of bacteria and endotoxin from the gut into mesenteric lymph nodes
- **e.** Significantly lower cost

2. Many **commercial formulas** are available to meet the individual needs of patients (Table 18-1).
   - **a.** Meal replacement formulas consist of whole protein, carbohydrates, and approximately 30% fat. The osmolarity ranges from 300–600 mOsm per liter, and caloric density is generally 1 kcal per milliliter. These formulas are well tolerated in patients with normal gastrointestinal function. However, whole proteins may not be well absorbed in patients with compromised gastrointestinal tracts and, this concentration of fat (especially LCT) can cause gastric retention and/or diarrhea in critically ill patients.
   - **b.** Elemental formulas
     - **(1)** Provide protein as amino acids or dipeptides, which are more easily absorbed than whole protein.
     - **(2)** The fat content is limited to 1–10% of the total calories, and a portion of this may be medium-chain triglycerides (MCT), which do not require emulsification by bile salts for their absorption. For this reason, improved gastric emptying and decreased diarrhea is often seen with these formulas.
     - **(3)** Amino acid formulas have a high osmolarity and may require dilution to avoid diarrhea. These formulas contain glutamine, which has been shown to have trophic effects on gut mucosa.
     - **(4)** Their cost is approximately 10 times the meal replacement formulas but only a fraction of parenteral formulas.
   - **c.** Modular diets can be formulated by combining pure sources of substrates such as protein, carbohydrate, and fat (specialized components such as branched chain amino acids [BCAA] and MCT are available) with specific amounts of electrolytes, minerals, and so forth. An individual formula can be mixed for each patient and can be as specific as parenteral admixtures. This process is time-consuming and thus expensive but still less costly than parenteral preparations.

B. Parenteral

1. **Peripheral parenteral nutrition (PPN)** admixtures are limited by their propensity to cause peripheral vein sclerosis. Solutions more concentrated than 600 mOsm per liter or with greater than 60 mEq per liter of KCl should be avoided. This limits the maximal concentration of PPN to approximately 0.5 kcal per milliliter. Few ICU patients will tolerate the amount of fluid required to deliver complete nutrition via this route. The most frequent indication for PPN is as a temporizing measure for patients in whom an alternative form of nutrition is planned within a few days.
2. **Total parenteral nutrition (TPN)** is indicated in patients who require nutrition (Table 18-2). Central venous catheter placement, with its attendant risks, is required.
3. **Three-in-one formulations** with protein, carbohydrate, and fat, administered via one 24-hour infusion container, result in substantial

Table 18-1. Commonly available enteral formulas

Product	Protein	Carbohydrate	Lipid	Concentration (kcal/ml)	Osmolarity (mOgm/L)
Meal Replacement Ensure (Ross)	Whole protein	Corn syrup, Maltodextrin, or cornstarch	LCT or LCT/MCT mixture	1	300–470
Osmolite (Ross) Isocal (Mead Johnson)	13–14% of calories	50–54% of calories	31–37% of calories		
Elemental	Free amino acids or free amino acids	Maltodextrin or cornstarch	LCT or LCT/MCT	1	500–630
Vivonex (Norwich Eaton) Vital (Ross)	Protein components (15–16% of calories)	Mixture (74–83% of calories)	2.0–10% of calories		

Table 18-2. Sample TPN formulas for typical clinical scenarios*

Clinical scenario	Nutritional goal (total kcal/g protein)	Volume (ml)	Protein (g)	Glucose (g)	Lipid (g)	Special considerations
50-kg man, severe ulcerative colitis	1,500/105	1,500	105	212	40	Serum K, PO_4, may decrease with refeeding
80-kg man with 10 kg postop fluid overload	1,000/70	1,000	70	210	—	Fluid (and nutrition) restricted until diuresis occurs; alkalosis may occur due to diuresis and NG losses
60-kg man, liver failure, tense ascites, stage II encephalopathy	1,500/60	1,500	60	240	50	Restrict protein; consider BCAA; restrict Na; monitor for worsening of fluid overload
50-kg man, renal failure	1,250/75	1,300	75	200	40	Restrict volume if oliguric; consider BCAA; restrict Na, K, Mg, PO_4; may require supplemental acetate

*These formulas are examples only and would require modifications for individual patients.

volume savings, fewer line interruptions (with fewer opportunities for bacterial contamination), and reduced nursing time.

IV. Organ failure considerations

A. Hepatic

1. Fluid overload may mask the true body weight and the extent of malnutrition.
2. Hepatic failure patients have been shown to be hypermetabolic per gram of lean body mass; thus, measurement with the metabolic cart may be necessary to obtain an accurate metabolic rate.
3. Strict volume and sodium restriction are usually required.
4. Protein restrictions secondary to encephalopathy may be necessary. BCAA are available both parenterally and enterally. Their use in hepatic encephalopathy remains controversial.

B. Renal

1. Volume restrictions require maximally concentrated parenteral solutions or enteral formulas.
2. Short-term protein restriction may be required during unstable periods, but chronic protein restriction is not advisable. Dialysis should be increased, if necessary, to allow at least 1 g of protein per kilogram of body weight.
3. BCAA may allow for more efficient amino acid utilization. Essential amino acid formulas are not recommended.
4. Ca^{++} should be generously supplemented. Mg^{+}, PO_4^{-}, and K^{+} must be restricted in anuric patients, but patients with nonoliguric renal failure often require modest Mg^{+}, PO_4^{-}, and K^{+} supplementation.

C. Cardiac patients require volume and sodium restrictions. However, nutrition is essential to cardiac muscle maintenance and function. If necessary, diuretic therapy should be increased to allow for the delivery of full nutritional therapy.

D. Pulmonary

1. The primary goal is to avoid overfeeding. Excess carbohydrate calories lead to net lipogenesis. The respiratory quotient (RQ) will rise above 1 when the carbohydrate calories exceed the energy expenditure.
2. Formulas with a high fat/carbohydrate ratio will lower the RQ further, but a minimum of 200 g of carbohydrate should always be supplied.

E. Obesity

1. In critically ill, obese patients, severe hypocaloric regimens (<50% estimated needs) may produce negative nitrogen balance.
2. A caloric goal of estimated (or measured) caloric needs less than 300–500 calories per day will promote both nitrogen balance and slow weight loss.
3. Glucose should be provided at 200–300 g per day.
4. Lipids are not routinely needed except in severely glucose-intolerant patients; obese patients metabolize their own fat stores, thus providing themselves with essential fatty acids.

F. Diabetes

1. Serum glucose control is of primary importance.
   - **a.** Begin with a glucose load of 100–150 g per day and increase slowly while titrating the insulin to maintain control.
   - **b.** For parenteral infusions, insulin should be added to the TPN solution (approximately 50% will adhere to the bag and tubing) and supplemented with subcutaneous doses as needed.
   - **c.** Patients on 24-hour enteral infusions should receive evenly distributed, subcutaneous insulin doses throughout the day and night.

2. Calorie and protein needs are identical to those of nondiabetic patients.

V. **Complications.** The transition from the fasting to the fed state involves a change in the hormonal status of the body. This can result in significant shifts in fluid, electrolyte, and nutrient concentrations. Some of the common pitfalls include:

A. **Total body fluid and sodium overload** secondary to the antinatriuretic effect of the increased insulin levels that accompany refeeding. Fluid and sodium should be increased gradually in susceptible patients, particularly those with severe marasmus (i.e., anorexia nervosa, cardiac cachexia), and diuretics administered if necessary.

B. **Decreased serum concentrations** of K^+ and PO_4^- as these ions shift intracellularly due to increased insulin levels. This can be prevented and/or corrected by supplementation in the nutritional mix.

C. **Hyperglycemia,** even in patients without a history of glucose intolerance. Frequent serum glucose determinations and insulin administration should prevent uncontrolled hyperglycemia.

D. **Hyperchloremic acidosis,** though less common with the current buffered amino acid solutions, can still occur when all cations are provided as a chloride salt. Provision of some of the Na^+ and K^+ as the acetate will prevent acidosis from developing.

E. **Hypoglycemia** can occur if infusions of hypertonic glucose are suddenly stopped. Infusion rates should be decreased gradually over 1–2 hours prior to stopping.

Suggested References

Baxter, J. K., and Bistrian B. R. Moderately hypocaloric nutrition in the critically ill, obese patient. *Nutr. Clin. Prac.* (publication pending).

Benotti, P. N., and Bistrian, B. R. Practical aspects and complications of total parenteral nutrition. *Crit. Care Clin.* 3:115, 1987.

Brimioulle, S., Vincent, J. L., Dufaye, P., et al. Hydrochloric acid infusion for treatment of metabolic acidosis: Effects on acid-base balance and oxygenation. *Crit. Care Med.* 13:738, 1985.

Lowell, J., and Blackburn, G. L. Preoperative Nutritional Assessment. In J. L. Cameron (ed.), *Current Surgical Therapy.* Toronto: BC Decker, 1989. Vol. 3.

Mascioli, E. A., and Bistrian, B. R. TPN in the patient with diabetes. *Nutr. Sup. Services* 3:12, 1983.

Mirtallo, J. M., Rogers, K. R., Johnson, J. A., et al. Stability of amino acids and the availability of acid in total parenteral nutrition solutions containing hydrochloric acid. *Am. J. Hosp. Pharm.* 38:1729, 1981.

Seidner, D. L., Mascioli, E. A., Istfan, N. W., et al. The effects of long chain triglyceride emulsions on reticuloendothelial system function in humans. *J. Parenter. Enteral Nutri.* 13:614, 1989.

Shanbogue, L. K. R., Chwals, W. J., Weintraub, M., et al. Parenteral nutrition in the surgical patient. *Br. J. Surg.* 74:172, 1987.

Shizgal, H. M., and Forse, R. A. Protein and calorie requirements with total parenteral nutrition. *Ann. Surg.* 192:562, 1980.

Sobrado, J., Moldawer, L. L., Pomposelli, J. J., et al. Lipid emulsions and reticuloendothelial system function in healthy and burned guinea pigs. *Am. J. Clin. Nutr.* 42:855, 1985.

Wolfe, R. R., Goodenough, R. D., Burke, J. F., et al. Response of protein and urea kinetics in burn patients to different levels of protein intake. *Ann. Surg.* 197:163, 1983.

Wolfe, R. R., O'Donnell, T. F., Jr., Stone, M. D., et al. Investigation of factors determining the optimal glucose infusion rate in total parenteral nutrition. *Metabolism* 29:892, 1980.

19

Infectious Diseases in the Intensive Care Unit

Daniel Shapiro

- I. Evaluation of the septic patient
  - A. Early recognition and treatment of sepsis
    1. Initial manifestations
    2. More subtle signs
    3. Abnormalities suggestive of changes in any organ system
    4. The most common types of ICU infections
  - B. A history and physical examination
  - C. Laboratory tests
    1. White blood cell (WBC) count and differential
    2. Blood cultures if bacteremia is suspected
    3. Further studies
    4. Gram's stain of suspicious secretions or drainage
    5. Other needed studies in a given patient
- II. Common infections in the ICU
  - A. Urinary tract infections
    1. Diagnosis
    2. Management
  - B. Respiratory tract infections
    1. Pneumonia
       - a. Community-acquired pneumonias
       - b. Hospital-acquired pneumonias
    2. Nosocomial pneumonia
    3. Diagnosis of pneumonia
    4. Management
    5. Problems associated with lower respiratory tract infections
  - C. Wound infections
    1. Incidence of postoperative wound infections
    2. Predisposing factors
    3. Diagnosis of wound infection
    4. Treatment
  - D. Bacteremia
    1. Secondary bacteremia
    2. Primary bacteremias
  - E. Further evaluation
    1. Appliance-related infection
    2. Decubitus ulcers
    3. Sinusitis
    4. Parotitis
    5. Prostatitis
    6. Biliary disease
    7. Subphrenic, intraabdominal, or pelvic abscess
    8. Clostridium difficile
    9. Unrecognized infection with the human immunodeficiency virus (HIV)
  - F. Noninfectious causes of fever
- III. Prevention of cross-infection
  - A. Strict hand-washing protocols
  - B. Spread from patient to patient or to hospital employees
    1. Complete precautions
    2. Contact precautions

Infectious diseases are among the major causes of morbidity and mortality in the ICU. The need to use invasive catheters and monitoring devices in critically ill patients treated with multiple antibiotics provides optimal opportunity for virulent, often multiple drug-resistant organisms to spread within the environment and to gain entry to the body. Many of these nosocomial infections are preventable and treatable. Strict protocols for care of wounds and skin, urinary tract catheters, ventilators, endotracheal tubes, intravascular cannulas, and other invasive devices can significantly decrease the incidence of nosocomial infections.

I. Evaluation of the septic patient

A. **Early recognition and treatment of sepsis** can have a profound effect on patient outcome. Sepsis must be considered in the differential diagnosis of any significant hemodynamic changes in an ICU patient.

1. **Initial manifestations** may include familiar signs of sepsis, such as chills, fever, diaphoresis, hypotension, and leukocytosis.
2. **More subtle signs** include tachypnea, acidosis, bleeding diatheses, thrombocytopenia, mental status changes, and elevated cardiac output.
3. **Abnormalities suggestive of changes in any organ system,** such as changes in chest radiograph, urinalysis, or liver function tests, may provide early clues to infection in these sites.
4. **Awareness of the most common types of ICU infections**—urinary tract infections (UTIs), pneumonia, wound infections, line sepsis, and bacteremia of unknown source—helps guide the initial search for sites of infection.

B. **A history and physical examination** should be performed in the patient with possible sepsis.

1. The history should take particular notice of conditions that may increase susceptibility to infections. These can range from an upper abdominal incision that might impair lower respiratory function to systemic immunosuppression. Recent invasive procedures, changes in medication, or specific clinical events such as aspiration should be particularly noted.
2. A brief physical examination should be performed, paying particular attention to lungs, abdomen, wounds (including decubiti), and catheter sites. Less frequently involved areas such as sinuses, salivary glands, oral cavity, prostate, pelvis, and rectum must be examined. If initial laboratory screening does not confirm infection in one of the most common sites, a reevaluation of the history and a more detailed physical examination can be helpful.

C. **Laboratory tests are essential** in the evaluation of the septic patient. Diagnostic studies should be designed to document a suspected site of infection while screening for other possible etiologies of the signs of sepsis. Initial tests in the septic patient in the ICU should include the following:

1. **White blood cell (WBC) count and differential.** Significant leukocytosis (>10,000/mm^3) often occurs in sepsis, although in some cases the WBC may be normal or low. Differential counts are frequently useful even in the absence of leukocytosis, since a shift to the left, atypical lymphocytosis, eosinophilia, or granulocytopenia may be significant.
2. **Blood cultures should always be performed if bacteremia is suspected,** preferably drawing two sets at different times from different sites. In patients with a suspected endovascular infection and in patients with prosthetic heart valves or vascular graft, three to five sets of blood cultures should be obtained. If Candidemia is suspected, lysis-centrifugation blood cultures, which are used by many hospital

laboratories, have a better yield for yeast than do routine blood cultures and should be obtained.

3. **Further studies** usually include the following:
   a. Chest radiograph
   b. Sputum or tracheal aspirate, if secretions are present, for Gram's stain and culture
   c. Gram's stain and culture of any purulent drainage
4. **Gram's stain of suspicious secretions or drainage** should be performed. The importance of this cannot be overstated since it may provide immediate answers concerning the presence or absence of bacterial infection, as well as the etiology of bacterial infection at a given site. In performing and examining a Gram's stain, select, if possible, that portion of the specimen that is grossly purulent. Do the test carefully, being particularly careful to decolorize adequately so that the nuclei of polymorphonuclear leukocytes (PMNs) are pink. Areas where PMNs are found in abundance should be examined under the oil-immersion lens for bacteria. The general nature of the predominant bacterial forms should be noted, observing not only the characteristic color on Gram's stain but the organisms' sizes, shapes, and relationships to each other. Even the observation of mixed flora, as opposed to a predominant pathogen, may be useful. The major groups that can be morphologically distinguished and the major therapeutic inferences that can be appropriately drawn include the following:
   a. **Gram-positive cocci**
      (1) **In chains:** Streptococci of all kinds. *Streptococcus pneumoniae* (pneumococcus) may appear in pairs (diplococci) or in chains. Major clinical problems are caused by enterococci that cannot be distinguished by appearance but may be inferred by the site or specimen examined (e.g., urine).
      (2) **In clusters:** If organisms are seen that are slightly larger than the streptococci and appear in clusters (bunch of grapes) or classically in tetrads, staphylococci must be suspected. The less pathogenic, coagulase-negative staphylococci, which are frequent skin colonizers, cannot be distinguished morphologically from *Staphylococcus aureus.* The anaerobic streptococci and staphylococci (*Peptococci*) have a Gram's stain appearance identical to aerobic organisms.
   b. **Gram-positive bacilli.** A wide variety of organisms may appear as gram-positive rods, whose size and shape range from small, variable diphtheroids (a frequent contaminant or skin organism) to the large "boxcar" bacilli of *Clostridium,* which is a component of normal stool. *Listeria,* which may be seen in meningitis, and *Bacillus* species are gram-positive rods. Except for the appearance of *Clostridium* in a wound or *Listeria* in cerebrospinal fluid, however, these are rarely useful determinants of therapy.
   c. **Gram-positive hyphae or large ovoid forms** may suggest fungi or yeast, such as *Candida.*
   d. **Gram-negative cocci.** A large number of gram-negative cocci may appear as part of the normal flora, either as a result of decolorization during staining or because many of these—for example, *Moraxella* (formerly *Branhamella*) *catarrhalis*—may also appear in normal throat flora. Two other species are pathogenic; both are gram-negative diplococci of characteristic "kidney bean" alignment. *Neisseria meningitidis* can be identified if it appears in cerebrospinal fluid; however, these are rarely useful determinants of therapy.
   e. **Gram-positive bacilli.** A large number of organisms appear as

gram-negative rods. The major subdivisions of clinical importance include the Enterobacteriaceae such as *Escherichia coli* and *Klebsiella*; the nonenteric gram-negative rods such as *Pseudomonas*; and the anaerobic gram-negative rods, including the *Bacteroides* species. In a few situations, tentative identification may be inferred on Gram's stain. In sputum or cerebrospinal fluid, for example, a small, variably shaped gram-negative rod, often approaching coccoid form (coccobacillary), may suggest *Haemophilus* infection. In most cases, however, gram-negative bacilli cannot be distinguished by Gram's stain, and inferences about antimicrobial therapy must be drawn from the clinical setting and prior culture results.

f. In nonsterile sites, such as sputum or many draining wounds, the problem is one of determining if there is a new organism or a predominant organism that is not part of the anticipated normal flora.

5. The results of prior studies or history and physical examination may suggest other needed studies in a given patient. For example, the patient who becomes febrile following a neurosurgical procedure should have an examination of spinal fluid in search of postoperative meningitis.

II. Common infections in the ICU. Specific knowledge concerning the most common infections found in the ICU is useful because the initial diagnosis of such infections and initial antibiotic decisions may have to be based on incomplete information. The risk of antibiotic treatment in acutely ill patients in the ICU must be considered. However, the danger of not treating a potentially fatal infection often outweighs the risk of a short course of antibiotics. Early treatment can sometimes be limited in spectrum, directed against organisms most likely to be found in suspicious sites. However, in immunocompromised patients, empiric broad-spectrum antibiotics are often indicated pending culture results and other diagnostic information. The pathogens involved in ICU infections include a wide variety of organisms. This range can be limited, however, by considering the specific organ or site involved. Additionally, each unit or institution may have its own flora with its own pattern of antibiotic susceptibility. Information from surveillance by infection control teams and published antibiotic sensitivity patterns for hospital pathogens can be very helpful. **The most common hospital-acquired infections** involve the urinary tract, respiratory tract, wounds, and bloodstream and should be considered first in the evaluation of septic patients in the ICU.

A. Urinary tract infections. The most commonly seen, though generally not the most severe, hospital and ICU infection is in the lower urinary tract. The majority of hospital-acquired UTIs can be related to instrumentation of the urinary tract; the risk of infection increases the longer an indwelling catheter is kept in place. Even a single bladder catheterization may carry a significant risk of infection, particularly in older, debilitated patients.

1. Diagnosis

a. The diagnosis of UTI can be established by the presence of pyuria and a urine culture yielding 100,000 or more bacteria per milliliter. Fewer bacteria can also be associated with infection. Bacteria seen on an unspun sample of urine correlate roughly with at least 100,000 bacteria per milliliter if the Gram's stain is performed immediately after obtaining the urine sample.

b. Infection in other sites must be excluded before ascribing signs of clinical sepsis to a UTI alone because asymptomatic bacteriuria or bladder colonization is quite common with increasing catheter time.

c. **The most common pathogen** in hospital-acquired UTIs is *E. coli,* followed by a variety of gram-negative bacilli, including *Pseudomonas aeruginosa,* as well as enterococci and *Candida.*

2. **Management**

a. In ICUs, should fever or evidence of septicemia present, parenteral therapy should be started. If the urine Gram's stain demonstrates gram-negative rods, a third-generation cephalosporin with good activity against *Pseudomonas aeruginosa,* as well as other gram-negative bacilli (such as ceftazidime), should be begun. If the Gram's stain is consistent with enterococci, ampicillin and gentamicin should be given. This regimen may be modified when culture and sensitivity results are available.

b. **The complications of UTIs should be considered.**

(1) **Acute pyelonephritis** may be suggested by fever, rigors, flank pain, and costovertebral angle tenderness. It can definitely be diagnosed only by the presence of WBC casts in the urine. The presence of any of the signs of pyelonephritis in an ICU patient, particularly fever or leukocytosis in association with pyuria and bacteriuria, should be treated with parenteral antibiotics.

(2) **Inappropriate therapy or urinary tract obstruction** may be suggested by persistent fever beyond 48–72 hours after the initiation of therapy, severe flank pain, hematuria, or deteriorating renal function. If this is clinically suspected, a renal ultrasound should be obtained; if hydronephrosis is found, percutaneous nephrostomy should be considered to drain any purulent collections proximal to the level of obstruction.

(3) **Bacteremia occurs in a small percentage of UTIs.** When clinically suspected or documented by a positive blood culture, broad-spectrum parenteral antibiotic coverage is mandatory until sensitivity data are obtained.

(4) **Acute prostatitis** can occasionally present as a recurrent UTI, with symptoms of dysuria, urgency, and frequency, and can appear as a complication of catheterization in male patients. It is commonly associated with a tender, boggy prostate gland. The organisms involved are most commonly gram negative or enterococci. In the setting of acute prostatitis, antibiotic penetration of the inflamed prostate is good. Prostatic abscess is a rare complication of prostatitis and may be difficult to diagnose, requiring transrectal ultrasonography or computerized tomography (CT). In addition to appropriate antibiotics, the abscess should be drained.

B. **Respiratory tract infections.** Pneumonia is the leading nosocomial infectious cause of death.

1. Pneumonia is either community acquired or hospital acquired.

a. **Community-acquired pneumonias** are often caused by penicillin-sensitive mouth flora or by specific organisms, such as pneumococcus, *Haemophilus influenzae, Mycoplasma pneumoniae, Chlamydia,* or *Legionella pneumophila.*

b. **Hospital-acquired pneumonias.** Intensive care patients are susceptible to colonization of their respiratory secretions with hospital flora, primarily aerobic gram-negative rods and *S. aureus.* This colonization occurs rapidly, usually with 24 hours. Thus, unless a patient has entered the ICU within 24 hours of hospital admission, colonization with hospital pathogens should be assumed, and any lower respiratory infection should be treated for in-hospital organisms. Recent studies have also suggested an association between gastric colonization and tracheal colonization and subsequent pneumonia. Elimination of gastric acidity with antacid therapy and H2-blockers increases gastric colonization and may be associated with an increased risk of pneumonia.

2. **Nosocomial pneumonia** is caused by a variety of organisms. The frequency of specific organisms varies among institutions and even among ICUs in the same institution.
   - **a.** Aerobic gram-negative rods such as *Klebsiella, E. coli, Enterobacter, Proteus, Serratia, Acinetobacter,* and *Pseudomonas* species, as well as *S. aureus,* a gram-positive organism, are usual organisms.
   - **b.** *Streptococcus pneumoniae* and *H. influenzae* are far less common in hospital-acquired than in community-acquired disease.
   - **c.** Anaerobic and viral infections are difficult to document, although they may play greater roles than is recognized.
   - **d.** *Candida albicans* identified on sputum Gram's stain usually results from mucosal candidiasis. It is rarely responsible for respiratory infection, with the exception of lung transplant recipients.
   - **e.** Organisms not recognizable on Gram's stain, such as *Mycoplasma, Legionella pneumophila, Mycobacterium tuberculosis,* and viruses, can cause pneumonia.
   - **f. In immunocompromised hosts,** a wide variety of organisms may cause pneumonia but usually cannot be recognized by Gram's stain. The etiologies of these vary with the underlying disease but most commonly include *Aspergillus* (particularly in neutropenic hosts and in patients with chronic granulomatous disease), *Pneumocystis carinii* and *Cryptococcus neoformans* (in AIDS patients and others with defects in cell-mediated immunity), *Nocardia* (in patients with defects in cell-mediated immunity and in patients with pulmonary alveolar proteinosis), and viral infections (in patients with defects in cell-mediated immunity).
3. **Diagnosis** of pneumonia is based on history, physical examination, and laboratory tests.
   - **a. History**
     - **(1)** The possibility of pneumonia will be raised by a history of underlying disorders, such as congestive heart failure, diabetes, alcoholism, chronic lung disease, AIDS, recent upper airway manipulation, and conditions predisposing to aspiration, such as drug overdose and seizures. Mechanical ventilation increases the risk of developing lower respiratory infection. The risk of infection increases with prolonged duration of intubation.
     - **(2)** Cough, sputum production, hemoptysis, fever, rigors, and diaphoresis are common signs of pneumonia.
     - **(3)** Pleuritic chest pain will occur with pleural involvement, although this is more common with a community-acquired pneumococcal or Group A streptococcal pneumonia.
   - **b. Physical examination**
     - **(1)** Pulmonary examination often reveals only wet rales initially, progressing in some pneumonias to signs of consolidation with dullness to percussion, bronchial breath sounds, and egophony.
     - **(2)** Cyanosis, tachypnea, and use of accessory muscles suggest significant respiratory distress. Unexplained dyspnea should raise the possibility of pneumonia in an ICU patient.
   - **c. Laboratory tests**
     - **(1)** Chest radiography may show a new or progressive infiltrate. However, other conditions such as pulmonary edema, atelectasis, hemorrhage, and pulmonary infarction may mimic pneumonia radiographically.
     - **(2)** Sputum Gram's stain is essential for suggesting a bacterial etiology and, thus, for determining the initial antibiotic coverage; however, its diagnostic accuracy is variable. In the pres-

ence of a few squamous cells (<10 cells/high-power field) and many neutrophils (>25 cells/high-power field), the findings on sputum Gram's stain are more significant.

(a) Several techniques can be used to help induce sputum production, including chest physical therapy, humidified air, ultrasonic nebulization, and nasotracheal suctioning.

(b) Transtracheal aspiration in nonintubated patients should be considered if noninvasive attempts to induce sputum fail. Relative contraindications include bleeding diatheses (including thrombocytopenia), hypoxemia, and hypercapnia. This is a potentially dangerous procedure, and complications include pneumothorax, hemorrhage, and cervical cellulitis.

(c) Sputum culture with sensitivity testing should be sent, ideally prior to the initiation of antibiotic therapy.

(d) In the immunocompromised host, bronchoscopy with transbronchial biopsy, percutaneous needle aspiration, or open lung biopsy should be considered.

4. **Management.** The clinical setting, history, physical examination, and chest radiograph will establish a presumptive diagnosis; however, only prior cultures and sputum Gram's stain will dictate the specific initial course of therapy. The major categories of etiologic organisms can often be determined by careful inspection of the Gram's stain. As culture and antibiotic sensitivity results become available, therapy can be altered. Nevertheless, the initial choice of antibiotics often has to be made on the basis of incomplete information. The Gram's stain of the most purulent material available will dictate the antibiotics used. If the secretions do not contain PMNs, they are probably not worth examining further, except in the severely granulocytopenic patient.

a. **Gram-positive cocci.** Their morphology should be noted.

(1) Tetrads and grapelike clusters suggest a staphylococcal infection; a penicillinase-resistant penicillin such as oxacillin or nafcillin should generally be used. First-generation cephalosporins, such as cefazolin, cephalothin, and cephapirin, are also highly effective agents. Neither the antistaphylococcal penicillins nor the cephalosporins are effective against methicillin-resistant *S. aureus* (so-called MRSA). If the patient is penicillin allergic or if MRSA is widely prevalent, vancomycin is the drug of choice. *Staphylococcus epidermidis* is rarely a significant pathogen in this site.

(2) Pairs of chains suggest a streptococcal infection. Penicillin G alone generally suffices. **If the sputum sample is inadequate to determine on Gram's stain the etiology of the pneumonia, narrow-spectrum treatment with an antistaphylococcal penicillin or with penicillin G is unacceptable therapy.**

b. **Gram-negative rods.** Most gram-negative rods can be treated adequately with a third-generation cephalosporin (or, in the penicillin-cephalosporin allergic patient, aztreonam). If *Pseudomonas aeruginosa* pneumonia is suspected, an antipseudomonal penicillin such as piperacillin or imipenem should be given with an aminoglycoside. In an ill ICU patient with a gram-negative pneumonia, empiric treatment with an antipseudomonal antibiotic and an aminoglycoside should be begun. If the organism subsequently isolated does not require an aminoglycoside for synergy or to prevent the development of resistance, the aminoglycoside should be stopped.

c. **Gram-positive mixed with gram-negative organisms.** If this is an adequate sample, it suggests aspiration of mixed mouth flora. This can present as pneumonitis or as a lung abscess due to a mixture of aerobic and anaerobic organisms from the oropharynx. For years, penicillin has been the mainstay of treatment of lung abscesses resulting from oropharyngeal anaerobes, but with the increasing resistance to penicillin of beta-lactamase-producing *Bacteroides* species, many authorities suggest penicillin G and either clindamycin or metronidazole for the initial treatment of serious anaerobic lung abscesses. In this setting, cultures (aerobic and anaerobic) should be performed on empyema fluid (if present) to confirm the diagnosis. If the patient has an aspiration pneumonitis and not a lung abscess, coverage should aim for both gram-negative rods and mouth anaerobes. Possible antibiotic combinations include imipenem, ticarcillin-clavulanate, or a third-generation cephalosporin plus clindamycin, or in penicillin-allergic patients, aztreonam plus clindamycin.

d. When no sputum is available, the choice of antibiotics depends on the bacterial flora of the ICU. If *Pseudomonas aeruginosa* and other resistant gram-negative rods (e.g., *Serratia, Acinetobacter*) are not common, the combination of a first-generation cephalosporin such as cefazolin or cephapirin along with an aminoglycoside is often used. However, in an ICU with a high incidence of pseudomonal infections, a combination of two antipseudomonal agents (such as ceftazidime, cefoperazone, imipenem, or piperacillin *with* tobramycin) with an antistaphylococcal agent added (except when imipenem is used, which has excellent activity against staphylococci) might be appropriate.

e. **Massive aspiration** of food or gastric contents does not invariably lead to pneumonia and should be managed with immediate and thorough endotracheal suctioning. Bronchoscopy and lavage with small amounts of saline should be performed if large particles cause airway obstruction. Corticosteroids and prophylactic antibiotics have not been demonstrated to affect mortality and may increase the rate of superinfection with resistant organisms. Thus, antibiotic usage should be determined by subsequent clinical status and sputum examination.

f. **Chest physical therapy** has traditionally been a mainstay in the initial treatment of all lower respiratory infections, particularly in patients with chronic lung disease and impaired clearance mechanisms.

5. Several problems can be associated with lower respiratory tract infections.

   a. **Bronchospasm** should be treated appropriately. The simultaneous administration of erythromycin with aminophylline or theophylline causes an increased serum theophylline level, which may result in toxicity. If erythromycin is given, dosing of the aminophylline or theophylline should be reduced and appropriate monitoring of serum levels performed.

   b. **Parenchymal destruction** is particularly common with infections due to *Klebsiella* species, *S. aureus,* and anaerobes but is unusual with pneumococcal infection. As damage progresses, **lung abscess, pneumothorax, empyema,** and even **bronchopleural fistula** can occur. Infrequently, vascular erosion can result in **pulmonary hemorrhage.** Contiguous spread can occasionally involve the pericardium, with resultant **purulent pericarditis.**

   c. **Pleural effusions** usually require thoracentesis, at least for diagnostic purposes. Most pleural effusions in the setting of cardiac, hepatic, or renal disease are transudative. Effusions due to inflammation and infection, in contrast, tend to be exudative. Local inflammation in adjacent tissues may cause a **parapneumonic effusion** without infection due to increased capillary permeability or lymphatic obstruction. **Empyema** is formed by the extension of infection to the pleural space.

(1) **Diagnostic thoracentesis** will help to distinguish transudates, parapneumonic effusions, and empyema, as well as identify other important causes of pleural effusions, such as malignancy, pulmonary infarction, connective tissue disease, or pancreatitis.

(a) Pleural fluid should be examined with Gram's stain and routine and anaerobic cultures. If the clinical setting is appropriate, acid-fast stains and cultures (with Cope needle biopsy of pleura), fungal mounts, and fungal cultures should be included. An empyema usually demonstrates organisms of Gram's stain, although they may be absent following prior antibiotic therapy.

(b) Chemical studies of serum and pleural fluid protein, glucose, lactic acid dehydrogenase (LDH), pH, and occasionally amylase should always be obtained. Exudative effusions have been defined by one of three criteria:

(i) Pleural fluid protein divided by serum protein greater than 0.5

(ii) Pleural fluid LDH divided by serum LDH greater than 0.6

(iii) Pleural fluid LDH greater than two-thirds of the upper limit of normal for serum LDH

An empyema, in contrast to a parapneumonic effusion, can be easily diagnosed with grossly purulent fluid but in borderline cases is suggested by a glucose less than 40 mg per deciliter or a pH less than 7.20 (with an arterial blood pH > 7.35).

(c) The pleural fluid WBC count and differential may be important in both the initial diagnosis and therapy.

(d) If tuberculosis is suspected, a purified protein derivative (PPD) should be placed. In addition to acid-fast smears and mycobacterial cultures noted in **(a)** sputum should be sent for acid-fast smear and mycobacterial culture. If other body sites are suspicious for tuberculosis infection (e.g., sterile pyuria), appropriate smears and cultures should be performed.

(e) If malignancy is suspected, pleural fluid cytology should be obtained.

(2) **Management** of parapneumonic effusions usually involves treatment of the underlying pneumonia alone. Empyemas nearly always require drainage. This eliminates a nidus of infection and may prevent the late development of restrictive lung disease caused by extensive pleural scarring. Some empyemas can be managed by serial thoracentesis and antibiotics, but the thicker the fluid is and the more destructive the organism is, the more likely they are to require thoracostomy. If the latter is unsuccessful, open thoracostomy drainage or decortication may be needed.

d. **Bacteremia** is clinically recognized in 5% of all nosocomial pneumonias. Its presence significantly increases mortality and the risk of metastatic infection. One of the common sites of metastatic infection, particularly in pneumococcal pneumonia, is the CNS. A lumbar puncture should be performed in all patients with signs suggestive of meningitis, such as mental status changes, meningismus, nausea, vomiting, or headache.

e. Precautions to prevent spread to other patients are required with some pneumonias, particularly staphylococcal, streptococcal, and tuberculous pneumonias.

C. **Wound infections**

1. The incidence of postoperative wound infections in many procedures can be reduced with prophylactic antibiotics. These should be used in selected clean and clean-contaminated cases and probably in all contaminated and dirty cases. The continuation of antibiotics for a prolonged period postoperatively has, in most cases, not been demonstrated to decrease rates of infection.
2. **Predisposing factors** are necrotic tissue, foreign bodies, accumulations of blood or serous fluids, and violation of aseptic technique.
3. **Diagnosis** of wound infection rests on the inspection of the surgical site and the search for purulent drainage or signs of cellulitis. Deep infection or infection within a hematoma may require aspiration and a search for PMNs and bacteria on the Gram's stain. The antibiotic used should be on the basis of pathogens likely to be present following a particular procedure and the known antibiotic sensitivities in a given institution. The most common wound pathogens are the aerobic gram-negative rods and *S. aureus*. A wide variety of other organisms, including enterococci, *Bacteroides,* anaerobic streptococci, *Clostridium* and *Candida,* and fungi will also appear, depending on the setting, source, and nature of the wound.
4. **Treatment**
   a. Some important distinctions can be made on Gram's stain of wound drainage or aspirated material.
      (1) **Gram-positive cocci in clusters** suggest staphylococci. Both *S. aureus* and coagulase-negative staphylococci can cause wound infections, and, thus, vancomycin should be considered pending culture results (since many coagulase-negative staphylococci are resistant to cephalosporins and to antistaphylococcal penicillins).
      (2) **Gram-positive cocci in chains** in abdominal or pelvic sites are suggestive of enterococci, and treatment with ampicillin or vancomycin is usually adequate. Imipenem is active against *Enterococcus (Streptococcus) faecalis,* but many isolates of *Enterococcus faecium* are resistant. Increasing resistance has been reported among the enterococci, and sensitivities of the organism may help guide therapy. When enterococci cause endocarditis, the addition of gentamicin (or streptomycin, depending on sensitivities) to ampicillin or penicillin G or vancomycin is mandatory.
      (3) **Gram-negative bacilli** require either an aminoglycoside or another agent with broad gram-negative coverage, such as imipenem or a third-generation cephalosporin, pending culture and sensitivity results.
   b. **Bowel anaerobes** may present in wounds (particularly abdominal or pelvic sites), requiring an agent such as metronidazole, clindamycin, imipenem, ticarcillin-clavulinic acid (Timentin), or ampicillin-sulbactam (Unasyn).

D. **Bacteremia** can occur as the result of infection in an extravascular site or as a primary bacteremia in which no other infection can be demonstrated.

1. **Secondary bacteremia** arises most commonly from the urinary tract, skin, lungs, and wounds.
2. **Primary bacteremias** are most commonly due to *S. aureus,* coagulase-negative staphylococci, *E. coli,* and *Klebsiella*. The focus of infection can be related to contaminated infusion apparatus or instru-

ments or, more commonly, to invasion around the site of the catheter insertion.

a. With fevers of unknown etiology, the changing of all lines should be considered, even without localized cellulitis or thrombophlebitis. In all such cases, cultures of blood and catheter tips should be obtained. Rarely, IV solutions can become contaminated. In such situations, cultures of the infusion solutions are positive.

b. Treatment of catheter-related sepsis generally requires removal of the catheter, followed by 2–4 weeks of IV antibiotics (4 weeks in the case of *S. aureus* to prevent endocarditis and other metastatic infections), depending on the organism and the clinical setting. The diagnosis of fungal sepsis may be difficult. The use of lysis-centrifugation blood cultures (Isolator, du Pont) and an ophthalmologic examination for *Candida* retinitis are important. The eye is the most common site of secondary infection with that organism.

c. Once bacteremia (or fungemia) has been documented, it is mandatory to obtain repeat blood cultures to document the clearance of the bacteremia (or fungemia) with therapy. If bacteremia persists despite a meticulous evaluation of urinary tract, lungs, wounds, and catheter sites, the search for a source has to be individualized and dictated by the clinical setting.

E. **If a patient has been evaluated for fever and none of the sources already noted has been identified,** begin again with a fresh look at the history and a careful repeat physical examination, paying particular attention to the following:

1. **Appliance-related infection.** Check all sites of lines and hardware. Have they remained for longer than 4 days? Consider empirically changing lines and culture of catheter tips.
2. **Decubitus ulcers.** Have these been unrecognized? Are they gangrenous or necrotic? Is there an underlying abscess or osteomyelitis? Do they require debridement or drainage?
3. **Sinusitis.** Does the patient have a nasotracheal or nasogastric tube in place (or a history of one) that might predispose to sinus outflow obstruction? If so, percussion for tenderness and sinus films or CT scan with sinus cuts may be helpful.
4. **Parotitis.** Does the patient have an enlarged, tender parotid or other salivary gland? Is the serum amylase elevated?
5. **Prostatitis.** Perform a rectal examination, particularly if an indwelling urethral catheter has been present. Is the prostate tender or boggy?
6. **Biliary disease.** Does the patient have occult cholecystitis or pancreatitis? Obtain liver function tests and amylase and a right upper quadrant ultrasound if this is suspected.
7. **Subphrenic, intraabdominal, or pelvic abscess.** The abdominal and pelvic examinations can be benign even in the presence of significant disease. Previous intraabdominal or gynecological surgery and bacteremia with an anaerobe are often clues to this diagnosis.
8. **Clostridium difficile** colitis is common in patients who have received prior antibiotics. Diagnosis is by identification of the toxin. Treatment is with oral metronidazole or oral vancomycin.
9. **Unrecognized infection with the human immunodeficiency virus (HIV)** can present as a fever. Obtaining a history of a risk factor for HIV infection (intravenous drug use, male homosexuality or bisexuality, transfusion or blood product recipient in the past, heterosexual contact with a member of a high-risk group including prostitutes, being from a country with a high incidence of heterosexual transmission) should prompt a request to the patient for an HIV antibody test.

F. **Noninfectious causes of fever,** common in ICU patients, include the following:

1. **Drug reaction.** This is most common with antibiotics, cardiac medications, chemotherapeutic agents, and antiseizure medications. Many other agents have been implicated in drug fevers. The minority of patients have eosinophilia, and some will have a rash. Resolution of the fever follows the discontinuation of the offending agent. It is always worthwhile to minimize the number of medications to only those that are required for the patient.
2. **Tissue necrosis**
3. **Atelectasis**
4. **Pulmonary emboli**
5. **Thrombophlebitis**

III. **Prevention of cross-infection**

A. **Strict hand-washing protocols** and constant awareness of the need for sterile technique are the most important means of preventing infection. In any ICU, infections result from the patient's own flora, as well as from the flora shed by or transmitted from hospital personnel via the hands.

B. **Many diseases have an increased likelihood to spread from one patient to another or to hospital employees.** Methods of containing or preventing spread have been incorporated into precaution manuals within each hospital. The most widely used scheme employs precautions that vary in type and intensity.

1. **Complete precautions** require a separate room and strict use of gowns, masks, and gloves.
2. **Contact precautions** interrupt transmission from major wounds or diseases that can be spread by droplets, as well as direct contact.
3. **Drainage and secretion precautions** are used for barrier protection for simple, small wounds.
4. **Respiratory precautions** are used for diseases spread by a truly airborne route.
5. **Enteric precautions** are needed for diseases spread by the fecal-oral route.
6. **Universal precautions** are now in place in order to protect against the possibility of transmitting HIV and other bloodborne agents. All blood, cerebrospinal fluid (CSF), synovial fluid, amniotic fluid, semen, vaginal secretions, or body secretions containing these fluids are considered potentially infectious.

IV. **Patients with HIV infection**

A. **Risk factors** are IV drug use, male homosexuality or bisexuality, prior blood transfusion or blood product use, sexual contact with a person at high risk, and being from a country (e.g., nations in central Africa, Haiti) where heterosexual transmission of the disease is common.

B. **Infection** with the virus follows sexual relations with an infected individual or exposure to contaminated blood or needles.

C. **Diagnosis** of HIV infection is made by a positive enzyme-linked immunosorbent assay (ELISA) test for antibody to HIV followed by Western blot confirmation. There is a period of time, or window, following primary infection in which the test for antibody to HIV is negative.

D. **Immunosuppression** follows the infection in a progressive manner. The time from initial infection to the development of clinically significant immunosuppression is on the order of years.

1. Measurement of the **CD4 count** (T-helper cell count) in patients infected with HIV allows a determination of the state of immunosuppression.
   a. A CD4 greater than 500 per cubic millimeter is not usually associated with symptoms.

b. A CD4 count of 200–500 per cubic millimeter may be associated with weight loss, malaise, oral thrush, or herpes zoster infection.
c. A CD4 count of less than 200 is associated with the development of life-threatening (and AIDS-defining) opportunistic infections and malignancies.

2. **Complications of HIV disease**
   a. **Pulmonary diseases**
      (1) ***Pneumocystis carinii* pneumonia,** the leading cause of mortality in AIDS patients. This pneumonia may present with a normal chest x ray in the setting of fever, dyspnea, and hypoxemia. Diagnosis is made by the identification of cysts in induced sputum specimens or bronchoalveolar lavage fluid. Treatment is a 21-day course of IV trimethoprim-sulfamethoxazole or pentamidine. In mild disease, aerosolized pentamidine can be given. In cases with PO_2 less than 75 mm Hg, corticosteroids should be given as well.
      (2) **Mycobacterium tuberculosis** is common in HIV-positive patients. In addition to pulmonary tuberculosis, extrapulmonary disease is common. Acid-fast smears and mycobacterial cultures should be sent on HIV-positive patients with pulmonary infiltrates. Given the increased risk of tuberculosis in this patient population, until a diagnosis is established, all HIV-positive patients with pulmonary infiltrates should be placed on respiratory precautions to guard against transmission of tuberculosis.
      (3) **Encapsulated bacteria,** including *Streptococcus pneumoniae* and *Haemophilus pneumoniae,* may cause pneumonia in this population.
      (4) **Cytomegalovirus** may cause disease.
      (5) **Fungal infection** by *Cryptococcus neoformans* and, with the proper geographic history, *Histoplasma capsulatum* or *Coccidium immitis.* Sputum or bronchoscopic specimens should be evaluated for fungi, and a serum cryptococcal antigen should be obtained in HIV-positive patients with pulmonary infiltrates.
      (6) **Kaposi's sarcoma** may cause pulmonary infiltrates. Patients often have evidence of disease elsewhere and may have a pleural effusion.
      (7) **Non-Hodgkin's lymphoma** may be present.
   b. **Neurologic complications**
      (1) **Toxoplasmosis** may cause single or multiple ring-enhancing lesions on CT scan; it may not be detected on CT scan, however.
      (2) **Lymphoma** may be radiologically identical to toxoplasmosis.
      (3) ***Cryptococcus neoformans*** may cause meningitis or, less commonly, an intracranial mass lesion.
      (4) **Tuberculosis** may cause meningitis or an intracranial mass lesion.
      (5) **Progressive multifocal encephalopathy** is a demyelinating disease.
      (6) **Cytomegalovirus retinitis** is the most common cause of blindness in AIDS patients. Treatment is with IV ganciclovir.
      (7) **Neurosyphilis** is common in these patients. Failures of standard regimens for primary and secondary syphilis have been reported; appropriate therapy for neurosyphilis is high-dose IV penicillin G.
      (8) **HIV** can cause an aseptic meningitis and an encephalopathy, which may progress to dementia.
   c. **Gastrointestinal complications,** in particular diarrhea, are common in HIV-positive patients. Stool should be sent for bacterial cultures and parasite examination. Etiologies for diarrhea include:

(1) **Salmonella infections.** Relapse following treatment is common, and life-long therapy with oral amoxicillin (if ampicillin sensitive) or ciprofloxacin should be considered.

(2) The parasite **cryptosporidum** can cause a massive diarrhea of many liters per day. Diagnosis is by examination of feces with a modified acid-fast stain. There is currently no effective treatment. Octreotide may be given subcutaneously in an effort to decrease the massive fluid loss.

(3) The parasite **isospora** can be treated with trimethoprim-sulfamethoxazole.

(4) **Cytomegalovirus** may cause disease diagnosed by obtaining positive viral cultures at sigmoidoscopy.

(5) **Other causes of diarrhea** include infection with *Campylobacter, Shigella, Giardia, Entamoeba histolytica,* and, in patients who have received antibiotics, *Clostridium difficile* toxin.

(6) Patients may develop **esophagitis** due to infection with *Candida* or cytomegalovirus.

d. **Fever workup** in an HIV-positive patient should include, in addition to the standard evaluation, a serum cryptococcal antigen, lysis-centrifugation blood cultures for mycobacteria (particularly common is *Mycobacterium avium-intracellulare*) and fungi, and, if a chest x ray is normal, an arterial blood gas to look for an A-a gradient that may be a clue to infection with *Pneumocystis carinii.* If the chest x ray or neurologic exam is abnormal or if diarrhea is present, appropriate attention should be directed to the abnormality. Many AIDS patients have Hickman or other catheters for the long-term administration of antibiotics. As with normal hosts, these can be fever sources.

e. **Other involved systems**

(1) **Hematologic with anemia** (often worsened by drugs including zidovudine [AZT, Retrovir] and trimethoprim-sulfamethoxazole); **thrombocytopenia** (often due to immune-mediated idiopathic thrombocytopenic purpura); and **leukopenia** (which is frequently worsened by ganciclovir and may be worsened by zidovudine).

(2) **Renal disease,** sometimes progressing to end-stage renal disease, particularly in IV drug users

(3) **Skin diseases** including **herpes simplex virus** infections, which may become resistant to acyclovir after long-term use

V. **Antibiotic selection.** The selection of antibiotic agents is an increasingly complex and sophisticated art and must take into consideration the organism, the certainty of the diagnosis, the site infected, and the state of the patient, as well as the toxicity, pharmacokinetics, and cost of the agent used. Initial hypotheses regarding etiologic agents can be made from the clinical status, Gram's stain, and prior cultures. As further information is obtained, an initial broad-spectrum approach can often be narrowed. Sensitivity patterns for many organisms vary from one hospital to another, particularly for gram-negative rods and *S. aureus*. Care should be taken in planning treatment of sites that may be relatively sequestered from blood-borne antibiotics. The most important example is cerebrospinal infection, which is ineffectively treated by many antibiotics. The following summary of the major antibiotics provides their usual indications, with some comments concerning the use of these agents and their pharmacology and side effects. The route of excretion must be carefully considered in the face of renal or hepatic insufficiency. For more details, refer to textbooks of infectious diseases and pharmacology, as well as recently published reviews.

A. **Penicillins. A history of an allergy to one penicillin agent should be considered before any member of this class is given. There is also some cross-reaction with cephalosporins.**

1. **Penicillin G and related agents**
   a. **Indications.** These penicillins are highly active against streptococcal species including *Streptococcus pyogenes* (group A streptococcus), *Streptococcus agalactiae* (group B streptococcus), and the viridans group of pneumoniae (except those isolates that are resistant to penicillin, which are rare). They are also the drugs of choice for treatment of *Neisseria meningitidis, Clostridium* species (except *C. difficile*), *Treponema pallidum, Pasteurella multocida, Actinomyces israelii,* and isolates of *S. aureus* (on the order of 10%) that do not produce penicillinase. They are active against the majority of mouth anaerobes; however, there has been a recent increase in isolates that produce a beta-lactamase and are therefore resistant to penicillin G.
   b. **Agents**
      (1) **Penicillin G**
         (a) Administration: IV, IM
         (b) Excretion: renal, minimal hepatic
         (c) Dose: 2.4–10.0 million units per day; up to 24 million units per day for CNS infections and endocarditis
         (d) Dosage interval: 4–6 hours; 2 hours for CNS infections
      (2) **Penicillin V**
         (a) Administration: PO
         (b) Excretion: renal
         (c) Dose: 1.0–2.0 g per day
         (d) Dosage interval: 6 hours
   c. **Caution:** Decreasing dosages are required with severe renal insufficiency.
   d. **Side effects.** Hypersensitivity is most common, with fever, rash, serum sickness, or anaphylaxis possible. Coombs-positive hemolytic anemia, thrombocytopenia, bone marrow depression, and seizures are uncommon. Long courses of high dosages are more often associated with bone marrow suppression. Central nervous system side effects are very uncommon, except in high dosages and with renal failure.
2. **Penicillinase-resistant penicillins**
   a. **Indications.** These are the agents of choice for methicillin-sensitive, penicillinase-producing *S. aureus*. They are slightly less active against some of the penicillin-sensitive organisms but are adequate to treat common aerobic gram-positive cocci. Enterococci, *Listeria,* and *Neisseria* are not effectively treated with these agents.
   b. **Agents**
      (1) **Nafcillin**
         (a) Administration: IV, IM
         (b) Excretion: hepatic, renal
         (c) Dose: 2–12 g per day
         (d) Dosage interval: 4–6 hours
      (2) **Oxacillin**
         (a) Administration: IV, IM
         (b) Excretion: renal, hepatic
         (c) Dose: 2–12 g per day
         (d) Dosage interval: 4–6 hours
      (3) **Methicillin** is no longer recommended due to potential renal toxicity.
      (4) **Cloxacillin and dicloxacillin**
         (a) Administration: PO
         (b) Excretion: renal, hepatic

(c) Dose: 1.0–3.0 g per day
(d) Dosage interval: 6 hours

c. **Caution:** Because of significant biliary excretion, reduction in dosage is required only in severe renal insufficiency.

d. **Side effects.** Interstitial nephritis and agranulocytosis have been associated with methicillin use and, less commonly, with the other agents. Hypersensitivity, cholestatic jaundice, elevated transaminases, thrombocytopenia, and Coombs-positive hemolytic anemia have been reported. Other complications may be shared with the penicillins.

3. **Extended-spectrum penicillins**

a. **Indications.** These agents are as effective as penicillin G in treating pneumococcal, streptococcal, and meningococcal infections, with some additional action against the gram-negative bacilli *Salmonella, Shigella, Proteus mirabilis,* and *E. coli*. Most strains of *H. influenzae* are susceptible, but a significant minority produce beta-lactamase and are resistant. They are active against *Listeria monocytogenes* and *Enterococcus* species (although some enterococci are resistant) and can be used as a single agent in the treatment of susceptible enterococcal UTIs. They have been used successfully in the treatment of gonococcal infections, but recently resistance has made them an undependable choice for this infection.

b. **Agents**

(1) **Ampicillin**
(a) Administrations: PO, IV, IM
(b) Excretion: renal, hepatic
(c) Dose: PO, 1–4 g per day; parenteral, 1–12 g per day
(d) Dosage interval: 4–6 hours

(2) **Amoxicillin**
(a) Administration: PO
(b) Excretion: renal, hepatic
(c) Dose: 0.75–1.5 g per day
(d) Dosage interval: 8 hours

c. **Caution:** Decreasing dosages are required in severe renal insufficiency.

d. **Side effects.** Hypersensitivity, rash, gastrointestinal effects (especially diarrhea), pseudomembranous colitis, leukopenia, transaminase elevation, convulsions, and nephropathy have been reported.

4. **Penicillins with extended activity against gram-negative bacteria**

a. **Indications.** These agents have increased activity against *Pseudomonas* species, *Proteus,* and other gram-negative bacilli such as *Enterobacter* and *Serratia. Klebsiella* species are often resistant. In serious pseudomonal infections, an aminoglycoside is usually added for synergy. Mezlocillin has somewhat broader coverage than carbenicillin or ticarcillin, with action against *Klebsiella* and anaerobes, particularly *B. fragilis*. Piperacillin has similar activity to mezlocillin. These agents should not be used as monotherapy in serious pseudomonal infections. These agents may cause an increase in bleeding time, which may be clinically significant (e.g., in a thrombocytopenic patient). Piperacillin and mezlocillin are active against *Enterococcus faecalis*. The activity of piperacillin against gram-positive cocci is similar to that of ampicillin.

b. **Agents**

(1) **Carbenicillin**
(a) Administration: PO, IV, IM

(b) Excretion: renal, hepatic
(c) Dose: PO, 4–8 tablets; parenteral, 400–500 mg/kg/day
(d) Dosage interval: PO, 6 hours; parenteral, 4–6 hours

(2) **Ticarcillin**
(a) Administration: IV, IM
(b) Excretion: renal, hepatic
(c) Dose: 150–300 mg/kg/day
(d) Dosage interval: 4–6 hours

(3) **Mezlocillin, azlocillin**
(a) Administration: IV, IM
(b) Excretion: renal, hepatic
(c) Dose: 6–18 g per day
(d) Dosage interval: 4–6 hours

(4) **Piperacillin**
(a) Administration: IV, IM
(b) Excretion: renal, hepatic
(c) Dose: 12–24 g per day

c. **Caution:** Dosages need to be reduced in moderate to severe renal insufficiency.

d. **Side effects.** Hypersensitivity, rash, fever, anaphylaxis, local phlebitis, elevated transaminases, nausea, neutropenia, hemolytic anemia, platelet dysfunction, hypokalemia, sodium overload, and nephropathy have been reported.

B. **Cephalosporins. No cephalosporin treats infections caused by methicillin-resistant staphylococci (including MRSA), enterococci, or *Listeria monocytogenes.* Cross-reacting allergic responses may occur in patients who are penicillin allergic.** With these limitations in mind:

1. **First-generation cephalosporins**

a. **Indications.** The drugs in this group have similar bactericidal actions against gram-positive cocci, including penicillinase-producing staphylococci, as well as many gram-negative bacilli, especially *E. coli, Klebsiella,* and indole-negative *Proteus.* These agents are not active against methicillin-resistant *Staphylococcus, Pseudomonas aeruginosa, Serratia marcescens,* or *Bacteroides fragilis* and should not be used for these organisms. The drugs in this class do not cross the meninges and thus have no role in the treatment of meningitis. Within this class, the most significant differences are those of cost. Blood levels of cefazolin are significantly higher for a given dosage than they are for cephalothin or cephapirin, and dosages generally need to be given only every 8 hours.

b. **Agents**

(1) **Cephalothin, cephapirin**
(a) Administration: IV, IM (painful)
(b) Excretion: renal, hepatic; renal for cephapirin
(c) Dose: 2–12 g per day
(d) Dosage interval: 4–6 hours

(2) **Cefazolin**
(a) Administration: IV, IM
(b) Excretion: renal
(c) Dose: 2–6 g per day
(d) Dosage interval: 6–8 hours

(3) **Cephalexin**
(a) Administration: PO
(b) Excretion: renal
(c) Dose: 1–2 g per day
(d) Dosage interval: 6 hours

c. **Caution:** Dosages need to be reduced in moderate to severe renal insufficiency.

d. **Side effects.** The cephalosporins cross-react with the penicillins in some patients. In the presence of a penicillin allergy, cephalosporins should be used circumspectly, depending on the nature of the penicillin allergy. Hypersensitivity, rash, fever, anaphylaxis, local phlebitis, gastrointestinal symptoms, hypoprothrombinemia, hemolytic anemia, hepatic dysfunction, leukopenia, thrombocytopenia, nephropathy, pseudomembranous colitis, and convulsions have been reported.

2. **Second-generation cephalosporins**

a. **Indications.** The drugs in this group have broader activity against gram-negative organisms. With the exception of cefuroxime, these agents do not reach therapeutic levels in the CSF. *Haemophilus influenzae,* including beta-lactamase-positive strains that are resistant to ampicillin, are sensitive to cefuroxime and cefaclor. The activity of cefamandole against beta-lactamase-positive *H. influenzae* is less than that of cefuroxime. Both cefuroxime and cefamandole are active against most gram-positive cocci (not enterococci or MRSA). Cefoxitin is less active against anaerobes than the other agents (although there are anaerobes resistant to this agent, and there are broader anaerobic agents). It is also active against *Neisseria gonorrhoeae* and is part of one of the treatment regimens for pelvic inflammatory disease. It is generally used in the treatment of intraabdominal and pelvic mixed aerobic-anaerobic infections, as well as in diabetic foot infections. It is often used with an aminoglycoside to improve gram-negative coverage. Cefotetan has a similar spectrum of activity to cefoxitin but has less activity against nonfragilis *Bacteroides* species. It is used in situations where cefoxitin can be used and has the advantage of less frequent dosing. Ceforanide and cefonicid are similar to cefamandole.

b. **Agents**

(1) **Cefoxitin**
- (a) Administration: IV, IM
- (b) Excretion: renal
- (c) Dose: 3–12 g per day
- (d) Dosage interval: 4–6 hours

(2) **Cefuroxime**
- (a) Administration: PO (axetil), IV, IM
- (b) Excretion: renal
- (c) Dose: PO, 0.5–1 g per day; parenteral 3–6 g per day
- (d) Dosage interval: PO, 12 hours; parenteral, 6–8 hours

(3) **Cefaclor**
- (a) Administration: PO
- (b) Excretion: renal
- (c) Dose: 0.75–2 g per day
- (d) Dosage interval: 6–8 hours

(4) **Cefotetan**
- (a) Administration: IV, IM
- (b) Excretion: renal
- (c) Dose: 2–4 g per day
- (d) Dosage interval: 12 hours

(5) **Cefamandole**
- (a) Administration: IV, IM
- (b) Excretion: renal
- (c) Dose: 2–18 g per day
- (d) Dosage interval: 4–6 hours

(6) **Ceforanide**
  (a) Administration: IV, IM
  (b) Excretion: renal
  (c) Dose: 1–2 g per day
  (d) Dosage interval: 12 hours
(7) **Cefonicid**
  (a) Administration: IV, IM
  (b) Excretion: renal
  (c) Dose: 1–2 g per day
  (d) Dosage interval: 24 hours

c. **Caution:** Dosages need to be reduced in moderate to severe renal insufficiency.

d. **Side effects.** Hypersensitivity reactions are most common, with rash, fever, eosinophilia, and anaphylaxis possible. Positive Coombs' test, granulocytopenia, thrombocytopenia, elevated prothrombin time, local phlebitis, pain at the injection site, diarrhea, abnormal liver function tests, nephropathy, pseudomembranous colitis, and disulfiramlike reactions with alcohol ingestion have been reported.

3. **Third-generation cephalosporins**

a. **Indications.** These agents are more active than first-generation cephalosporins against gram-negative bacilli. These are the cephalosporins with activity against *Pseudomonas aeruginosa*. They are often active against gram-negative bacilli that are resistant to other antibiotics. These agents are highly active against *H. influenzae* and *N. gonorrhoeae* (including beta-lactamase-producing strains). They have variable activity against anaerobes and are often less active than first-generation cephalosporins against gram-positive cocci. The most active agents against gram-positive cocci are cefotaxime, ceftriaxone, and ceftizoxime (which has more activity against *Bacteroides* than the other agents). The agents with the greatest activity against *Pseudomonas aeruginosa* are ceftazidime and cefoperazone. Ceftriaxone is the drug of choice for gonococcal infection. These agents (except for cefoperazone) penetrate well into the CSF and can be used in the treatment of bacterial meningitis. Since none of the agents is active against *Listeria monocytogenes,* the addition of ampicillin is recommended when this is a possible cause of the meningitis. Bleeding complications occur with these agents, in part due to the overall poor nutritional status of many of the patients who receive these agents. Moxalactam has a high frequency of bleeding complications associated with its use and is not recommended. In infections with *Pseudomonas aeruginosa* and other multiple-resistant gram-negative organisms, the addition of an aminoglycoside (tobramycin or gentamicin) is suggested. Cefixime and oral cephalosporin have limited activity against *S. aureus* but otherwise have activity similar to that of ceftizoxime. Although there is debate on the point, cefoperazone (which contains a methylthiotetrazole side chain) may be more likely to cause bleeding complications than the other agents in this class.

b. **Agents**

(1) **Cefoperazone**
  (a) Administration: IV
  (b) Excretion: hepatic, renal
  (c) Dose: 3–12 g per day
  (d) Dosage interval: 6–8 hours

(2) **Ceftazadime**
   (a) Administration: IV, IM
   (b) Excretion: renal
   (c) Dose: 3–6 g per day
   (d) Dosage interval: 8 hours

(3) **Cefotaxime**
   (a) Administration: IV, IM
   (b) Excretion: renal
   (c) Dose: 3–12 g per day
   (d) Dosage interval: 6–8 hours

(4) **Ceftizoxime**
   (a) Administration: IV, IM
   (b) Excretion: renal
   (c) Dose: 4–12 g per day
   (d) Dosage interval: 8–12 hours

(5) **Ceftriaxone**
   (a) Administration: IV, IM
   (b) Excretion: renal, hepatic
   (c) Dose: 2–4 g per day
   (d) Dosage interval: 12 hours

(6) **Cefixime**
   (a) Administration: PO
   (b) Excretion: renal
   (c) Dose: 0.4 g per day
   (d) Dosage interval: 24 hours

c. **Caution:** Dosages need to be reduced in moderate to severe renal insufficiency for cefotaxime.

d. **Side effects.** Hypersensitivity reactions are most common, with rash, fever, eosinophilia, and anaphylaxis possible. Local phlebitis, positive Coombs' test, anemia, thrombocytosis, neutropenia, elevated transaminases, diarrhea, nausea, pain at injection sites, azotemia, and a disulfiramlike reaction with alcohol ingestion have been reported. The use of vitamin K supplementation may decrease the probability of bleeding in patients with poor nutritional status who are on lengthy courses of these agents.

C. Carbapenems

1. **Indications.** The only carbapenem that is available in the United States is imipenem. It is given in combination with cilastatin, an inhibitor of a renal peptidase. This is the broadest-spectrum antibiotic available and possesses activity against virtually all gram-positive species (except *Enterococcus faecium, JK Corynebacterium,* methicillin-resistant *S. aureus,* and methicillin-resistant coagulase-negative staphylococci), most gram-negative organisms (except for *Pseudomonas* [now called *Xanthomonas*] *maltophilia,* some *Pseudomonas cepacia,* and *Flavobacterium*), and anaerobes (except for *Clostridium difficile*). It does not treat *Chlamydia trachomatis*. It has excellent activity against most strains of *Pseudomonas aeruginosa,* although some multiple-drug-resistant species are resistant, and emergence of resistance has been documented during therapy in cystic fibrosis patients. As with other antibiotics, an aminoglycoside should be given in addition to this agent in patients with *Pseudomonas aeruginosa* pneumonia. This agent can be used in the treatment of serious infections (e.g., polymicrobial intraabdominal infections), where regimens containing several drugs would otherwise be used. The compound, which contains a beta-lactam, may cross-react in patients allergic to other beta-lactam agents. There has not been extensive experience in using this agent in the treatment of bacterial meningitis, and other agents are preferred.

2. **Agent: Imipenem**
   a. Administration: IV, IM
   b. Excretion: renal
   c. Dose: 2 g per day
   d. Dosage interval: 6–8 hours
3. **Caution:** Dosages need to be reduced in renal insufficiency. Seizures occur, most often in patients with abnormal renal function who receive inappropriately high doses of this agent.
4. **Side effects.** Hypersensitivity, seizures, confusion, myoclonus, rash, diarrhea, pseudomembranous colitis, elevations in liver function tests, leukopenia, phlebitis, and oliguria have been reported.

D. Monobactams

1. **Indications.** Aztreonam, the sole member of this class of drugs that is currently available, has activity that is limited to gram-negative bacilli. There is essentially no activity against gram-positive or anaerobic bacteria. It acts in a manner similar to the penicillins, cephalosporins, and imipenem in that it affects the cell wall of bacteria by binding to penicillin-binding proteins. It is active against many strains of *Pseudomonas aeruginosa,* but many strains are resistant to this agent. There is said to be less likelihood of a cross-reaction in patients who are allergic to penicillin. Thus, this agent can be given cautiously in penicillin-allergic patients. This has a spectrum of activity that is similar to that of third-generation cephalosporins, except that there is no gram-positive coverage with this agent. It is not an aminoglycoside and is synergistic with aminoglycosides against some gram-negative rods. It is best used when for allergic reasons a third-generation cephalosporin cannot be used (with the understanding that no gram-positive coverage is provided by this agent).
2. **Agent: Aztrenonam**
   a. Administration: IV
   b. Excretion: renal
   c. Dose: 3–8 g per day
   d. Dosage interval: 6–8 hours
3. **Caution:** Dosages should be reduced in renal insufficiency. If there is any chance of a gram-positive infection, another agent must be given as well.
4. **Side effects.** Superinfection with gram-positive cocci, rash, elevated liver function tests, pseudomembranous colitis, and phlebitis have been reported.

E. Combination beta-lactamase inhibitors and beta-lactam agents

1. **Indications.** The addition of a beta-lactamase inhibitor to ampicillin, amoxicillin, and ticarcillin broadens the spectrum of coverage to beta-lactamase-producing bacteria, including *S. aureus* (but not methicillin-resistant *S. aureus*), *Haemophilus influenzae, Branhamella catarrhalis,* anaerobes, and many *E. coli* and *Klebsiella* organisms that are resistant to the parent compound. The addition of clavulanate does not result in sensitivity to ticarcillin-clavulanate in ticarcillin-resistant *Pseudomonas aeruginosa* since the beta-lactamase produced is not inhibited by clavulanate. These agents are most commonly used to treat mixed aerobic/anaerobic infections, including diabetic foot and intraabdominal and gynecologic infections. These agents can be used in the treatment of pneumonia due to susceptible organisms. Amoxicillin-clavulanate can be given for the treatment of chronic bronchitis. In serious intraabdominal infections, these agents are often combined with an aminoglycoside. They are superb drugs for anaerobic infections.

2. **Agents**
   (1) **Ticarcillin-clavulanate**
      (a) Administration: IV
      (b) Excretion: renal, hepatic
      (c) Dose: 12.4–18.6 g per day
      (d) Dosage interval: 4–6 hours
   (2) **Ampicillin-sulbactam**
      (a) Administration: IV, IM
      (b) Excretion: renal, hepatic
      (c) Dose: 6–12 g per day
      (d) Dosage interval: 6 hours
   (3) **Amoxicillin-clavulanate**
      (a) Administration: PO
      (b) Excretion: renal
      (c) Dose: 0.75–1.5 g per day
      (d) Dosage interval: 8 hours
3. **Caution:** Dose reduction in renal insufficiency is required with ticarcillin-clavulanate.
4. **Side effects.** Diarrhea is common with amoxicillin-clavulanate. Other side effects are those of the parent compound.

F. Quinolones

1. **Indications.** These antibiotics have broad gram-negative rod activity against urinary pathogens and are often active against enterococci; thus, they can be used in the management of UTIs. Ciprofloxacin, which now has an IV formulation, has been used in the treatment of pulmonary infections with susceptible organisms. Of note, the activity of these agents against the pneumococcus and anaerobes is limited. Thus, quinolones should not be given in cases of community-acquired pneumonia, aspiration pneumonia, or acute sinusitis. There is also a significant failure rate when this drug is used to treat *S. aureus* and *Pseudomonas aeruginosa* pneumonia. Bacterial causes of diarrhea (including *Salmonella, Shigella,* and *Campylobacter*) have been successfully treated with norfloxacin (which is not intended for systemic infections) and with ciprofloxacin. Oral therapy with ciprofloxacin has been used to treat soft tissue infections and osteomyelitis. It is worth checking sensitivities to ciprofloxacin in the setting of infection with a highly resistant gram-negative rod (e.g., *Pseudomonas aeruginosa* pneumonia) that requires a second effective antibiotic. Some strains of methicillin-resistant *S. aureus* are sensitive to ciprofloxacin. In settings where patients have severe allergies to vancomycin, it is worthwhile to determine the sensitivity of the isolate to ciprofloxacin. In addition, gonococcal infections are susceptible to ciprofloxacin. These agents, which affect DNA gyrase, should not be used in pregnant women or in children.
2. **Agents**
   a. **Ciprofloxacin**
      (1) Administration: PO, IV
      (2) Excretion: renal, hepatic
      (3) Dose: PO, 0.5–1.5 g per day
      (4) Dosage interval: 12 hours
   b. **Norfloxacin**
      (1) Administration: PO
      (2) Excretion: renal, hepatic
      (3) Dose: 0.8 g per day
      (4) Dosage interval: 12 hours
   c. **Ofloxacin**
      (1) Administration: PO
      (2) Excretion: renal

(3) Dose: 0.4–0.8 g per day
(4) Dosage interval: 12 hours

3. **Caution:** Dosages need to be reduced in renal insufficiency. These agents may cause an increase in serum theophylline concentrations.
4. **Side effects.** Nausea, vomiting, elevated liver function tests, dizziness, headache, rash, leukopenia

G. **Vancomycin**

1. **Indications.** Vancomycin is active against most gram-positive bacteria, including *S. aureus* (the drug of choice for methicillin-resistant strains), coagulase-negative staphylococci, and enterococci. It has minimal activity against gram-negative bacteria. The oral form is effective in treating pseudomembranous colitis caused by *C. difficile* but cannot be used for any systemic effect even though there may be a small amount of absorption that is significant only in the presence of renal insufficiency.
2. **Agent: Vancomycin**
   (a) Administration: PO, IV
   (b) Excretion: renal
   (c) Dose: PO, 0.5 g per day; IV, 1–2 g per day
   (d) Dosage interval: 12 hours
3. **Caution:** Dosages need to be reduced even in mild renal insufficiency. Serum levels should be obtained. Levels less than or equal to 10 μg per milliliter and peak levels of 20–30 μg per milliliter are preferred.
4. **Side effects.** Hypersensitivity reactions with rash, fever, eosinophilia, and anaphylaxis are possible. Rapid infusion (over less than 45 minutes) has been associated with hypotension and urticarial lesion. These reactions do not usually represent hypersensitivity reactions; the drug can be administered again slowly, usually without further sequelae. Local phlebitis, ototoxicity, nephrotoxicity, neutropenia, and peripheral neuropathy have been reported.

H. **Erythromycin and clindamycin**

1. **Indications.** Erythromycin is active against many gram-positive organisms, particularly streptococcal and staphylococcal species, *Corynebacterium diphtheriae,* as well as *Bacteroides, Mycoplasma pneumoniae, Legionella species,* and *Chlamydia trachomatis.* Clindamycin has similar activity against gram-positive organisms, although it is inactive against the enterococcus. Clindamycin is more active against anaerobes than erythromycin, but *C. difficile* is resistant. Clindamycin is also active against the parasite *Toxoplasma gondii.*
2. **Agents**
   a. **Erythromycin**
      (1) Administration: PO, IV
      (2) Excretion: hepatic, renal
      (3) Dose: PO, 1–2 g per day; IV, 1–4 g per day
      (4) Dosage interval: 6 hours
   b. **Clindamycin**
      (1) Administration: PO, IV, IM
      (2) Excretion: hepatic, renal
      (3) Dose: PO, 600–1,800 mg per day; IV, IM, 600–2,700 mg per day
      (4) Dosage interval: PO, 6 hours; parenteral, 8 hours
3. **Caution:** Dosages should be reduced in hepatic insufficiency.
4. **Side effects.** Hypersensitivity reactions such as fever, rash, eosinophilia, and anaphylaxis can occur with either agent. Erythromycin can cause cholestatic hepatitis (primarily with the estolate form), elevated transaminases, epigastric distress, pain at injection site, local phlebitis, transient ototoxicity, stomatitis, pseudomembranous colitis, hemolytic anemia, and increased theophylline effect. Clinda-

mycin has been associated with diarrhea, pseudomembranous colitis, transaminase elevation, Stevens-Johnson syndrome, granulocytopenia, thrombocytopenia, and local phlebitis.

I. Tetracyclines

1. **Indications.** The tetracyclines have a wide spectrum of activity against gram-positive and gram-negative bacteria but have largely been replaced by other antibiotics. They remain useful agents for *Rickettsia, Chlamydia, Nocardia, Borrelia, Mycoplasma,* and *Vibrio vulnificus* and, accordingly, are used infrequently in an ICU setting.
2. **Agents**
   - a. **Tetracycline, oxytetracycline, and chlortetracycline**
     - (1) Administration: PO, IV
     - (2) Excretion: renal, hepatic
     - (3) Dose: 1–2 g per day
     - (4) Dosage interval: 6 hours
   - b. **Doxycycline**
     - (1) Administration: PO
     - (2) Excretion: hepatic
     - (3) Dose: 0.1–0.2 g per day
     - (4) Dosage interval: 12–24 hours
   - c. **Minocycline**
     - (1) Administration: PO
     - (2) Excretion: hepatic, renal
     - (3) Dose: 0.2 g per day
     - (4) Dosage interval: 12 hours
3. **Caution:** Dosages of tetracycline and oxytetracycline need to be reduced in moderate to severe renal insufficiency.
4. **Side effects.** Gastrointestinal irritation is common. Hypersensitivity reactions, phototoxicity, hepatic toxicity (fulminant acute fatty liver necrosis in pregnant women, rarely), renal failure, tooth discoloration in children, local thrombophlebitis from IV administration, leukocytosis, and vestibular toxicity (especially with minocycline) have been observed. This family of drugs is best avoided in pregnant women and in small children.

J. Chloramphenicol

1. **Indications.** Chloramphenicol is a broad-spectrum agent with activity against *H. influenzae, N. meningitidis, S. typhi,* and *Rickettsia,* as well as anaerobes and many gram-positive and gram-negative bacteria. It is not frequently used because of the rare side effect of aplastic anemia and because other potentially less toxic agents can almost always be found that are appropriate for the clinical situation.
2. **Agent: Chloramphenicol**
   - a. Administration: PO, IV
   - b. Excretion: renal (after hepatic metabolism)
   - c. Dose: PO, 1.5–3 g per day; IV, 2–4 g per day
   - d. Dosage interval: 6 hours
3. **Caution:** Dosages should be reduced in hepatic insufficiency
4. **Side effects.** Idiosyncratic aplastic anemia is rare (incidence of 1 in 25,000 to 1 in 40,000). Dose-related pancytopenia is usually reversible and can be detected by serial testing of hematologic parameters, including the reticulocyte count, iron, and iron-binding capacity. Other reactions include hypersensitivity, hemolytic anemia, gastrointestinal irritation, and optic neuritis, as well as fatal "gray syndrome" in neonates. Therefore, chloramphenicol is not safe for use in pregnancy.

K. Metronidazole

1. **Indications.** Metronidazole is a useful agent in anaerobic infections,

with activity against most anaerobic bacteria and many protozoa such as *Trichomona, Giardia,* and *Entamoeba.* It should not be used as a sole agent in lung or brain abscess because of the likely presence of microaerophilic streptococci, which are not sensitive to metronidazole. The addition of, for example, penicillin covers these organisms as well. It is often used with an agent active against gram-negative bacilli in the treatment of intraabdominal infections. This agent can be used as a less expensive alternative to oral vancomycin in cases of pseudomembranous colitis due to *C. difficile.*

2. **Agent: Metronidazole**
   a. Administration: PO, IV
   b. Excretion: renal (after hepatic metabolism)
   c. Dose: PO, 1,500 mg per day; IV, 15 mg per kilogram loading dose followed by 30 mg/kg/day
   d. Dosage interval: PO, 8 hours; IV, 6 hours
3. **Caution:** Dosages should be reduced in renal insufficiency.
4. **Side effects.** Gastrointestinal irritation, metallic taste, glossitis, stomatitis, furry tongue, disulfiramlike reaction with alcohol ingestion, dizziness, vertigo, ataxia, peripheral neuropathy, and neutropenia have been reported.

L. Sulfonamides

1. **Indications.** The sulfonamides exert a wide spectrum of activity against both gram-positive and gram-negative bacteria but have few indications in the ICU other than in the treatment of pneumonia due to *Pneumocystis carinii* with trimethoprim-sulfamethoxazole. Nocardiosis and toxoplasmosis often require the use of these drugs. One organism that is frequently resistant to virtually all antimicrobials except for trimethoprim-sulfamethoxazole is *Xanthomonas (Pseudomonas) maltophilia.* Trimethoprim-sulfamethoxazole is also indicated for the treatment of *Listeria monocytogenes* infections meningitis in penicillin-allergic patients.
2. **Agents**
   a. **Sulfisoxazole**
      (1) Administration: PO
      (2) Excretion: renal
      (3) Dose: 4–6 g per day
      (4) Dosage interval: 4–6 hours
   b. **Sulfadiazine**
      (1) Administration: PO
      (2) Excretion: renal
      (3) Dose: 2–4 g per day
      (4) Dosage interval: 4–8 hours
   c. **Sulfamethoxazole**
      (1) Administration: PO
      (2) Excretion: renal
      (3) Dose: 2–3 g per day
      (4) Dosage interval: 8–12 hours
   d. **Trimethoprim-sulfamethoxazole**
      (1) Administration: PO, IV
      (2) Excretion: renal
      (3) Dose: PO, 4 tablets or 3 double-strength tablets per day; IV (based on trimethoprim component) 8–10 mg/kg/day, 20 mg/kg/day for *Pneumocystis carinii*
      (4) Dosage interval: PO, 12 hours; IV, 6 hours
3. **Caution:** Dosages should be reduced in moderate and severe renal insufficiency. Adequate hydration to maintain a urinary output

greater than or equal to 1,200 ml per day is necessary to prevent crystallization in the urine, particularly with sulfadiazine. These agents interact with sulfonylureas to cause an increased hypoglycemic effect.

4. **Side effects.** Hypersensitivity reactions, hemolytic anemia, agranulocytosis, thrombocytopenia, aplastic anemia, eosinophilia, peripheral neuritis, arthritis, and psychiatric disorders have been reported.

M. Aminoglycosides

1. **Indications.** These agents are active primarily against the aerobic gram-negative bacilli. Streptomycin and gentamicin have limited use against enterococci and other streptococci, in combination with a penicillin or with vancomycin. Tobramycin and gentamicin have similar activity, although tobramycin tends to be more active against *Pseudomonas aeruginosa* and gentamicin tends to be more active against *Serratia* species. Amikacin is often active against nosocomial gram-negative organisms resistant to the other aminoglycosides and is reserved from standard use at many institutions for this reason. Streptomycin is generally confined to the use of tuberculosis, plague, tularemia, and brucellosis. Netilmicin has activity that is similar to that of gentamicin and tobramycin. These agents do not cover anaerobes. In an ICU setting (particularly in an NPO patient) IV amikacin can be used as an antituberculous drug instead of IM streptomycin. These agents do not penetrate well into the CSF.
2. **Agents**
   a. **Tobramycin and gentamicin**
      (1) Administration: IV, IM
      (2) Excretion: renal
      (3) Dose: 1.5 mg per kilogram loading dose; then 3–5 mg per day (in normal renal function)
      (4) Dosage interval: 8 hours (depending on renal function)
   b. **Amikacin**
      (1) Administration: IV, IM
      (2) Excretion: renal
      (3) Dose: 7.5 mg per kilogram loading dose; then 15 mg/kg/day in normal renal function
      (4) Dosage interval: 8 hours (depending on renal function)
   c. **Netilmicin**
      (1) Administration: IV, IM
      (2) Excretion: renal
      (3) Dose: 4–6.5 mg/kg/day (in normal renal function)
      (4) Dosage interval: 8 hours (depending on renal function)
3. **Caution:** Renal function must be monitored carefully before and during use of aminoglycosides, with dosages reduced for renal insufficiency. Dosages should be decreased in the elderly even in the setting of a normal serum creatinine. Serum drug levels should be monitored. Trough levels under 2 μg per milliliter and peak levels of 4–8 μg per milliliter are considered therapeutic for tobramycin, gentamicin, and netilmicin. For amikacin, trough levels of less than or equal to 5 μg per milliliter and peak levels of 15–25 μg per milliliter are desirable. In general, if the peak level is too high, the dosage should be reduced. If the trough level is too high, the dosage interval should be increased. Lower doses of gentamicin should be given in the setting of treatment of enterococcal or streptococcal endocarditis, when the agents are given for synergy.
4. **Side effects.** The aminoglycosides have significant nephrotoxicity, causing an acute tubular necrosis that is usually reversible. Ototoxicity with vestibular and auditory dysfunction is also common. Neuro-

muscular blockade can occur in patients treated with succinylcholine, drugs related to curare and magnesium, and in patients with myasthenia gravis. Hypersensitivity reactions are relatively rare.

N. Antituberculous drugs

1. **Indications.** These drugs are indicated for the treatment of infection with *Mycobacterium tuberculosis* and for certain other mycobacterial diseases. Rifampin has broad activity against other infectious agents and is often used with erythromycin in the treatment of *Legionella* infections and in close contacts of patients with meningococcal disease. The diagnosis of tuberculosis is made difficult by the slow growth of the organism, and the initiation of antituberculous therapy is often made before culture data confirm the diagnosis. Since the development of resistance occurs during therapy with a single drug, the treatment of active disease should include a minimum of two drugs (more if resistance is suspected, as in patients who have received previous antituberculous therapy or are from areas of the world in which drug resistance is common). Treatment must continue for many months to prevent relapse. In an ICU setting, amikacin in appropriate doses is sometimes given IV instead of streptomycin to treat tuberculosis. The dosages that follow are for the treatment of tuberculosis.

2. **Agents**

   a. **Isoniazid (INH)**
      (1) Administration: PO, IM; IV possible
      (2) Excretion: hepatic, renal (minor)
      (3) Dose: 5–10 mg/kg/day, up to 300 mg per day
      (4) Dosage interval: 24 hours

   b. **Rifampin**
      (1) Administration: PO, IV
      (2) Excretion: hepatic
      (3) Dose: 600 mg per day
      (4) Dosage interval: 24 hours

   c. **Ethambutol**
      (1) Administration: PO
      (2) Excretion: renal
      (3) Dose: 15–25 mg/kg/day for 2 months followed by 15 mg/kg/day
      (4) Dosage interval: 24 hours

   d. **Pyrazinamide**
      (1) Administration: PO
      (2) Excretion: renal, hepatic
      (3) Dose: 25 mg/kg/day
      (4) Dosage interval: 24 hours

   e. **Streptomycin**
      (1) Administration: IM
      (2) Excretion: renal
      (3) Dose: 0.75–1 g per day for 2–3 months; then 15 mg/kg/day, 2–3 times per week
      (4) Dosage interval: 24 hours

3. **Caution:** Liver function tests should be performed prior to the initiation of therapy for treatment with isoniazid, rifampin, and pyrazinamide. Liver function tests should be repeated if symptoms develop while on isoniazid and rifampin, and monthly while on pyrazinamide. A baseline and the monthly visual acuity and red-green vision tests should be performed for patients undergoing therapy with ethambutol. A baseline and monthly audiogram should be performed on patients treated with streptomycin. Uric acid should be checked if a gouty attack occurs in patients on pyrazinamide. Isoniazid, rifampin, and pyrazinamide require dose reduction in hepatic failure, and streptomycin (or amikacin), pyrazinamide, ethambutol, and, to a

lesser degree, isoniazid require dose reduction in renal failure. Isoniazid can cause an increase in Dilantin toxicity, and numerous drug interactions (including a decrease in the plasma levels of corticosteroids, oral contraceptives, barbiturates, sulfonylureas, theophylline, verapamil, digoxin, and propranolol) can occur with rifampin.

4. **Side effects.** Elevations in transaminases occur with isoniazid, rifampin, and pyrazinamide. Frank hepatitis may occur with these agents, which may be life threatening. Patients with preexisting liver disease should not receive pyrazinamide. Neuropathy can occur with isoniazid, and pyridoxine is often given with this agent in an effort to reduce the risk of neuropathy. Fever and a lupuslike syndrome are other side effects of isoniazid. Rifampin causes an orange color in body fluids and can cause fever, flushing, interstitial nephritis, and eosinophilia. The side effects of streptomycin are noted under the aminoglycosides. The most significant side effect of ethambutol is retrobulbar neuritis, with a decrease in visual acuity or color vision. The major toxicities of pyrazinamide are hepatotoxicity and hyperuricemia.

O. Pentamidine

1. **Indications.** The major use of pentamidine isethionate is for the treatment and prophylaxis of pneumonia due to *Pneumocystis carinii*. The drug is indicated in the prophylaxis of HIV-infected individuals with less than 200 CD4 cells per cubic millimeter. The drug, when given for the treatment of *Pneumocystis carinii* pneumonia, is usually reserved for patients who do not tolerate trimethoprim-sulfamethoxazole therapy. Intravenous use is preferred to IM use because of the risk of local reactions following IM injection.
2. **Agent: Pentamidine**
   - **a.** Administration: IV, IM, aerosol
   - **b.** Excretion: renal
   - **c.** Dose: IV, 4 mg/kg/day; aerosol, 600 mg in 6 ml sterile water (aerosol as therapy for mild pneumonia), 300 mg per month (aerosol as prophylaxis)
   - **d.** Dosage interval: daily; monthly for prophylaxis
3. **Caution:** Dosages should be reduced in renal failure.
4. **Side effects.** Hypotension, nephrotoxicity, neutropenia, nausea, vomiting, rash, hypoglycemia followed by hyperglycemia, liver function abnormalities, pancreatitis, hypocalcemia, and thrombocytopenia can occur with parenteral use.

P. Antifungal agents

1. **Indications.** These agents are used in the treatment of infections due to fungi. There is an evolving literature due to the introduction of agents such as fluconazole, which has good activity against *Candida albicans* and *Cryptococcus neoformans*. Itraconazole, which is not yet available, appears to have good activity against many *Aspergillus isolates*. Recommendations regarding the use of specific antifungal agents may have to be modified as new information becomes available. Amphotericin B is the drug of choice for most invasive fungal infections, including aspergillosis, mucormycosis (zygomycosis), cryptococcosis (although fluconazole can play a role in mild cryptococcal meningitis in AIDS patients), blastomycosis (in disseminated disease or if ketoconazole therapy fails), histoplasmosis in an immunocompromised host or with CNS involvement, candidemia (although there may be a role for fluconazole), meningitis due to coccidiomycosis, and extracutaneous sporotrichosis. Ketoconazole, which requires an acid pH for absorption, can be used in the treatment of many cases of blastomycosis, histoplasmosis, coccidiomycosis, mucocutaneous candidiasis, and certain dermatophytes. Fluconazole,

which does not require an acid pH in gastric contents for absorption, is excreted in the urine and can be used to treat most candidal urinary tract infections. Potential uses for this agent include candidemia, cryptococcal disease, vaginal candidiasis, and mucocutaneous candidiasis. In severe infections such as cryptococcal meningitis, 5-flucytosine is often given with amphotericin B.

2. **Agents**
   a. **Amphotericin B**
      (1) Administration: IV
      (2) Excretion: nonrenal; poorly understood
      (3) Dose: varies with infecting agent and site
      (4) Dosage interval: 24 hours
   b. **Ketoconazole**
      (1) Administration: PO
      (2) Excretion: hepatic
      (3) Dose: 200–800 mg per day
      (4) Dosage interval: 12–24 hours
   c. **Fluconazole**
      (1) Administration: PO, IV
      (2) Excretion: renal
      (3) Dose: 100–200 mg per day
      (4) Dosage interval: 24 hours
   d. **Flucytosine**
      (1) Administration: PO
      (2) Excretion: renal
      (3) Dose: 150 mg/kg/day
      (4) Dosage interval: 6 hours
3. **Caution:** Amphotericin B is nephrotoxic, and serum blood-urea nitrogen and creatinine, as well as potassium and magnesium, should be followed during therapy (they predictably rise). Saline loading decreases the risk of amphotericin B nephrotoxicity. In order to absorb ketoconazole, the gastric pH must be acidic. Thus antacids and H2-blockers will interfere with its absorption. In achlorhydric patients, this can be overcome by administering oral Coca-Cola with the ketoconazole. Dosages of fluconazole and 5-flucytosine should be decreased in renal insufficiency.
4. **Side effects.** With amphotericin B, fever, chills, nausea, vomiting, and hypotension often occur. Premedication with acetaminophen (650–1,300 mg PO), diphenhydramine (25–50 mg PO or IV), and in some cases hydrocortisone (25–50 mg IV) may help prevent these symptoms. Other possible side effects are ventricular fibrillation, seizures, anaphylaxis, hypokalemia, hypomagnesemia, and anemia. Ketoconazole may rarely cause a severe hepatitis and commonly causes an increase in transaminases. Other side effects are gynecomastia, adrenal insufficiency, nausea, vomiting, and decreased libido. Fluconazole can also cause transaminase elevation, headache, nausea, vomiting, and skin rash. Ketoconazole and fluconazole interact with other drugs, including warfarin, phenytoin, and benzodiazepines in which the drug effect of these agents is increased. The most common side effects of 5-flucytosine are hematologic (particularly in patients with renal dysfunction), hepatotoxicity, and gastrointestinal symptoms.

Q. Antiviral agents

1. **Indications.** Acyclovir is indicated in the treatment of infections with herpes simplex and varicella-zoster virus infections. Ganciclovir has documented efficacy in the treatment of cytomegalovirus (CMV) retinitis in AIDS patients and is often used in other severe CMV

infections. Zidovudine (AZT; Retrovir) is indicated in the treatment of HIV-positive patients with CD4 counts of less than 500 cells per cubic millimeter. Although the data have not established efficacy, it is often given to health care providers following needle-stick accidents resulting in exposure to HIV. Ribavirin can be given as an aerosol to patients with respiratory syncytial virus infection and IV in infections caused by several of the hemorrhagic fever viruses. Amantadine can be given for prophylaxis against influenza A infection or during the first 20 hours of infection with this agent.

2. **Agents**
   a. **Acyclovir**
      (1) Administration: PO, IV
      (2) Excretion: renal
      (3) Dose: PO, 1,000 mg per day (herpes simplex), 4,000 mg per day (varicella-zoster, compromised host)
      (4) Dosage interval: PO, 5 doses per day; IV, every 8 hours
   b. **Ganciclovir**
      (1) Administration: IV
      (2) Excretion: renal
      (3) Dose: 10 mg/kg/day (induction), 6 mg/kg/day (maintenance)
      (4) Dosage interval: 12 hours (induction), 24 hours (5 days/week) during maintenance therapy
   c. **Zidovudine (AZT, Retrovir)**
      (1) Administration: PO
      (2) Excretion: renal
      (3) Dose: 500 mg per day
      (4) Dosage interval: every 4 hours, 5 times per day
   d. **Amantadine**
      (1) Administration: PO
      (2) Excretion: renal
      (3) Dose: 200 mg per day
      (4) Dosage interval: 12 hours
   e. **Ribavirin**
      (1) Administration: aerosol, IV
      (2) Excretion: hepatic, renal
      (3) Dose: aerosol, 1.1 g per day; if IV ribavirin is required for treatment of a viral hemorrhagic fever, contact the Centers for Disease Control immediately.
      (4) Dosage interval: administer aerosol for 12–18 hours per day for 3–7 days
3. **Caution:** Dosage of acyclovir must be decreased in patients with renal insufficiency. Adequate hydration should be ensured to prevent crystallization of acyclovir within the kidney. Dosage of zidovudine should be reduced in patients with renal insufficiency. Dosage of amantadine should be reduced in renal insufficiency.
4. **Side effects.** Side effects of acyclovir include fatigue, vertigo, rash, and diarrhea when given orally. The IV preparation may be associated with phlebitis, elevation of creatinine, seizures, hallucination, and delirium. The major side effect of ganciclovir is hematologic (leukopenia, thrombocytopenia), although rash and elevated liver function tests occur. Zidovudine may cause anemia, leukopenia, headache, malaise, nausea, vomiting, and myalgias. Amantadine may cause symptoms referable to the CNS, including tremors, hallucinations, and confusion, as well as rash and nausea. Ribavirin may cause anemia, conjunctivitis, and rash.

Selected References

Bartlett, J. G. *Pocketbook of Infectious Disease Therapy.* Baltimore: Williams and Wilkins, 1991.

Mandell, G. L., and Douglas, R. G., Jr. (eds.). *Principles and Practice of Infectious Diseases.* New York: Churchill Livingstone, 1990.

Rubin, R. H., and Young, L. S. (eds.). *Clinical Approach to Infection in the Immunocompromised Host.* New York: Plenum, 1988.

Sanford, J. P. *Guide to Antimicrobial Therapy 1991.* West Bethesda, MD: Antimicrobial Therapy, 1991.

20

Bleeding Disorders in the Intensive Care Unit

Alan Lichtenstein

C. Von Willebrand's disease
  1. Clinical manifestations
  2. Therapy
D. Fibrinogen defects
  1. Afibrinogenemia
  2. Hypofibrinogenemia
  3. Dysfibrinogenemia

In the past several years, there have been important advances in the recognition and treatment of acquired bleeding disorders. This chapter focuses on diagnosis and management of acquired and congenital coagulation defects, with emphasis on recent advances in therapy.

I. **The hemostatic mechanism.** Clinicians may best approach the bleeding patient by considering the three essential elements of the hemostatic system: vascular integrity, platelets, and the coagulation cascade.
   A. **Vascular integrity.** Injury to the blood vessel wall exposes the subendothelial connective tissue, which stimulates platelet adhesiveness and aggregation.
   B. **Platelets.** A platelet plug forms at the site of vascular injury. In addition, the platelet surface membrane initiates the intrinsic coagulation cascade and facilitates the interaction of the coagulation factors.
   C. **Coagulation cascade.** The coagulation factors are serine proteases that circulate in the plasma as inactive proenzymes. The coagulation cascade can be activated by tissue factor, a phospholipid that is released from cell surface membranes of injured tissues. The two activation sequences of the coagulation cascade are called the intrinsic and extrinsic pathways. The intrinsic pathway begins intravascularly with endothelial damage and is evaluated by the activated partial thromboplastin time (aPTT). The extrinsic pathway is initiated by extravascular tissue phospholipid released with tissue damage and is evaluated by the prothrombin time (PT) (Fig. 20-1). These two pathways meet at the level of factor X and then share a final common pathway.

II. **Diagnostic approach to the bleeding patient**
   A. **History and physical examination**
      1. **History.** The patient or family should be questioned about any previous bleeding episodes, such as epistaxis or hemarthrosis. A history of excessive bleeding following common surgical procedures such as circumcision, tonsillectomy, or dental extraction is significant when considering inherited coagulation disorders. A family history of bleeding abnormalities and a history of drug ingestion should be sought.
      2. **Physical examination.** The patient is inspected for evidence of petechiae, ecchymoses, or bleeding sites. The patient should also be examined for evidence of systemic disease that may impair hemostasis.
   B. **Laboratory evaluation** (Tables 20-1 and 20-2). The tests of the coagulation system include the following:
      1. **Prothrombin time (PT)** measures extrinsic and common pathway function and is used as an initial screening test. Results are reported in seconds along with a control specimen. The PT is prolonged by deficiencies in factors II (prothrombin), V, VII, and X and fibrinogen. The normal value is usually 11–12 seconds.
      2. **Activated partial thromboplastin time (aPTT)** measures the intrinsic and common pathway activity. By adding previously surface-activated factors XII and XI, the test becomes more standardized and reproducible than the older PTT test. The aPTT is prolonged by deficiencies in HMW kininogen, prekallikrein, factors II, V, VIII, IX, X, XI, XII, and fibrinogen and by inhibitors of coagulation such as heparin, fibrin split products, and "lupus" inhibitor. The normal value is 25–37 seconds.
      3. **Whole-blood clotting time (Lee-White method)** uses the glass surface of the test tube to activate factor XII, thus triggering the intrinsic system. The lack of reproducibility makes this test difficult to interpret. It has been replaced by more reliable measurements. It should never be used for screening purposes.

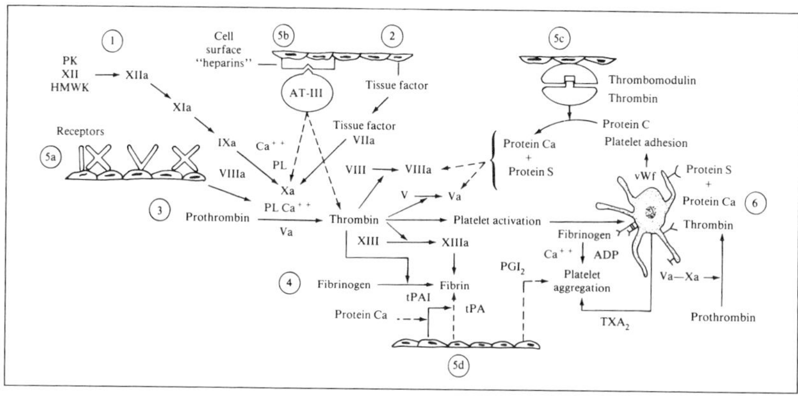

Fig. 20.1. Reactions of blood coagulation, platelet activation, and hemostasis. Solid lines indicate reactions that promote blood coagulation, platelet activation, and hemostasis. Dotted lines represent inhibitory mechanisms or regulatory mechanisms of the hemostatic process. Components of the hemostatic system are numbered 1–6. The coagulation scheme comprises numbers 1–4. Number 1 shows the pathway of blood coagulation. Prekallikrein (PK), factor XII, and high-molecular-weight kininogen (HMWK) form a complex on negatively charged surfaces that activates factor XII, which in turn initiates the activation of other coagulation proteins. Number 2 shows the pathway of blood coagulation that involves the interaction of tissue factor with factor VII to form factor VIIa, which converts factor X to factor Xa. Number 3 is the common pathway of blood coagulation, the generation of prothrombin to thrombin, by the complex of factor Xa, phopholipid (PL), calcium, and another nonenzymatic cofactor, factor Va. The thrombin that is generated has several important roles in hemostasis: the conversion of fibrinogen to fibrin, the activation of factor VIII and factor V by proteolytic cleavage, platelet activation, and the conversion of factor XIII to an activated form that cross-links polymerized fibrin. Number 4 is the conversion of fibrinogen to fibrin. Numbers 5a–d shows the known contributions of endothelial cells to the hemostatic process. Number 5a shows receptors for factors IX, V, and X on endothelial cells. These receptors play a role in the formation of thrombin on endothelial surface. Number 5b is a regulatory mechanism of hemostasis in which proteoglycans interact with antithrombin III (AT-III) to inhibit the generation of thrombin. Number 5c shows another mechanism of modulating thrombin generation, regulating the hemostatic mechanism in which thrombin binds to a receptor on the endothelial surface called thrombomodulin. Number 5d shows two mechanisms of inhibition of the hemostatic mechanism. One mechanism is the release of the prostacyclin (PGI_2), which is a vasodilator and potent inhibitor of platelet aggregation. The second mechanism is a release of tissue plasminogen activator (tPA) that binds to plasminogen bound to fibrin and causes fibrinolysis. Number 6 shows the platelet contribution to hemostasis in which von Willebrand's factor (vWF) causes platelet adhesion to the subendothelium through the glycoprotein lb. Platelet aggregation occurs when fibrinogen binds to its receptor in the presence of adenosine diphosphate and calcium. Aggregation is promoted by the endoperoxide thromboxane A_2. Protein S in the presence of activated protein C can modulate various coagulation factor reactions on the platelet surface. (Modified from Medical Knowledge Self-Assessment Program VIII, American College of Physicians, Hematology, Part B, Book 3, Copyrighted by American College of Physicians, Philadelphia, 1988.)

Table 20-1. Screening laboratory tests in selected hemostatis disorders

Clinical bleeding	aPTT	PT	TCT	Bleeding time	Platelet count	Possible defects	Tests to confirm
Absent	Abnormal	Normal	Normal	Normal	Normal	HMW kininogen, prekallikrein, factor XII, lupus inhibitor	Factor XII assay
Present	Abnormal	Normal	Normal	Normal	Normal	Factor XI, IX, VIII	Factor XI, IX, or VIII assay
Present	Abnormal	Abnormal	Normal	Normal	Normal	Factor V, X, II, coumadin, vitamin K deficiency, mild liver disease	Factor V, X, or II assay Liver function studies
Present	Normal	Abnormal	Normal	Normal	Normal	Factor VII	Factor VII assay
Present	Abnormal	Normal	Normal	Abnormal	Normal	von Willebrand's disease	vWF:Ag, vWF ristocetin cofactor activity, ristocetin Factor VIII multimers
Present	Abnormal	Abnormal	Abnormal	Abnormal	Normal	Afribronogenemia	Fibronogen assay
Present	Normal	Normal	Normal	Abnormal	Abnormal	Thrombocytopenia	Platelet count
Present	Normal	Normal	Normal	Abnormal	Normal	Qualitative platelet disorder (aspirin, thrombasthenia, Bernard-Soulier syndrome)	Thromboelastography, platelet aggregation studies, platelet adhesion studies
Present	Normal	Normal	Normal	Normal	Normal	Factor XIII	Factor XIII assay
Present	Abnormal	Abnormal	Abnormal	Abnormal	Abnormal	DIC, severe liver disease	Fibrin split products

Modified from G. C. White, V. J. Marder, R. W. Colman, et al. Approach to the Bleeding Patient. In R. W. Colman, J. Hirsch, V. J. Marder, and E. W. Salzman (eds.), *Hemostasis and Thrombosis—Basic Principles and Clinical Practice* (2d ed.). Philadelphia: Lippincott, 1987.

Table 20-2. Screening tests for bleeding patients

Test	Normal value
Peripheral blood smear	Normal RBC morphology
Platelet count	150,000–350,000/mm^3
PT	Control ± 2 seconds
aPTT	25–37 seconds
Bleeding time	3–9 minutes
ACT	90–120 seconds
Thrombin time (TT)	15 seconds
Reptilase time	14–21 seconds
Euglobulin lysis time	90 minutes–6 hours
Platelet aggregation	2–10 minutes
Fibrinogen	200–400 mg/dl
Fibrin split products	> 1:4
Specific factor assays	1 unit/ml

4. **Activated coagulation time (ACT)** standardizes surface activation by adding celite to evaluate the intrinsic and common pathway. The ACT is readily performed at the bedside. A sufficient number of platelets is required to supply the phospholipid for coagulation protein interaction. The normal value is 90–120 seconds.
5. **Thrombin time (TT)** measures the time it takes exogenous thrombin to convert fibrinogen to fibrin. The TT is prolonged by a number of factors, including hypofibrinogenemia, abnormal fibrinogen, fibrin split products (FSPs), myeloma proteins, and heparin. The TT can be normal even in the presence of a severe coagulopathy that affects the coagulation pathway leading up to, but not including, the conversion of fibrinogen to fibrin. The normal value is approximately 15 seconds.
6. **Reptilase time** is useful for determining if heparin or other thrombin inhibitors are present in the plasma being tested. The normal value is 14–21 seconds.
7. **Platelet count** measures the concentration of platelets in whole blood. Normal values are 150,000–350,000 per cubic milliliter.
8. **Bleeding time** is used as a screening test for disorders of platelet function, both congenital and acquired, and for von Willebrand's disease. A blood pressure cuff is inflated on the upper arm to a pressure of 40 mm Hg. A spring-loaded device is used to make a single 1–2-mm-deep incision in the forearm. At 30-second intervals, drops of blood that have exuded from the wound are absorbed into a piece of filter paper until bleeding ceases. Normal values are 3–9 minutes. With normal platelet function, as the platelet count falls below 100,000 per cubic milliliter, the bleeding time increases linearly so that at a platelet count of 50,000 per cubic milliliter, the bleeding time is approximately 15 minutes.
9. **Fibrinogen concentration** in plasma can be determined by laboratory analysis. Normal values are 200–400 mg per deciliter.
10. **Fibrin split products** are present in serum during consumption coagulopathies such as disseminated intravascular coagulation (DIC). Normal values are negative titers at dilutions greater than 1:4.
11. **Thromboelastography (TEG)** is a method that measures the shear elasticity of a blood clot from the time when the first fibrin strands are formed to the completion of the clot formation, including fibrinolysis.

TEG records the activity of whole blood coagulation with measurements made of reaction time, maximum amplitude, coagulation time, clot formation rate, and blood clot lysis time. The reaction time is closely related to aPTT. The maximum amplitude is a reflection of platelet function and factor XIII activity. The rate of clot formation reflects the function of fibrinogen.

C. **Vascular abnormalities.** If there are no detectable abnormalities in platelet or coagulation factors, the clinician should suspect a problem with vascular integrity.

III. **Acquired bleeding disorders** (Table 20-3)

A. **Platelet disorders** are common in critically ill patients. These can be characterized as quantitative or qualitative. A patient who has undergone major surgery, head injury, or other trauma should have the platelet count maintained above 50,000–100,000 per cubic millimeter, depending on the type of surgery, adequacy of hemostasis, and clinical

Table 20-3. Disorders associated with disseminated intravascular coagulation

Infection
- Gram-negative endotoxemia with hypotension or shock
- Severe gram-positive septicemia
- Ricketsial infections (Rocky Mountain spotted fever)
- Viral infections (herpes, dengue, yellow fever)
- Louse-borne infections (typhus)
- Malaria (*Plasmodium falciparum*)
- Subacute bacterial endocarditis

Complications of pregnancy and delivery
- Gram-negative sepsis
- Abruptio placentae
- Amniotic fluid embolism
- Retained dead fetus
- Toxemia

Pediatric disorders, especially in the newborn

Malignant diseases
- Metastatic carcinoma (prostate, pancreas, lung, stomach, colon, breast)
- Leukemia, especially acute promyelocytic leukemia

Liver diseases (cirrhosis, acute hepatic necrosis)

Complications of surgery: extracorporeal circulation

Critical tissue damage
- Brain tissue destruction
- Massive trauma
- Heat stroke
- Extensive burns

Adult respiratory distress syndrome (ARDS)

Miscellaneous
- Hemolytic transfusion reactions
- Vasculitis (collagen disease, TTP, hemolytic-uremic syndrome)
- Aneurysms
- Giant hemangioma
- Snake bite envenoming (saw-scaled viper, Russell's viper)
- Rewarming after hypothermia
- Insertion of LeVeen peritonovenous shunts
- Tissue rejection after organ transplantation

Modified from J. E. Ansell. Acquired Bleeding Disorders. In J. M. Rippe, R. S. Irwin, J. S. Alpert, and J. E. Dalen (eds.), *Intensive Care Medicine*. Boston: Little, Brown, 1985.

status. The oncology patient receiving chemotherapy, however, generally is not given platelets until counts fall below 10,000–20,000 per cubic millimeter, at which point the incidence of spontaneous bleeding increases dramatically. The presence of an adequate platelet count does not ensure proper function; uremia, cardiopulmonary bypass, or drug therapy may result in defective platelet function. The bleeding time is a test of both platelet function and platelet number and is normally 3–9 minutes. It will be elevated with abnormal platelet function or decreased numbers of platelets.

1. **Quantitative platelet disorders (thrombocytopenia)** (Table 20-4)
   a. Decreased or ineffective thrombopoiesis. Decreased platelet production may be due to a number of causes:

Table 20-4. Drugs associated with thrombocytopenia

Acetaminophen	Meperidine
Acetazolamide	Meprobamate
Aminopyrine	Mercurial diuretics
Amrinone	Methyldopa
Antazoline	Nitroglycerin
Barbiturates	Novobiocin
Bismuth	Organic hair dyes
Carbamazepine	*p*-aminosalicylic acid
Carbutamide	Paramethadione
Centulin	Penicillin
Cephalothin	Phenacetin
Chlorothiazides	Phenylbutazone
Chlorpheniramine	Potassium iodide
Chlorpromazine	Prednisone
Chlorpropamide	Prochlorperazine
Chloroquine	Promethazine
Codeine	Propylthiouracil
Desipramine	Pyrazinamide
Dextroamphetamine sulfate	Quinidine
Diazepam	Reserpine
Diazoxide	Rifampin
Digoxin and digitoxin	Spironolactone
Disulfiram	Streptomycin
Ergot	Stibophen
Erythromycin	Sulfamethazine
Ethylchlorvinyl	Sulfonamides
Gold Salts	Tetracycline
Heparin	Tetraethylammonium (TEA)
Hydantoin	Thiourea
Hydroxychloroquine	Trimethadione
Insecticides	Turpentine
Iopanoic acid (Telepaque)	Valproate sodium
Isoniazid	Xylocaine

Modified from M. E. Rybak. Thrombocytopenia. In J. M. Rippe, R. S. Irwin, J. S. Alpert, and J. E. Dalen (eds.), *Intensive Care Medicine*. Boston: Little, Brown, 1985.

(1) Marrow aplasia. Primary aplastic anemias such as Fanconi's anemia, as well as secondary aplastic anemias caused by drugs (methotrexate, chloramphenicol, phenylbutazone, gold, benzene, trimethoprim-sulfamethoxazole, captopril, cimetidine, tolbutamide, chlorpropamide, thiazides, and estrogens), can cause thrombocytopenia.

(2) Bone marrow infiltration (leukemias, other malignancies, myelofibrosis)

(3) Infections (non-A/non-B hepatitis, infectious mononucleosis, influenza, tuberculosis, measles, or measles vaccination)

(4) Nutritional disorders. Folate or vitamin B_{12} deficiency

(5) Ethanol. Alcohol ingestion causes thrombocytopenia and shortens platelet survival. Nutritional deficiencies are also common in alcoholics.

(6) Congenital syndromes such as Wiskott-Aldrich syndrome, Bernard-Soulier syndrome, and May-Hegglin anomaly are characterized by thrombocytopenia.

(7) Miscellaneous causes of thrombocytopenia are cyclic thrombocytopenia, thrombopoietin deficiency, and paroxysmal nocturnal hemoglobinuria.

b. **Shortened platelet survival.** Accelerated platelet destruction is classically divided into immunologically and nonimmunologically mediated causes.

(1) Immunologically mediated causes of accelerated platelet destruction as idiopathic thrombocytopenic purpura (ITP), autoimmune disorders (e.g., systemic lupus erythematosus), lymphoproliferative disorders (e.g., chronic lymphocytic leukemia), and some infections (e.g. infectious mononucleosis) produce autoantibodies that are directed against platelet membrane antigens. Increased gamma G immunoglobulin (IgG) and complement levels are frequently present, which can aid in the diagnosis. Alloantibodies can cause thrombocytopenia in several situations. These antibodies are responsible for destroying transfused platelets, as well as causing posttransfusion purpura.

(2) Drug-induced thrombocytopenia is often immunologically mediated. A partial list of drugs implicated in thrombocytopenia is shown in Table 20-4. Heparin-induced thrombocytopenia has been reported to occur in 2–30% of all patients on heparin. The disorder is idiosyncratic and is not dose related.

(3) Some malignancies, such as ovarian carcinoma, basal cell carcinoma, adenocarcinoma of the prostate, breast cancer, and squamous cell carcinomas of the lung and vagina, have been implicated as causes of immunologically mediated thrombocytopenia.

(4) Nonimmunologically mediated causes of accelerated platelet destruction include DIC, thrombotic thrombocytopenic purpura (TTP), the hemolytic-uremic syndrome, extracorporeal circulation, indwelling vascular prostheses, and pregnancy-induced hypertension (PIH).

(5) Abnormal distribution of platelets occurs with hypersplenism. As much as 90% of the total body platelet mass may be sequestered in the spleen with hypersplenism. Causes of hypersplenism include cirrhosis, portal hypertension, Gaucher's disease, myeloproliferative diseases, and chronic hemolytic anemias, such as hereditary spherocytosis.

2. **Qualitative platelet disorders.** Poorly functioning platelets, even when present in normal quantity, may be responsible for a bleeding disorder. The platelet reactions of adhesion, release, and aggregation may be affected individually or, more frequently, together.
   a. Drugs are the most common cause of qualitative platelet disorders. Some of the drugs associated with platelet dysfunction are antibiotics (penicillins, nitrofurantoin, hydroxychloroquine), antihistamines (diphenhydramine), antiinflammatory agents (aspirin, nonsteroidal antiinflammatory drugs, corticosteroids), antithrombotic agents (heparin, dextrans), calcium channel blockers (verapamil), serotonin antagonists, alpha-blocking agents (phentolamine), beta-blocking agents (propanolol), antipsychotic agents (phenothiazines), tricyclic antidepressants, tranquilizers, vasodilators (sodium nitroprusside, nitroglycerin), xanthine derivatives (theophylline, caffeine, dipyridamole), ethanol, and clofibrate.
   b. Myeloproliferative disorders such as essential thrombocythemia, chronic myelogenous leukemia (CML), and myelofibrosis with myeloid metaplasia are commonly associated with qualitative platelet defects. Usually platelet release or platelet aggregation is diminished.

B. **Coagulation disorders** (see Fig. 20-1). Coagulation factor deficiencies can develop due to production defects, accelerated destruction, massive blood replacement (dilution), or inhibitors of coagulation. Levels of the various clotting factors required for safe surgical hemostasis are listed in Fig. 20-1.

1. **Production defects.** Defects in the production of coagulation factors can be attributed to vitamin K deficiency, liver disease, or a combination of the two.
   a. **Vitamin K deficiency.** Severely malnourished patients who are being given broad-spectrum antibiotics that suppress the flora of the intestinal tract commonly develop vitamin K deficiency. This can also occur in patients with fat malabsorption due to biliary disease. The deficiency of vitamin K causes decreased synthesis of the vitamin K–dependent coagulation factors (II, VII, IX, and X).
      (1) Characteristic laboratory abnormalities in vitamin K deficiency include a prolonged PT (due to rapid decline of factor VII) and a gradual prolongation of the aPTT (due to a decline of factor IX).
      (2) Therapy depends on the severity of the coagulopathy and the need for rapid correction of the defect. Parenteral vitamin K (10 mg IV over 10 minutes or 10 mg IM or 10 mg subcutaenously [SC]) will correct the PT in 12–24 hours. This dosage is usually repeated daily for 3 days. If rapid correction is needed (e.g., hemorrhagic gastrointestinal bleeding, emergency surgery), transfusion of 2 units of fresh-frozen plasma is indicated. This will immediately correct the PT by replacing the vitamin K–dependent factors. The administration of DDAVP (desmopressin) has been reported to be associated with significant improvement in the levels of factors VII, VIII, IX, XI, and XII, as well as shortening the bleeding time and causing the appearance of larger molecular weight von Willebrand factor (vWF) multimers in the plasma.
   b. **Liver disease** in its advanced stages commonly produces a coagulopathy. This is due to decreased coagulation factor synthesis, production of abnormal factors, increased factor consumption, thrombocytopenia, or, rarely, primary fibrinolysis. Since most

coagulation factors are produced in the liver, liver disease usually causes multiple factor deficiencies. The vitamin K–dependent factors (II, VII, IX, and X) are most vulnerable to hepatic dysfunction and are the first affected (particularly factor VII). Fibrinogen concentration is not depressed until end-stage liver failure.

2. **Accelerated destruction of coagulation factors** may occur in certain bleeding disorders. **Disseminated intravascular coagulation** is an acquired defect of coagulation that occurs when normal homeostatic mechanisms fail. It is never a primary disease but rather a syndrome that occurs during the course of another disease. DIC represents systemic activation of the coagulation system, resulting in excess thrombin generation and secondary plasmin formation. It is important to recognize that the fibrinolytic system is also activated simultaneously. Fibrinolysis and coagulation may be occurring at quite different rates. If the thrombin effect is dominant, thrombosis and ischemic tissue damage will dominate the clinical picture. If the fibrinolytic pathway is predominant, diffuse bleeding will occur. Thrombin and activated factor XIIa convert plasminogen to plasmin, the primary lytic enzyme that cleaves both fibrinogen and fibrin, forming fibrinogen/fibrin split products (FSPs are also called fibrin degradation products). If these FSPs are not removed by the reticuloendothelial system, which can occur in hepatic failure or hypoperfusion, they can become potent inhibitors of clot formation. A list of disorders associated with DIC is found in Table 20-3.
   a. Diagnosis of DIC. Bleeding can occur from IV sites, the gastrointestinal tract, venipuncture sites, or surgical wounds. Thrombosis may produce vascular insufficiency and organ dysfunction when intravascular clot formation occurs. Decreased urine output, worsening hypoxemia, or altered mental status may be the first evidence of DIC. Skin manifestations include petechiae, purpura, purpura fulminans, gangrene, and acral cyanosis. DIC can also be a silent syndrome, detected only when an abnormal coagulation test is found.
   b. Laboratory investigation of DIC may be difficult because there is no single test pathognomonic of it. A number of tests are needed to characterize the spectrum of abnormalities in vascular integrity, platelets, coagulation cascade, and clot lysis, which can arise with DIC. Early diagnosis may prompt an earlier search for a reversible cause and may prevent complications. Laboratory tests useful in the diagnosis of DIC are:
      (1) Platelet count decreases early in DIC. The exact incidence of thrombocytopenia in DIC is debatable. However, the platelet count does decrease to less than 100,000 per milliliter in 80% of patients with acute DIC. Moderate thrombocytopenia (platelet counts of 50,000–150,000/ml) frequently occurs in septic patients without evidence of DIC. In septic patients with severe thrombocytopenia (platelet count $<$ 50,000/ml), there usually is other laboratory evidence of DIC. The platelet count is useful to follow serially to assess the activity of the process.
      (2) Fibrinogen levels may vary with different diseases. Therefore, it is the trend in the fibrinogen level that is important to follow to support the diagnosis and assess the activity of the process. However, a fibrinogen level less than 160 mg per deciliter without concomitant liver disease is highly suggestive of DIC.

(3) Prothrombin time. A prolonged PT is usually seen with DIC.
(4) Peripheral blood smears. Examination may reveal fragmented red blood cells suggestive of a microangiopathic hemolytic anemia, with schistocytes occurring in 10–30% of patients with DIC.
(5) Fibrin split products. Although FSPs occur in a variety of disease states, they must be elevated to entertain a diagnosis of DIC (although FSPs may decrease late in the process as fibrinogen is consumed). The FSP assay normally is negative at greater than 1:4 dilution.
(6) Thrombin time. Although early in DIC the TT is variable, with severe DIC the TT is prolonged.

c. Treatment of DIC. The most important component in the treatment of DIC is identification and treatment of the underlying disease.
(1) Platelets and clotting factors should be administered if they are depleted and clinically evident bleeding is taking place. Clotting factors, normally having a half-life of several hours, are rapidly consumed in DIC.
(2) Cryoprecipitate is rich in fibrinogen, factor VII, and factor XIII. Factors V, VIII, and fibrinogen are rapidly depleted in DIC. Cryoprecipitate is useful to replace factor VII and fibrinogen, being administered to maintain the fibrinogen level at or above 100 mg per deciliter.
(3) Fresh-frozen plasma can be given to replace coagulation factors. It also provides important inhibitors of coagulation such as antithrombin III (AT-III), alpha$_2$ antiplasmin, heparin cofactor II, protein C, protein S, C1-inhibitor, and alpha$_2$-macroglobulin. Because of rapid factor depletion, it may be necessary to administer fresh-frozen plasma every 6–8 hours, depending on the coagulation test results. Blood samples for clotting studies should be drawn approximately 20 minutes after replacement factor administration to monitor replacement therapy.
(4) Heparin. The use of heparin in the treatment of DIC is highly controversial. In certain specific circumstances, such as promyelocytic leukemia or purpura fulminans, it has shown to be useful. In other situations, such as transfusion reactions, amniotic fluid embolism, septic abortion, or retained dead fetus, its use has been suggested by some authors, but the recommendation is by no means universal. Platelet and factor deficiencies should be corrected before and during heparin administration. Heparin exerts its effect by acting on antithrombin III to allow more effective binding to prothrombin. Since AT-III is depleted in DIC, fresh-frozen plasma should be given when heparin is administered to ensure its effectiveness. Heparin should be given in low dosages initially (500–1000 units/hour) without a bolus, subsequently increasing the dosage as dictated by its effects on the coagulation cascade (e.g., aPTT). Large doses may be necessary; resistance to its effects is common with DIC. If it is effective, the platelet count and fibrinogen level should increase.

3. **Primary fibrinolysis.** The fibrinolytic system is activated at the same time the coagulation system is triggered. In certain situations, however, the fibrinolytic system can be activated independently, and abnormal fibrinolysis can occur. Uncontrolled fibrinolysis can result in a severe hemorrhagic disorder. Situations where primary fibrin-

olysis may occur are urologic surgery (especially of the prostate gland which may release urokinase), streptokinase or urokinase infusion to treat intravascular clots, open heart surgery with extracorporeal circulation, pelvic surgery, and liver disease. DIC must be excluded when considering the diagnosis of primary fibrinolysis. Epsilon aminocaproic acid (EACA, Amicar) could cause diffuse intravascular thrombosis if used in a patient with DIC.

a. Important distinguishing features that can be helpful in differentiating primary or secondary fibrinolysis are:

(1) Platelet count is usually normal in primary fibrinolysis but decreased in DIC.

(2) On peripheral smear, a microangiopathic hemolytic appearance with fragmented red blood cells strongly suggests DIC but is not present in primary fibrinolysis.

(3) Euglobulin lysis time, which measures the rate of fibrin clot lysis time, is a simple and rapid test used for accelerated fibrinolysis detection. In patients with DIC, FSPs often prevent clot formation and can make the test difficult to interpret. The euglobulin lysis time may be normal or shortened in DIC. A normal euglobulin lysis time excludes the diagnosis of primary fibrinolysis.

b. Treatment. First and foremost, the underlying disease process must be treated. EACA stops fibrinolysis by inhibiting plasminogen activation; however, it does increase the risk of intravascular thrombosis. EACA is eliminated by the kidney; therefore, the dosage may need to be adjusted in patients with renal insufficiency. A loading dose of 5 g can be administered orally or IV, followed by 1 g per hour until clinical bleeding stops. The coagulation cascade must be monitored. EACA is contraindicated in the presence of intravascular clotting or hematuria. A hematologist should be consulted before its use.

4. Cardiopulmonary bypass often leads to coagulopathies whose etiology is multifactorial. Some of its causes are inadequate heparin neutralization, postneutralization rebound effect of heparin, functional platelet defects, activation of factor XII, DIC, and excessive fibrinolysis. Surgical bleeding always needs to be considered because surgical reexploration would be necessary.

5. Massive blood replacement can cause pathologic bleeding as large quantities of donor blood are given due to the poor survival of labile coagulation factors and platelets during storage. The remaining platelets and coagulation factors in the circulation are diluted by the homologous blood products. Many empiric protocols have been suggested for fresh-frozen plasma and platelet administration during massive transfusion. The empiric transfusion of blood products without laboratory confirmation of decreased clotting factors or platelets is unwarranted in most circumstances and places the patient at risk for contracting infectious diseases from homologous blood transfusion of perhaps unnecessary blood products. During truly massive exsanguination of greater than 1 blood volume, empiric transfusion of fresh-frozen plasma and platelets is justified. For lesser amounts of blood loss, objective laboratory evidence of a coagulopathy (thrombocytopenia or elevated PT or aPTT) should be required before transfusion of fresh-frozen plasma or platelets is initiated.

C. Inhibitors of coagulation. Several endogenous and exogenous substances act as inhibitors of the coagulation cascade.

1. Antibodies to specific factors. Antibodies to factor VIII are the most common, occurring in 10–20% of all patients with hemophilia. They may also occur with autoimmune disorders (e.g., systemic lupus erythematosus, rheumatoid arthritis). Hemophiliacs with inhibitors are notoriously difficult to treat as hemophiliacs rapidly raise their antibody titers with factor VIII administration. Inhibitors have been described against factors IX, V, VII, XI, XII, and XIII, as well as vWF and fibrinogen.

2. **Antibodies to phospholipid.** This is known as lupus anticoagulant and is present in as many as 10% of patients with systemic lupus erythematosus. A similar inhibitor has been demonstrated in a number of other disease states or with drug administration (e.g., procainamide, hydralazine, chlorpromazine). The clinical significance of this inhibitor is minimal; most patients do not have increased bleeding tendencies unless a concomitant coagulation defect exists.
3. **Fibrin split products** interfere with the polymerization of the fibrin monomer.

D. **Heparin.** Heparin is frequently employed in the treatment of patients with thromboembolic disease.

1. Heparin administration by continuous infusion causes fewer bleeding problems than by intermittent bolus doses. Treatment is initiated with 5,000 units administered as an IV bolus, followed by an infusion, initially at 1,000 units per hour. The subsequent dose is titrated against the aPTT (which should be obtained before heparin administration) at 2–4-hour intervals until the desired aPTT is obtained, and then daily. Dosage should be adjusted to maintain the aPTT at 1.5–2.0 times control value. Multiple factors affect heparin requirements:
   a. Heparin half-life varies with the dose of heparin. When 100, 400, or 800 units per kilogram of heparin are administered IV, the half-life of the anticoagulant activity is approximately 1, 2, and 3 hours, respectively.
   b. Heparin is metabolized in the liver but can be excreted by the kidney with large dosages. Dosages may have to be reduced with hepatic or renal dysfunction.
   c. Ongoing embolism of thrombi requires more heparin to prolong aPTT.
   d. DIC may induce resistance to heparin by releasing platelet factor IV from destroyed platelets to exert an antiheparin effect.
2. **Complications of heparin therapy**
   a. **Hemorrhage** is the most common. Stools, urine, nasogastric drainage, and sputum should be checked periodically for the presence of blood.
   b. **Thrombocytopenia.** Mild thrombocytopenia occurs in 2–30% of patients. It results from heparin-induced platelet aggregation and can occur within 2 hours to 2 days after administration. Severe thrombocytopenia with significant bleeding is rare, occurring in 1–2% of patients. It is due to formation of heparin-dependent antiplatelet antibodies and develops within 2–15 days. Bovine lung heparin appears to cause thrombocytopenia more frequently than other forms.

IV. **Congenital bleeding disorders**

A. **Hemophilia A.** Hemophilia A ("classical hemophilia") is an X-linked recessive disorder of coagulation caused by decreased circulating levels of procoagulant factor VIII (also known as factor VIII:C or antihemophilic factor). The metabolic defect in hemophilia A is not the absence of factor VIII but a molecular defect in its procoagulant portion. It is the most common congenital bleeding disorder, occurring in 1 in 10,000 males.

1. **Clinical manifestations.** The severity of bleeding in hemophilia is related to the circulating levels of factor VIII; levels less then 1% normal are characterized as severe hemophilia, factor VIII levels

between 1% and 5% normal are characterized as moderate hemophilia, and factor VIII levels greater than 5% normal are characterized as mild hemophilia. Since platelet function is normal with hemophilia, it is the maintenance stage of hemostasis that shows a defect. Therefore, hemarthrosis, bruises, ecchymoses, and intramuscular and subcutaneous hematomas, hematuria, epistaxis, and gingival hemorrhage are the most common manifestations of the disorder. Intracranial bleeding is relatively rare, but it is the single major cause of death in hemophilia. Gastrointestinal bleeding is rare in hemophilia. If it occurs, anatomical lesions need to be excluded.

2. **Therapy.** For life-threatening bleeding (intracranial hemorrhage, major trauma, severe hemarthrosis) or surgery, 40–50 units factor VIII per kilogram is required to yield 0.8–1.0 units factor VIII per milliliter plasma (80–100% of normal factor VIII levels). At least 1 week of maintenance of minimal factor VIII levels is necessary. For a major nonlife-threatening hemorrhage (advanced joint bleeding, tongue or pharyngeal hematoma, head trauma without neurologic deficit), 25 units factor VIII per kilogram should be given to yield 0.5 unit factor VIII per milliliter plasma (50% of normal factor VIII levels). Subsequent doses are often required. For mild hemorrhages (severe epistaxis, early joint bleeding, dental bleeding), 15 units factor VIII per kilogram should be given to yield 0.3 unit factor VIII per milliliter plasma (30% of normal factor VIII levels). A useful rule of thumb is that every unit of factor VIII per kilogram transfused will raise the plasma factor VIII level by 2% (0.02 unit factor VIII per milliliter). Factor VIII maintenance is given by infusion at least every 12 hours (its half-life is 8–12 hours).
3. **Choice of product.** Cryoprecipitate contains 70–100 units of factor VIII in 10–40 ml of volume. Factor VIII concentrate contains 1000 units of factor VIII in a volume of 30–100 ml.

B. **Hemophilia B (factor IX deficiency, Christmas disease).** Hemophilia B is an X-linked recessive disorder of coagulation caused by decreased circulating levels of procoagulant factor IX:C. The average hemophilia B patient has a milder degree of deficiency of factor IX:C than the corresponding deficiency of factor VIII:C, seen with hemophilia A.

1. **Clinical manifestations** are indistinguishable from hemophilia A.
2. **Therapy.** The minimal level of factor IX necessary for adequate hemostasis is 0.1–0.25 unit per milliliter plasma (10–25% normal). Life-threatening hemorrhages require 60 units per kilogram to yield 0.6 unit factor IX per milliliter plasma (60% normal). Major hemorrhage requires 40 units per kilogram to yield 0.4 unit factor IX per milliliter plasma (40% normal). Mild hemorrhage requires 20 units per kilogram to yield 0.2 unit factor IX per milliliter plasma (20% normal). A simple rule of thumb is that every unit of factor IX per kilogram transfused will raise the plasma factor IX level by 1% (0.01 unit factor IX/ml). One-half of the initial dose needs to be repeated every 24 hours to maintain the level above 40% normal for several days and then above 20% of normal for at least 7–10 days in life-threatening hemorrhages. When giving FFP, 1 ml FFP per kilogram will raise factor IX levels by 1.7%.
3. **Choice of product.** Fresh-frozen plasma (single donor preferably) is still used as a source of factor IX when bleeding is minor or baseline levels are relatively high. Prothrombin complex concentrate (factor IX concentrate) is the treatment of choice for patients with severe or life-threatening hemorrhage. If factor IX concentrate is given, 5–10 units of heparin per milliliter of reconstituted factor IX concentrate or 5,000 units of heparin subcutaneously every 12 hours should be given to prevent deep venous thrombosis.

C. **von Willebrand's disease** is a hereditary bleeding disorder. Type I von Willebrand's disease leads to mild symptoms since patients have a certain amount of functional vWF. Type II variants often have severe bleeding disorders. The most severe homozygous form of the disease is quite rare. vWF is required for normal platelet aggregation in vivo, as well as for adhesion of platelets to the subendothelium to occur.

1. **Clinical manifestations.** In most patients, a mild hemorrhagic disorder exists, with frequent epistaxis, easy bruising, menorrhagia, and prolonged bleeding after dental extractions. Rarely, hemarthrosis and gastrointestinal bleeding can develop. The diagnosis is made if a prolonged bleeding time, elevated aPTT, and low levels of factor VIII:C occur with normal PT or platelet count. The prevalence of von Willebrand's disease is approximately 1 per 25,000 population.
2. **Therapy.** DDAVP (0.3–0.4 μg/kg) causes a rapid 3–20-fold increase in factor VIII levels in plasma. Cryoprecipitate provides a source of both factor VII and vWF and should be used in patients refractory to DDAVP or with severe coagulopathies. Patients with severe von Willebrand's disease often have a less dramatic response to DDAVP. The utility of fresh-frozen plasma is limited by the volume load that transfusion of sufficient levels of vWF would place on the circulation. Factor VIII concentrate should not be used because it lacks the high molecular weight multimers of vWF necessary for hemostasis. In women in whom menorrhagia is the greatest problem, oral contraceptives have been found to be quite effective in controlling this type of bleeding.

D. **Fibrinogen defects.** Congenital fibrinogen defects are rare coagulation disorders that reflect absent or defective protein synthesis.

1. **Afibrinogenemia** is a bleeding disorder in which fibrinogen is not synthesized. The hemorrhagic tendency is particularly severe during the neonatal period and childhood. Umbilical cord bleeding is usually the first symptom. PT, aPTT, TT, and reptilase time are infinitely prolonged. The thromboelastographic tracing is a straight line. Bleeding time is also prolonged.
2. **Hypofibrinogenemia** is also due to a defect in fibrinogen synthesis, except that some fibrinogen is produced. Treatment for hypofibrinogenemia consists of maintenance of fibrinogen levels of 50–100 mg per deciliter (the normal level of fibrinogen is 200–400 mg/dl). The half-life of transfused fibrinogen is about 3–4 days.
3. **Dysfibrinogenemias** are disorders due to qualitative defects in the fibrinogen molecule. Many varieties of the disorder exist, with different defective fibrinogen molecules produced. Some varieties lead to clinical bleeding; others are asymptomatic. Laboratory tests in which fibrinogen is converted to fibrin (e.g., PT, aPTT, TT, and reptilase time) are elevated. Bleeding time can be normal. Serum levels of fibrinogen are usually 20–80 mg per deciliter. Treatment, when necessary, consists of fibrinogen repletion with fresh-frozen plasma, cryoprecipitate, or fibrinogen concentrate.

Selected References

Bang, N. U. Diagnosis and Management of Thrombosis. In W. C. Shoemaker, S. Ayres, A. Grenvik, et al. (eds.), *Textbook of Critical Care* (2d ed.). Philadelphia: W. B. Saunders, 1989.

Bell, W. R., and Royall, R. M. Heparin-associated thrombocytopenia: A comparison of three heparin concentrations. *New Engl. J. Med.* 303:902, 1980.

Clouse, L. H., and Comp, P. C. The regulation of hemostasis: The protein C system. *New Engl. J. Med.* 314:1298, 1986.

Coller, B. S. von Willebrand Disease. In R. W. Colman, J. Hirsch, V. J. Marder, and E. W. Salzman (eds.), *Hemostasis and Thrombosis—Basic Principles and Clinical Practice* (2d ed.). Philadelphia: Lippincott, 1987.

Girolami, A., DeMarco, L., Dal Bo Zanon, R., et al. Rarer quantitative and qualitative abnormalities of coagulation. *Clin. Haematol.* 14:385, 1985.

Gralnick, H. R., and Rick, M. E. Danazol increases factor VIII and factor IX in classic hemophilia and Christmas disease. *New Engl. J. Med.* 308:1393, 1983.

Harker, L. A., and Slichter, S. J. The bleeding time as a screening test for evaluation of platelet function. *N. Engl. J. Med.* 287:155, 1972.

Holmberg, L., and Nilsson, I. M. von Willebrand disease in factor VIII/vWF and platelet formation and function in health and disease. *Ann. N.Y. Acad. Sci.* 509:461, 1987.

Hougie, C. Hemophilia and Related Conditions—Congenital Deficiencies of Prothrombin (Factor II), Factor V, and Factors VII to XII. In W. J. Williams, E. Beutler, A. J. Erslev, and M. A. Lichtman (eds.), *Hematology* (3d ed.). New York: McGraw-Hill, 1983.

Kang, Y. G., Martin, D. J., Marquez, J., et al. Intraoperative changes in blood coagulation and thrombelastographic monitoring in liver transplantation. *Anesth. Analg.* 64:888, 1985.

Kanter, R. K., and Oski, F. A. The Acutely Bleeding Child. In W. C. Shoemaker, S. Ayres, A. Grenvik, et al. (eds.), *Textbook of Critical Care* (2d ed.). Philadelphia: W. B. Saunders, 1989.

Kasper, C. K., and Dietrich, S. L. Comprehensive management of haemophilia. *Clin Haematol.* 14:489, 1985.

Levine, P. H. Clinical Manifestations and Therapy of Hemophilias A and B. In R. W. Colman, J. Hirsch, V. J. Marder, and E. W. Salzman (eds.), *Hemostasis and Thrombosis—Basic Principles and Clinical Practice* (2d ed.). Philadelphia: Lippincott, 1987.

Mahajan, S. L., Myers, T. J., and Baldini, M. G. Disseminated intravascular coagulation during rewarming following hypothermia. *J.A.M.A.* 245:2517, 1981.

Mannuccio, P. M., Remuzzi, G., Pusineri, F., et al. Deamino-8-D-arginine vasopressin shortens the bleeding time in uremia. *New Engl. J. Med.* 308: 8, 1983.

Rybak, M. E. Thrombocytopenia. In J. M. Rippe, R. S. Irwin, J. S. Alpers, and J. E. Dalen (eds.), *Intensive Care Medicine.* Boston: Little, Brown, 1985.

Tolman, K. G., and Cohen, A. Accidental hypothermia. *Can. Med. Assoc. J.* 103:1357, 1970.

Weinstein, M., Ware, J. A., and Salzman, E. Changes in von Willebrand factor during cardiac surgery: Effect of desmopressin acetate. *Blood* 71:1648, 1988.

Williams, W. J. Classification of Disorders of Hemostasis. In W. J. Williams, E. Beutler, A. J. Erslev, and M. A. Lichtman (eds.), *Hematology* (3d ed.). New York: McGraw-Hill, 1983.

21

Transfusion Principles

Alan Lichtenstein and Charles Huggins

Transfusion of blood products is a common occurrence in the ICU population. This chapter reviews the principles and the practices of blood product transfusion.

I. Blood component therapy: the major use of blood for transfusion

A. Blood component or derivative administration accomplishes:

1. Blood volume restoration
2. Oxygen transport improvement
3. Correction of bleeding (using platelets, fresh-frozen plasma, cryoprecipitate, or factor VIII or IX concentrate)
4. Support of neutropenic and thrombocytopenic patients, maximizing utilization of limited blood resources

B. Single-unit donations are collected in presterilized and interconnected plastic bag systems, enabling closed sterile separation into components without violating the system. The once-common problems of bacterial and pyrogenic contamination are thus practically eliminated.

C. The most widely used preservative is citrate-phosphate-dextrose with saline-adenine-glucose-mannitol added to the packed red blood cells (Adsol, Nutricel). Blood can be safely stored in this preservative for 42 days. Some blood banks use the older citrate-dextrose-phosphate adenine (CPDA-1) solutions.

1. The solution CPDA-1 allows storage of whole blood or red blood cells (RBCs) at 4°C for 35 days, with 70% survival of the infused cells 24 hours following transfusion.
2. Citrate-phosphate-dextrose (CPD) and anticoagulant-citrate-dextrose (ACD) allow storage for 21 days.

D. Each unit of whole blood contains approximately 450 ml of donor blood with 63 ml of anticoagulant. The storage lesion consists of progressive decreasing cell viability, increasing acidosis, decreased adenosine triphosphate (ATP) levels, hyperkalemia, and increased RBC oxygen affinity associated with decreased 2,3-DPG.

II. Available blood components

A. Packed RBCs are most frequently used for correcting anemia. They should be used to correct deficiencies in oxygen transport. **No decision to transfuse patients with RBCs should be made on the basis of an arbitrary level of hematocrit.** For many years, physicians transfused patients to a hematocrit of 30%. The theoretical basis for this practice was the observation that oxygen delivery of blood is maximal at a hematocrit of 30%. (The decrease in oxygen content as one dilutes blood from a hematocrit of 45% down to 30% is more than offset by the increase in cardiac output caused by the decrease in viscosity during isovolemic hemodilution.) (Figure 21-1). The fallacy in the argument to transfuse to a hematocrit of 30% lies in the slope of the oxygen delivery curve. Oxygen delivery at a hematocrit of 25% is still 92% of the oxygen delivery at a hematocrit of 30%. The oxygen delivery at a hematocrit of 20% is still 90% that of a hematocrit of 30%. Clearly, most patients tolerate hematocrits of 20% or even less as long as they are normovolemic. The decision to transfuse with RBCs should be on the basis of a patient's clinical condition or index of oxygen delivery, not any arbitrary level of hematocrit. An additional concern is that a clinician could be placed in a compromising legal position if a patient contracted hepatitis or human immunodeficiency virus (HIV) from a transfusion that was given to treat a specific hematocrit in an otherwise stable patient.

1. The size and hematocrit of each unit of packed RBCs may vary, depending on the donor. More than 80% of the plasma is removed, resulting in a final hematocrit of 70–80% for CPDA-1 containing units or 52–60% for Adsol containing units.

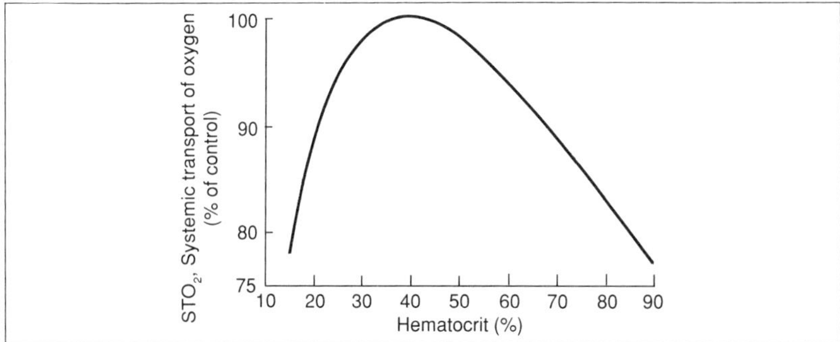

Fig. 21-1. The Relationship of Systemic Oxygen Transport to Hematocrit

2. Packed RBC units contain virtually all of the oxygen-carrying capacity of whole blood in about half the volume, reducing the potential problem of circulatory overload.
3. Partial removal of isoagglutinins by removal of the plasma permits elective transfusion of non-ABO identical red cell units that are crossmatch compatible (e.g., the use of O-negative "universal donor" units to group A or B patients, group A or B units to group AB recipients).
4. Storage time is identical to whole blood containing the same preservative.
5. Packed RBCs are recommended for all uses that require increased oxygen-carrying capacity.
6. Leukocyte-poor RBCs are prepared by a variety of methods, including filtration and centrifugation. They are sometimes effective for patients with previous nonhemolytic febrile reactions mediated by leukocyte antibodies. Freeze-thaw storage and washing also effectively remove most leukocytes. RBCs may be irradiated to prevent graft vs. host disease in immunocompromised recipients.
7. Washed RBCs are prepared by multiple saline washes of packed RBCs. They are physiologically similar to packed RBCs, but excess potassium and ammonia are removed with the plasma.
8. Several long-term storage freezing methods are used to preserve RBCs. Present methods allow storage up to 10 years with maintenance of original levels of ATP and 2,3-diphophoglycerate (DPG).
9. **Washed RBCs and deglycerolized RBCs** are similar products suspended in 0.2% dextrose-saline, with a shelf life of 24 hours once prepared.
   a. Nonhemolytic-related febrile reactions are reduced in both preparations by removing leukocyte elements.
   b. Both are expensive and must be used for appropriate indications.
   c. Neither product has been demonstrated to reduce the risk of hepatitis.
10. During anemia, packed RBCs remain the component of choice.

B. **Platelet concentrates** are prepared from single-unit donations or by platelet phoresis. Platelet units in breathable polyolefin containers can be stored for up to 5 days at 20–24°C, with constant agitation to help maintain pH.
   1. Platelets are indicated for patients bleeding due to thrombocytopenia (platelet count < 50,000) or abnormal platelet function.
      a. Prophylactic platelet infusions should be considered in surgical patients with platelet counts under 50,000 and in acutely ill non-

surgical patients with counts under 10,000 because of the risk of serious hemorrhage.

   b. The adult dose is 4–10 units infused slowly. The standard dose at the Massachusetts General Hospital is 6 units.

   c. One unit of platelets will raise the platelet count approximately 7,000 in a 70-kg patient.

2. Each unit is stored in 50 ml of donor plasma; thus, approximately 300 ml of plasma accompanies each adult dosage.

3. Each platelet pheresis donation contains the equivalent of 5–6 single platelet units. When patients are refractory to platelet transfusions, platelet pheresis donors may be selected on the basis of human leukocyte antigens for a specific recipient.

4. ABO and Rh(D) compatibility is not necessary unless gross RBC contamination is present. Rh(D) sensitization may occur and should be avoided in Rh-negative females with child-bearing potential.

5. Platelets may be pooled into a single transfer bag or administered as single units. Filters with pore sizes less than 170 μm (microaggregate filters) should not be used because they remove a significant number of platelets.

6. Limitations

   a. Conditions such as idiopathic thrombocytopenia purpura or disseminated intravascular coagulation with accelerated platelet destruction may not respond to platelet infusions.

   b. The short half-life of platelets may necessitate repeated transfusions.

   c. Hepatitis and HIV risk is always present.

   d. Nonhemolytic transfusion risks are similar to other component preparations.

C. Whole blood historically was considered the treatment of choice for massive hemorrhage, although it is rarely available now except for autologous units. Homologous whole blood is probably never indicated. Whole blood storage results in the rapid loss of labile clotting factors.

1. Platelet and granulocyte functions are lost after 24 hours.

2. Coagulation factor V is reduced to 50% activity after 14 days.

3. Coagulation factor VIII is reduced to below 50% activity after 24 hours.

III. Plasma

A. Fresh-frozen plasma

1. Fresh-frozen plasma is isolated from whole blood within 6 hours of collection and then frozen. Seventy percent or more of the original procoagulant activity is preserved in this manner when the plasma is used within 24 hours of thawing. The usual unit contains about 250 ml of anticoagulated plasma and can be stored up to 1 year at −18°C or lower.

2. Fresh-frozen plasma is indicated for patients bleeding from multiple clotting-factor deficiencies, secondary to liver disease, massive transfusion, patients with antithrombin III deficiency who require heparin therapy, patients with C1 esterase inhibitor deficiency with life-threatening laryngeal edema, defibrination syndromes and congenital coagulation deficiencies for which no specific factor concentrate is available, such as deficiencies of factor V, VIII, or XI.

   a. Coumadin anticoagulation can be quickly reversed with 2 units of fresh-frozen plasma (for example, in patient requiring emergency surgery). If time permits, it is preferable to reverse the coumadin with vitamin K or the passage of a few days, rather than subject the patient to the hazard of HIV or hepatitis infection.

   b. Two units of fresh-frozen plasma raise the level of circulating procoagulants by approximately 20% and fibrinogen by about 52 mg per deciliter in adult patients. Twenty percent of normal is sufficient for coagulation in surgical patients. Each millimeter of donor fresh-frozen plasma contains 1 unit of each coagulation factor.

c. Fresh-frozen plasma should **not** be used for colloid volume expansion except in patients undergoing massive blood loss and replacement. This use of fresh-frozen plasma purely for colloid volume expansion is specifically renounced by the National Institutes of Health.

B. **Platelet-rich plasma** is prepared by a soft spin of whole blood providing both procoagulant and platelet activity. It is most often prepared by cell-saver devices via intraoperative phlebotomy, and used later in the operation for transfusion.

C. **Cryoprecipitate** is prepared by thawing fresh-frozen plasma slowly at 4°C. The cold precipitated protein is recovered and can then be refrozen at −18°C and stored up to 1 year. It is a concentrated source of fibrinogen, factor VIII:C, factor VIII:vWF, and factor XIII.

1. Indications include factor VIII or XIII deficiencies, von Willebrand's disease, fibrin glue preparations, a supply of fibronectin, and hypofibrinogenemic conditions for which the specific factors can be provided without large volume increases.
2. The risks of hepatitis and HIV infection are similar to those with plasma products. However, it is important to realize that no purification techniques are used in its preparation to remove viral particles.
3. ABO compatibility is not required.
4. The infusion rate should be rapid through a filter. If the thawed cryoprecipitate is not used immediately, it may be stored for no more than 6 hours at 1–8°C.
5. Each 10–40 ml bag of cryoprecipitate contains approximately 80–120 units of factor VIII:C, 40–70% of the von Willebrand's factor present in the initial unit of fresh-frozen plasma, 20–30% of the initial factor XIII, and 250 mg of fibrinogen.

D. **Factor VIII—poor plasma** is the product remaining after cryoprecipitate removal (see sec. **C.**). Identical to single donor plasma, it can be used for congenital clotting deficiencies not involving factors V, VIII or XIII.

E. **Human factor VIII concentrate** is prepared from pooled plasma that is lyophilized.

1. Indications include home administration by hemophilia A patients for minor hemorrhages and for patients with low titer factor VIII inhibitors (levels less than 10 Bethesda units per milliliter). At refrigerator temperatures, it is stable and freeze dried.
2. Because it is pooled plasma product (made from thousands of donors), the risk of acquiring hepatitis after its administration is great. Various methods of heat pasteurization and solvent-detergent treatment are employed to reduce this risk. Factor VIII concentrate produced via recombinant DNA technology is presently undergoing clinical evaluation. No present treatment procedures completely eliminate the risk of hepatitis.
3. Isoagglutinins to red cell antigens A and B are present. These may accumulate during a prolonged course of therapy and cause hemolysis in patients of blood groups A, B, and AB.
4. It is not a good source of the important large molecular weight multimers of von Willebrand's factor.
5. It is an efficient source of factor VIII as each 20–100 ml reconstituted product contains 1000 units of factor VIII:C.
6. A disadvantage is cost (approximately $55–90 per 1000-unit vial wholesale cost).

F. **Porcine factor VIII concentrate** is prepared from highly purified porcine plasma.

1. The sole indication is for use in patients with classical hemophilia A who have developed inhibitors against factor VIII:C.

2. Hepatitis risk is nonexistent.
3. Allergic reactions are possible since this is a nonhuman product.

G. **Factor IX complex or prothrombin complex (Konyne, Proplex, Profilnine)** is a lyophilized preparation obtained by fractionation of pooled plasma by absorption with ion exchanges or inorganic chemicals. It contains factors II, VII, IX and X.
1. The main indication is factor IX deficiency or hemophilia B (Christmas disease).
2. Other indications are acquired hypoprothrombinemia, factor X deficiency, and coumadin overdose.
3. The risk of viral transmission of hepatitis or HIV is **extremely high,** although present concentrates are heat treated to reduce this risk. No present treatment procedures completely eliminate the risk of hepatitis.
4. Thromboembolic problems are common with administration. To combat this, 5–10 units of heparin should be added to each milliliter of reconstituted prothrombin complex. Patients with liver disease or antithrombin III deficiency should not receive prothrombin complex.

H. **Coagulation factor IX (AlphaNine®)** is a lyophilized preparation obtained by fractionation of pooled plasma first into cryoprecipitate, then into prothrombin complex, and finally via absorption with resins and prolonged heat treatment into coagulation factor IX.
1. Coagulation factor IX is 16–20 times more pure than the prothrombin complex from which it is derived.
2. It contains undetectable levels of factor II and VII, and less than 10 units of factor X per 100 units for factor IX.
3. Mean half life of this preparation is 21 hours.
4. It causes substantially less activation of the hemostatic system than prothrombin complex concentrate.
5. A disadvantage is cost ($1300–1500 per 1000-unit vial wholesale cost) as compared to prothrombin complex ($150–350 per 1000-unit vial wholesale cost).

I. **Antithrombin III concentrate** is a lyophilized preparation prepared from pooled plasma that is heat treated to reduce the risk of transmission of viral disease.
1. The main indication is to treat congenital antithrombin III deficiency with its related thrombotic complications. It should be given when the blood antithrombin III level is less than 75% of normal. Its half-life is approximately 60–70 hours.
2. If a patient is receiving heparin therapy, the dosage may need to be lowered after receiving antithrombin III concentrate to reduce the risk of bleeding.

IV. **Blood derivatives** differ from blood components in that (1) they require extensive processing facilities, (2) they are derived from large pools of donor plasma, (3) clotting factors are removed, and (4) they do not carry the risk of clinical hepatitis. Blood derivatives include the following:

A. **Serum albumin** is prepared from pooled human plasma that is heat treated and sterilized to eliminate viral and bacterial contamination. The albumin fraction is the major plasma component and is available as 5% solution in saline (250 ml) and 25% solution in distilled water (25–50 ml). Both solutions are isotonic and contain small amounts of stabilizers; they can be stored for 5 years at 2–10°C.
1. Indications for 5% albumin include hypovolemia from plasma loss, non-hemorrhagic shock if the total protein is less than 52 grams per liter, protein losing nephropathy with hypotension, hemolytic disease of the newborn to bind indirect bilirubin during exchange transfusion, and hypotension after paracentesis. Emergency administration in hemorrhagic shock is also appropriate until definitive blood ther-

apy is available. Advantages of 5% albumin over other volume expanders are controversial.

2. Twenty-five percent albumin has an oncotic equivalent 5 times that of plasma, sequestering large amounts of interstitial fluid and increasing blood volume out of proportion to the amount infused. This preparation has been used in the treatment of burn patients, cerebral edema, and the exchange transfusion of newborns, but its efficacy is unproved.

B. **Plasma protein fraction (PPF),** 5% solution, consists of 88% albumin as well as 12% alpha and beta globulins not contained in albumin preparations.

1. Hypotension may occur following rapid infusion due to vasoactive contaminants.
2. Hepatitis and HIV risk is negligible.
3. Compatibility testing is not required since no ABO antibodies are present.
4. Indications are the same as for serum albumin.

C. **Immune serum globulin (ISG)** is a sterile preparation of pooled gamma-globulin products containing specific antibody titers against diphtheria, hepatitis A, measles and polio.

1. Immune serum globulin is used for maintenance therapy of immunodeficient patients, to treat selected patients with acute or chronic idiopathic thrombocytopenic purpura, or for prophylaxis following exposure to measles, hepatitis A, polio, rubella and varicella.
2. Immune serum globulin is administered IV or IM. The dosage is stated in the package insert for each batch.
3. Side effects include local irritation and, rarely, anaphylaxis.
4. Active hepatitis B immunization sometimes occurs, but clinical hepatitis and HIV infection does not.

D. **Hyperimmune serum globulin** is obtained from individuals with high antibody titers against rabies, mumps, tetanus, pertussis, or hepatitis B and is used for prophylaxis of individuals exposed to these agents. Zoster and vaccinia-immune globulins are useful for immunodeficient patients and are available from the Centers for Disease Control in Atlanta, Georgia. Zoster-immune serum is also available from many blood banks. Side effects and complications of hyperimmune serum globulin are identical to ISG.

E. **Rh(D) immune globulin (RhoGAM™, MICRhoGAM™)** is a hyperimmune globulin used in obstetrics to block the immune response to the small amounts of Rh-incompatible blood infused as a result of delivery, ectopic pregnancy, or abortion. One standard dosage vial (300 μg) given to each Rh(D)-negative mother following exposure will prevent sensitization to 15 ml of fetal blood. One "micro-dosage" vial (50 μg) is protective for abortion, miscarriage, ectopic pregnancy, vaginal hemorrhage, or abdominal trauma during the first 12 weeks of pregnancy. A standard dose vial should be used after amniocentesis or when Rh-positive platelets are given to Rh-negative recipients of childbearing age. HIV or hepatitis transmission has not been reported with this product.

V. **Red blood cell antigens** were first described in 1900 by Landsteiner. Nearly 400 blood groups are currently known. Most are inherited through single genes in simple Mendelian patterns; only a few account for the vast majority of hemolytic transfusion reactions.

A. **The ABO antigens** are the major blood groups. Anti-A and anti-B antibodies are found in the serum of all normal individuals over the age of 6 months who lack the corresponding RBC antigen (Table 21-1). Other blood group antibodies may appear in the absence of known exposure, but their origin is unclear, and they are seldom clinically significant.

B. **The Rh system** comprises more than 30 antibodies, the most important of which is the Rh(D) system. Rh(D) sensitization is seldom the cause of major hemolytic reactions in adults but is responsible for hemolytic disease of the newborn.

C. Minor blood group antigens infrequently produce intravascular hemolytic reactions but are commonly involved in extravascular hemolysis and shortened RBC life. Antibodies to other minor blood group antigens are most often found in recipients with multiple past transfusions or pregnancies.

D. Antibodies in donor blood are seldom clinically significant, although hemolysis of recipient RBC can occur with infusion of large amounts of untyped group O whole blood or plasma. Donor antibodies against white cell antigens may produce leukoagglutination reactions and respiratory distress.

VI. **Compatibility testing,** intended to prevent hemolytic transfusion reactions, involves **typing** both donor and recipient cells for ABO and Rh(D) antigens while **testing** the recipient's serum for RBC alloantibodies, which react with the donor's RBCs.

A. Typing determines the recipient's blood type (ABO and Rh). Blood typing alone results in a 99.8% chance of a compatible transfusion.

B. The **screen** involves testing the recipient's serum against two or more samples of commercially available RBCs known to contain the antigens involved in most transfusion reactions. The addition of an antibody screen results in a 99.94% chance of a compatible transfusion.

C. The major **crossmatch** tests the recipient's serum against samples of the donor's RBCs and is more time-consuming and expensive than the screen. Crossmatching is used to set up blood where there is a high probability that it will actually be infused. The addition of a crossmatch results in a 99.95% chance of a compatible transfusion.

D. For situations where the likelihood of transfusion is low, the type and screen is most cost-effective.

E. Compatibility testing can be waived when blood is needed in an emergency situation. However, administered blood must always be ABO compatible. In a dire emergency, group O Rh-negative blood can be given to prevent exsanguination. After 2–4 units of group O Rh-negative blood are given, subsequent transfusions during the acute episode should continue with group O Rh-negative blood to prevent hemolysis.

VII. **Adverse effects of transfusions** from blood products range from minor pruritis to hemolysis and cardiovascular collapse. Life-threatening complications are rare but often unpredictable; therefore, blood products should be given for specific reasons and potential adverse effects must be considered. Most fatal reactions are due to clerical and laboratory errors. Thorough checking of each blood component prior to infusion is the only way to reduce the incidence of severe sequelae. The long-term sequelae of transfusion of

Table 21-1. ABO blood group system

Blood group	Antigen on RBC	Antibody in serum	Selection of RBCs for transfusion	Selection of plasma for transfusion
0	None	Anti-A, anti-B	0	0, A, B, or AB
A	A	Anti-B	A or O	A or AB
B	B	Anti-A	B or O	B or AB
AB	AB	None	AB, A, B, or O	AB

blood products are much harder to quantitate. The more common problems follow:

A. **Viral hepatitis** is the most common infectious disease transmitted by blood transfusion. The incidence has been estimated to be 0.4–1.0% per unit transfused. Approximately 10% of posttransfusion hepatitis is hepatitis B (HBV), and most of the remainder is non-A, non-B.
   1. The clinical presentation of HBV ranges from nonsymptomatic to a rapidly fatal fulminant disease occurring 50–180 days after receiving blood. Recovery without sequelae is most common, but chronic infection occurs in up to 10% of adults and a much higher proportion of children.
   2. Chronic HBV is most often an asymptomatic carrier state characterized by continued hepatitis B surface antigen (HBsAg) titers but may progress to postnecrotic cirrhosis.
   3. The history of chronic non-A, non-B viral infections is unknown. A high percentage of patients are thought to develop chronic liver disease.
   4. Transfusion-related hepatitis A does not occur.
   5. Viral hepatitis treatment is symptomatic. Hepatitis B hyperimmune globulin is partially effective for **prophylaxis** in patients with known exposure, although all banked blood is tested for HBsAg.
   6. Immune serum globulin may reduce the severity of symptoms in non-A, non-B infection but does not prevent the disease.
   7. Immunization for HBV in populations at risk is recommended. A recombinant DNA-derived vaccine is available that itself carries no risk of viral transmission.

B. **Infectious diseases.** The once-common transmission of bacterial and parasitic diseases via transfusion has been nearly eliminated by storing blood for 72 hours at 4°C.
   1. **Syphilis.** The routine, required serologic testing is of limited efficacy, with numerous false-positives and false-negatives. Spirochetes survive poorly in stored banked blood, however, so transmission of syphilis is virtually eliminated after storing blood for 72 hours at 4°C.
   2. **Malaria** parasites survive storage and should be considered with posttransfusion spiking fevers.
   3. **Cytomegalovirus (CMV)** and **Epstein-Barr virus** have been transmitted via transfusion, producing self-limited febrile illness. Blood may be screened for CMV in neonates or organ transplant patients.
   4. **Trypanosomiasis, leishmaniasis, toxoplasmosis, filariasis, brucellosis, Colorado tick fever, Q fever, Chagas disease, babesiosis, kala-azar, and salmonellosis** rarely have been transmitted or reported.
   5. **Acquired immune deficiency syndrome (AIDS)** has been implicated as a transfusion-associated syndrome, produced by HIV type 1 (HIV-1). Serologic testing for HIV-1 is part of blood screening which has reduced **but not eliminated,** the risk of AIDS transmission. The latest estimates of the risk of transmission of AIDS by a seronegative unit of blood lie between 1 in 40,000 and 1 in 200,000. A second HIV (HIV-2) can also be spread via blood transfusion.
   6. Low-level **bacterial contamination** of fresh blood is not uncommon. Although units are sterile when cultured at 24 hours, the highest risk is with platelet products stored at room temperature. Gross bacterial contamination is rare.

C. **Transfusion reactions** occur immediately or within a few hours of transfusion and are categorized according to the severity of the syndrome.
   1. **Category I reactions** are the most common, characterized by urticaria and pruritis; they are not considered life threatening. The

etiology is unclear, although antibodies to plasma components are suspected. Treatment consists of slowing the infusion rate, administering antihistamines, and observing symptoms. If improvement does not occur within 30 minutes, the transfusion must be stopped and managed as a category II reaction. Category I reactions are the only reactions in which the blood product administration can be continued. They occur in 3% of patients receiving blood products. These reactions typically do not occur until the patient has received at least 1/2 unit of whole blood or 1/2 unit of packed RBCs.

2. **Category II reactions** are associated with antibodies to plasma components, white blood cells, or platelets, as well as infrequent bacterial contamination or pyrogens.
   - **a.** Symptoms include agitation, palpitations, dyspnea, headache, chills, fever and urticaria. Moderate tachycardia without hypotension may occur.
   - **b.** Treatment consists of stopping the transfusion, checking for clerical errors, and returning the remaining blood to the blood bank along with fresh blood and urine samples to be checked for hemoglobin, bilirubin and haptoglobin. Visual inspection of the serum may reveal gross hemolysis.
   - **c.** Further treatment is symptomatic with parenteral antihistamines and antipyretics.
3. **Category III reactions** are life threatening and associated with intravascular hemolysis, gross bacterial contamination, or anaphylactoid reactions.
   - **a.** Obvious signs and symptoms include agitation, confusion, headache, flank pain, chest pain, red urine, chills, fever, tachycardia, hemorrhage, and cardiovascular collapse. General anesthesia or unconsciousness will conceal many symptoms; unexplained bleeding may be the only sign of a problem.
   - **b.** Treatment consists of stopping the blood infusion and providing cardiovascular and respiratory support as described in Chapter 11. The blood bag must be sent to the blood bank along with fresh samples of blood and urine.
   - **c.** The serum should be examined for hemolysis.
   - **d.** Urine output must be maintained with the use of fluids, diuretics, and hemodynamic support. Consideration should be given to alkalinizing the urine to avoid renal damage from free hemoglobin.
   - **e.** Follow-up should include consideration for possible disseminated intravascular coagulation or renal failure (see Chaps. 20 and 25).
   - **f.** Compatible blood products may be administered as required.
   - **g.** The signs of a serious hemolytic transfusion reaction **always** occur during transfusion of the first 100 ml of the blood product.
4. **Pulmonary edema** may occur following transfusions.
   - **a.** Most cases are due to fluid overload and can be prevented with proper administration rates and diuretics as needed.
   - **b.** Noncardiac pulmonary edema is thought to be due to passively transfused antibodies to granulocytes that produce inflammatory activation and sequestration of aggregates in the pulmonary vasculature.
     - **(1)** Fever, dyspnea, hypoxemia, and cyanosis may occur.
     - **(2)** The transfusion must be stopped and supportive therapy instituted, including intubation and mechanical ventilation as required. Transient hypoxemia may be a major problem. However, most cases resolve without specific therapy with 24 hours.

D. Anaphylactoid reactions are characterized by cardiopulmonary collapse following blood administration and are uncommon (see Chap. 11).

1. They are usually unpredictable and associated with the following:
   a. Donor antibodies to leukocytes from parturition or prior transfusions.
   b. Congenital immune globulin A (IgA) deficiency. These patients have immune globulin G (IgG) antibodies to IgA, a normal component of blood products.
2. It may be difficult to distinguish anaphylactoid reactions from category III reactions except by the absence of hemolysis and the rapid onset of symptoms after the blood infusion. Signs and symptoms include the following:
   a. Nausea, agitation, unconsciousness.
   b. Hypotension, tachycardia, cardiovascular collapse.
   c. Wheezing, dyspnea.
3. Treatment consists of stopping the transfusion and immediately resuscitating the patient as outlined in Chapter 11.
4. If further blood components are required, washed or deglycerolized cells should be used.
5. Blood from known IgA-deficient individuals is often difficult to obtain. Therefore, autologous transfusion or washed cells should be considered for these individuals. The Red Cross has IgA-deficient fresh-frozen plasma.

E. **Delayed transfusion reactions** include delayed hemolysis, hemosiderosis, graft versus host disease, posttransfusion purpura, alloimmunization to various blood antigens, and depression of the immune response to cancer, which may become apparent hours to months after transfusion.
1. Alloimmunization occurs to some degree with pregnancy or previous transfusion. When RBC antibodies form, a delayed hemolytic reaction may occur, manifested only by a decreased RBC survival time, although occasionally hemoglobinemia and renal failure occur.
2. **The onset of delayed hemolysis** is often insidious. Unexplained fever with increased bilirubin and unexplained anemia 1–2 weeks after transfusion may be the presenting symptom.
3. Antibodies to leukocytes are thought to be the cause of most febrile nonhemolytic reactions, including posttransfusion purpura resulting from formation of platelet antibodies.
4. Graft versus host blastogenesis may occur from transfusion of lymphocytes into immunocompromised hosts unless the blood is first irradiated. Irradiation does not affect RBC or platelet survival.
5. Hemosiderosis is common in patients chronically receiving multiple infusions of RBC preparations with resultant hepatic, cardiac, and endocrine failure.
6. Blood transfusion is associated with an **increased risk of cancer recurrence.** Five-year recurrence-free survival rates in colorectal and lung cancer patients who received blood transfusions have been shown to be significantly reduced over similar patients who did not receive transfusions.

VIII. **Massive transfusion** is defined as a rapid administration of over 1.5 blood volumes for hemorrhagic shock. Patients requiring massive transfusions often suffer from cardiovascular instability, metabolic abnormalities, and dilutional coagulopathy (Fig. 21-2).

A. Common metabolic problems include abnormalities in potassium, oxygen affinity, acid-base equilibrium, temperature, and calcium.
1. **Hyperkalemia** is rare in adults but may be a problem in neonates. Hyperkalemia may be an indicator of intravascular hemolysis or renal failure.
2. **Hypokalemia** is common and may be accentuated with deglycerolized or washed RBC administration.

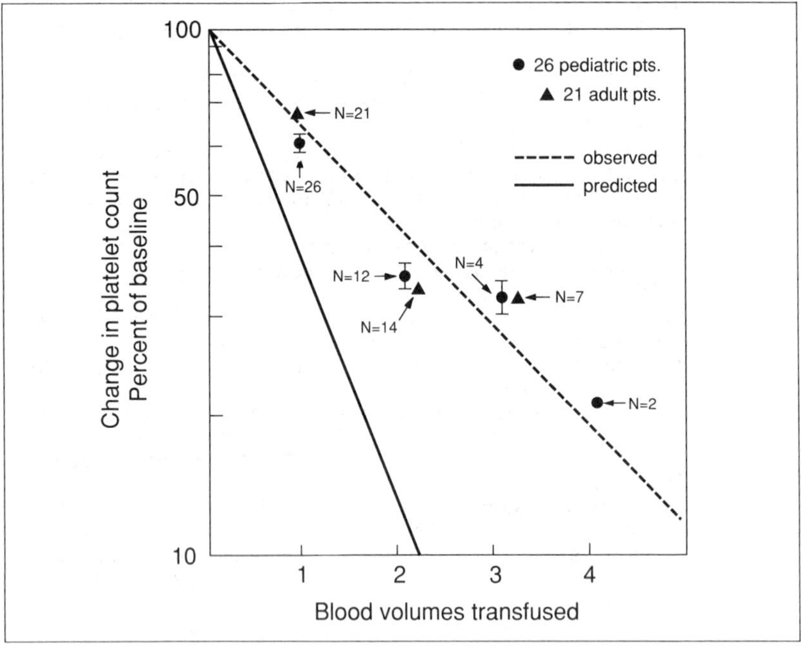

Fig. 21-2. The effect of massive blood transfusion on platelet count. Modified from Coté CJ, Liu LMP, Szyfelbein SK, Goudsouzian NG, Daniels AL: Changes in serial platelet counts following massive blood transfusion in pediatric patients. *Anesthesiology. 62:197–201, 1985.*

3. **Acidosis,** if present, is secondary to shock with lactate production.
4. **Alkalosis** may occur hours to days following massive transfusions due to metabolism of citrate to bicarbonate.
5. **A higher oxygen affinity** characterizes stored blood, but is clinically insignificant.
6. **Hypothermia can be prevented with the use of blood warmers.**
7. **Hypocalcemia** from citrate with massive transfusions is uncommon in adult patients with normal hepatic function, although it may occur when the infusion rate exceeds 1.5 ml/kg/minute. Electrocardiographic monitoring of the Q-T interval with appropriate IV calcium administration may be required.

B. Dilution of platelets and plasma clotting factors to the point of producing clinical bleeding is not usually seen until at least 1.5 blood volumes have been transfused (Fig. 21-2).

1. Prothrombin time (PT), activated partial thromboplastin time (aPTT), and platelet count **must be evaluated** and fresh-frozen plasma or platelets administered if necessary.
   - **a.** Routine fresh-frozen plasma and platelet administration should be avoided.
   - **b.** Platelet count should be maintained above 50,000–70,000, if possible, in surgical patients. Eight to 10 units of platelets should be administered with each 1.5–2.0 blood volumes if bleeding is a problem.

C. Pulmonary dysfunction may occur after massive transfusion. The exact mechanism remains unknown but may represent pulmonary leukostasis from a leukoagglutinin reaction.

IX. **Transfusion filters** are commercially available and are recommended for use with blood product administration. These include the following:

A. The **standard filter** is an 80 or 140 μm filter and is included in most transfusion sets.

B. The 20 or 40 μm **microaggregate filter.** Unfiltered blood does contain a significant amount of possibly harmful debris that is removed with 20 or 40 μm filters. Microscopic aggregates consisting of platelets, leukocytes, and fibrin are known to form and are removed by microaggregate filters at the expense of slower transfusion rates and higher cost. These microaggregates, however, have not been conclusively linked to any harmful effects (e.g., pulmonary dysfunction). Microaggregate filters are recommended for massive transfusion when the slower infusion rates can be tolerated.

Selected References

Aledort, L. M. Cryoprecipitate revisited. *Transfusion* 28:295, 1988.

Barrera, J. M., Bruguera, M., Ercilla, M. G., Sanchez-Tapias, J. M., Gil, M. P., Costa, J., Gelabert, A., Rodes, J., and Castillo, R. Incidence of non-A, non-B hepatitis after screening blood donors for antibodies to hepatitis C virus and surrogate markers. *Ann. Intern. Med.* 115:596, 1991.

Bourke, D. L., and Smith, T. C. Estimating allowable hemodilution. *Anesthesiology* 41:609, 1974.

Brettler, D. B., Alter, H. J., Dienstag, J. L., Forsberg, A. D., and Levine, P. H. Prevalence of hepatitis C virus antibody in a cohort of hemophilia patients. *Blood* 76:254, 1990.

Choo, Q. L., Kuo, G., Weiner, A. J., Overby, L. R., Bradley, D. W., and Houghton, M. Isolation of a cDNA clone derived from a blood-borne non-A, non-B viral hepatitis genome. *Science* 244:359, 1989.

Cote, C. J., Drop, L. J., Hoaglin, D. C., Daniels, A. L., and Young, E. T. Ionized hypocalcemia after fresh frozen plasma administration to thermally injured children: effects of infusion rate, duration, and treatment with calcium chloride. *Anesth. Analg.* 67:152, 1988.

Cote, C. J., Liu, L. M., Szyfelbein, S. K., Goudsouzian, N. G., and Daniels, A. L. Changes in serial platelet counts following massive blood transfusion in pediatric patients. *Anesthesiology* 62:197, 1985.

Cuthbert, J. A. Hepatitis C. *Am. J. Med. Sci.* 299:346, 1990.

Gettinger, A. Rational use of blood products and alternative fluids. 39th Annual Refresher Course Lectures, American Society of Anesthesiologists, 112:1, 1988.

Goodnough, L. T., and Shuck, J. M. Risks, options, and informed consent for blood transfusion in elective surgery. *Am. J. Surg.* 159:602, 1990.

Kasper, C. K., and Dietrich, S. L. Comprehensive management of haemophilia. *Clin. Haematol.* 14:489, 1985.

Klienman, S., and Secord, D. Risk of human immunodeficiency virus (HIV) transmission by anti-HIV negative blood. *Transfusion* 28:499, 1988.

Kuo, G., Choo, Q. L., Alter, H. J., Gitnick, G. L., Redeker, A. G., Prucell, R. H., Miyamura, T., Dienstag, J. L., Alter, J. J., Stevens, C. E., Tegtmeier, G. E., Bonino, F., Colombo, M., Lee, W. S., Kuo, C., Berger, K., Shuster, J. R., Overby, L. R., Bradley, D. W., and Houghton, M. An assay for circulating antibodies to a major etiologic virus of human non-A, non-B hepatitis. *Science* 244:362, 1989.

Little, A. G., Wu, H. S., Ferguson, M. K., Ho, C. H., Bowers, V. D., Segalin, A., and Staszek, V. M. Perioperative blood transfusion adversely affects prognosis of patients with stage I non-small-cell lung cancer. *Am. J. Surg.* 160:630, 1990.

Mannuccio, P. M., Bauer, K. A., Gringeri, A., Barzegar, S., Bottasso, B., Simoni, L., and Rosenberg, R. D. Thrombin generation is not increased in the blood of hemophilia patients after the infusion of a purified factor IX concentrate. *Blood* 76:2540, 1990.

Miller, P. H., O'Connell, J., Leipold, A., and Wenzel, R. P. Potential liability for transfusion-associated AIDS. *J.A.M.A.* 253:3419, 1985.

Miller, R. D. Complications of massive blood transfusions. *Anesthesiology* 39:82, 1973.

Miller, R. D., Robbins, T. O., Tong, M. J., and Barton, S. L. Coagulation defects associated with massive blood transfusions. *Ann. Surg.* 174:794, 1971.

NIH Consensus Conference: Fresh-frozen plasma indications and risks. *J.A.M.A.* 253:551, 1985.

NIH Consensus Conference: Perioperative red blood cell transfusion. *J.A.M.A.* 260:2700, 1988.

NIH Consensus Conference: Platelet transfusion therapy. *J.A.M.A.* 257:1777, 1987.

Oberman, H. A., Barnes, B. A., and Friedman, B. A. The risk of abbreviating the major crossmatch in urgent or massive transfusion. *Transfusion* 18:137, 1978.

Pisciotto, P. T., ed. *Blood Transfusion Therapy: A Physician's Handbook,* 3rd ed. Arlington, VA: American Association of Blood Banks, 1989.

Polesky, H. F., and Hanson, M. R. Transfusion-associated hepatitis C virus (non-A, non-B) infection. *Arch. Pathol. Lab. Med.* 113:232, 1989.

Rosenberg, S. A., Seipp, C. A., White, D. E., and Wesley, R. Perioperative blood transfusions are associated with increased rates of recurrence and decreased survival in patients with high-grade soft-tissue sarcomas of the extremities. *J. Clin. Oncol.* 3:698, 1985.

Saxena, S., Korula, J., and Shulman, I. A. A review of donor alanine aminotransferase testing. Implications for the blood donor and practitioner. *Arch. Pathol. Lab. Med.* 113:767, 1989.

Schimpf, K., Mannucci, P. M., Kreutz, W., Brackmann, H. H., Auerswald, F., Ciavarella, N., Mosseler, J., DeRosa, V., Kraus, B., Brueckmann, C., Mancuso, G., Mittler, U., Haschke, F., and Morfine, M. Absence of hepatitis after treatment with a pasteurized factor VIII concentrate in patients with hemophilia and no previous transfusions. *N. Eng. J. Med.* 316:918, 1987.

Walker, R. H. What is a Clinically Significant Antibody? In H. F. Polesky and R. H. Walker. *Safety and Transfusion Practices.* College of American Pathologists, 1982, Pp. 79–94.

22

Intensive Care Unit Management of Adult Patients Following Orthotopic Liver Transplantation

Gary J. Vorsanger, William F. Eckhardt, and Charles E. Cook

I. Preoperative evaluation
- **A. Factors predisposing to electrolyte disturbances**
- **B. Factors predisposing to excessive bleeding**
  1. **Thrombocytopenia**
  2. **Portal hypertension**
  3. **Clotting factor deficiencies**
  4. **Previous abdominal surgery or peritonitis**
  5. **Fibrinolysis**
  6. **Corticosteroids**
  7. **Type of liver disease**
- **C. Hemodynamic considerations**
  1. **Preoperative fluid status**
  2. **Cirrhosis**
  3. **Preexisting coronary artery or valvular heart disease**
- **D. Pulmonary considerations**
  1. **Intrapulmonary shunting**
  2. **Atelectasis**
  3. **Encephalopathy**
  4. **Chronic obstructive pulmonary disease**
- **E. Renal considerations**
  1. **Chronic renal insufficiency (CRF)**
  2. **Hepatorenal syndrome**
  3. **Immunosuppressive therapy**

II. Surgical technique
- **A. Stage I: Preanhepatic phase, preparation for hepatectomy**
  1. **Incision**
  2. **Dissection**
  3. **Preparation for veno-venous bypass**
  4. **Arrival of the donor liver**
- **B. Stage II: Anhepatic phase**
  1. **Veno-venous bypass**
  2. **Hepatectomy**
  3. **Insertion of donor liver**
- **C. Stage III: Postanhepatic phase**
  1. **Reperfusion**
  2. **Hepatic artery anastomosis**
  3. **Biliary reconstruction**
  4. **Abdominal closure**

III. Stage I: Intraoperative problems
- **A. Preanhepatic phase**
  1. **Incision**
  2. **Monitoring of coagulation status**
  3. **Calcium**
- **B. Stage II: Anahepatic phase**
  1. **Veno-venous bypass**
  2. **Hepatectomy**
  3. **Insertion of the donor liver**
- **C. Stage III: Postanhepatic phase**
  1. **Reperfusion**

2. **Hepatic artery anastomosis**
3. **Biliary reconstruction**
4. **Closure**

IV. Postoperative ICU care following liver transplantation

A. **Initial evaluation**

B. **Postoperative complications**

1. **Cardiovascular**
2. **Temperature homeostasis**
3. **Pulmonary**
4. **Metabolic**
5. **Coagulation**
6. **Hepatic dysfunction**
7. **Central nervous system**
8. **Renal function**
9. **Infectious disease**
10. **Nutrition**
11. **Pain management**

Orthotopic liver transplantation (OLT) is being performed with increasing frequency throughout the United States. It is estimated that 5,000 of the 20,000 people who die each year of primary liver disease could benefit from hepatic transplantation (Brown). According to data from the Mayo Clinic, the following types of liver disease result in end-stage liver failure and qualify for possible transplantation: chronic active hepatitis (CAH), 29%; primary sclerosing cholangitis (PSC), 27%; primary biliary cirrhosis (PBC), 24%; and other, 11% (Kahan, 1989).

I. **Preoperative evaluation.** This should include a complete history, physical examination, and review of laboratory data as they relate to the pathophysiology of end-stage liver disease.

A. **Factors predisposing to electrolyte disturbances.** Ascites is frequently found and may be due to portal hypertension and/or hypoalbuminemia. Despite total body fluid excess, patients are frequently intravascularly volume depleted, which can lead to secondary hyperaldosteronism, hyponatremia, and hypokalemia. Hypocalcemia from intestinal malabsorption and vitamin deficiency may occur. In addition, malnutrition may result in hypophosphatemia, hypomagnesemia, and hypoglycemia.

B. **Factors predisposing to excessive bleeding**

1. **Thrombocytopenia.** This is frequently associated with splenomegaly secondary to portal hypertension. Petechiae may be noted on physical examination, and a platelet count with possible bleeding time should be part of the routine laboratory screen.
2. **Portal hypertension.** Gastroesophageal varices and internal hemorrhoids may complicate bleeding. Physical examination may reveal a "caput medusa," a form of portal-systemic shunt, noted on the anterior abdominal wall.
3. **Clotting factor deficiencies.** These patients may present with epistaxis, gastrointestinal bleeding, or hemarthrosis. Laboratory tests may reveal a prolonged prothrombin time (PT) or partial thromboplastin time (PTT).
4. **Previous abdominal surgery or peritonitis.** The presence of adhesions can lead to excessive bleeding and complicate the surgical procedure.
5. **Fibrinolysis.** Sepsis may lead to fibrinolysis. In addition, fibrin split products may be elevated in end-stage liver disease due to decreased clearance.
6. **Corticosteroids.** Steroid therapy may be used to treat patients with chronic active hepatitis, systemic lupus erythematosus, or previous transplantation. Corticosteroids may be implicated in causing increased capillary fragility.
7. **Type of liver disease.** Patients with chronic active hepatitis may tend to bleed more readily during live transplantation. Patients with CAH have been shown to require twice as much cryoprecipitate and 20% more platelets than patients with PSC or PBC (Rettke, 1989b).

C. **Hemodynamic considerations**

1. **Preoperative fluid status.** Patients may be intravascularly volume depleted, especially if receiving chronic diuretic therapy for ascites. Pulmonary artery catheterization may guide fluid management.
2. **Cirrhosis.** Patients with end-stage liver disease may exhibit a hyperdynamic circulatory response manifested by increased cardiac output, decreased systemic vascular resistance, elevated heart rate, and low mean arterial blood pressure with normal central venous pressure (CVP) and pulmonary capillary wedge pressures (PCWP).
3. **Preexisting coronary artery or valvular heart disease.** Fluid shifts during liver transplantation and electrolyte changes, partic-

ularly during reperfusion, can be profound and may worsen myocardial ischemia.

D. **Pulmonary considerations**

1. **Intrapulmonary shunting** can result in hypoxemia.
2. **Atelectasis.** The presence of ascites (with elevated intraabdominal pressure), as well as the use of surgical-retracting devices such as the Omni retractor, may prevent full expansion of lower lung segments. This can be treated with increased tidal volume and positive end-expiratory pressure (PEEP).
3. **Encephalopathy.** Central nervous system dysfunction seen in end-stage liver disease may alter ventilation and lead to hyperventilation and respiratory alkalosis.
4. **Chronic obstructive pulmonary disease (COPD).** Patients with underlying lung disease may have more complicated intraoperative and postoperative management and may have difficulty weaning from mechanical ventilation. We recommend obtaining preoperative chest radiographs, room air arterial blood gases, and pulmonary function tests on all patients awaiting liver transplantation.

E. **Renal considerations**

1. **Chronic renal insufficiency (CRF),** which can be exacerbated by hypovolemia, diuretic therapy. and nephrotoxic drugs
2. **Hepatorenal syndrome.** Circulating factors from patients with end-stage liver disease can lead to reversible renal failure. Virtually all of these patients have both ascites and oliguria. Laboratory tests can suggest this diagnosis: a normal urine sediment; no proteinuria; urine sodium less than 10 mEq per liter, urine/plasma creatinine ratio greater than 30:1, and the urine/plasma osmolality ratio greater than 1.0.
3. **Immunosuppressive therapy.** Cyclosporine can cause nephrotoxicity, especially for repeat transplants.

II. **Surgical technique.** A complete description of surgical techniques for adult liver transplantation is beyond the scope of this text. However, a brief overview of the procedure, as performed in the Massachusetts General Hospital, follows. The procedure is divided into stages, and intraoperative complications occurring during each phase are presented as a guide to postoperative care.

A. **Stage I: Preanhepatic phase, preparation for hepatectomy**

1. **Incision.** A bilateral, subcostal incision with midline extension in a cephalad direction is used. This incision crosses both sets of epigastric vessels and includes removal of the xiphoid process. As the peritoneum is entered, ascites may be released, and hemodynamic instability may occur.
2. **Dissection.** The recipient's liver, inferior vena cava, hepatic artery, common bile duct, and portal structures are dissected free.
3. **Preparation for veno-venous bypass.** Use of veno-venous bypass allows decompression of the portal venous system, decreases intraoperative blood loss, and minimizes the intestinal engorgement that can occur with portal venous occlusion. There is no requirement for systemic anticoagulation; standard systems employ heparin-bonded polyvinyl chloride (PVC) tubing to connect cannulae in the portal vein and femoral vein to a turbine pump and inflow cannula in the left axillary vein. Potential flow rates range from 2–13 liters per minute, with an average range of 2–4 liters per minute. Potential problems associated with veno-venous bypass include hypothermia, thrombocytopenia (due to platelet adhesion to the bypass tubing), venous air embolism, clotting in the bypass tubing, or hemorrhage secondary to accidental decannulation (Plevak, 1989).

4. **Arrival of the donor liver.** The donor liver and its blood vessels are resected en bloc from the heparinized donor, and a preservative solution is perfused through the liver prior to placing it on ice. In the past, Euro-Collins solution was used; it permitted a cold ischemia time of 6–8 hours. More recently, the University of Wisconsin (UW) solution has been developed; it provides for a mean preservation time greater than twice that of the Euro-Collins and may approach 24–30 hours. In one study, use of the UW solution provided a lower retransplantation rate and improved 1-month survival rates (Ritter, 1989). Once the donor liver has arrived, it is inspected, and the portal structures are dissected free.

B. Stage II: Anhepatic phase

1. **Veno-venous bypass.** Cannulation of the portal vein is performed, and initiation of veno-venous bypass is begun. It is important to avoid hypovolemia prior to initiation of bypass; otherwise, hypotension and hemodynamic instability may occur.
2. **Hepatectomy.** The inferior vena cava (IVC), hepatic artery, and common bile duct are cross-clamped and resected. At this point, venous return is dependent on flow through the superior vena cava (SVC), veno-venous bypass circuit, and azygous vein. The diseased liver is then removed.
3. **Insertion of donor liver.** The cold donor liver is placed in the abdominal cavity, and anastomosis of the supra- and intrahepatic IVC are begun. Once the anastomoses are completed, flow is begun via the IVC, and veno-venous bypass is terminated. The bypass cannulae are removed, and anastomosis of the portal vein is started.

C. Stage III: Postanhepatic phase

1. **Reperfusion.** Reperfusion of the liver occurs when the IVC and portal vein are unclamped. This can be a period of hemodynamic instability; hypothermia, metabolic acidosis, hypocalcemia, and hyperkalemia may occur.
2. **Hepatic artery anastomosis.** Hepatic artery reconstruction is performed. Although this blood vessel provides only 20–30% of total hepatic blood flow, it provides up to 50% of oxygen requirements.
3. **Biliary reconstruction.** The donor gallbladder is removed. If the recipient had a functioning hepatic duct, a primary choledochostomy may be performed over a T-tube. Otherwise, a Roux-en-Y with a choledochojejunostomy is created. A cholangiogram is performed to verify patency of the biliary tree, and femoral and axillary venotomies are repaired.
4. **Abdominal closure.** The axillary, femoral, and abdominal incisions are closed, after anchoring several drains and the T-tube. Interrupted wire sutures and a subcuticular closure is performed.

III. Intraoperative problems

A. Stage I: Preanhepatic phase

1. **Incision.** Patients with portal hypertension may suffer from excessive bleeding when incisions cross enlarged epigastric blood vessels. In addition, peritoneal incision in patients with ascites may lead to a sudden decrease in arterial blood pressure and central venous pressure (CVP). To cope with this problem, most centers use some form of rapid transfusion device. There are several commercially available models, and in general they are capable of transfusing blood products at a rate of 1,000–1,500 ml per minute. We use a custom-designed rapid infusion system consisting of a cardiotomy reservoir, high-pressure PVC tubing, roller pump, warming bath, and bubble detector. Other centers have reported success using autotransfusion systems to decrease demand on hospital blood banks and to reuse some of the patient's blood, thereby decreasing exposure to possible blood-

borne contaminants such as cytomegalovirus (CMV), non-A, non-B hepatitis, and human immunodeficiency virus (HIV) (Rettke, 1989a).

2. **Monitoring of coagulation status.** Patients with end-stage liver disease frequently have a coagulopathy. At many institutions, this is monitored with sequential determination of platelet count, PT, PTT, or activated clotting time (ACT). Some institutions also employ use of thromboelastography to assess coagulation status. Thromboelastography measures sheer elasticity of a blood clot from initial fibrin deposition to final clot formation. As such, coagulation time and quality of clot formation are assessed. Different patterns are generated depending on the problem with coagulation (thrombocytopenia or functional platelet defect versus factor deficiency, for example).
3. **Calcium.** In a hemodynamically unstable patient requiring massive transfusion during the preanhepatic phase, hypocalcemia may become a significant problem due to citrate chelation of calcium.

B. Stage II: Anhepatic phase

1. **Veno-venous bypass.** Initiation of veno-venous bypass can lead to hemodilution as the cardiotomy reservoir is primed with 2 units of packed red blood cells (RBCs), 2 units of fresh-frozen plasma, and 500 ml of normal saline solution (mean overall hematocrit of approximately 28). This stage can be associated with continued blood loss and necessitates careful hemodynamic monitoring. Hypotension can be caused by hypovolemia, venous air emboli (from the pump or open blood vessels), inadequate output from the pump, or formation of thromboemboli in the pump circuit. Myocardial depression leading to hypotension may be caused by hypocalcemia, hypothermia, or citrate intoxication from rapid transfusion. The last may require measuring frequent ionized calcium levels and repletion by frequent boluses of calcium chloride.
2. **Hepatectomy.** Many individuals have described profound hypoglycemia occurring during the anhepatic phase. This hypoglycemia is believed to be secondary to absent hepatic glycogenolysis and gluconeogenesis along with decreased insulin clearance. This has not been a major problem in our experience; we usually see glucose levels rise only to the range of 200–400 mg%. Thrombocytopenia may occur during this phase; platelets are frequently bound to the walls of the veno-venous bypass tubing.
3. **Insertion of the donor liver.** Hypothermia may become a significant problem during this phase of the procedure because the donor liver is ice cold and approximately 40–50% of the cardiac output is flowing through the unheated tubing of the veno-venous bypass shunt. After completion of the IVC anastomosis, the portal cannula is clamped, and the portal venous anastomosis is completed. Venous air emboli are a potential problem if they enter the portal vein during decannulation or the axillary vein from the bypass pump.

C. Stage III: Postanhepatic phase

1. **Reperfusion.** Reestablishment of hepatic perfusion is the most difficult phase of the operation. The donor liver is cold, acidotic, and hyperkalemic (from inactivity of the Na-K ATPase pump), and profound hemodynamic changes may accompany mixing of this perfusate solution with the systemic circulation. Blood temperature may fall 1–3°C, accompanied by cardiac arrhythmias, which may range from atrial irritability to ventricular tachycardia and fibrillation. A postreperfusion syndrome has been described; it consists of sinus or junctional bradycardia accompanied by hypotension. Other metabolic changes include hyperkalemia, hypocalcemia, and metabolic acidosis. Potential therapeutic maneuvers at this time include IV calcium chloride, IV sodium bicarbonate, atropine or beta-1 agonists for

mild bradycardia, and epinephrine or Levophed (norepinephrine) for hypotension. If cardiovascular collapse occurs, a brief round of cardiopulmonary resuscitation may be required to push this bolus of perfusate through the heart. Sources of bleeding at this time include:

a. Bleeding from one of the vascular anastomoses

b. A consumptive coagulopathy secondary to activation of the fibrinolytic system

c. Release of heparin from the donor liver may be a theoretical concern. A controversy exists regarding the treatment of patients with a consumptive coagulopathy. Some centers treat this using alpha amino-caproic acid (Amicar). This may present a significant problem because the leading cause of patient morbidity is pulmonary thromboembolism.

2. Hepatic artery anastomosis. Hepatic artery blood flow provides 20–30% of total liver blood flow but delivers 50% of the oxygen required for normal metabolism. As liver function improves, so does hepatocellular homeostasis. Whereas hyperkalemia was a problem during the anhepatic stage, it is often necessary to supplement the patient with potassium during this phase, especially if the urine output has been brisk. Functioning hepatocytes will activate the Krebs cycle and thus metabolize citrate. Citrate is metabolized to bicarbonate, which may cause a metabolic alkalosis. This is cleared by the kidneys over the subsequent 48 hours. Important signs of a functioning graft are a falling potassium, a stable or elevated total calcium, and a normal or slightly decreased ionized calcium. Other monitors of graft function include bile production, a decrease in plasma glucose to normal, and increased urine output (especially in patients with preoperative hepatorenal syndrome).

3. Biliary reconstruction. In general, two alternative alternatives exist: choledochojejunostomy or choledochocholedochostomy. Either the donor gallbladder is removed and a primary choledochocholedochostomy over a T-tube is performed, or a Roux-en-Y with a choledochojejunostomy is created. A cholangiogram is undertaken to check for patency.

4. Closure. A final check for hemostasis is performed, hemodynamics are optimized, and the patient is readied for transport to the ICU.

IV. Postoperative ICU care following liver transplantation. The information in this section is a distillation of the experience at both the Massachusetts General Hospital and the Mayo Clinic. We have divided the ICU experience into changes occurring during the first postoperative day, as well as those occurring on postoperative days 2 and 3. Patients stay an average of 48–72 hours in our ICU and are transferred to a specialized postoperative transplantation unit. At the Mayo Clinic, patients stay 4–9 days in the ICU.

A. Initial evaluation. On admission to the ICU, oral report is given to the ICU staff (residents, fellows, and visits) and nurses. The full preoperative history is discussed, as well as the intraoperative course, with special attention given to complications (e.g., oliguria) and recent laboratory tests (e.g., complete blood count [CBC], coagulation studies, and electrolytes). Initial ICU evaluation should include physical examination, hemodynamics, ventilatory data, blood gases, CBC, clotting studies, thrombelastograph (if used), glucose, electrolytes, blood-urea nitrogen (BUN) and creatinine, abdominal circumference, bile output via T-tube, and output from surgical drains. **Common medications** used in the ICU include:

1. Cyclosporine, need to monitor renal function

2. Cyclophosphamide, need to follow CBC

3. **Steroids**
4. **Antacids/H2 blockers,** to prevent gastrointestinal bleeding
5. **Antibiotics** for bowel coverage and to suppress gram-negative organisms
6. **Dopamine,** for renal perfusion at 2–5 μg/kg/minute
7. **Narcotics.** Analgesia is often provided by patient-controlled analgesia (PCA).

B. Postoperative complications

1. **Cardiovascular**

a. **First 24 hours**

(1) Patients are usually hemodynamically stable.

(2) **Patients are often hypothermic (93–96°F),** and the cold-induced vasoconstriction often increases both blood pressure and systemic vascular resistance (SVR). PA filling pressures are
often low-normal, and fluid in the postoperative period is frequently administered in the form of colloid—generally albumin and fresh-frozen plasma (the latter if clotting studies are abnormal).

(3) Patients often exhibit a mild tachycardia.

(4) With rewarming, blood pressure and SVR decrease, and PA filling pressures begin to increase in response to maintenance fluid infusion and to increasing discomfort as anesthesia wears off.

(5) Cardiac output generally increases.

(6) Inotropic medications are rarely needed. Dopamine is used to augment renal function, and hypotension is treated with volume (if urine output is decreased and filling pressures are low), pressors (epinephrine or norepinephrine), or calcium chloride are used if hypocalcemia is present.

b. **Postoperative days 2 and 3**

(1) **Hypertension** is common. Patients are usually treated with a combination of hydralazine, nitroglycerin, sodium nitroprusside, and labetalol.

(2) **Cyclosporine** may precipitate or exacerbate hypertension.

(3) **Hypertension** may lead to an increased risk of intracranial hemorrhage in patients.

2. **Temperature homeostasis**

a. **First 24 hours.** Hypothermia is associated with hemodynamic instability and potential cardiac arrhythmias. Hypothermia may worsen a preexisting coagulopathy.

b. **Postoperative days 2 and 3.** Normal body temperature; occasionally hyperthermic, if septic

3. **Pulmonary**

a. **First 24 hours.** The patient is intubated and mechanically ventilated until the effects of general anesthesia and muscle relaxation have worn off. Positive end-expiratory pressure is often used to prevent atelectasis. Patients are usually extubated within 24 hours, pending successful completion of standard extubation criteria. Following this, a program of chest physiotherapy, incentive spirometry, and deep-breathing exercises is used. Abnormal postoperative chest radiograph findings may include bilateral infiltrates in up to 22% of patients, with a differential diagnosis of:

(1) Volume overload

(2) Congestive heart failure

(3) Infection

(4) Respiratory distress syndrome

(5) Some combination of (1)–(4)

(6) If infiltrates persist beyond the immediate postoperative period, flexible bronchoscopy and bronchoalveolar lavage should be used to establish a diagnosis. If nondiagnostic, some centers would consider an open lung biopsy. Data from the Mayo Clinic reveal that 12% of their patients had pneumonia at the time of ICU admission. Forty percent of those infections were caused by cytomegalovirus or *Pneumocystis carinii,* with only 10% being due to gram-negative or fungal sources.

b. **Postoperative days 2 and 3.** Following extubation, it is common for routine chest radiographs to reveal pleural effusions and an elevated right hemidiaphragm. If a large pleural effusion is associated with respiratory compromise, a thoracentesis may be performed. If atelectasis occurs, accompanied by respiratory deterioration and an elevated A-a gradient, reintubation and mechanical ventilation should be considered.

4. **Metabolic**

a. **First 24 hours**

(1) **Glucose.** Hyperglycemia is common during the immediate postoperative period. Approximately 10% of patients require insulin therapy, usually for serum glucose levels exceeding 500 mg%. Hypoglycemia can be due to hypoperfusion, as well as overzealous insulin administration.

(2) **Acid-base.** Metabolic alkalosis is common following an initial metabolic acidosis. The etiologies for metabolic alkalosis include loss of gastric fluid via surgical drains and nasogastric tubes, diuretic effect, glucocorticoid excess, potassium and chloride effect, and delayed metabolism of citrate to bicarbonate. Treatment includes appropriate volume expansion and replacement and correction of electrolyte abnormalities. Acetazolamide may be considered for refractory metabolic alkalosis.

b. **Postoperative days 2–3.** Continue treatment as described in **4.a.**

5. **Coagulation**

a. **First 24 hours.** On the patient's arrival in the ICU, a coagulation profile is sent to determine the adequacy of intraoperative replacement. This should include the following: hemoglobin, PT, PTT, platelet count, fibrinogen level, and a thrombelastograph (if available). Appropriate replacement with packed red cells, fresh frozen plasma, cryoprecipitate, and platelets is administered as needed. Although patients with chronic active hepatitis tend to have greater preoperative clotting abnormalities, there is little difference in use of blood products when compared with patients with primary biliary sclerosis or primary sclerosing cholangitis. Thrombocytopenia is treated when patients reach a platelet count in the range of 20,000–50,000 because they are at greater risk for hemorrhage.

b. **Postoperative days 2 and 3.** Data from the Mayo Clinic suggest the following postoperative transfusion requirement over the first 48 hours:

Packed RBCs: 6.6 ± 9.9 units
Fresh-frozen plasma: 7.4 ± 9.8 units
Cryoprecipitate: 6.6 ± 13.6 units
Platelets: 8.5 ± 15.4 units

If patients are negative for cytomegalovirus, blood products are transfused after filtering with white blood cell filters. Postoperative blood loss is assessed by serial hematocrits, changes in abdominal circumference, surgical drain output, and need for blood products.

6. Hepatic dysfunction

a. Signs of adequate function in a transplanted graft

(1) Improving liver function tests
(2) Adequate bile production
(3) No evidence of coagulopathy

b. Graft dysfunction: signs and symptoms

(1) Metabolic acidosis
(2) Absence of bile production
(3) Hypoglycemia
(4) Deteriorating liver function tests
(5) Persistent coagulopathy
(6) Disseminated intravascular coagulation
(7) Encephalopathy
(8) Renal failure

c. Graft dysfunction: etiology

(1) **Preoperative**

(a) Unrecognized donor hypoxia
(b) Prolonged organ ischemic time
(c) Poor perioperative perfusion (e.g., technical problems with the portal vein, hepatic artery, or IVC anastomoses)

(2) **Postoperative**

(a) Hepatic artery thrombosis
(b) Budd-Chiari syndrome (hepatic or portal vein thrombosis)
(c) Bile duct obstruction
(d) Acute rejection

d. Graft dysfunction: diagnostic studies

(1) Doppler ultrasound to evaluate the size of hepatic blood vessels
(2) Arteriography, the gold standard by which to evaluate patency of hepatic blood vessels
(3) Abdominal computerized tomography or magnetic resonance imaging. A diffuse decrease in signal attenuation may signify acute rejection or diffuse infection. Localized abnormalities in the liver parenchyma suggest infection or vascular dysfunction.
(4) Biliary system evaluation: Standard methods include T-tube cholangiography, transhepatic cholangiography, and endoscopic cholangiographic pancreatography.

e. Graft dysfunction: need for retransplantation. No recovery of liver function within 48 hours; acute hepatic necrosis caused by hepatic artery thrombosis.

7. Central nervous system. Factors affecting postoperative level of consciousness

a. Hepatic encephalopathy, especially with graft failure
b. Hypoglycemia
c. Seizure with postictal state; avoid hyponatremia and hypoglycemia
d. Drug toxicity: cyclosporine, residual anesthetic effect
e. Intracranial hypertension: may occur with graft failure and may be manifested by seizures, depressed level of consciousness, or frank coma
f. Cerebrovascular accident—either embolic or thrombotic
g. Intracranial hemorrhage—a potential problem in patients with uncontrolled hypertension in association with thrombocytopenia or coagulopathy
h. Meningitis/encephalitis: always a potential problem in immunosuppressed patients and the major reason that preoperative bacteremic sources, such as cholecystitis, intraabdominal abscess, pneumonia, and infected dental caries, must be identified and treated

i. Venous air embolus, which can result in mental status changes if it resulted in hypotension and, thus, cerebral hypoperfusion or if it involved cerebral arterial embolization via a patent or probe-patent foramen ovale as in paradoxical embolization. This can occur intraoperatively and postoperatively (e.g., by central venous line disconnection or air entrainment during CVP line removal).

8. **Renal function.** Postoperative renal function will reflect preexisting renal insufficiency and be exacerbated by hypovolemia, diuretic use, and nephrotoxic drugs (cyclosporine and antibiotics). Renal arterial perfusion is dependent on adequate blood pressure and cardiac output. If urine output decreases postoperatively:
   a. Give **volume,** if PA filling pressures are low.
   b. Consider a **diuretic** (Lasix, mannitol, or a Lasix/mannitol drip)
   c. Follow **BUN, creatinine, urine sodium and osmolality.** Check urine for casts, macro- or microscopic blood, and myoglobin. Adjust nephrotoxic **drug doses** (antibiotics, H2 blockers, and cyclosporine). **Hemodialysis** may be necessary in 4–8% of patients.

9. **Infectious disease.** Since patients are immunocompromised, meticulous attention to sterile technique is critical. Many institutions use prophylactic antibiotics for bowel coverage, but these patients are at risk for both the usual organisms (e.g., *Streptococcus faecalis, Pseudomonas aeruginosa*) and atypical pathogens (e.g., cytomegalovirus, *Pneumocystis carinii*). Routine blood cultures, as well as surveillance cultures of sputum, urine, bile, and oropharyngeal secretions, should be followed. Invasive monitors are usually removed on the first or second postoperative day, and any remaining monitors or IV catheters are carefully checked each day. Despite these precautions, recent studies have suggested that the incidence of postoperative septic shock may approach 17%.

10. **Nutrition.** Patients are initially kept NPO, and members of the nutritional support team are advised regarding use of central hyperalimentation, as these patients often are malnourished preoperatively. Controversy surrounds the use of branched chain amino acid preparations as a means to limit encephalopathy. They are currently restricted to patients with marginal liver function or hepatic encephalopathy.

11. **Pain management.** Either PCA or parenteral narcotics are given as needed. There are few patients who would qualify for epidural analgesia; many have a preoperative or postoperative coagulopathy that theoretically would place them at greater risk for epidural hemorrhage.

Selected References

Brown, R., Jr. *Anesthesia and Transplantation Surgery.* Philadelphia: F. A. Davis Company, 1987.

Carmichael, F. J., Lindop, M. J., and Farman, J. V. Anesthesia for hepatic transplantation: Cardiovascular and metabolic alterations and their management. *Anesth. Analg.* 64:108, 1985.

deGroen, P. C. Cyclosporine: A review and its specific use in liver transplantation. *Mayo Clin. Proc.* 64:680, 1989.

Eid, A., Steffen, R., Poraykom, K., et al. Beyond 1 year after liver transplantation. *Mayo Clin. Proc.* 64:446, 1989.

Grenvik, A., and Gordon, R. Postoperative care and problems in liver transplantation. *Transplant. Proc.* 19:26 (Suppl. 3), 1987.

Kahan, B. D. Cyclosporine. *New Engl. J. Med.* 321:1725, 1989.

Kang, Y., Aggarwal, S., and Freeman, J. A. Update on anesthesia for adult liver transplantation. *Transplant. Proc.* 19:7, 1987.

Krom, R. A. F., Wiesner, R. H., Rettke, S. R., et al. The first 100 liver transplantations at the Mayo Clinic. *Mayo Clin. Proc.* 64:84, 1989.

Plevak, D. J., Southorn, P. A., Narr, B. J., and Peters, S. G. Intensive-care unit experience in the Mayo Liver Transplantation Program: The first 100 cases. *Mayo Clin. Proc.* 64:433, 1989.

Rettke, S. R., Janossy, T. A., Chantigan, R. C., et al. Hemodynamic and metabolic changes in hepatic transplantation. *Mayo Clin. Proc.* 64:232, 1989.

Rettke, S. R., Chantigan, R. C., Janossy, T. A., et al. Anesthesia approach to hepatic transplantation. *Mayo Clin. Proc.* 64:224, 1989.

Ritter, D. M., Owen, C. A., Jr., Bowie, E. J. W., et al. Evaluation of preoperative hematology-coagulation screening in liver transplantation. *Mayo Clin. Proc.* 64:216, 1989.

23

Critical Care of Obstetric Patients

Lee Adlestein

I. Physiologic and anatomic changes in normal pregnancy
- **A. Cardiovascular system**
- **B. Respiratory system**
- **C. Central nervous system**
- **D. Hematologic system**
- **E. Gastrointestinal system**
- **F. Renal system**

II. Pharmacologic considerations in pregnant patients
- **A. Pharmacokinetic and pharmacodynamic alterations**
- **B. Placental transfer of drugs**
- **C. Drugs of special interest**
  - **1. Tocolytics**
    - **a. Terbutaline and ritodrine**
    - **b. Magnesium sulfate**
    - **c. Calcium channel blockers**
    - **d. Cyclooxygenase inhibitors**
  - **2. Oxytocics**
    - **a. Oxytocin (Pitocin)**
    - **b. Methylergonovine (Methergine) and ergonovine (Ergotrate)**
    - **c. Prostaglandin F2**
  - **3. Vasopressors**

III. Management of specific problems
- **A. Supine hypotensive syndrome**
- **B. Preeclampsia**
  - **1. Eclampsia**
  - **2. Diagnosis**
  - **3. Effects on specific organ systems**
    - **a. Cardiovascular**
    - **b. Central nervous system**
    - **c. Renal**
    - **d. Hepatic**
    - **e. Hematologic**
  - **4. HELLP syndrome**
  - **5. General management goals in preeclampsia**
  - **6. Antihypertensive therapy**
    - **a. Hydralazine**
    - **b. Labetalol**
    - **c. Sodium nitroprusside**
  - **7. Fluid management**
  - **8. Treatment of eclamptic seizures**
- **C. Amniotic fluid embolism**
  - **1. Pulmonary embolism**
  - **2. Disseminated intravascular coagulation**
  - **3. Uterine atony**
    - **a. Clinical features**
    - **b. Diagnosis**
    - **c. Treatment**
- **D. Acute fatty liver of pregnancy**
- **E. Peripartum cardiomyopathy**
- **F. Hyperemesis gravidarum**
- **G. Bupivacaine cardiotoxicity**

H. Postpartum hemorrhage
  1. Uterine atony
  2. Cervical, vaginal, or perineal lacerations
  3. Retained placental fragments
  4. Submucosal uterine fibroids
  5. Placental implantation site in the lower uterine segment
  6. Uterine inversion
  7. Uterine rupture
  8. Coagulation abnormalities
  9. Abnormal placentation

I. Sheehan's syndrome

Advances in perinatal intensive care have reduced the number of serious complications associated with several diseases unique to pregnancy. Nevertheless, the hypertensive disorders of pregnancy and several other less common diseases remain a substantial cause of maternal and fetal morbidity and mortality. A thorough understanding of the physiologic and anatomic changes of normal pregnancy, as well as what is known regarding the pathophysiology of these diseases, is essential to effect a favorable outcome for both mother and fetus.

I. **Physiologic and anatomic changes in normal pregnancy.** All maternal organ systems are significantly altered beginning in the first trimester and lasting well into the postpartum period.

A. **Cardiovascular system.** Blood volume begins to increase as early as the fifth week of gestation and increases by as much as 50% by the thirty-second week. Blood volume remains at this level until term. An increase in plasma volume in excess of the increase in red cell mass leads to a physiological anemia of pregnancy. Increases in cardiac output parallel the increases in blood volume during the first 32 weeks of pregnancy, reaching levels 50% above the nonpregnant state. Following a slight decline in the third trimester, cardiac output reaches its maximum level during the second stage of labor and the immediate postpartum period owing to transfusion of blood sequestered in the placenta during contractions, as well as increased maternal catecholamine levels during labor. Arteriolar dilatation due to the endocrine changes of pregnancy results in decreases in systemic vascular resistance and mean arterial blood pressure. Normal parturients are less responsive to vasopressor and chronotropic agonists, possibly related to a down-regulation of adrenergic receptors. Venous pressure, although normal in the upper half of the body, may be significantly elevated in the lower extremities and epidural space owing to the partial or complete obstruction of the iliac veins and inferior vena cava by the gravid uterus, particularly in the supine position.

B. **Respiratory system.** Oxygen consumption is increased by 20% at rest and up to 100% during labor. The gravid uterus impinges significantly on the diaphragm during the third trimester, leading to decreased functional residual capacity and consequent decreases in oxygen reserves. Airway closure may occur, resulting in increases in intrapulmonary shunt. All of these changes contribute to the rapidity of oxyhemoglobin desaturation commonly seen when the parturient is rendered apneic. Carbon dioxide production increases in proportion to the increases in oxygen consumption but is more than compensated for by increases in tidal volume and respiratory rate. Minute ventilation is increased by 70% at term, and blood gas analysis reflects a partly compensated respiratory alkalosis. Elevated progesterone levels resulting in an increased ventilatory drive is the suspected etiology for the hyperventilation.

C. **Central nervous system.** Cerebrospinal fluid (CSF) pressure is significantly increased during labor. Uterine contractions may produce CSF pressures as high as 23 cm H_2O, with pressure rising to as much as 70 cm H_2O during the voluntary pushing efforts associated with the second stage of labor. Decreased dosages of all anesthetic agents are required in pregnancy. The minimum alveolar concentration (MAC) of inhaled anesthetics is decreased, and neuronal sensitivity to local anesthetics is increased. Both of these effects may be related to elevated progesterone levels.

D. **Hematologic system.** Changes in plasma volume and red cell mass have been discussed. An increase in the absolute neutrophil count occurs. Although absolute numbers of lymphocytes remain unchanged during pregnancy, there is a depression of lymphocyte function with a resultant defect in cell-mediated immune response. Virtually all coagulation factors are increased in normal pregnancy, with fibrinogen levels rising to a range of 400–650 mg per deciliter in late pregnancy. Platelet count is increased slightly, although thrombocytopenia may occasionally be seen during the course of normal pregnancy. A milieu best described as a hypercoagulable state exists, and thrombotic events occur more frequently in pregnancy. The oxyhemoglobin binding curve of maternal hemoglobin is shifted rightward to a p50 of 30.2 mm Hg, enhancing oxygen unloading to maternal tissues and fetal hemoglobin.

E. **Gastrointestinal system.** Through alterations in smooth muscle activity, progesterone decreases gastrointestinal motility and reduces lower esophageal sphincter pressure. Placental gastrin release promotes maternal gastric acid secretion. The gravid uterus impinges on the stomach and elevates intragastric pressure. All of these alterations facilitate the occurrence of and increase the severity of gastroesophageal reflux or aspiration pneumonitis.

F. **Renal system.** Aldosterone secretion is increased in pregnancy, and renal plasma flow increases considerably. Glomerular filtration rates are increased by 50% above prepregnant values by the sixteenth week of gestation. Creatinine clearance is increased, and serum measurements of creatinine and blood-urea nitrogen (BUN) are decreased. Glycosuria is common in pregnancy, possibly under the influence of elevated levels of cortisol and human placental lactogen. This, along with the mechanical obstruction created by the gravid uterus, results in an increased incidence of urinary tract infections.

II. Pharmacologic considerations in pregnant patients

A. **Pharmacokinetic and pharmacodynamic alterations.** With the 7–10-liter increase in total body water (TBW) associated with term pregnancy, the volume of distribution of drugs dispersed in extracellular fluid or TBW is increased. It should be remembered that measurement of TBW in a pregnant woman includes the fetus, amniotic fluid, and placenta, which together account for nearly half of the overall increase in TBW. Albumin, the most important drug-binding protein, is reduced in concentration by 0.5–1.0 g per deciliter in pregnancy. As a result of increased blood volume, however, the total amount of circulating albumin is virtually unchanged. Globulins are increased in pregnancy and are important in binding certain drugs. The placenta has a tremendous capacity for biotransformation of certain molecules, particularly the steroid hormones. The fetal liver is capable of metabolizing many drugs, including anticonvulsants, ethanol, diazepam, meperidine, and halothane.

B. **Placental transfer of drugs.** Passive diffusion of small molecules is the primary mechanism by which placental transfer occurs. In general, drugs that are poorly protein bound, relatively un-ionized, and soluble in lipid membranes and have a molecular weight of less than 600 d cross the placenta with relative ease. It is important to recognize that many of the agents used to produce sedation, analgesia, and anesthesia possess many of these properties. Since the pH of fetal blood is significantly below that of maternal blood during labor, it is possible that any drug that behaves as a weak base (e.g., amide local anesthetics) may become protonated, trapped, and perhaps concentrated in the fetus. The clinical significance of this possibility has not been established, but the relationship should be borne in mind in settings where significant plasma levels of drug may occur under conditions of fetal acidemia.

C. **Drugs of special interest**

1. **Tocolytics.** Preterm labor is one of the primary causes of perinatal mortality. Tocolytics include several classes of drugs used to delay the onset of labor or to slow or arrest active labor to allow for fetal

maturation. Relative contraindications to their use include prolonged rupture of membranes, suspected chorioamnionitis, severe preeclampsia requiring delivery, or fetal distress.

a. **Terbutaline and ritodrine.** These beta-adrenergic agonists, having predominantly beta-2 effects, are the most commonly used tocolytics. Uterine smooth muscle relaxation is produced by activation of adenyl cyclase. Predictable side effects of these drugs include vasodilation, tachycardia, and bronchodilation. Arrhythmias and angina pectoris are sometimes seen. Metabolic effects of these drugs include increased glycogenolysis and gluconeogenesis resulting in hyperglycemia. Hypokalemia may also occur owing to two mechanisms: **(1)** hyperglycemia-stimulating, insulin-mediated intracellular potassium flux and **(2)** direct beta-2 receptor-mediated translocation of potassium from plasma to cells. Pulmonary edema occurs in up to 5% of patients being treated with these drugs. The etiology is poorly understood but may involve myocardial ischemia due to unfavorable effects of beta-1 stimulation on myocardial oxygen balance or fluid overload related to the propensity of these drugs to stimulate antidiuretic hormone (ADH) release.

b. **Magnesium sulfate** is an effective tocolytic agent although used most commonly in the treatment of preeclampsia/eclampsia. Magnesium interferes with the process of excitation-contraction coupling in uterine smooth muscle and results in a decrease in the force and frequency of contractions. Side effects include hypotension due to vasodilation, nausea, impairment of cardiac conduction, and skeletal muscle weakness. Most side effects are dose related and can be avoided by closely monitoring serum levels and clinical signs, particularly deep tendon reflexes. Magnesium is eliminated by the kidneys. Hypermagnesemia retards acetylcholine release at the motor end plate and decreases the sensitivity of the muscle to stimulation. Close surveillance must be maintained for signs of respiratory muscle weakness. Both depolarizing and nondepolarizing muscle relaxants are potentiated by hypermagnesemia. Magnesium crosses the placenta and may result in neonatal hypotension and flaccidity.

c. **Calcium channel blockers. Nifedipine,** the only calcium channel blocker employed clinically for tocolysis, is usually prescribed when a contraindication to beta sympathomimetics or magnesium sulfate exists. Side effects include hypotension, reflex tachycardia, and postpartum uterine atony, which may be unresponsive to oxytocin.

d. **Cyclooxygenase inhibitors.** These agents, which include aspirin and nonsteroidal antiinflammatory agents, are rarely used tocolytics because of their hazardous fetal side effects. Prostaglandins are found in blood and amniotic fluid and increase during labor, augmenting uterine contraction and serving to soften the cervix. Cyclooxygenase inhibitors may lead to premature closure of the ductus arteriosus in the fetus if used after 28 weeks gestation. Impairment of platelet function and reduction in glomerular filtration rate are additional problematic side effects of this class of drug.

2. **Oxytocics.** These frequently used drugs are employed to induce or augment labor, to facilitate placental expulsion, and to induce uterine smooth muscle contraction for controlling postpartum bleeding caused by an atonic uterus. There are three groups of oxytocic drugs, each having distinct actions on the uterus and cardiovascular system.

a. **Oxytocin (Pitocin).** A synthetic 8–amino acid peptide that increases the force and frequency of myometrial contraction. Oxytocin has complex cardiovascular effects; in small doses it has a transient vasodilator effect and may produce hypotension, tachycardia, and occasionally dysrhythmias. At larger doses, a biphasic effect on BP may be seen, consisting of transient hypotension followed by a 15–35% increase in BP. Oxytocin exhibits some ADH-like activity, and cases of dilutional hyponatremia, cerebral edema, and convulsions have been attributed to the use of large doses of the drug along with liberal administration of IV fluids.

b. **Methylergonovine (Methergine)** and **ergonovine (Ergotrate)** are ergot alkaloids that are potent vasoconstrictors in both myometrial and peripheral arterioles. Used in small doses, these drugs increase the force and frequency of uterine contraction and permit normal relaxation between contractions; larger doses may produce uterine tetany. The use of these ergot alkaloids is restricted to the control of postpartum hemorrhage. These drugs should be avoided in hypertensive patients or patients in whom the avoidance of hypertension is necessary. The dose is usually 0.2 mg intramuscularly; the drug should never be given IV, as it may precipitate a hypertensive crisis.

c. **Prostaglandin F2.** Historically used to induce midtrimester abortions, this agent may be used as a third-line drug to stimulate postpartum uterine contraction. The drug is given intramuscularly or intramyometrially and is associated with frequent side effects, including pyrexia, wheezing, nausea, and vomiting.

3. **Vasopressors.** If the usual steps to correct hypotension (fluids, left uterine displacement, Trendelenburg position) fail, the use of vasoconstrictors may become necessary. The uteroplacental vasculature is supplied with alpha-adrenergic receptors that may reduce uteroplacental blood flow if a pure alpha-agonist is used to restore maternal BP. Although an evolving body of evidence suggests that phenylephrine may not represent the threat to the fetus that was once thought, ephedrine, a mixed alpha- and beta-adrenergic agonist, is still recommended as the first-line drug in treating hypotension in parturients. Maternal cardiac disease wherein increases in heart rate or contractility may be deleterious (e.g., severe mitral stenosis or idiopathic hypertrophic subaortic stenosis, respectively) are conditions where phenylephrine may be judiciously used as a first-line drug.

III. Management of specific problems

A. **The supine hypotensive syndrome** merits special mention due to its frequency of occurrence and its potential for harm to both mother and fetus. The syndrome occurs in 10% of parturients beginning in the second trimester and results from aortic and/or inferior vena cava obstruction from the gravid uterus when the patient lies supine. The problem is usually easily relieved by shifting the axis of the uterus to the left by placing a roll or pillow under the patient's right hip, by turning the patient to a decubitus position, or by having the patient sit up. Occasionally right uterine displacement mitigates the problem more effectively. Since uteroplacental blood flow may itself be compromised by aortic compression from the gravid uterus, the supine position should be avoided despite seemingly reassuring maternal BP values.

B. **Preeclampsia** is a hypertensive disorder of late pregnancy associated with proteinuria and edema and sometimes accompanied by abnormalities of coagulation or liver function. When preeclampsia is accompanied by convulsions that cannot be attributed to a preexisting seizure disorder, the disease is termed eclampsia.

1. **Eclampsia.** Preeclampsia occurs in 5–10% of all pregnancies, usually presents after the twentieth week of gestation, and is significantly more common in the primigravid. Although characterized by multiorgan system involvement, the syndrome resolves completely in

the very early postpartum period. The etiology and pathophysiology of preeclampsia remain obscure, although speculation is abundant. Most current theories implicate an immunologic incompatibility between mother and placenta as the inciting event, leading to vasculitic involvement of the placenta and maternal organs. Placental ischemia develops and results in the release of placental renin, which in turn increases circulating angiotensin II levels. Preeclamptics also exhibit an exquisite sensitivity to angiotensin II and norepinephrine not seen in normal pregnancy and probably related to abnormalities in the ratios of prostaglandins in vascular endothelium. Other abnormalities of vascular endothelium may mediate the loss of vascular integrity, aggregation of platelets, and deposition of fibrin that collectively constitute the final common pathway of organ damage in this disorder.

2. **Diagnosis.** The diagnosis of preeclampsia can be confounded by the presence of essential hypertension, since the two disorders may coexist. Preeclampsia is considered to be present when hypertension (defined as two BP measurements taken > 6 hours apart) reveal systolic BP greater than 140 mm Hg (or > 30 mm Hg above prepregnant values) or diastolic BP greater than 90 mm Hg (or > 15 mm Hg above prepregnant values), along with either proteinuria (>300 mg/24 hours) or generalized edema. Preeclampsia is termed severe if the blood pressure exceeds 160 mm Hg systolic or 100 mm Hg diastolic or when any of the following conditions exists:
   a. More than 5 g proteinuria in 24 hours
   b. Oliguria (<400 ml/24 hours)
   c. Epigastric or right upper quadrant (RUQ) pain
   d. Visual or cerebral disturbances
   e. Pulmonary edema

3. **Effects on specific organ systems**
   a. Cardiovascular. In severe preeclampsia, intravascular volume may be reduced by 30–40%, yet total body water is increased as a result of a generalized increase in vascular permeability and the formation of edema. Total peripheral resistance is increased, as is sensitivity to exogenous catecholamines. Central venous pressure in preeclampsia is usually low and varies inversely with the severity of the hypertension. Hemodynamic studies of preeclamptics have demonstrated widely varying ventricular function curves, ranging from hyperdynamic to depressed function. A significant discrepancy may exist between right- and left-sided filling pressures in severe preeclampsia. A small subset of patients may develop overt left ventricular failure and pulmonary edema. Noncardiogenic pulmonary edema is sometimes seen, presumably as a consequence of increased vascular permeability and/or decreased plasma oncotic pressure.

   b. Central nervous system. Increased irritability exists. The onset of convulsions is usually preceded by premonitory signs, which may include headache, hyperreflexia, and abdominal pain. The genesis of eclampsia is thought to be more likely related to cerebral vasospasm and/or thrombotic occlusion of the cerebral microcirculation than to a hypertensive encephalopathy. Coma may develop even in the absence of seizures.

   c. Renal. Glomerular filtration rate and creatinine clearance are reduced. A characteristic swelling of glomerular cells, termed endotheliosis, occurs. Proteinuria results from injury to renal vascular endothelium.

   d. Hepatic. Epigastric pain may be due to periportal hemorrhages, generalized hepatic edema, subcapsular hematoma, or, rarely, spontaneous hepatic rupture. Hepatocellular damage may result in elevations in serum transaminases and abnormalities in synthetic function.

e. **Hematologic.** Thrombocytopenia (<150 K) occurs in 15% of preeclamptics and 30% of eclamptics and reflects increases in platelet consumption. In addition, a qualitative platelet defect may be present. A low-grade consumptive coagulopathy and primary fibrinolysis commonly occurs.

4. The combination of **h**emolysis, **e**levated **l**iver enzymes, and **l**ow **p**latelets is a relatively common variant presentation of severe preeclampsia (**HELLP syndrome**). Occasionally, these may be the initial or dominant manifestations of preeclampsia with little or no hypertension or proteinuria, leading to confusion about the diagnosis. Nausea, vomiting, and RUQ pain are the most common complaints presented in this disorder. Once the diagnosis of HELLP syndrome is established, prompt delivery of the fetus is usually undertaken. It may be necessary to correct coagulation defects prior to delivery. The nadir in platelet count and peak in liver function test abnormalities is seen 24–36 hours postpartum.

5. **General management goals in preeclampsia.** The goals of management in preeclampsia consist of **(1)** improvement of the circulation through judicious volume replacement and treatment of vasospasm, **(2)** correction of acid-base, electrolyte, and coagulation abnormalities, **(3)** reduction in CNS irritability and the prevention of eclamptic seizures, and **(4)** control of hypertension.

   Magnesium sulfate remains the cornerstone in the pharmacologic therapy of preeclampsia owing to its long safety record, well-established therapeutic ranges and ease of assay, and effects as a combined anticonvulsant and vasodilator. The loading dose is 2–4 g IV over 15 minutes, followed by an infusion of 1–3 g per hour. The infusion rate is reduced with renal insufficiency. The therapeutic range is 4–8 mEq per liter. Levels of 7–10 mEq per liter result in loss of the patellar reflex. Levels in excess of 10 mEq per liter may result in respiratory depression and heart block. In the event of an overdose, calcium gluconate is recommended as an agent for reversing the deleterious effects of hypermagnesemia. Eclampsia presents in the postpartum period in approximately 20% of cases, and it therefore is recommended that magnesium therapy be continued for a minimum of 24 hours following delivery.

6. **Antihypertensive therapy.** A subset of patients require additional, more potent antihypertensive therapy.

   a. **Hydralazine** acts through direct arteriolar dilatation to produce a peak antihypertensive effect 10–20 minutes after IV administration. It is unlikely to produce a precipitous fall in BP, and its duration of action is several hours. Uterine blood flow is maintained as long as hypotension is avoided. Reflex tachycardia and postural hypotension are common side effects. The somewhat slow onset of action of hydralazine limits its use in acute hypertensive crises. Dose is 5–10 mg IV q15min as needed (maximum usually 20–40 mg).

   b. **Labetalol** has been used safely in pregnancy in doses up to 1 mg per kilogram. The problem of reflex tachycardia is minimal with this combined alpha- and beta-adrenergic antagonist. Uterine blood flow is maintained. Doses of 10 mg IV q5–10min are usually well tolerated.

   c. **Sodium nitroprusside,** a supremely potent, easily titrated direct vasodilator, may be used in treating hypertensive crises in parturients. A concern regarding fetal cyanide toxicity (the fetal liver has less thiosulfate substrate for rhodanese detoxification of cyanide than the maternal liver) dictates that its use be reserved for levels of hypertension of immediate threat to the mother and that the duration of the infusion be short.

7. **Fluid management.** The classic hemodynamic profile of severe preeclampsia is one of reduced intravascular volume, low right- and left-sided filling pressures, high systemic vascular resistance, and normal or hyperdynamic cardiac function. Evidence suggests, however, that many preeclamptics, depending on the severity and duration of their disease, may vary considerably from this profile. Moreover, up to 25% of preeclamptics have been shown to have a significant discrepancy between right- and left-sided filling pressures. These data, coupled with fears of precipitating pulmonary or cerebral edema with fluid loading, have led to controversies regarding fluid management. Figure 23-1 depicts a reasonable method for managing the oliguric preeclamptic. Therapy and monitoring must be individualized. and if a confusing picture exists (e.g., low central venous pressure [CVP] and pulmonary edema or high CVP and oliguria), a pulmonary artery catheter may be required to guide therapy. This management strategy presupposes that causes for hypoxemia other than pulmonary edema have been considered and ruled out.
8. **Treatment of eclamptic seizures.** Attention must simultaneously be directed to treating the seizure and maintaining adequate ventilation and oxygenation through bag-mask ventilation or endotracheal intubation. Increments of diazepam 2.5–5 mg or thiopental 50–100 mg, may be used for initial control of the seizure. For the longer term, magnesium sulfate 2–4 g IV loading dose over 15 minutes, followed by an infusion of 1–2 g per hour (guided by periodic serum levels) is the therapy of choice.

C. **Amniotic fluid embolism** has a reported incidence of 1 case per 20,000 deliveries and accounts for approximately 10% of all maternal mortality. A recent review suggests that a mortality rate of 86% exists in identified amniotic fluid embolism. In order for amniotic fluid to enter the maternal circulation, two separate events must occur: **(1)** rupture of membranes and **(2)** laceration of endocervical veins or development of open sinusoids at the uteroplacental margins. Rapid cervical dilatation may lead to endocervical tears. When membranes rupture and the fetal head tamponades the cervix, uterine contractions push amniotic fluid into the circulation. Placental abruption or incipient uterine rupture also may allow the transgression of amniotic fluid into the circulation. Amniotic fluid embolism usually occurs during labor but has also been seen following intraamniotic injection of hypertonic saline for abortion or during transcervical evacuation of uterine contents during the first and second trimesters of pregnancy. There are three common **mechanisms of injury.**

1. **Pulmonary embolism,** a combination of mechanical (obstructive) and vasospastic processes, leads to cardiopulmonary collapse. This may include a sudden decrease in left atrial filling due to the accumulation of intraamniotic debris in the pulmonary capillaries and severe pulmonary hypertension related to both the vascular obstruction and the vasoconstrictive effects of eicosanoic molecules found in amniotic fluid. Ventilation-perfusion (V/Q) mismatch occurs and results in hypoxemia.
2. **Disseminated intravascular coagulation.** Amniotic fluid embolism commonly incites a consumptive coagulopathy through the liberation of thromboplastinlike substances contained in placental tissues and amniotic fluid with consequent activation of the extrinsic clotting pathway.

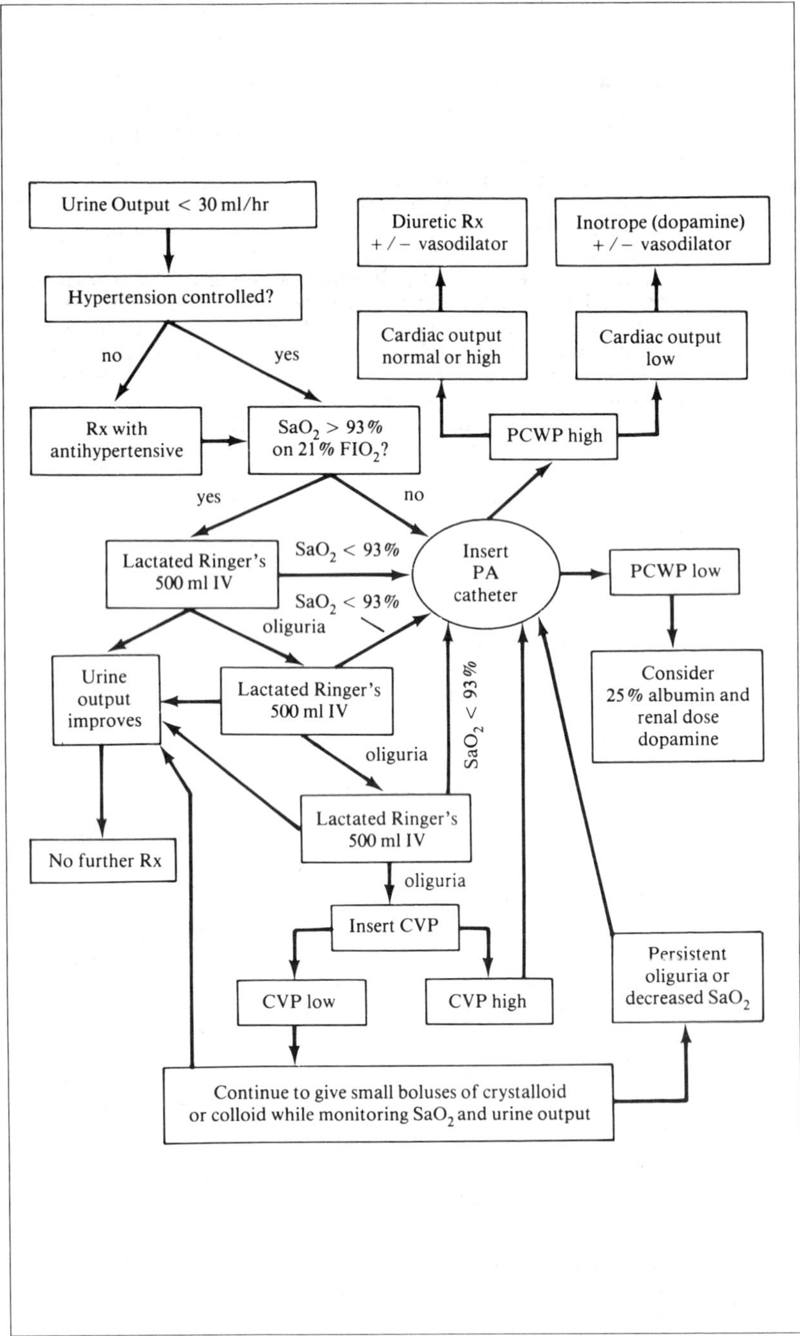

Fig. 23-1. Management of oliguria in preeclampsia

3. **Uterine atony,** caused by hypotension, hypoxemia and poor uterine perfusion, contributes to postpartum hemorrhage.
   a. **Clinical features.** A prodrome of chills, diaphoresis, coughing, and tachypnea is often seen. In severe cases, these signs are quickly followed by respiratory distress, cyanosis, cardiovascular collapse, and unconsciousness.
   b. **Diagnosis.** Fetal squamous cells, amorphous debris, lanugo, or fat from fetal vernix may be found in the maternal circulation. The ECG may show signs of right ventricular strain; tachycardia is usually present. The coagulation profile may show evidence of thrombocytopenia, prolongation of clotting times, and the presence of fibrin degradation products. The chest radiograph may be normal. Differential diagnosis includes thrombo- or air embolism, bronchoaspiration, or local anesthetic toxicity.
   c. **Treatment is supportive.** The uterus should be evacuated as soon as possible to facilitate effective aggressive maternal cardiopulmonary resuscitation. Volume replacement in the setting of shock, along with the administration of red cells, plasma, platelets, and cryoprecipitate based on the coagulation profile, are frequently needed. If the patient survives the embolic and coagulation problems, recovery is usually complete and without sequelae.

D. **Acute fatty liver of pregnancy** is an extremely uncommon disease of unknown etiology that may complicate the third trimester of pregnancy. It is characterized by the accumulation of microvesicles of fat in the hepatic parenchyma and once carried with it a maternal mortality rate of up to 85%. Recent estimates of maternal and fetal mortality as low as 20% have been attributed to earlier recognition of the disease and improvements in intensive supportive treatment. Its presentation is usually between the thirtieth week and early postpartum period, with symptoms of headache, anorexia, nausea and vomiting, malaise, abdominal pain, and jaundice. The time of onset of the disease is similar to that of preeclampsia, and like preeclampsia, it may be accompanied by hypertension, peripheral edema, and proteinuria. Unlike preeclampsia, however, the disease frequently progresses rapidly to fulminant hepatic failure with encephalopathy and coagulopathy. In contrast with acute hepatitis, the disease typically has a shorter prodrome, and abdominal pain, typically epigastric, is a predominant symptom. Hypoglycemia, portal hypertension, and gastrointestinal bleeding occur frequently. Supportive, aggressive treatment of hepatic failure with correction of coagulopathy, control of hypoglycemia, and treatment of encephalopathy is salutary. Most agree that early delivery of the fetus is singularly effective in halting the course of the disease.

E. **Peripartum cardiomyopathy** is an uncommon disease resulting in idiopathic cardiac failure in the last month of pregnancy or the first 6 postpartum months. It occurs in patients with no prior history of cardiac disease. Signs of left ventricular failure may occur indolently or present in a sudden, fulminant fashion. Diagnostic tests reveal evidence of a dilated cardiomyopathy. The overall mortality rate is 30–60%. Management parallels the severity of the cardiomyopathy, ranging from the use of diuretics and afterload reducing agents for moderate symptoms to endotracheal intubation, positive end-expiratory pressure, and inotropic support for severe left ventricular failure accompanied by pulmonary edema. If the patient survives, the recurrence rate in subsequent pregnancies is 50–80%.

F. **Hyperemesis gravidarum** is a disorder characterized by excessive nausea and vomiting during pregnancy. Its reported incidence is 3.5 cases per 1,000 deliveries. Typically seen in the first trimester, the disease is self-limiting and never extends beyond the duration of the pregnancy, although it may recur in subsequent pregnancies. If symptoms are severe, serious fluid and electrolyte abnormalities may occur. Abnormalities of liver function including jaundice may occur due to malnutrition. The etiology of hyperemesis gravidarum is unknown. Its clinical manifestations include frequent and sustained vomiting (usually 4–8 weeks in duration), resulting in significant dehydration and weight loss. Oliguria, ketonuria, hypochloremic metabolic alkalosis, and hemoconcentration are commonly seen. Other disorders, including peptic ulcer disease, intestinal obstruction, cholecystitis, and hydatidiform mole, may mimic hyperemesis gravidarum and should be ruled out. The principal underlying treatment is fluid and electrolyte replacement and the judicious use of antiemetics. Volume deficits in these patients may be considerable, and special attention should be paid to deficiencies in B vitamins and trace elements.

G. **Bupivacaine cardiotoxicity** is a devastating problem associated with epidural analgesia in labor. There is overwhelming evidence that the pregnant patient is more sensitive to the cardiodepressant effects of bupivacaine. High plasma levels of bupivacaine may occur as a result of an excessive dose or inadvertent venous injection. Direct myocardial depression accompanied by ventricular arrhythmias, including ventricular tachycardia and ventricular fibrillation, is common. Aggressive control of respiratory or metabolic acidosis is of vital importance since the cardiodepressant actions of bupivacaine are potentiated under these conditions. Bretylium is the drug of choice in treating ventricular arrhythmias. Electrical cardioversion may be safely performed in pregnant patients. Very large doses of epinephrine and atropine may be required. When resuscitating these patients, it should be kept in mind that the binding of bupivacaine to cardiac tissue is prolonged, and several hours of cardiopulmonary resuscitation may be required. Emergent cesarean section may be necessary to facilitate maternal resuscitation. Since closed-chest compressions may be ineffective in maintaining an adequate circulation during an extended cardiac arrest, serious consideration should be given to open chest cardiac massage or cardiopulmonary bypass if the appropriate resources are available.

H. **Postpartum hemorrhage** remains the third most common cause of maternal death (preceded by pulmonary embolism and hypertensive disorders of pregnancy). Following placental separation, the site of previous attachment is a bed of open blood vessels that have no significant muscular coat and, hence, are unable to constrict. For hemorrhage to cease, the myometrium must contract and tamponade the bleeding. This explains the concern that the uterus remain firmly contracted postpartum and accounts for the importance of uterine atony as a cause of postpartum bleeding. The cardinal steps in the management of significant postpartum hemorrhage consist of prompt restoration of circulatory volume, replacement of red cells and coagulation factors, and the control of specific bleeding sites. Postpartum hemorrhage has diverse etiologies:

1. **Uterine atony** contributes to over 90% of cases of postpartum bleeding and is the most frequent antecedent to maternal hemorrhagic death. Risk factors include overdistension of the uterus from multiple gestations, fetal macrosomia, chorioamnionitis, or polyhydramnios. Multiparity, prolonged labor, recent tocolytic use, and concomitant hypertensive disorder of pregnancy are also risk factors. Prolonged induction of labor by oxytocin may lead to a downregulation of myometrial oxytocin receptors with consequent hyporesponsiveness to oxytocin. Management consists of aggressive intravascular volume replacement, firm massage of the uterus, and the administration of oxytocic agents. Recalcitrant bleeding may require surgical or embolic interruption of uterine blood supply or hysterectomy.

2. **Cervical, vaginal, or perineal lacerations** from traumatic natural or instrumental deliveries are the second most common cause of excessive maternal blood loss. Previous perineal operations, including episiotomy, present fibrous obstructions and predispose to lacerations. Inspection for lacerations should be carried out when vaginal bleeding occurs despite a firm, contracted uterus.
3. **Retained placental fragments** can contribute to both early and late (6–10 days postpartum) hemorrhage and serve as a nidus for endometritis. If suspected early, the fragments can easily be removed by means of digital or forceps extraction immediately following delivery. Dilatation and curettage may be employed after the uterus has contracted. Placenta accreta (see **9**) is suspected if the placental fragments cannot be removed.
4. **Submucosal uterine fibroids** may prevent uniform uterine contraction and contribute to bleeding.
5. **Placental implantation site in the lower uterine segment** is an area of insufficient musculature to contract effectively. This is typically seen in placenta previa wherein the placenta encroaches on or overlies the cervical os. Since most patients with placenta previa undergo cesarean delivery, it may be possible to visualize and ligate individual bleeding sites. Hypogastric artery ligation or embolization or hysterectomy may be necessary for uncontrollable bleeding.
6. **Uterine inversion** may cause overwhelming hemorrhage and exsanguination. It usually occurs immediately after the third stage of labor. It is associated with an atonic uterus and with the use of excessive fundal pressure or traction on the umbilical cord during delivery. This catastrophic situation warrants the immediate manual reduction of the inversion. If the diagnosis is made after the inverted uterus has had time to contract, reduction may be impossible without uterine relaxation, usually brought about by deep general anesthesia with a halogenated volatile agent. Vigorous restoration of circulatory volume must be carried out early to allow the patient to tolerate such an anesthetic. After the inversion is reduced, the uterus is massaged and oxytocics are given.
7. **Uterine rupture** is often unrecognized and accounts for approximately 50% of all maternal hemorrhagic deaths. It typically presents as antepartum bleeding and severe lower abdominal pain accompanied by fetal distress but may first achieve recognition as postpartum hemorrhage, particularly in the setting of attempted vaginal delivery following prior cesarean section. Contributory factors include the presence of a uterine scar, excessive oxytocin use, prolonged labor, forceps delivery, or the performance of intrauterine fetal version maneuvers. Therapy is directed at volume resuscitation and operative repair.
8. **Coagulation abnormalities.** Preexisting coagulopathies have an obvious permissive role in determining the extent of peripartum bleeding. Severe clotting abnormalities related to preeclampsia or maternal liver disease should be corrected prior to delivery. Placental abruption and amniotic fluid embolism may incite a consumptive coagulopathy through release of tissue thromboplastin into the circulation and activation of the extrinsic clotting pathway.
9. **Abnormal placentation.** Placenta accreta occurs when the chorionic villi penetrate the endometrium without an intervening decidua basalis and may attach directly to the myometrium. Absent this physiologic line of cleavage, the placenta tears during separation and massive bleeding may result. In placenta increta, the villi extend into the myometrium, reaching or even penetrating the uterine serosa. These abnormalities of placentation are strongly associated with pla-

centa previa and prior uterine surgery and may take their origin at sites of uterine scar. These disorders must be suspected when no plane of placental cleavage can be found or where a small area of placenta cannot be detached. If efforts to detach the placenta are unsuccessful and hemorrhage continues, hysterectomy should be considered. Conservative measures such as uterine packing are ill advised.

I. **Sheehan's syndrome,** a syndrome of acute ischemic necrosis of the anterior pituitary gland, may occur in a minority of patients after severe postpartum hemorrhage. Prolactin-secreting cells are usually the first to be affected, and the diagnosis should be suspected if lactation fails to occur.

Selected References

Benedetti, T. J., Kates, R., and Williams, V. Hemodynamic observations in severe preeclampsia complicated by pulmonary edema. *Am. J. Obstet. Gynecol.* 152:330, 1985.

Berkowitz, R. *Critical Care of the Obstetric Patient.* New York: Churchill-Livingston, 1983.

Cotton, D., and Clark, S. (eds.) *Clinics in Perinatology—Critical Care in Obstetrics.* 1986.

Crosby, E. T. Obstetrical anaesthesia for patients with the syndrome of haemolysis, elevated liver enzymes and low platelets. *Can. J. Anaesth.* 38:227, 1991.

Danforth, D. *Obstetrics and Gynecology* (6th ed.). New York: Harper & Row, 1990.

Datta, S. *Anesthetic and Obstetric Management of High Risk Pregnancy.* Toronto: C. V. Mosby, 1991.

Datta, S., and Ostheimer, G. *Common Problems in Obstetric Anesthesia.* Chicago: Yearbook Medical Publishers, 1987.

Friedman, S. A. Preeclampsia: A review of the role of prostaglandins. *Obstet. Gynecol.* 71:122, 1988.

James, F., III, Wheeler, A. S., and Dewan, D. *Obstetric Anesthesia: The Complicated Patient* (2d ed.). Philadelphia: F. A. Davis, 1988.

Joyce, T. H., III, Debnath, K. S., and Baker, E. A. Preeclampsia—Relationship of CVP and epidural anesthesia. *Anesthesiology* 51:S297, 1979.

Kaplan, M. Acute fatty liver of pregnancy. *N. Engl. J. Med.* 313:367, 1985.

Lindheimer, M., and Katz, A. Hypertension in pregnancy. *N. Engl. J. Med.* 313:675, 1985.

Voulgaropoulos, D., Johnson, M., and Covino, B. Local anesthetic toxicity. *Sem. Anesth.* 9:8, 1990.

Wright, J. Anesthetic considerations in preeclampsia and eclampsia. *Anesth. Analg.* 63:590, 1983.

24

Postanesthesia Unit Care of Healthy Patients

S. A. Grace and John D. Wasnick

The postoperative care of healthy patients following routine surgery represents an extension of the principles and the practices of critical care medicine into the recovery room. Airway compromise, respiratory embarrassment, and hemodynamic instability occur with high frequency in both the ICU and postanesthesia care unit (PACU) populations. Critical care physicians must be cognizant of the goals and the practices of the PACU in assisting the PACU team in the management of postoperative complications.

I. **General assessment.** Upon patient arrival in the PACU, an immediate assessment of the patient's condition is made by the PACU nurse.

A. **Airway.** The majority of patients arrive from the operating room extubated. The PACU nurse will confirm that the airway is patent and free of debris, and that the patient is breathing easily. Occasionally patients are found to have a potentially life-threatening airway obstruction. Signs of airway obstruction include:

1. Lack of air movement
2. Tracheal tug
3. Discoordination of breathing pattern
4. Cyanosis

Causes of airway obstruction/apnea include

1. Residual anesthesia effects
2. Excessive narcotization
3. Airway edema

Therapy is directed at reestablishing the airway. Interventions include:

1. Bag/mask ventilation
2. Oral/nasal airway or reintubation
3. Reversal of residual narcotic
4. Racemic epinephrine/steroids to decrease airway edema

No matter what the etiology of airway obstruction, therapy is directed at restoring airway patency and patient ventilation.

B. **Breathing.** After ensuring airway patency, attention is next focused on the pattern of breathing. Often patients in the immediate postoperative period hypoventilate as a consequence of:

1. Residual inhalational anesthetics
2. Narcotic analgesics
3. Hypothermia

If hypoventilation is noted, the patient must be carefully monitored. Assisted ventilation with bag-mask and/or reintubation may be warranted. If residual narcotic analgesics are believed to be a contributing factor, the judicious interval administration of naloxone (0.04 mg IV) will stimulate respiration without depriving the patient of analgesia. Hypoventilation is characterized by carbon dioxide retention and respiratory acidemia. Postoperative hypercarbia can occur as a consequence of:

1. Decreased ventilation
2. Increased carbon dioxide production

Most frequently, diminished ventilation is the source of an elevated carbon dioxide tension. Nevertheless, rarely elevated PCO_2 may result from increased carbon dioxide production. Conditions that increase carbon dioxide production include:

1. Malignant hyperthermia
2. Thyrotoxicosis
3. Hyperalimentation with elevated respiratory quotient

Tachypnea in the postoperative period may reflect:

1. Hypoxemia
2. Anxiety
3. Pain

It is imperative that the patient who presents with a rapid respiratory rate (>30) be carefully examined. Hypoxemia must be ruled out as a possible etiologic factor of the patient's tachypnea before ascribing rapid breathing to anxiety or to pain. **Diagnostic interventions include:**

1. Pulse oximetry
2. Arterial blood gas
3. Chest x ray

The possible etiologies of postoperative hypoxemia include:

1. Decreased FIO_2
2. Decreased ventilation
3. Ventilation-perfusion abnormality (V/Q)
4. Absolute shunt

In general, the patient who is tachypnic and hypoxemic is most likely suffering from a V/Q abnormality. Conditions producing such an imbalance include:

1. Pneumothorax
2. Pulmonary edema
3. Atelectasis
4. Pulmonary embolism
5. Pneumonia

Supportive therapy is directed at restoring oxygenation either by increasing FIO_2 or providing assisted ventilation. Ultimately treatment is aimed at correction of the underlying problem producing hypoxemia.

C. **Circulation.** Having ensured a patent airway and stable breathing pattern, the PACU nurse next assesses the circulation by determining BP and heart rate. Specific problems in hemodynamic stability are discussed later in **III.**

D. **Neurologic.** The patient is assessed as to level of consciousness. The nurse asks the patient to follow simple commands and to state his or her name. If the patient has had neurosurgery, the PACU neurologic examination is expanded to serve as a serial test of neurologic function. In this way, the PACU nurse can detect any sudden deterioration that might herald intracranial catastrophe.

E. **Goals of PACU care.** The purpose of the PACU is to provide an environment in which the patient can be closely observed following anesthesia and surgery. The PACU staff provide the necessary support with which the patient can be safely returned to the surgical ward. Patients may be discharged from the PACU when they are:

1. Awake and responsive
2. Hemodynamically stable
3. Adequately ventilating
4. Given appropriate analgesia

When the patient meets these criteria, the PACU nurse informs the anesthesiologist that the patient is ready for discharge. The anesthesiologist evaluates the patient, and if he or she is in agreement with the PACU nurse, the patient is discharged to the floor.

II. Specific considerations

A. Cardiovascular

1. Hypertension. Postoperative hypertension is frequently seen in the PACU.

a. Etiology

(1) Preexisting hypertension
(2) Pain
(3) Anxiety
(4) Bladder distention
(5) Hypercarbia
(6) Hormonal response to surgical stress

b. Therapy must be individualized. Hypertension as a consequence of pain, anxiety, bladder distention, and hypercarbia should be treated by directing therapy at the underlying cause. Postoperative hypertension occurs frequently in patients with preexisting high BP. It is imperative that the patient resume his or her outpatient antihypertensive medical regimen as soon as possible in the postoperative period. Should IV antihypertensive medications be required in the PACU the guidelines in Table 24-1 may be employed.

2. Hypotension. Only two conditions produce hypotension: **decreased cardiac output** and **decreased peripheral vascular tone.**

a. Etiology. The hypotensive patient is assessed as follows:

1. Airway patency
2. Breathing
3. Circulation (BP, heart rate)
4. Level of mentation. If the patient is unconscious, airway protection is mandatory.
5. Review anesthetic record: intraoperative ischemia, blood loss, fluid replacement
6. Physical examination: bleeding, abdominal distention, sympatholysis, ECG, arterial blood gases, chest x ray

While undergoing the assessment, the patient is given supplemental oxygen and usually a fluid bolus. If the patient remains hypotensive following a fluid challenge, additional monitoring is warranted:

1. Arterial line
2. Foley catheter
3. If patient has a history of ventricular failure or evidence of ongoing myocardial ischemia, pulmonary artery cannulation may be necessary.
4. Diagnosis of ongoing hypotension centers on calculating the patient's stroke volume and knowledge of pulmonary capillary occlusion pressure (PCOP) (Fig. 24-1).

Table 24-1. Guide to the treatment of postoperative hypertension

Heart rate	BP	Therapy
↑	↑	Beta-blockers (esmolol, propanolol, labetalol)
↓	↑	Vasodilators (nifedipine, hydralazine, Nipride)
⇃↾	Myocardial ischemia	Nitroglycerin, beta-blockers

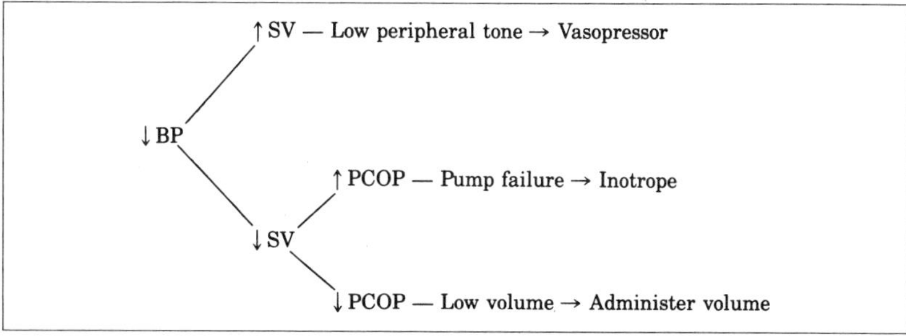

Fig. 24-1. Management of perioperative hypertension.

b. **Therapy**
   (1) **Hypovolemia:** volume administration
   (2) **Ventricular failure**
      (a) Relieve myocardial ischemia
      (b) Inotropic support
      (c) Mechanical assist device (intraaortic balloon pump)
   (3) **Low peripheral tone,** which is commonly seen in patients with septicemia, chemical or traumatic sympatholysis, and hepatic disease. Treatment centers on the restoration of blood pressure with pressor agents (phenylephrine, norepinephrine).

3. **Tachycardia** may be considered as being primary or secondary.
   a. **Primary tachycardia:** supraventricular dysrhythmias, atrial fibrillation, atrial flutter, ventricular tachycardia. Diagnosis is by ECG.
   b. **Secondary tachycardia:** sinus tachycardia, secondary to:
      (1) Anemia
      (2) Hypovolemia
      (3) Hypercarbia
      (4) Pain/anxiety
      (5) Bladder fullness
      (6) Fever
      (7) Sepsis
      (8) Hypotension
   c. **Therapy.** Treatment is directed at correcting the primary or secondary causes of tachycardia.
4. **Bradycardia**
   a. Types of bradycardia
      (1) **Primary bradycardia:** second and third degree heart block, sick sinus syndrome
      (2) **Secondary bradycardia:** sinus bradycardia secondary to:
         (a) Hypertension
         (b) Vagal tone
         (c) Drug effects (anticholinesterases, narcotics)
         (d) Sympatholysis
   b. **Therapy.** The therapy is guided toward correcting the underlying cause. If hemodynamic instability ensues, treatment is with atropine, pressors, and mechanical pacing.
5. **Myocardial ischemia.** Chapter 8 contains a detailed discussion of the diagnosis and treatment of perioperative myocardial ischemia. More perplexing than the management of myocardial ischemia is the approach to the asymptomatic, previously healthy patient who develops ECG changes in the postoperative period.

a. **Etiology.** Postoperative ECG changes may occur as a consequence of:
   (1) Electrolyte abnormalities
   (2) Hypothermia
   (3) Neurocardiac interrelationships
   (4) Myocardial ischemia

b. **Therapy.** Because postoperative myocardial ischemia is generally silent in character, it becomes difficult to determine whether postoperative ECG changes are benign or whether they signal ongoing myocardial ischemia. The following approach may be employed in managing postoperative ECG changes:
   (1) Assess total patient: vital signs, history, physical, operative course.
   (2) Correct electrolyte abnormalities.
   (3) Warm the patient.
   (4) Repeat the ECG. ST-segment changes, arrhythmias, and premature ventricular contractions are ominous; T wave changes are of less concern.
   (5) If ECG changes persist, use a trial of IV nitroglycerin (TNG). Begin IV TNG infusion until BP is decreased by 20% systolic. Do not induce relative hypotension by this trial. Repeat the ECG. If ECG changes improve, then they are most likely of ischemic origin. If no change is noted in the ECG and the patient is asymptomatic, the ECG changes are most likely benign. The TNG may be discontinued and the patient discharged to a monitored floor bed.
   (6) A cardiology consultation is often helpful in providing postoperative follow-up.
   (7) Always err on the side of caution in managing post-operative ECG changes.

B. **Respiratory care.** Frequently patients arrive in the PACU intubated, requiring ventilatory support. Anesthetists may elect to leave patients intubated for a number of reasons.

1. Residual anesthetics
2. Narcotization
3. Poor reversal neuromuscular blockade
4. Preexistent medical illness (chronic obstructive pulmonary disease, etc.)
5. Intraoperative complications

Patients who arrive intubated are assessed in the same manner as those who are not in need of respiratory support. The anesthetist explains the rationale for leaving the patient intubated, and a plan is agreed upon as to what interventions are needed to wean the patient from mechanical ventilation.

C. **Decreased urine output.** Low urine output is defined as being less than 0.5 cc/kg/hour.

1. **Etiology.** The causes of low urine output may be characterized as being:
   a. **Prerenal:** hypovolemia, low cardiac output, hypotension
   b. **Renal:** acute tubular necrosis, ischemic/toxic nephric injury
   c. **Postrenal.** Mechanical obstruction to urine flow (kinked Foley catheter, urethral obstruction)
2. **Diagnosis.** Low urine output in the routine recovery room patient is frequently due to inadequate intraoperative fluid replacement.
3. **Therapy.** A fluid bolus is the first-line therapy. Should urine output remain low, additional diagnostic and therapeutic interventions are required. (See Chap. 25.)

D. Delirium/slow awakening. Often patients are noted to be excessively somnolent compared to the norm in the immediate postoperative period. In evaluating the patient with slow arousal following general anesthesia the following steps are taken:

- **a.** Review the history; physically examine the patient.
- **b.** Review the intraoperative anesthesia record.
- **c.** Review the recovery room record.
- **d.** Rule out sources of slow awakening:
  - **(1) Airway-breathing-circulation abnormality.** Ensure vital signs are stable.
  - **(2) Drug effects** of residual anesthetics, narcotization, alcohol intoxication, or other preoperative substance abuse
  - **(3) Neurologic** (subarachnoid hemorrhage, cerebral ischemia, etc.)

Selected References

Feeley, T. W. The Post Anesthesia Care Unit. In R. D. Miller (ed.), *Anesthesia*, 3d ed. New York: Churchill-Livingstone, 1990.

Morris, R. W., Euchman, A., Warren, E. L. et al. The prevalence of hypoxemia detected during recovery from anesthesia. *J. Clin. Monitor* 4:16, 1988.

Cullen, D. J., and Cullen, B. L. Post anesthesia complications. *Surg. Clin. N.A.* 55:987, 1975.

25

Acute Renal Failure

Christopher O'Connor

I. Pathogenesis
  A. Back diffusion
  B. Tubular obstruction
  C. Abnormal renal blood flow
  D. Decreased glomerular filtration coefficient
II. Differential diagnosis of causes of acute renal failure
  A. Renal ischemia
  B. Nephrotoxins
  C. Less common causes
    1. Urinary tract obstruction
    2. Renal vascular emboli
    3. Acute interstitial nephritis
    4. Urate nephropathy
    5. The hepatorenal syndrome
    6. Acquired immunodeficiency syndrome
    7. Infrequent causes
III. Risk factors
IV. Evaluation of patients with acute renal failure
  A. History and physical examination
  B. Examination of the urine
    1. Proteinuria
    2. Casts
  C. Blood
    1. Nonoliguric ATN
    2. Early urinary tract obstruction, acute glomerulonephritis, or renal emboli
    3. Preexisting renal disease
    4. Diuretic administration
  D. Imaging techniques
    1. Plain film of the abdomen
    2. Ultrasound
    3. Intravenous pyelography (IVP)
    4. Antegrade pyelography
    5. Renal scans
    6. Angiography
    7. Computerized tomography scan
  E. Renal biopsy
V. Management of acute renal failure
  A. Prevention
    1. Mannitol
    2. Loop diuretics
      a. Nephrotoxic drug exposure
      b. Prevention of acute renal failure in transplanted cadaveric kidneys
      c. Hemoglobinuria and myoglobinuria
      d. Urate nephropathy
      e. Radiocontrast agents
      f. Jaundice
      g. Cardiac and vascular surgery
    3. Dopamine
  B. Early drug therapy of acute renal failure

1. Recommendations
   a. Mannitol
   b. Furosemide
2. Dopamine

C. Management of complications of acute renal failure
1. Volume overload
   a. Eliminating excess fluid administration
   b. Dialysis
2. Hyponatremia
3. Metabolic acidosis
   a. Sodium bicarbonate
   b. Dialysis
4. Hyperkalemia
   a. Calcium gluconate
   b. Sodium bicarbonate
   c. Glucose and insulin
   d. Sodium polystyrene sulfonate (Kayexalate)
   e. Dialysis
5. Hypermagnesemia
6. Hyperphosphatemia
7. Anemia
8. Altered mental status
9. Decreased drug elimination
10. Pericarditis
11. Bleeding abnormalities
    a. Dialysis
    b. Cryoprecipitate
    c. Red blood cell transfusions
    d. Estrogen-progesterone therapy and recombinant erythropoietin
12. Immunoincompetence

VI. Dialysis
A. Hemodialysis
1. Advantages
2. Disadvantages

B. Peritoneal dialysis
1. Advantages
2. Disadvantages

C. Continuous arteriovenous hemofiltration (CAVH)

VII. Nutritional support

VIII. Postoperative management of patients with chronic renal failure
A. Volume status
B. Hyperkalemia
C. Infections
D. Pericarditis
E. Access complications
F. Postoperative bleeding
G. Drug dosages

Acute renal failure is a syndrome characterized by a rapid deterioration in renal function that results in the accumulation of nitrogenous wastes. In the general hospital population, up to 5% of patients develop renal failure during their hospital stay, and up to 20% of those in the ICU have this complication. The importance of this problem is dramatized by the fact that almost half of all patients who develop acute renal failure do not survive, a figure that has not changed significantly in the past 30 years. Mortality is especially high when multiorgan failure accompanies renal insufficiency. In addition, the highest mortality associated with acute renal failure approaches 80% in patients after gastrointestinal or open heart surgery. Hence, critical care physicians must be familiar with the diverse clinical settings in which renal failure is likely to develop and be knowledgeable in the management of its many complications. The general management of patients with acute renal failure is outlined in this chapter.

I. **Pathogenesis.** The literature in this area is extensive and conflicting. Several theories have been proposed in an attempt to elucidate the mechanism responsible for the decreased glomerular filtration rate (GFR) seen in acute renal failure. In all probability, multiple mechanisms are operative in any given patient.
   A. **Back diffusion.** Glomerular filtration is normal, but as a result of injury to proximal tubular cells, solute and water are extensively reabsorbed, resulting in oliguria and uremia.
   B. **Tubular obstruction.** Necrotic debris causes tubular obstruction. Intratubular pressures increase and act to oppose filtration across the glomerulus, resulting in a decrease in GFR.
   C. **Abnormal renal blood flow.** Abnormalities in renal blood flow and normal glomerular capillary pressures have been proposed to explain the failure of filtration seen in acute renal failure. Laboratory studies have confirmed that total renal blood flow is reduced, afferent and efferent glomerular arteriolar resistances are increased, and glomerular plasma flow is decreased. However, other recent studies have shown that maintenance of normal renal blood flow by volume expansion does not result in improved GFR.
   D. **Decreased glomerular filtration coefficient.** Glomerular micropuncture data suggest that the filtration properties of the glomerular capillary membrane are decreased after acute ischemic injury.

II. **Differential diagnosis of causes of acute renal failure.** The causes of acute renal failure can be classified as those secondary to prerenal, intrarenal, and postrenal factors, a useful classification in that each implies a specific therapy (Table 25-1). Most cases of acute renal failure in the ICU are due to the following:
   A. **Renal ischemia** after periods of renal hypoperfusion occurs in hemorrhagic, cardiogenic, and septic shock; with acute burns; following renal transplant; and with temporary intraoperative interruption of renal blood flow, as in surgery involving the abdominal aorta.
   B. **Nephrotoxins**
      1. **Aminoglycoside antibiotics**
      2. **Radiocontrast agents**
      3. **Free hemoglobin or myoglobin,** seen after massive transfusion, intravascular hemolysis, or rhabdomyolysis
      4. **Amphotericin B**
      5. **Cis-platinum**
   C. **Less common causes** of acute renal failure need to be considered, particularly because several of these entities can be successfully treated.
      1. **Urinary tract obstruction** can be caused by bilateral urethral obstruction, unilateral obstruction of a single functioning kidney, or

Table 25-1. Causes of acute renal failure

Prerenal	Intrinsic renal disease	Postrenal
Hypovolemia Volume redistribution Impaired cardiac function Renovascular Hepatorenal syndrome	Acute tubular disease ischemic (postshock) Sepsis (postoperative) Toxins Contrast dye Drugs, heavy metal pigment Calcium, urate Acute glomerulorephritis Interstitial nephritis Vascular Emboli Vasculitis Intrarenal thrombosis Thrombotic thrombocytopenic purpura	Ureteral obstruction Intrinsic Extrinsic Bladder, outlet obstruction Urethral obstruction

Adapted from Ellison, D. H., and Bia, M. J. Acute renal failure in critically ill patients. *J. Int. Care Med.* 2:8, 1987.

bladder outlet obstruction. The presence of anuria or alternating oliguria and polyuria is especially suggestive of obstruction.

2. **Renal vascular emboli** can arise from the heart in patients with rheumatic heart disease, prosthetic valves, atrial fibrillation, or myocardial infarction or from the arterial vasculature. Emboli from the aorta most commonly occur during aortic surgery or angiography. Large emboli usually produce flank pain and hematuria; microvascular emboli are often silent.
3. **Acute interstitial nephritis** may be suggested by the presence of fever, rash, peripheral eosinophilia, and eosinophiluria. It is a hypersensitivity reaction, most frequently seen with penicillins, cimetidine, nonsteroidal antiinflammatory drugs, and sulfonamides.
4. **Urate nephropathy** is most commonly seen in patients being treated for hematologic malignancies who have not been pretreated with allopurinol.
5. **The hepatorenal syndrome** is seen in patients with cirrhosis and other forms of severe liver disease. It is associated with progressive azotemia and oliguria. Hepatorenal syndrome has a mortality approaching 95%.
6. **Acquired immunodeficiency syndrome (AIDS).** Acute renal failure is not uncommon in critically ill patients with AIDS since they are frequently exposed to ischemic and nephrotoxic insults, including sepsis, severe hypovolemia, and nephrotoxic antibiotics. In addition, a newly described syndrome or AIDS-associated nephropathy, characterized by proteinuria, glomerulosclerosis, and rapidly deteriorating renal function that leads to end-stage kidney disease in several weeks, further accounts for the rising incidence of acute renal failure in this patient population.
7. **Infrequent causes**
   a. Malignant hypertension
   b. Disseminated intravascular coagulation (DIC)
   c. Vasculitis

d. Rapidly progressive glomerulonephritis
e. Severe hypercalcemia
f. Multiple myeloma

III. **Risk factors.** Several factors have been identified that render an individual more susceptible to the development of acute renal failure: intravascular volume depletion, advanced age, preexisting renal insufficiency, and possibly diabetes mellitus. All appear to increase the risk from nephrotoxic agents, such as contrast dye and aminoglycoside antibiotics.

IV. **Evaluation of patients with acute renal failure.** The first evidence of impaired renal function is often oliguria. Because the management of oliguria resulting from volume depletion is radically different from the management of early acute renal failure, a thorough evaluation of the oliguric patient is essential.

A. **History and physical examination.** This should be carefully performed, eliciting evidence for recent fluid losses (third space, GI, or renal losses) and reviewing fluid balance and daily weights. Attention to signs of hypovolemia (postural changes, poor skin turgor) or volume overload (gallop rhythm, peripheral or sacral edema, jugular venous distention), along with measurements of central venous pressure, pulmonary capillary wedge pressure, and cardiac output when indicated, should help assess the adequacy of intravascular volume. **Hypovolemia** is the most frequent cause of prerenal azotemia. The response to a fluid challenge frequently helps to differentiate early acute renal failure from prerenal azotemia. This can usually be done rapidly and safely while other tests are pending. Normal saline or lactated Ringer's solute, 250–500 cc infused over 15 minutes, will rapidly increase intravascular volume while minimizing the total fluid infused.

B. **Examination of the urine. Urinalysis,** though rarely diagnostic, is a simple test that provides considerable information.

1. **Proteinuria,** although usually associated with glomerular lesions, can also be seen with tubular injury. Glomerular lesions allow large proteins to pass into the urine and most frequently result in significant proteinuria, usually 3–4 or more, by routine dipstick testing. Normally only small proteins are filtered through the glomerulus, and these are reabsorbed by the tubules. Tubular dysfunction accounts for the presence of mild proteinuria (1–2 or more) in acute tubular necrosis.

2. **Casts** in the urinary sediment provide insight into recent events in the nephron. They are composed of gellike aggregates of Tamm-Horsfall protein molecules and contain cellular elements present in the tubules at the time of aggregation.

a. **Hyaline casts** contain no cells and are generally seen with acidosis and dehydration. Their presence suggests prerenal azotemia.

b. **White blood cells (WBC) and WBC casts** reflect inflammatory lesions and are seen in pyelonephritis and acute intestinal nephritis. In the latter condition, eosinophil casts may be seen.

c. **Red blood cell (RBC) casts** are indicative of a glomerular lesion and are frequently seen with glomerulonephritis, malignant hypertension, and occasionally renal artery emboli.

d. **Granular casts,** which contain degenerating renal tubular cells, are commonly seen in acute renal failure secondary to ischemic injury or nephrotoxins. In hemoglobin and myoglobin-related acute renal failure, these casts are frequently pigmented.

C. **Blood.** A positive dipstick test for blood without RBCs suggests hemoglobinuria or myoglobinuria. The former will be associated with pink plasma. The supernatant of a spun specimen of blood will be clear with myoglobin-induced renal failure.

Urinary diagnostic indexes are tests of urine composition that may help in differentiating prerenal azotemia from acute tubular necrosis (ATN). When oliguria is secondary to prerenal causes, the urine reflects intact tubular mechanisms of salt and water conservation. The urine is concentrated, containing only small amounts of sodium and chloride; hence, urine-plasma ratios of creatinine and urea are high. In contrast, tubular function is usually deranged in acute renal failure, reflected in an abnormal urinary concentrating ability. The urine therefore is isotonic, with considerable quantities of sodium. The fractional excretion of sodium (FEna) and the renal failure index (RFI) are generally felt to be the most useful indexes in evaluating acute azotemia. Table 25-2 contrasts indexes typically seen in prerenal states with those encountered in intrarenal and postrenal causes of renal failure. Despite the utility of urinary indexes, they are occasionally nondiagnostic, and there are specific limitations to their use:

1. **Nonoliguric ATN.** The FEna may be low and resemble that seen with prerenal azotemia. In addition, low values for FEna have been reported in acute renal failure following acute burns, contrast dye exposure, sepsis, and cardiac or liver failure (Brezis, 1986).
2. **Early urinary tract obstruction, acute glomerulonephritis, or renal emboli.** In these entities, GFR may be abnormal while tubular function remains intact. The elaboration of a concentrated urine in these settings is an appropriate response to the decrease in GFR. With persistent obstruction, tubular function becomes abnormal, and the urinary indexes will then resemble those seen with ATN.
3. **Preexisting renal disease** frequently affects salt and water homeostatic mechanisms and makes interpretation of urine electrolytes difficult.
4. **Diuretic administration** specifically interferes with tubular reabsorption and invalidates interpretation of urine electrolytes and renal concentrating mechanisms.

D. **Imaging techniques.** Often additional tests are necessary to help delineate the cause of acute renal failure, although their primary utility in the ICU setting is to exclude obstruction and renal trauma.

Table 25-2. Urine and serum diagnostic indexes

	Prerenal	Renal	Postrenal
Urine (Na)	<10 mEq/L	>20 mEq/L	>20 mEq/L
Urine (CL)	<10 mEq/L	>20 mEq/L	
FEna	<1%	>2%	>2%
Urine osmolarity	>500	<350	<350
Urine/serum (creatinine)	>40	<20	<20
Renal failure index (RFI)	<1%	>2%	>2%
Urine/serum (urea)	>8	<3	<3
Serum (BUN)/creatinine	>20	=10	=10

FEna = (Una/Pna) ÷ (Ucr/Pcr) × 100.
RFI = Una ÷ (Ucr/Pcr).
FEna = fractional excretion of sodium.
RFI = renal failure index.
Una = urine concentration of sodium.
Pna = plasma concentration of sodium.
Ucr = urine concentration of creatinine.
Pcr = plasma concentration of creatinine.

1. **A plain film of the abdomen** can assess kidney size and shape and may be a clue to the presence of chronic renal failure when bilateral small kidneys are seen. It will also detect urinary calculi.
2. **Ultrasound** is the most valuable initial radiologic study to exclude obstruction and is easily performed in the ICU. If the obstruction has been present for less than 24 hours, however, the test may be normal.
3. **Intravenous pyelography (IVP)** is indicated only when renal trauma is suspected. It otherwise has no role in the evaluation of acute renal failure.
4. **Antegrade pyelography** allows for exact localization of urinary tract obstruction. When performed with percutaneous nephrostomy, the obstructed kidney will be drained.
5. **Renal scans** may be helpful for the diagnosis of renovascular disease or acute rejection in a transplanted kidney.
6. **Angiography** evaluates the arterial system.
7. **Computerized tomography (CT) scan** provides anatomic information when renal trauma is suspected.

E. **Renal biopsy.** The use of renal biopsy in the initial evaluation of acute renal failure is controversial. The following have been suggested as possible indications for renal biopsy: no clear etiology, evidence of glomerular disease or interstitial nephritis, when a systemic disease is suggested (e.g., systemic lupus erythematosus), or with prolonged renal failure.

V. Management of acute renal failure

A. **Prevention.** There is extensive literature regarding the use of various prophylactic measures to reduce the occurrence of acute renal failure. These include the use of diuretics such as mannitol and furosemide, dopamine, calcium channel blockers, ATP-$MgCl_2$, and simple volume loading prior to the ischemic or nephrotoxic insult. None has been conclusively shown to be of benefit despite experimental data supporting their use. The efficacy of those agents most thoroughly evaluated will be discussed, as well as the clinical situations in which their use in preventing renal failure seems justified. An awareness of these clinical settings is important since data derived from experimental data support their use.

1. **Mannitol** is an inert sugar that is freely filtered at the glomerulus and not reabsorbed by the tubules, thus causing a marked diuresis even in the presence of hypovolemia. By maintaining a high tubular flow rate, intratubular obstruction may be overcome and a beneficial effect on GFR seen. In addition, mannitol dilates the renal vasculature and causes an increase in renal blood flow, an effect partly mediated by changes in renal prostaglandins. Although in human clinical studies mannitol uniformly increases urine output, the protective effect against renal failure has not been confirmed. As a result of these experimental data, mannitol has been used prophylactically in aortic surgery and as therapy for oliguria in a variety of settings. The widespread clinical use of mannitol is based on anecdotal observations, the strong belief of many clinicians that it is efficacious, and the absence of significant adverse reactions to the drug.
2. **Loop diuretics** such as furosemide differ from other classes of diuretics in that they increase renal blood flow. Animal studies suggest that the combination of an increase in renal blood flow and solute excretion (thereby preventing intratubular obstruction) is necessary for an agent to be protective when given prior to experimentally induced renal failure. Both mannitol and furosemide exert these effects. However, the weight of clinical evidence suggests that the **prophylactic** use of mannitol or furosemide may be beneficial only in the following settings:

a. **Nephrotoxic drug exposure.** The nephrotoxicity of cis-platinum and amphotericin B may be reduced by concurrent therapy with mannitol.

b. **Prevention of acute renal failure in transplanted cadaveric kidneys.** The incidence of ATN following renal transplantation is 20–40%. Several reports have suggested that the use of hydration and the infusion of mannitol just prior to arterial clamp removal may diminish the incidence of ATN in the transplanted kidney.

c. **Hemoglobinuria and myoglobinuria** are usually treated by alkalizing the urine and inducing a brisk diuresis. This may prevent intratubular precipitation and can be accomplished by IV fluids, sodium bicarbonate, and diuretics.

d. **Urate nephropathy,** usually seen during chemotherapy for hematologic malignancies, may be prevented by the maintenance of a high urine flow induced by fluids and diuretics. In addition, pretreatment with allopurinol can prevent the rise in serum urate levels.

e. **Radiocontrast agents.** Adequate hydration prior to exposure to these agents and the concurrent administration of mannitol, furosemide, or both, may diminish the frequency of acute renal failure.

f. **Jaundiced patients** undergoing biliary tract surgery have a 10% incidence of postoperative renal failure due to poorly defined mechanisms. The results of earlier studies supporting the use of prophylactic mannitol in this patient population have been countered by recent reports failing to document a protective effect of intraoperative mannitol administration.

g. **Cardiac and vascular surgery** are high-risk surgical settings where the incidence of renal failure may approach 20%. Up to 25% of patients undergoing emergency repair of abdominal aortic aneurysms manifest significant renal dysfunction postoperatively (Brezis, 1986). Despite conflicting data, there is no clearly documented benefit from the use of prophylactic diuretics in this setting. Some authors recommend a trial of mannitol when other attempts to produce a diuresis have failed.

3. **Dopamine** in low dosages directly dilates the renal vasculature, increases renal blood flow, and promotes a diuresis. It is widely used in the treatment of oliguria and has been shown to increase urine output and sodium excretion. One study was able to demonstrate a slight increase in creatinine clearance in oliguric patients receiving dopamine, but this has not been a consistent finding, and there are no data to suggest that such treatment has any effect on the frequency of development of acute renal failure or on the rate of recovery of renal function in established renal failure.

B. **Early drug therapy of acute renal failure.** The value of diuretics in the **early** stages of acute renal failure, as well as in cases of established renal failure, has received considerable attention in the literature. No prospective randomized trials have been performed, nor does the current literature allow a firm conclusion to be made regarding their efficacy. Clinically, furosemide, in varying dosages up to 3 g per day, has been used in patients with **early** acute renal failure in an attempt to increase urine output. It has been proposed that such use may convert oliguric to nonoliguric renal failure. Although **spontaneous** nonoliguric renal failure has a lower mortality than oliguric renal failure, data from studies on the outcome of **diuretic-induced** nonoliguric renal failure are inconclusive. In trials evaluating high-dose furosemide therapy for established renal failure, results are conflicting. Most suggest a significant increase in urine output, and some report a reduction in the number of dialysis treatments needed. Few, however, report any improvement in recovery of renal function or any effect on mortality.

1. **Recommendations.** The absence of clear-cut evidence that mannitol, furosemide, and dopamine are efficacious in the early treatment of acute renal failure makes it difficult to make specific recommendations. However, since the toxicity of these drugs is minimal when used in appropriate dosages and because the conservative management of fluid therapy may be simplified in patients who do respond, the following guidelines are suggested:
   a. **Mannitol,** 12.5–25 g IV, may be given prophylactically prior to renal ischemia (i.e., before aortic cross-clamp or prior to massive intraoperative hemorrhage) or when other attempts to maintain hemodynamic stability in these high-risk surgical settings have failed to produce adequate urine output (Levinsky, 1988). It may be tried at similar dosages in patients with early acute renal failure when administered within the first 48 hours of renal insult.
   b. **Furosemide,** 80–320 mg IV, may be given initially to patients with early acute renal failure in an attempt to induce a diuresis and limit the progression of azotemia. Doses of 40–80 mg IV q6h may be administered to those with established renal failure when an increase in urine output is necessary for fluid management. Rarely, high-dose therapy may cause ototoxicity. Diuretics should be used **only** when hypovolemia has been corrected. Therapy should be discontinued if urine output does not respond significantly or if urine output is adequate without diuretics.
2. **Dopamine,** in dosages of 1–4 μg/kg/minute IV, may be administered to patients with early acute renal failure unresponsive to diuretics. Limited data from uncontrolled studies suggest an augmented diuretic response when dopamine is used in conjunction with furosemide. It may also improve urine output in critically ill patients with prerenal oliguria unresponsive to fluid administration. It should be discontinued if unacceptable tachycardia occurs or if there is no response.

C. **Management of complications of acute renal failure.** The management of acute renal failure is similar to that of chronic renal failure. Critically ill patients with acute renal failure frequently have other injuries that may result in an altered metabolic state, hemodynamic instability, and other organ system failure, all of which can complicate management. In health, the kidneys maintain normal intravascular volume, osmolality, and pH; eliminate excess potassium, phosphorus, magnesium, many pharmacologic agents, and endogenous wastes; and produce hormones that are important in the maintenance of normal levels of serum calcium and the production of erythrocytes by the bone marrow. A variety of problems can arise when the kidneys are unable to perform their normal functions.

1. **Volume overload.** In patients with acute renal failure who have a stable caloric intake, weight loss should average 0.2–0.3 kg per day due to catabolism. Fluids should be administered to equal urine output plus insensible losses, as well as losses from other sources, such as abdominal or nasogastric drains. However, most patients who develop acute renal failure in the ICU (1) have multiple intravascular catheters that require a finite infusion to maintain patency, (2) receive a large number of drugs, including antibiotics, antacids, and vasoactive agents, and (3) often receive IV hyperalimentation. All of these add to the total fluid burden and further predispose to volume overload. Treatment modalities include:
   a. **Eliminating excess fluid administration.** Specific recommendations include (1) utilizing low flow, constant flush systems on

pressure-monitoring catheters, and infusion pumps on all other intravascular catheters, (2) concentrating all drugs to the limit of their solubility, and (3) scrupulously avoiding unnecessary fluid administration.

b. **Dialysis** is an efficient means of fluid removal if the previously mentioned measures are unsuccessful in preventing volume overload.

2. **Hyponatremia** may develop during the course of acute renal failure due to defective renal-concentrating mechanisms. When present, it reflects an excess of free water and the need for more aggressive fluid restriction. Conversely, a rising serum sodium suggests the need for greater free water intake.

3. **Metabolic acidosis** results from the endogenous production of organic acids. These are normally produced at a rate of 1 mEq/kg/day but may be produced in much greater quantities in catabolic, critically ill patients. The serum bicarbonate may fall at a daily rate of 2 mEq per liter or more. Treatment is usually unnecessary unless the bicarbonate level falls below 15 mEq per liter. Aggressive correction of severe acidosis may precipitate acute hypocalcemia and tetany due to rapid lowering of ionized calcium levels by bicarbonate. Management includes:

   a. **Sodium bicarbonate.** pH can usually be maintained in the normal range with 44–88 mEq per day.

   b. **Dialysis** may be necessary when acid production is very high or when volume overload limits the amount of sodium bicarbonate that can be administered.

4. **Hyperkalemia** is a potentially life-threatening complication of acute renal failure. Hyperkalemia results in distinct ECG changes. Peaking of the T waves and shortening of the QT interval are usually the earliest changes, followed by prolongation of the PR interval and decreasing amplitude of the P wave. As hyperkalemia progresses, depression of the ST segment and widening of the QRS complex follows, eventually resulting in a sine-wave configuration. Treatment depends on the degree of hyperkalemia and the severity of ECG changes. The presence of a widened QRS complex is an indication for prompt treatment with IV calcium, bicarbonate and glucose, and insulin. Less pronounced changes such as T-wave peaking may be managed with cation exchange resins. Treatment guidelines include:

   a. **Calcium gluconate,** 1–2 ampules (10–20 cc) of a 10% solution, given IV over 2–5 minutes, directly antagonizes the effect of potassium on the myocardium.

   b. **Sodium bicarbonate,** 50–100 mEq IV, will partly reverse the acidosis and together with glucose and insulin will cause a redistribution of potassium into cells.

   c. **Glucose and insulin,** 1–2 ampules of 50% dextrose in water and 10 units of regular insulin IV, should be given with bicarbonate. The onset of effect for this intervention is within minutes.

   d. **Sodium polystyrene sulfonate (Kayexalate)** is a sodium potassium ion exchange resin given via the GI tract that directly removes potassium from the body. Approximately 1 mEq of potassium is exchanged for each mEq of sodium per gram of sodium polystyrene sulfonate; 25–50 g, given with 100 cc of a 20% sorbitol solution, may be given orally or as a retention enema. Sodium polystyrene sulfonate may be given for less urgent situations; it should be also given **concurrently** with the above therapy for more severe hyperkalemia.

   e. **Dialysis** will rapidly remove excess potassium.

5. **Hypermagnesemia** can cause depressed mental status and muscle weakness but rarely occurs unless supplemental magnesium is administered. This is most commonly seen with the use of magnesium-containing antacids.
6. **Hyperphosphatemia** is common in acute renal failure. Although phosphorus has no known toxic effects, in excess it acts to lower serum calcium concentration. Phosphorous binding antacids (Amphojel, AlternaGEL) are usually given to lower phosphorus and maintain calcium in a normal range. Severe hypophosphatemia has occurred with their overzealous use.
7. **Anemia** in patients with acute renal failure is multifactorial in origin. Erythropoietin is produced by the kidney and stimulates erythrocyte production in the bone marrow. Absence of this hormone probably contributes to the anemia seen in acute renal failure. Although patients with chronic renal failure usually tolerate a hematocrit in the low 20s, acutely ill patients with acute renal failure require a higher level.
8. **Altered mental status** with renal failure is due to retention of endogenous wastes. Manifestations range from tremor, myoclonus, asterixis, and frank seizures to lethargy, disorientation, and coma. In critically ill patients, other metabolic derangements may also affect the CNS. Dialysis usually results in an improved mental status when obtundation is due to uremia.
9. **Decreased drug elimination.** A large number of drugs are eliminated by the kidneys, including several muscle relaxants and such potentially toxic agents as the aminoglycoside antibiotics and digoxin. Therefore, the dosage of all drugs excreted by the kidney should be adjusted when renal function is depressed. It is important to remember that the serum creatinine concentration reflects GFR only in the steady state. Therefore, early in acute renal failure, the serum creatinine concentration will not reflect GFR. It is safest to assume that the creatinine clearance is zero at this point and adjust drug dosages accordingly.
10. **Pericarditis** occurs with uremia for unknown reasons. Both cardiac tamponade and infective pericarditis are potential complications. Patients should be examined daily for the presence of a pericardial friction rub, and cardiac tamponade should be suspected if unexplained cardiovascular decompensation occurs. Many physicians consider pericarditis to be an indication for emergency dialysis.
11. **Bleeding abnormalities** are common in patients with acute renal failure and are generally attributed to abnormal platelet function and possibly to factor VIII dysfunction. Management of bleeding problems includes the following:
    a. **Dialysis** occasionally corrects the platelet abnormality.
    b. **Cryoprecipitate,** 10 units IV, and desmopressin acetate (DDAVP), 0.3–0.4 μg per kilogram IV or intranasally, have been reported to be efficacious in bleeding disorders in uremic patients.
    c. **Red blood cell transfusions** may improve the bleeding time in uremic patients since bleeding is more frequent when the hematocrit is below 30.
    d. **Estrogen-progesterone therapy and recombinant erythropoietin** are promising new treatment alternatives for uremic bleeding.
12. **Immunoincompetence.** Infectious complications are responsible for the majority of deaths in patients with acute renal failure. The ability to fight infection is impaired with uremia. To complicate the situation, the usual manifestations of infection may be blunted with uremia. Recommended procedures to minimize infectious complications include the following:

a. Scrupulous attention to aseptic technique in the placement and care of all intravascular catheters
b. Avoidance of urethral catheters when possible
c. Routine surveillance of blood, urine, and sputum cultures
d. Frequent dialysis has been suggested by some to decrease the incidence of infectious complications, but its use is controversial.
e. Prophylactic antibiotics are not beneficial and should be avoided.

VI. **Dialysis.** Dialysis should be instituted when more conservative measures fail to control the manifestations of acute renal failure (see **V.C**). Most authors agree that dialysis should be initiated before the blood-urea nitrogen (BUN) reaches 100 mg per deciliter or the creatinine rises to 8–10 mg per deciliter. In severely catabolic patients, more frequent and aggressive dialysis may be necessary. Several methods of dialysis are available, each with specific advantages and disadvantages, although there exist no randomized prospective trials comparing the clinical efficacy of one method to another.

A. **Hemodialysis** utilizes an extracorporeal circuit in which blood is pumped through a dialysis cartridge under pressure and returned to the patient. The dialysis cartridge brings blood in contact with dialysate via a semipermeable membrane permitting exchange of toxic solutes by diffusion. The concentrations of electrolytes, buffers, and glucose in the dialysis solutions are adjusted according to the metabolic requirements of each patient.

1. **Advantages**
   a. **Rapid** removal of large quantities of fluid and correction of metabolic acidosis and hyperkalemia due to its efficient clearance
   b. **Short** treatment times
   c. **Beneficial** for severely catabolic patients
2. **Disadvantages**
   a. **Hemodynamic** instability. Hypotension is a frequent complication of hemodialysis in critically ill patients. This is usually treated with crystalloid or colloid administration, which may undermine fluid removal.
   b. **Requires vascular access.** High flow rates are necessary for effective dialysis. This most frequently requires insertion of a large catheter into a central vein or surgical creation of an arteriovenous fistula.
   c. **Disequilibrium syndrome.** Characterized by confusion, restlessness, gastrointestinal symptoms, or seizures, this syndrome is most common during the initial dialysis and may be related to hyperosmolarity of cells in the CNS. Treatment is largely preventive using slow dialysis during the early phases of therapy.

B. **Peritoneal dialysis** utilizes the peritoneal membrane for exchange of solutes and fluids, allowing exchange of toxic substances from the patient to the infused dialysate by means of diffusion.

1. **Advantages**
   a. Minimal hemodynamic instability
   b. Technically simple
   c. Avoidance of anticoagulation
2. **Disadvantages**
   a. Potentially inadequate removal of toxic products in severely catabolic patients
   b. Risk of peritonitis
   c. Limited use in patients after recent abdominal surgery, where multiple abdominal drains are in place, or in the presence of paralytic ileus
   d. Intraabdominal dialysate may interfere with ventilation, especially in patients with limited pulmonary function.
   e. Hyperglycemia

C. **Continuous arteriovenous hemofiltration (CAVH),** a relatively new technique for the treatment of acute renal failure that is especially suitable for critically ill patients too hemodynamically unstable for hemodialysis and with contraindications to peritoneal dialysis. This technique has applications for the treatment of patients with fluid overload or persistent oliguria. It requires arteriovenous access, usually via the femoral vessels, and involves delivery of blood to an extracorporeal hemofilter at a rate determined by the patient's own systemic BP without the use of a blood pump, as in hemodialysis. Unlike hemodialysis, where diffusion governs solute removal, solute loss in CAVH occurs by convection. When the hydrostatic pressure across the synthetic membrane of the filter exceeds osmotic pressure, an ultrafiltrate is formed composed of plasma water and nonprotein-bound solutes, which passes into a collection device. As water and solutes are removed, clear nonuremic fluid (usually a modified saline solution similar to plasma) is administered to the patient at the venous end of the access, resulting in net removal of fluid and solutes. In this manner, uremic toxins, potassium, and excess fluid may be removed without the cardiovascular changes associated with hemodialysis. Filtration rates up to 14 liters per day can be achieved with average net fluid losses of 1–3 liters per day. Continuous arteriovenous hemofiltration has been likened to "exchange transfusion" of the extracellular space. Figure 25-1 outlines this system. This technique has been recommended for the following groups of patients:

1. Hemodynamically unstable postoperative patients with renal failure
2. Where peritoneal dialysis is contraindicated
3. Those with cardiogenic shock and pulmonary edema where rapid fluid removal is desired
4. Where the administration of parenteral hyperalimentation is limited due to volume overload
5. Those with massive fluid overload or diuretic unresponsive oliguria

It is **not** recommended for patients with acute renal failure in whom the correction of uremia, hyperkalemia, or metabolic acidosis is the primary concern.

VII. **Nutritional support** is an important ancillary measure in critically ill patients with acute renal failure. Providing adequate nutritional support for these patients is complicated by the need for volume restriction and the concern that supplemental protein may result in the production of additional nitrogenous wastes. Carbohydrates have a protein-sparing effect, and when administered with essential amino-acid preparations, nutritional supplements can be provided that do not significantly elevate the BUN level. Hyperalimentation may be instituted early in the hope that prevention of malnutrition decreases the complications associated with acute renal failure.

VIII. **Postoperative management of patients with chronic renal failure.** Patients with chronic renal failure (CRF) maintained on hemodialysis are frequently seen in the ICU following surgery. Studies have suggested that up to one-third of patients on home dialysis required major operations during a 3-year period. Nevertheless, mortality is usually low. Problems arising from cardiovascular disease, diabetes mellitus, and vascular access complications are common in patients with CRF. Finally, procedures unique to this patient population, including nephrectomy, renal transplantation, and urologic reconstructive procedures, increase the frequency with which these patients come to the operating room. Issues pertinent to the management of these individuals in the postoperative setting include:

A. **Volume status.** Careful monitoring of intake and output, daily weights, and often central venous and pulmonary capillary wedge pressure mea-

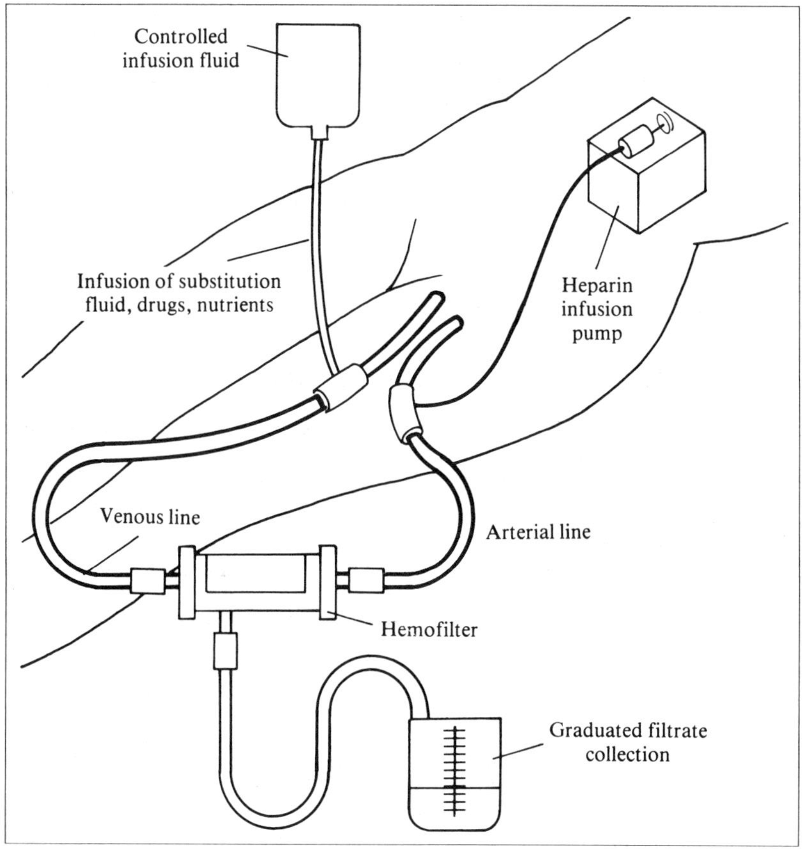

Fig. 25-1. CAVH using femoral artery and vein accesses.

surements are necessary to ensure adequate circulatory stability. Fluids are administered as balanced salt solutions according to the electrolyte concentration of those fluids lost. Some authors recommend that dialysis be performed for 2 consecutive days prior to surgery utilizing minimal heparinization and removing adequate volume to establish optimal fluid homeostasis and blood pressure control. Transfusion can be accomplished during the next-to-last dialysis session prior to surgery to allow for elimination of excess potassium. If possible, dialysis is withheld for 48 hours after surgery to minimize the risk of bleeding.

B. **Hyperkalemia** is a **common,** potentially lethal, and preventable postoperative phenomenon in patients with CRF. Tissue trauma, metabolic acidosis, and concurrent infections all predispose to significant hyperkalemia following major surgery. Frequent determinations of potassium levels should be performed and appropriate therapy instituted if hyperkalemia develops (see **V.C**).

C. **Infections** are more common in these patients due to the immunosuppressive effects of uremia. Wound healing is often prolonged, and subsequent wound infections are frequent.

D. **Pericarditis** appears to be a frequent occurrence postoperatively, yet early detection by careful and timely clinical assessment should minimize the potential hemodynamic consequences of this complication.

E. **Access complications** may accompany major surgery in patients on hemodialysis. Clotting of the vascular access site, presumably as a result of low blood flow during surgery, may occur in the immediate postoperative period.

F. **Postoperative bleeding** is uncommon if adequate preoperative hemodialysis was performed.

G. **Drug dosages** should be adjusted for all medications requiring renal excretion.

Selected References

Bartlett, R. H., Botch, J., Geronemus, R., et al. Continuous arteriovenous hemofiltration for acute renal failure. *Trans. Am. Soc. Artif. Intern. Organs* 34:67, 1988.

Bennett, W., Aronoff G. R., Morrison, G., et al. Drug prescribing in renal failure: Dosing guidelines for adults. *Am. J. Kidney Dis.* 3:155, 1983.

Brezis, M., Rosen, S., and Epstein, F. H. Acute Renal Failure. In B. M. Brenner and F. C. Rector (eds.), *The Kidney*. Philadelphia: W. B. Saunders, 1986.

Burnier, M., and Schrier, R. W. Protection from acute renal failure. *Adv. Exp. Med. Biol.* 212:275, 1987.

Corwin, H. L., and Bonventre, J. V. Acute renal failure in the intensive care unit. *Int. Care Med.* 14:10, 1988.

Ellison, D. H., and Bia, M. J. Acute renal failure in critically ill patients. *J. Int. Care Med.* 2:8, 1987.

Gubern, J. M., Sancho, J. J., Simó, J., and Sitges-Sorra, A. A randomized trial on the effect of mannitol on postoperative renal function in patients with obstructive jaundice. *Surgery* 103:39, 1988.

Hesdorffer, C. J., Milne, J. F., Meyers, A. M., et al. The value of Swan-Ganz catheterization and volume loading in preventing renal failure in patients undergoing abdominal aneurysmectomy. *Clin. Nephrol.* 28:272, 1987.

Kasiske, B. L., and Kjellstrand, C. M. Perioperative management of patients with chronic renal failure and postoperative acute renal failure. *Urol. Clin. North Am.* 10:35, 1983.

Levinsky, N. G., and Bernard, D. B. Mannitol and Loop Diuretics. In B. M. Brenner and J. J. Lazarus, (eds.), *Acute Renal Failure*. Philadelphia: W. B. Saunders, 1988.

Remuzzi, G. Bleeding in renal failure. *Lancet* 1:1205, 1988.

Solez, K. Pathogenesis of acute renal failure. *Int. Rev. Exp. Pathol.* 24:277, 1983.

von Valenberg, P. L. J., Hoitsma, A. J., Tiggeler, R. G. W. L., et al. Mannitol as an indispensable constituent of an intraoperative hydration protocol for the prevention of acute renal failure after renal cadaveric transplantation. *Transplantation* 44:784, 1987.

Wagner, K., and Neumayer, H. Prevention of delayed graft function in cadaver kidney transplants by diltiazam: Outcome of two prospective randomized clinical trials. *J. Cardiovasc. Pharm.* 10:S170, 1987.

26

Acid-Base Disturbance

William J. Mazzei and Christopher O'Connor

- I. Theoretic considerations
  - A. Oxidation of carbohydrate and fat
  - B. Concentration of bicarbonate, PCO_2, ratio of concentrations of bicarbonate to carbon dioxide, and normal arterial values
  - C. Acidosis and alkalosis
- II. Clinical acid-base measurement
  - A. Temperature
    - 1. Blood gas determinations
    - 2. Metabolism of blood gas sample
  - B. Heparin mixtures
  - C. Air bubbles
  - D. Measurement technique
- III. Acid-base disturbances
  - A. The four primary acid-base disorders
    - 1. Examine the pHa
    - 2. Examine the $PaCO_2$
    - 3. Calculate expected compensatory responses
  - B. The decision to treat any acid-base disturbance
  - C. Metabolic acidosis
    - 1. Differential diagnosis
    - 2. Evaluation of metabolic acidosis
    - 3. Treatment of metabolic acidosis
  - D. Metabolic alkalosis occurs because of an accumulation of alkali or loss of acid
    - 1. Differential diagnosis
      - a. Chloride responsive
      - b. Chloride unresponsive
    - 2. Evaluation of metabolic alkalosis
    - 3. Treatment of metabolic alkalosis
  - E. Respiratory acidosis
    - 1. Differential diagnosis
    - 2. Evaluation of respiratory acidosis
    - 3. Treatment of respiratory acidosis
  - F. Respiratory alkalosis occurrence
    - 1. Differential diagnosis
      - a. Hyperventilation
      - b. Reduced carbon dioxide production
    - 2. Evaluation of respiratory alkalosis
    - 3. Treatment
  - G. Mixed disorders
    - 1. Diagnosis of a mixed disorder
    - 2. Search for etiology
    - 3. Treatment

Acid-base distributions are an ever-present concern in the management of the ICU patient. To function properly, the body has an elaborate system of buffers to maintain pH homeostasis. Acid-base management is reviewed in this chapter.

I. Theoretic considerations

A. Oxidation of carbohydrate and fat yields carbon dioxide and water. Hydration of carbon dioxide yields carbonic acid, which exists in equilibrium with hydrogen ion and bicarbonate. Approximately 22,000 mEq of carbon dioxide is produced each day. In addition, metabolism of sulfur-containing amino acids and incomplete oxidation of carbohydrates and fat yield approximately 70 mEq of acid other than carbonic acid. Since these represent a much smaller acid load than carbon dioxide, the major determinant of serum pH is the equilibrium between carbon dioxide and hydrogen ion-bicarbonate:

$$CO_2 + H_2O = H_2CO_3 = H^+ + HCO_3^- \tag{1}$$

Solving for H^+, one obtains the familiar Henderson-Hasselbalch equation:

$$pH = pK + \log \frac{(HCO_3^-)}{a \times PCO_2} \tag{2}$$

where

HCO_3^- = concentration of bicarbonate
PCO_2 = partial pressure of carbon dioxide
a = solubility coefficient of carbon dioxide

B. Points of note concerning the variables in equation 2

1. The concentration of bicarbonate is set by the kidneys with adjustments requiring 2–3 days for a new steady state to arise.
2. The PCO_2 is set by the lungs, with adjustments requiring only minutes for equilibrium.
3. The ratio of concentrations of bicarbonate to carbon dioxide determines pH; thus, two of the three variables must be known ((HCO_3^-), PCO_2, or pH) to describe the acid-base status.
4. Normal arterial values

pH: 7.38–7.45
PCO_2: 36–45 mm Hg
(HCO_3^-) = 22–27 mEq per liter

C. Acidosis and alkalosis refer to processes that cause acid and alkali to accumulate. Acidemia and alkalemia refer to the actual pH present in the patient—the former applying with pHa less than 7.38, the latter with pHa greater than 7.45. Although the terms are often interchanged, this is not a proper usage because a patient may be acidic while an alkalosis is occurring or alkalemic while an acidosis is occurring.

II. Clinical acid-base measurement.

Several artifacts may affect acid-base measurements.

A. Temperature. Correction for the nonnormothermic patient

1. Blood gas determinations are carried out on blood samples at 37°C regardless of the patient's temperature. The values determined in a normothermic patient will be different from those in the nonnormothermic patient because of the change in water dissociation constant and carbon dioxide and oxygen solubility coefficients with temperature (i.e., the pH of the hydrogen ion–hydroxide ion neutrality point and the solubility of carbon dioxide and oxygen decrease as temperature rises). Examples of this effect in a febrile patient and a hypothermic patient are given below:

Measured (37°C)	Actual for patient At 40°C	Actual for patient At 30°C
PaO_2 = 60	PaO_2 = 74.5	PaO_2 = 37
$PaCO_2$ = 24	$PaCO_2$ = 27.3	$PaCO_2$ = 18
pHa = 7.41	pHa = 7.38	pHa = 7.51

It is controversial whether clinical decisions should be based on the measured values at 37°C or on the temperature-corrected values. Although pH changes with temperature, the ratio of intracellular concentrations of hydroxide ion to hydrogen ion does not. Furthermore, charges on protein molecules do not change with temperature, and ionization of protein molecules may be more important for cellular function than pH. Also, the shift in the oxyhemoglobin dissociation curve with temperature tends to offset any apparent change in PaO_2 caused by temperature alone. In the example (patient at 40°C), although the "actual" PaO_2 is higher than the PaO_2 at 37°C, the rightward shift in the oxyhemoglobin curve makes the oxygen saturation about the same for both temperatures.

2. Metabolism in an uncooled blood gas sample will decrease the PaO_2 and raise the $PaCO_2$ by about 3 mm Hg per minute. Therefore, any sample not immediately analyzed should be stored in ice before sending it to the laboratory.

B. **Heparin** should be adequately mixed with the blood gas sample in order to be an effective anticoagulant. This requires vigorous rolling of the syringe after a sample is obtained, particularly with a preheparinized syringe (i.e., heparin is deposited along the syringe wall). Aqueous heparin added to standard syringes used for blood gases is acidic (pH = 5) and has equilibrated with air; thus, excessive amounts of heparin will artifactually lower the pH and adjust the measured blood gas values toward room air (PO_2 = 150 mm Hg, PCO_2 = 0).

C. **Air bubbles,** as with heparin, adjust the blood gas values toward that of air.

D. **Measurement technique**

1. Electrodes are used to measure pH, PO_2, and PCO_2 directly. The PCO_2 electrode is usually the least precise; thus, measurement error should be suspected if rapid changes in PCO_2 occur without concomitant changes in pH (Table 26-1).
2. A variety of techniques are used to measure total carbon dioxide concentration. The measurements obtained may vary between techniques by as much as 4 mEq per liter, an important factor if different devices are used to analyze blood gases in one hospital.

Table 26-1. Mean whole body response equations for simple acid-base disturbances

Disorder	Equation*
Metabolic acidosis	$\Delta PaCO_2 \approx 1.2\ \Delta[HCO_3^-]$
Metabolic alkalosis	$\Delta PaCO_2 \approx 0.7\ \Delta[HCO_3^-]$
Respiratory acidosis	
Acute	$\Delta[H^+] \approx 0.75\ \Delta PaCO_2$
Chronic	$\Delta[H^+] \approx 0.30\ \Delta PaCO_2$
Respiratory alkalosis	
Acute	$\Delta[H^+] \approx 0.75\ \Delta PaCO_2$
Chronic	$\Delta[HCO_3^-] \approx 0.5\ \Delta PaCO_2$

*$[HCO_3^-]$ in mEq/L; $PaCO_2$ in mm Hg; H^+ in nmol/L. Between pH 7.2–7.6, each 10-nmol/L increase in H^+ decreases pH approximately 0.1.

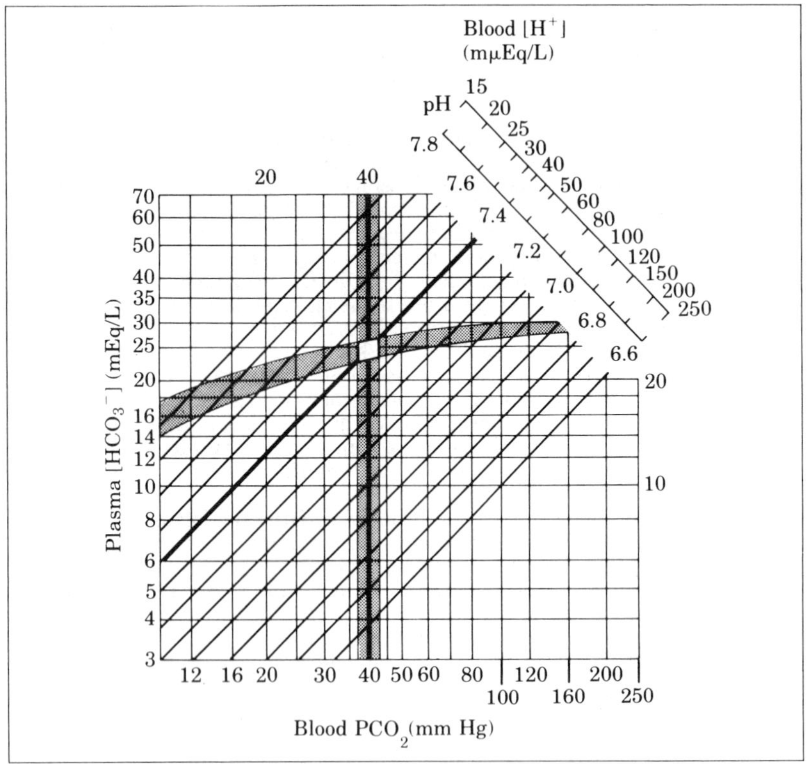

Fig. 26-1. Acid-base nomograph. This plot is a three-coordinate graph of the Henderson-Hasselbalch equation and represents all possible patient acid-base states (see text).

III. Acid-base disturbances

A. The four primary acid-base disorders are metabolic acidosis, metabolic alkalosis, respiratory acidosis, and respiratory alkalosis. In the spontaneously breathing patient, each of these disorders provokes a compensatory response that attempts to correct the pHa toward normal. Except for simultaneous respiratory acidosis and alkalosis, it is possible to have two or more simultaneous disorders. In evaluating a patient's acid-base status, one must determine which (if any) primary disorder is occurring, whether an appropriate level of compensation exists, and whether more than one disorder is occurring. After obtaining an arterial blood gas, one approach to acid-base evaluation is the following:

1. **Examine the pHa.** This informs one whether the sum of all disease processes is producing acidemia or alkalemia.
2. **Examine the $PaCO_2$.** If it is less than 36 mm Hg, respiratory alkalosis is occurring; if it is greater than 44 mm Hg, respiratory acidosis is occurring.
3. **Calculate expected compensatory responses.** This may be done using the equations in Table 26-1. Our preference is to do this graphically, using Figures 26-1 and 26-2.
   a. Plot the blood gas on Figure 26-1. This is a quick check on the

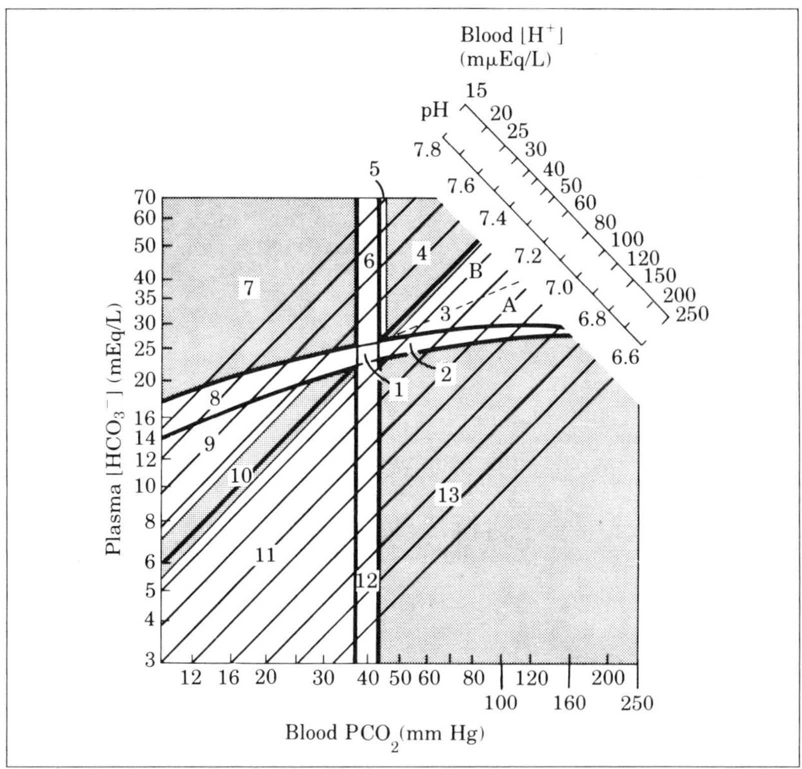

Fig. 26-2. Acid-base disturbances. The shaded areas represent the ranges of $PaCO_2$–bicarbonate relationships characteristic of acid-base disorders. Plotting the pH, PCO_2, and bicarbonate concentration from a blood gas on the graph will show which disorder or combination of disorders is occurring (see text). *1* = normal; *2* = respiratory acidosis; *3* = respiratory acidosis (compensated); *A* = acute; *B* = chronic; *4* = respiratory acidosis and metabolic alkalosis (mixed); *5* = metabolic alkalosis (compensated); *6* = metabolic alkalosis; *7* = respiratory alkalosis and metabolic alkalosis (mixed); *8* = respiratory alkalosis; *9* = respiratory alkalosis (compensated); *10* = metabolic acidosis and respiratory alkalosis (mixed); *11* = metabolic acidosis (compensated); *12* = metabolic acidosis; *13* = metabolic acidosis and respiratory acidosis (mixed).

accuracy of the blood gas reported, for if the gas cannot be plotted on this graph, at least one of the three variables (pHa, $PaCO_2$, or bicarbonate concentration) is in error. For example, if the pHa is 7.20 and $PaCO_2$ is 70 mm Hg, the bicarbonate concentration must be about 27 mEq per liter. If it is not within approximately 3 mEq per liter, a calculation error was made at the blood gas laboratory or the values have been recorded incorrectly.

b. Plot the blood gas on Figure 26-2. This plot separates the allowable values of pHa, $PaCO_2$, and bicarbonate concentration into zones that represent normal values, single simple disorders without compensation, simple disorders with appropriate compensation, and mixed disorders. In compensating for a single disorder, the pHa is corrected toward, but never equal to, 7.4. Thus, a normal pHa with an abnormal $PaCO_2$ implies two primary disorders (see areas 4 and 10 in Fig. 26-2).

c. Simultaneous metabolic acidosis and alkalosis could produce blood gas values in the normal range. Also, two separate disease processes, both causing either metabolic acidosis or alkalosis, are not differentiated in Figure 26-2. An approach to such mixed disorders is discussed in **G.**

B. The decision to treat any acid-base disturbance revolves around the pHa value, as marked variations in $PaCO_2$ and bicarbonate concentration are tolerated by the body. Table 26-2 shows the consequences of acidemia and alkalemia. Details for treatment are discussed in **C, D, E, F,** and **G.**

C. Metabolic acidosis results from accumulation of acid or loss of alkali. Pure metabolic acidosis implies a lowered serum bicarbonate level with a normal $PaCO_2$ (see area 12 in Fig. 26-2). In the spontaneously breathing patient, however, hypocapnia occurs because the body attempts to correct the pH with a compensatory respiratory alkalosis (see area 11 in Fig. 26-2).

1. Differential diagnosis: anion gap. By examining the anion gap, which equals $(Na^+) - ((Cl^-) + (HCO_3^-))$, one can separate a metabolic acidosis into one of two types:
   - **a.** Increased anion gap (>12) or normochloremic acidosis. This may be caused by the following:
     - (1) Toxic intake (e.g., methanol, ethylene glycol, salicylates, or paraldehyde)
     - (2) Increased acid production (e.g., starvation ketosis, diabetic ketoacidosis [DKA], alcoholic ketoacidosis, lactic acidosis)
     - (3) Decreased acid excretion (e.g., renal failure)
   - **b.** Normal anion gap, or hyperchloremic acidosis. Etiologies include the following:
     - (1) Bicarbonate loss (often with hypokalemia) (e.g., renal tubular acidosis, diarrhea, carbonic anhydrase inhibitor administration, or ureteral diversions)
     - (2) Hydrogen ion accumulation without an increase in unusual anions, often with normal or increased serum potassium (e.g., early renal failure, hydrochloride or potassium chloride administration, or hydronephrosis)
   - **c.** In some instances, the anion gap may be misleading in analyzing acid-base disorders. The following list comprises other causes of

Table 26-2. Consequences of acidemia or alkalemia

Site	Acidemia	Alkalemia
Cardiovascular	↓ Myocardial contractility Arrhythmias ↓ Arteriolar resistance	Arrhythmias
Neurologic	Lethargy Confusion	Paresthesias Tetany
Hematologic	Hyperkalemia Rightward shift in oxyhemoglobin dissociation curve	Hypokalemia Leftward shift in oxyhemoglobin dissociation curve
Bone	Osteomalacia	
Renal	Nephrocalcinosis Nephrolithiasis	
Pulmonary	↑ Pulmonary vascular resistance	↓ Pulmonary vascular resistance

↑ = increased; ↓ = decreased.

increases or decreases in the anion gap that are not necessarily related to acidosis.

(1) Factors increasing anion gap (other than acidosis): decreased nonsodium cation concentrations (hypokalemia, hypocalcemia, hypomagnesemia: especially if all three are present), laboratory error (falsely increased sodium, falsely decreased chloride or bicarbonate), hyperalbuminemia (transient, seen with albumin infusion)

(2) Factors decreasing anion gap: increased nonsodium cation concentration (hyperkalemia, hypercalcemia, hypermagnesemia), retention of abnormal cation (immunoglobulin G [IgG], globulin, tris[hydroxymethyl] amino methane [TRIS] buffer, lithium), decreased unmeasured anion (hypoalbuminemia), laboratory error (falsely decreased sodium, falsely increased chloride or bicarbonate)

2. Evaluation of metabolic acidosis

a. Measurement of arterial blood gas and serum electrolytes allows separation of a metabolic acidosis into the normal or increased anion gap type. Etiology is further defined:

(1) **History:** inquiring about toxic ingestion, diabetes, urologic surgery, or intraoperative hypotension or renal disease

(2) **Physical examination:** checking for hypoperfusion, adequacy of urine output, and excessive GI fluid loss

(3) **Medication review:** looking for carbonic anhydrase inhibitors or iatrogenically delivered acid loads

(4) **Laboratory tests:** blood-urea nitrogen (BUN), creatinine, urine pH, serum glucose, and ketones to establish the presence of renal failure or ketoacidosis of diabetic or another type. Other laboratory tests that are occasionally useful are serum lactate and alcohol levels and a toxic screen for ingested substances.

b. Lactic acidosis is the most common metabolic acidosis seen in the postoperative critical care setting. Since lactate levels are usually slow to return from the laboratory, lactic acidosis must be suspected in the presence of an increased anion gap once ketosis, uremia, or ingestion has been ruled out. A vigorous search for continuing tissue hypoxia should then be undertaken.

3. Treatment of metabolic acidosis

a. If possible, the underlying cause rather than the acidosis itself should be treated.

b. The precise pHa below which a metabolic acidosis should be treated is an individual judgment. Most clinicians treat an acute pHa less than 7.2. In acutely ill patients, treatment may be initiated at a higher pHa in the following situations:

(1) Impending or ongoing cardiovascular compromise

(2) The presence of marked compensatory hyperventilation

(3) A continuing decline in pHa without identification of the cause of the metabolic acidosis

c. To treat metabolic acidosis, sodium bicarbonate is given parenterally. The initial dose of bicarbonate may be estimated by the following equation:

$$HCO_3^- \text{ deficit in mEq} = (\text{body weight in kg}) \times (0.4) \times (\text{desired } [HCO_3^-] - \text{actual } [HCO_3^-])$$

This is based on the estimated apparent space of distribution of bicarbonate, which is twice as large as the normal extracellular fluid volume. In severe acidosis, with serum bicarbonate values less than 5 mEq per liter, this apparent space may approach 70% of body weight, and it is suggested that the equation be adjusted to reflect this increased space (e.g., 0.7 × body weight in kg). Only one-third to one-half of the calculated dosage should be administered and can be given as follows: 1 ampule of 7.5% $NaHCO_3^-$.

(1) Adding the desired amount of sodium bicarbonate to a volume of crystalloid and infusing it over 3 hours. This method is useful if the source of the acidosis has been removed or if the rate of acid accumulation is not unacceptably rapid.

(2) Intravenous bolus of either the entire ampule or in incremental pushes over several minutes. This is useful in the urgent situation or when fluid restriction is required.

d. Alkali therapy should be targeted to raise serum bicarbonate to no higher than 12–14 mEq per liter; this minimizes the potential risks of rapid parenteral bicarbonate administration (see **g**).

e. In lactic acidosis, it is impossible to define a rate of bicarbonate administration accurately since the rate of lactic acid production is so variable. One must therefore rely on frequent measurements of a patient's acid-base status and response to alkali therapy to determine the subsequent amount of bicarbonate needed.

f. Repeat arterial blood gases should be obtained with ongoing clinical assessment before further replacement is given.

g. Several caveats must be remembered when correcting metabolic acidosis with IV bicarbonate:

(1) Rapid increases in pHa in the patient with an underlying potassium deficit may lead to fatal hypokalemia due to intracellular movement of potassium. Potassium replacement must occur along with correction of acidosis in any patient with a low serum potassium or intracellular potassium deficit.

(2) An extremely low pHa (7.1) may be seen in diabetic ketoacidosis. Controversy exists as to the utility of bicarbonate therapy in this patient population. It has been suggested that bicarbonate be administered to those with severe acidosis (serum bicarbonate of 6–8 mEq/L) in an amount to repair the deficit partially (bicarbonate of 10–12 mEq/L). In those with uncomplicated diabetic ketoacidosis of moderate severity (HCO_3^- >10 mEq/L) and adequate renal function, bicarbonate therapy may be withheld (Cohen, 1982). Rather, the pHa should be followed as insulin, saline, potassium, and IV fluids are infused.

(3) A rapid increase in osmolarity with bolus injection may produce systemic vasodilation.

(4) Large infusions may produce fluid overload, provoke heart failure, or lead to life-threatening hyperosmolarity, hypernatremia, or both. Diuretics may lessen the risk of fluid overload. When renal failure is present, dialysis may be indicated.

h. Recent evidence suggests that a disparity between arterial and mixed venous blood gas determinations may frequently exist in patients during cardiopulmonary arrest. Because significant venous hypercapnia and acidemia may be present in these settings while only modest arterial acidosis is evident, it has been suggested that both central venous and arterial blood samples be measured in assessing acid-base equilibrium (Androgue, 1989). In addition, the use of bicarbonate may contribute to this observed venous hypercapnia. Recent recommendations by the American Heart Association have discouraged its use in cardiopulmonary resuscitation.

D. Metabolic alkalosis occurs because of an accumulation of alkali or loss of acid.

1. Differential diagnosis. Clinically, metabolic alkalosis may be separated into chloride-responsive and chloride-unresponsive types (i.e., responsive or unresponsive to administration of saline).

a. **Chloride responsive** (i.e., volume loss, urinary chloride concentration <10 mEq/L). Causes include the following:
   (1) Vomiting or nasogastric suctioning
   (2) Diuretic therapy
   (3) High-dose carbenicillin or penicillin therapy (where unreabsorbed anions cause hydrogen ion excretion)
   (4) Chloride-wasting diarrhea (rare, as diarrhea usually causes loss of HCO_3 and metabolic acidosis, as noted in **C.1.b.(1)**)
   (5) Villous adenoma

b. **Chloride unresponsive** (i.e., normovolemic, urinary chloride concentration >**20 mEq/L).** Causes include the following:
   (1) Excess mineralocorticoid effect: hyperaldosteronism, Cushing's syndrome, administration of steroids with mineralocorticoid effects, Bartter's syndrome, licorice ingestion, carbonoxolone administration
   (2) Excess alkali: alkali administration, milk-alkali syndrome, massive blood transfusion (citrate in blood is metabolized to carbon dioxide and water, leading to excessive HCO_3)

2. **Evaluation of metabolic alkalosis.** Measurement of serum and urine chloride will generally distinguish between the two major categories of metabolic alkalosis. Subsequent physical examination should disclose any sites of volume loss or lead to a suspicion of excess endogenous steroids. A review of medications may suggest iatrogenically induced chloride depletion or steroid-alkali administration. A morning cortisol level will confirm the diagnosis of excessive circulation steroids.

3. **Treatment of metabolic alkalosis**

a. Correction of the underlying disorder should first be attempted.

b. Unlike acidemic states, pHa above which a metabolic alkalosis should be treated remains unclear. This partly reflects the fact that there is no definite pHa above which sudden cardiovascular compromise is likely to occur. Furthermore, the underlying etiologies often present problems that are more dangerous than the alkalosis itself (e.g., hypovolemia producing hypotension; excessive steroids leading to diabetes and immunocompromised state). In the absence of a defined etiology for metabolic alkalosis or in the presence of a known but uncorrectable cause of metabolic alkalosis, the following guidelines may be used to justify treatment:
   (1) Cardiovascular compromise
   (2) Hypokalemia, especially in the presence of arrhythmias or digitalis therapy
   (3) Neurologic symptoms; paresthesias, tetany
   (4) Respiratory failure. The aim is to increase respiratory drive by lowering pHa. The value of this intervention remains controversial.

c. **Chloride-responsive states.** The initial therapy should be normal saline infusion until normovolemia is established, as judged by adequate urine output. This permits the kidney to excrete excess sodium bicarbonate and correct the alkalosis. Once normovolemia has been established, acetazolamide may be used (see **d**). If there is concomitant potassium depletion, potassium chloride may be added to normal saline, using 40–80 mEq per liter via a peripheral line or up to 120 mEq in 250 ml via a central line. The maximum rate of infusion is about 20 mEq per hour centrally. Continuous ECG monitoring should accompany potassium infusions.

d. **Chloride-unresponsive states.** Acetazolamide may be used to increase urinary excretion of bicarbonate. The starting dose is 250 mg IV every other day, up to 375 mg once a day for 2 days, alternating with a day of rest (intermittent dosage is required to allow the kidney to recover from the inhibitory effect of acetazolamide). Acetazolamide will cause a potassium-wasting diuresis, so both intravascular volume status and potassium level must be monitored.

e. **With renal failure,** sodium bicarbonate may not be easily excreted by the kidney. Also, fluid overload may be a problem. Hydrochloric acid (HCl) may be administered centrally to correct alkalosis. The dosage is calculated as follows:

$$\text{HCl required} = HCO_3^- \text{ excess} = (\text{body weight in kg}) \times (0.4) \times (\text{desired } [HCO_3^-] - \text{actual } [HCO_3^-])$$

Half the dose is administered over 3 hours, using a central line and a maximal concentration of 125 mEq per 250 ml.

E. **Respiratory acidosis** results when alveolar ventilation is insufficient to excrete metabolically produced carbon dioxide. Most commonly, this is due to inadequate ventilation with normal carbon dioxide production. There are several situations, however, where excessive carbon dioxide production, with inability to increase ventilation appropriately, is the underlying abnormality.

1. **Differential diagnosis is extensive** (see Chaps. 1–3).
   a. Inadequate ventilation with normal carbon dioxide production
      (1) Central depression, either drug induced or secondary to respiratory center diseases
      (2) Neuromuscular disorders, as in cervical spinal pathway interruption, neuropathies (e.g., Guillain-Barré syndrome, polio, diphtheria), myopathies, or neuromuscular junction disorders (e.g., myasthenia gravis, residual neuromuscular junction blockade, anticholinergic overdose, hypokalemia, hypermagnesemia)
      (3) Thoracic cage abnormalities
      (4) Upper airway obstruction, as with a kinked or occluded endotracheal tube, tracheal compression (following neck surgery or trauma), tumor or edema, laryngospasm, or a thoracic aortic aneurysm
      (5) Extraparenchymal intrathoracic disease, as with a pleural effusion, pneumo- or hemothorax, pleural scarring, or mesothelioma
      (6) Pulmonary parenchymal diseases
      (7) Massive obesity
      (8) Inadequate ventilator settings
   b. Excess carbon dioxide production with inability to increase ventilation adequately
      (1) Hypermetabolic states, such as fever, malignant hyperthermia, sepsis, or shivering
      (2) Glucose infusion greater than metabolic requirements (with fat synthesis increasing respiratory quotient)
2. **Evaluation of respiratory acidosis.** Details relevant to distinguishing among the etiologies are discussed in Chapters 2 and 3. The basic approach is to separate pulmonary disorders from extrapulmonary disorders by history, physical examination, electrolytes, complete blood count, sputum Gram's stain, and chest radiograph. In intubated patients, respiratory equipment should be examined to ensure adequacy of ventilation and absence of tubing leaks, kinks, or excessive mechanical dead space (with rebreathing).

3. **Treatment of respiratory acidosis** is aimed at improving ventilation. Acutely, this may be done by mask ventilation followed by endotracheal intubation with mechanical ventilation of the patient (see Chap. 1). If the patient is already intubated, the ventilator setting should be increased. Definitive therapy for the underlying disorder should then be instituted. In pure respiratory acidosis (i.e., without an accompanying metabolic acidosis), a low pHa should not be treated with bicarbonate, as this will only increase the carbon dioxide load that needs to be eliminated.

F. **Respiratory alkalosis occurs** when ventilation is greater than required for carbon dioxide production. There are multiple causes, although in the ICU the most common etiology is hyperventilation by mechanical ventilator. This often occurs postoperatively when a patient's carbon dioxide production is reduced because of hyperthermia, residual anesthesia, and residual muscle paralysis. It can also be seen as a compensatory response to hypoxemia.

1. **Differential diagnosis**
   a. **Hyperventilation** can be seen with excess mechanical ventilation. In the spontaneously breathing patient, it can occur with hypoxemia, anxiety, CNS disorders, administration of certain hormones or drugs (e.g., salicylates, catecholamines, doxapram, progesterone, analeptics), sepsis, hyperthyroidism, pregnancy, hepatic insufficiency, mild pulmonary edema, or metabolic acidosis.
   b. **Reduced carbon dioxide production** can be seen with hypothermia (in the absence of shivering), paralysis, drug overdose, or residual general anesthesia.
2. **Evaluation of respiratory alkalosis**
   a. In patients with pure respiratory alkalosis whose breathing is mechanically controlled, ventilator settings should be decreased before further evaluation is undertaken. If oxygenation is adequate when the $PaCO_2$ has been adjusted to normal, further studies are not needed. If the patient is hypoxemic, a search for causes of respiratory failure should be undertaken (see Chaps. 2 and 3).
   b. If hypoxia is not present in the spontaneously breathing patient, then the respiratory alkalosis is probably secondary to a centrally mediated stimulus. The alkalosis is usually an incidental finding and seldom requires further workup, although it may be a sign of one of the aforementioned disease processes. If hypoxemia is present, a search for the causes of respiratory compromise should be undertaken.
3. **Treatment is accomplished** by decreasing controlled ventilation in mechanically ventilated patients. (Hypothermic patients require increased ventilation with rewarming.) For patients breathing spontaneously, only the underlying disorder should be treated, although rebreathing in a paper bag may help the patient hyperventilating due to anxiety neurosis.

G. **Mixed disorders.** With the exception of simultaneous respiratory acidosis and alkalosis, any combination of the aforementioned primary acid-base disorders can exist. In addition, concurrent disease processes may produce multiple metabolic acid-base disorders with opposing or additive effect on pHa.

1. **Diagnosis of a mixed disorder** requires both arterial blood gases and serum electrolytes. As discussed in **III.A,** use of the pHa and $PaCO_2$ distinguishes acidemia from alkalemia and determines whether respiratory acidosis or alkalosis is present. Plotting of blood gas values on Figure 26-2 differentiates compensatory responses to primary disorders from true mixed disorders. Combined respiratory and metabolic disorders are easily distinguished in this manner. Simultaneous metabolic acidosis and alkalosis or concurrent meta-

Table 26-3. Mixed metabolic acid-base disorders

	Metabolic acidosis		Metabolic alkalosis plus metabolic acidosis		
	High AG	Normal AG	High AG	Normal AG	Mixed high and normal AG, metabolic acidosis
K^+	Nl	Nl	↓	↓	Nl
Cl^-	Nl	↑	↓	Nl	↑
HCO_3^-	↓	↓	Nl	Nl	↓
pH	↓	↓	Nl	Nl	↓

↑ = increased; ↓ = decreased; AG = anion gap; Nl = normal.

bolic acidosis of the increased and normal anion gap type are not distinguished on Figure 26-2. Table 26-3 summarizes the electrolyte changes that may help diagnose these mixed disorders. Two trends are evident in this table:

a. An elevated anion gap implies metabolic acidosis, even if the pHa is normal. Thus, except for the conditions listed in **C.1.c,** a search for the cause of acidosis should be undertaken if the anion gap is elevated.

b. Metabolic alkalosis is usually associated with a reduced serum potassium and chloride level. When such an alkalosis is combined with a metabolic acidosis of the high anion gap type, hypokalemia and hypochloremia will result with an elevated anion gap. However, when such a metabolic alkalosis is combined with a normal anion gap acidosis, all laboratory values except potassium tend to return to normal.

2. Once the types of primary disorders are established, the search for the etiology is continued as previously described in **III** for primary disorders.

3. Treatment is aimed at the underlying disease processes. Two primary disorders producing canceling effects on pHa will lessen the urgency to treat the acid-base disturbance itself. Conversely, two disorders producing additive effects on pHa may require treatment before diagnostic studies are completed.

Selected References

Androgué, H. J., Rashad, M. N., Gorin, A. B., et al. Assessing acid-base status in circulatory failure. Differences between arterial and central venous blood. *N. Engl. J. Med.* 320:1312, 1989.

Beck, L. H. (ed.). Symposium on body fluid and electrolyte disorders. *Med. Clin. North Am.* 65:321, 1981.

Cohen, J. J., and Kassirer, J. P. *Acid-Base.* Boston: Little, Brown, 1982.

Emmett, M., and Narns, R. G. Clinical use of the anion gap. *Medicine* 56:38, 1977.

Gabow, P. A., Kaehny, W. D., Fennessey, P. V., et al. Diagnostic importance of an increased serum anion gap. *N. Engl. J. Med.* 303:854, 1980.

Hanson, G. C., and Wright, P. L. *The Medical Management of the Critically Ill.* London: Academic Press, 1978.

Leaf, A. L., and Cotran, R. S. *Renal Pathophysiology.* New York: Oxford University Press, 1976.

Morris, L. R., Murphy, M. B., and Kitabchi, A. E. Bicarbonate therapy in severe diabetic ketoacidosis. *Ann. Intern. Med.* 105:836, 1986.
Muzock, B. A. Controversies in lactic acidosis: Implications in critically ill patients. *J.A.M.A.* 258:497, 1987.
Narins, R. G., and Emmett, M. Simple and mixed acid-base disorders: A practical approach. *Medicine* 59:161, 1980.
Oh, M. S., and Carroll, H. J. The anion gap. *N. Engl. J. Med.* 297:814, 1977.

Appendix

Approach to Acid-Base Disorders: Case Studies

The following case histories have been selected to illustrate the approach to acid-base disturbances. By utilizing the information presented in this chapter, including pertinent clues from the clinical history, calculation of expected compensatory responses, plotting of blood gas values on Figures 26-1 and 26-2, and guides to therapy, a solution to most acid-base problems can be easily obtained. In approaching these problems, one should, in a stepwise fashion, (1) examine first the pH, then the PCO_2 and HCO_3^-, and finally calculate the anion gap; (2) note whether the patient is acidemic or alkalemic; (3) calculate the expected compensatory responses using Table 26-1 and determine if the disorder is simple or mixed; (4) arrive at a conclusion regarding the cause(s) of the acid-base imbalance. The case studies illustrate these basic principles. For each case summary, apply these four steps and establish the nature of the acid-base imbalance.

Case Study 1

The patient is a 45-year-old man with progressive renal failure, admitted to the hospital because of weakness and lethargy. On examination, his blood pressure was 180/110 and respirations 22 per minute. The following admission laboratory values were obtained:

Na	135 mEq/L	Cr	14 mg/dl
K	5.4 mEq/L	pH	7.32
Cl	101 mEq/L	PCO_2	24 mm Hg
HCO_3	12 mEq/L	anion gap	22 mEq/L
BUN	155 mg/dl		

This patient is acidemic based on his pH. Since the PCO_2 is 24 mm Hg and the HCO_3^- is 12 mEq/L (normal 24–25), a metabolic acidosis is present. The anticipated compensatory change in the PCO_2 is $[PCO_2] = 1.2 \times [HCO_3^-]$ or 1.2×12 mEq/L = 14 mm Hg or roughly an expected PCO_2 of 26 mm Hg, an appropriate degree of secondary hypocapnia—hence, a simple metabolic acidosis. The anion gap of 22 mEq/L is high (normal 10–12 mEq/L) and consistent with the known diagnosis of chronic renal failure.

Case Study 2

A 71-year-old man was admitted to the hospital complaining of anorexia, abdominal pain, and vomiting. An upper GI series demonstrated gastric outlet obstruction associated with peptic ulcer disease. A nasogastric tube was inserted, intermittent suction begun, and large volumes of fluid were removed. Subsequent laboratory values revealed:

Na	141 mEq/L	pH	7.52
K	3.0 mEq/L	PCO_2	52 mm Hg
Cl	86 mEq/L	[H]	30 mEq/L
HCO_3^-	42 mEq/L	anion gap	13 mEq/L

Adapted with permission from J. J. Cohen and J. P. Kassirer. *Acid-Base.* Boston: Little, Brown, 1982, pp. 415–446.

This man is alkalemic. The elevated PCO_2 and HCO_3^-, in contrast to Case Study 1, confirm a metabolic alkalosis. The compensatory rise in PCO_2 would approximate (0.7) (HCO_3^-) or (0.7) (18), approximately a 13 mm Hg increase in PCO_2, nearly equivalent to the observed PCO_2 of 52 mm Hg. Thus, a simple metabolic alkalosis is present. Had the urinary chloride concentration been measured, it would be less than 10 mEq/L, establishing this as a chloride responsive alkalosis secondary to extensive nasogastric suction. Treatment with IV sodium chloride and supplemental potassium chloride will enhance renal bicarbonate excretion, correct hypokalemia, replete intravascular volume, and restore normal acid-base equilibrium.

Case Study 3

A 48-year-old man with insulin-dependent diabetes mellitus presented to the emergency ward with a two-day history of chest pain, anorexia, and nausea. He had recently stopped his insulin injections. On admission he was hypotensive, tachycardic, mildly tachypnic, and complaining of chest pain. His skin was cool, and an ECG showed evidence of a large anterior wall myocardial infarction. Admission laboratory values were as follows:

Na	128 mEq/L	BUN	35 mg/dl
K	5.9 mEq/L	Cr	1.8 mg/dl
Cl	92 mEq/L	pH	7.41
HCO_3^-	8 mEq/L	PCO_2	14 mm Hg
glucose	520 mEq/L	PaO_2	50 mm Hg
lactate	13 mEq/L	[H]	39 mEq/L
ketones	2+	anion gap	28 mEq/L

The acid-base status is normohydria, with a pH within the normal range. The low bicarbonate indicates the existence of a metabolic acidosis, confirmed by the elevated anion gap. The anticipated decrement in the PCO_2 would be 1.2 × HCO_3^-; or 1.2 × 16 = 19; or a PCO_2 of 21 mm Hg. This is higher than the measured PCO_2 and is evidence for a greater degree of hyperventilation than that expected for a normal compensatory response to the acidemia. Hence, the diagnosis is the coexistence of a respiratory alkalosis, presumably on the basis of severe chest pain and hypoxemia, yielding a mixed acid-base disorder. The elevated anion gap is likely a result of the lactic acidosis accompanying cardiogenic shock; diabetic ketosis also contributes a minor degree of unmeasured anions. When the values for pH, PCO_2, and HCO_3^- are plotted on the nomogram depicted in Figure 26-2, they fall within zone 10, a mixed metabolic acidosis and respiratory alkalosis.

Case Study 4

An elderly man with chronic hypertension on diuretic therapy was found comatose on the street and brought to the emergency ward. On examination, the patient was severely hypotensive, tachycardic, and obtunded. He was immediately intubated and ventilated. Subsequent evaluation revealed sepsis from pneumococcal peritonitis. Hypotension persisted despite high-dose vasopressors. Initial laboratory data revealed:

Na	139 mEq/L	anion gap	39 mEq/L
K	3.9 mEq/L	pH	6.86
Cl	84 mEq/L	PCO_2	81 mm Hg
HCO_3^-	16 mEq/L	$[H^+]$	138 mEq/L

This patient is clearly acidemic with a dangerously low pH. A metabolic acidosis, as demonstrated by a low HCO_3^- and an elevated anion gap, is occurring concurrently with a respiratory acidosis, reflected in a markedly elevated PCO_2. In addition, an element of metabolic alkalosis is evident because the increase in anion gap (AG = 27 mEq/L) is not matched by the modest decrement in the HCO_3^- and was much higher than normal in the absence of a metabolic acidosis, thus masking the true fall in the serum HCO_3^-; hence, a triple acid-base disturbance is the diagnosis. The acidemia was a consequence of lactate accumulation from septic shock, and carbon dioxide retention from CNS depression. The alkalosis may have been precipitated by chronic diuretic use and diminished oral intake. Mechanical ventilation and bicarbonate therapy, in addition to therapy directed at the underlying infection, are indicated. Figure 26-2 does not distinguish between a simultaneous metabolic acidosis—alkalosis or concurrent metabolic acidosis of the normal and elevated anion gap type. Clinical clues from the history and laboratory tests, as well as a knowledge of the expected changes in HCO_3^-, PCO_2 and anion gap, will help clarify these complex disturbances.

27

Neonatal Resuscitation

James K. Alifimoff

I. Pediatric resuscitation
- **A. Basic life support (BLS)**
  - **1. Airway/breathing**
  - **2. Circulation**
- **B. Advanced life support**
  - **1. Occurrence and resuscitation of cardiac arrest in children**
  - **2. Administration of drugs and fluids**
  - **3. Drugs for pediatric ALS**
    - **a. Oxygen**
    - **b. Epinephrine**
    - **c. Sodium bicarbonate**
    - **d. Cardiac output in infants**
    - **e. Glucose**
    - **f. Isoproterenol**
    - **g. Calcium**
    - **h. Ventricular fibrillation**
  - **4. Defibrillation of the pediatric patient**
    - **a. Size of electrode paddles**
    - **b. Electrode interface**
    - **c. Defibrillation settings**
    - **d. Children on digoxin**

II. Newborn resuscitation
- **A. Temperature regulation**
- **B. Assessment of the newborn**
- **C. Apgar score**
- **D. Intervention based on Apgar score**
  - **1. Apgar score 8–10**
  - **2. Apgar score 5–7**
  - **3. Apgar score 3–4**
  - **4. Apgar score 0–2**
- **E. Specific resuscitative measures**
  - **1. Airway**
  - **2. Breathing**
    - **a. Bag and mask ventilation**
    - **b. Endotracheal intubation**
  - **3. Technique of endotracheal intubation**
  - **4. Cardiac compressions**
  - **5. Drugs and fluids administration**
    - **a. Technique of umbilical vein cannulation**
    - **b. Epinephrine atropine and lidocaine administration**
  - **6. Neonatal ALS drugs**
    - **a. Epinephrine**
    - **b. $NaHCO_3$**
    - **c. Dextrose**
    - **d. Calcium and atropine**
    - **e. Naloxone**
  - **7. Hypovolemia**
    - **a. Hypovolemia consideration**
    - **b. Symptoms and signs of hypovolemia**
    - **c. Correction of suspected intravascular volume deficit**

Significant anatomical as well as physiological differences between adults and children have direct bearing on how resuscitation is performed in these groups of patients. In contrast to the adult population, cardiac arrest in neonatal patients is rarely a primary event; rather, it is usually due to hypoxemia as a result of airway obstruction from a variety of etiologies. For this reason, securing an airway and providing adequate ventilation are the primary concerns. For the purposes of this chapter, neonates are less than 1 month of age, infants are from 1 month to 1 year of age, and children are from 1 to 8 years of age. Children over 8 years of age may be treated as described in Chapter 6.

I. Pediatric resuscitation

A. Basic life support (BLS)

1. Airway/breathing

a. Open the airway using head-tilt, neck-lift, or chin support. Care should be taken not to hyperextend the neck in infants as this may obstruct the airway.

b. Ventilation can initially be performed with a bag and appropriately sized mask at a rate of 30 breaths per minute in infants and 20 breaths per minute in children. If gastric distention inhibits adequate bag-mask ventilation, intubate the trachea, and then place an orogastric tube to decompress the stomach.

c. In children, the narrowest portion of the trachea is subglottic as compared to the level of the vocal cords in adults. Thus, in children, an oversized endotracheal tube (ETT) will pass through the vocal cords only to meet obstruction at the cricoid cartilage. Appropriately sized ETTs are given in Table 27-1.

d. Due to the short distance from vocal cords to carina, it is important to auscultate breath sounds bilaterally to detect mainstem bronchial intubation, particularly in infants and neonates. Table 27-2 provides a useful guide to ETT position.

2. Circulation. To determine pulselessness in infants, the brachial or femoral artery is palpated rather than the carotid because the infant's short neck makes palpation of this artery difficult. In children, either the carotid or the femoral is suitable.

a. In infants, the heart is lower in the mediastinum than previously appreciated. To locate the appropriate position to perform cardiac compression, a line is drawn between the nipples, and compressions are performed one finger breadth below this line. For children, the correct hand position is determined as it is in adults.

b. The tips of two fingers are sufficient for performing compressions in infants. Alternatively, the infant's chest may be encircled with the hands and the sternum compressed with both thumbs. The latter

Table 27-1. Endotracheal tube sizes

Age	Size (internal diameter, mm)
Premature	
<1,250 g	2.5
1,250–3,000 g	3.0
Full term newborn–12 months	3.5
12–20 months	4.0
2 years	4.5
>2 years	$\frac{\text{Age (yr)} + 16}{4}$

Table 27-2. Endotracheal tube position

Age	Endotracheal tube position at alveolar ridge (cm)
Full term	8–9
3–12 months	10
12–24 months	12
>2 yrs	$\frac{\text{Age (yrs)} + 12}{2}$

technique is probably more effective. In either case, remember to place the infant on a firm, flat surface.

c. Respective rates and depth of compression during BLS–cardiopulmonary resuscitation (CPR) as well as compression-ventilation ratios are presented in Table 27-3. An important difference between CPR in the adult and pediatric populations is the need to interrupt compressions systematically to allow for ventilation in pediatric patients. The use of this **programmed breath** avoids hypoventilation, which may occur when chest compressions compete with ventilation in small patients.

B. Advanced life support (ALS)

1. The majority of pediatric cardiac arrests are in infants. Although the most common etiology is respiratory obstruction with secondary cardiac arrest, the principles of resuscitation are the same as those in adults, and it is important to approach all arrests with a similar therapeutic scheme. The first step is always the prompt initiation of BLS-CPR. Intravenous access is then established, and drugs are administered. Drug doses in milligram per kilogram, however, must be recalculated according to the regimens detailed below.

2. **Administration of drugs and fluids**

   a. Drugs and fluids may be administered through a peripheral IV or central venous pressure (CVP) line or by intraosseous or endotracheal injection.

   b. In children, peripheral IVs may be started in the median basilic, antecubital, or cephalic veins of the upper extremity, although these may be difficult to cannulate in obese patients. Scalp veins are the least desirable because attempted cannulation can interfere with BLS-CPR. As an alternative, the femoral vein allows access to the central circulation when a catheter of suitable length is used. Saphenous vein cutdowns can be quickly performed by skilled individuals. Sites of central venous access are the same as in adults.

Table 27-3. Pediatric cardiopulmonary resuscitation

Age	Ventilations	Compressions/ minute	Ventilation-compression ratio	Depth (inches)
Neonate	40–60	120	1:3	0.5–0.75
Infant	20–24	100–120	1:5	0.5–1.0
Young child (1–4 yrs)	20	100	1:5	1.0–1.5
Older child (>4 yrs)	16	80	1:5	1.5–2.0

c. Intraosseous injection is another method of vascular access that can allow for volume expansion as well as drug administration. A styletted spinal or bone marrow needle is inserted into the anterior tibial bone marrow to gain access to the circulation.

d. As in adults, atropine, epinephrine, and lidocaine may be administered endotracheally. Dilution of these drugs in up to 10 ml of sterile saline (depending on the size of the child) will ensure a volume sufficient to reach the alveoli. **$NaHCO_3$ and $CaCl_2$ should never be administered in this manner.**

e. Intracardiac administration of drugs is not recommended during external cardiac compressions. Endotracheal administration avoids the risks of pneumothorax and intramyocardial injection.

3. **Drugs for pediatric ALS**

   a. **Oxygen.** All patients should be ventilated with 100% oxygen during resuscitation. Although the potentially toxic effects of oxygen on the lungs and retina are of concern, oxygen should never be withheld or used in a concentration of less than 100% during resuscitation.

   b. **Epinephrine,** when used in large doses as recommended, primarily produces an alpha adrenergic response that results in vasoconstriction and enhancement of systemic as well as coronary perfusion pressures. It is indicated for asystole, bradyarrhythmias, electromechanical dissociation, and ventricular fibrillation (VF).
      (1) Initial dose of 0.01 mg per kg IV or by ETT (0.1 ml/kg of 1:10,000 solution)
      (2) Repeat q5min.

   c. **Sodium bicarbonate.** After adequate ventilation and administration of epinephrine, $NaHCO_3$ may be given when there is documented acidosis or prolonged cardiac arrest.
      (1) Initial dose of 1 mEq per kilogram for IV or intraosseous administration
      (2) Repeat doses of 0.5 mEq per kg q10min.
      (3) If arterial blood gases (ABGs) are available, subsequent doses should be calculated according to the base deficit.

   d. Cardiac output in infants is rate dependent due to their noncompliant ventricles. Thus, **atropine** is indicated in the treatment of bradycardia (heart rate less than 80), even in the absence of hypotension. It may also be used in asystole. **Since bradycardia is often the result of hypoxemia, adequacy of ventilation and oxygenation should always be ensured.** Initial dose of 0.02 mg/kg IV, IM, or by ETT, with a minimum dose of 0.1 mg to avoid paradoxical bradycardia.

   e. **Glucose** is important in resuscitation of pediatric patients, and a rapid blood glucose concentration should be obtained during resuscitation; however, treatment of suspected hypoglycemia should not await determination of blood glucose concentration. Administer 0.5–1.0 g per kilogram of 25% dextrose in water or 10% dextrose in water (2–4 ml/kg of 25% dextrose in water or 5–10 ml/kg of 10% dextrose in water).

   f. **Isoproterenol** may be used to treat persistent or refractory bradyarrhythmias. Initial rate is 0.1 μg/kg/minute and titrated to effect.

   g. **Calcium** is used for the treatment of documented or suspected hypocalcemia. Additionally, it is used for antagonizing the effects of hyperkalemia, hypermagnesemia, and calcium channel blocker overdose.

   h. **Ventricular fibrillation is rare** in the pediatric population and should prompt consideration of metabolic causes such as hypoxemia, hypothermia, hypoglycemia, or calcium and potassium abnormalities. **Lidocaine** is administered for ventricular tachycardia or if VF does not immediately respond to countershock.

(1) Initial dose of 1 mg per kilogram IV or by ETT or intraosseous infusion

(2) Repeat dose may be administered in 10 minutes and a continuous infusion started at a rate of 20–50 μg/kg/min.

4. **Defibrillation of the pediatric patient.** Heart block and bradyarrhythmias, rather than VF, are the usual causes of cardiac arrest in pediatric patients. For this reason, defibrillation should be performed only when ECG monitoring shows VF.
   - **a.** Size of electrode paddles. Since the propagated current is directly proportional to the size of the defibrillating electrode, the largest possible diameter that allows reasonable separation should be used. In infants, a 4.5-cm electrode is adequate; an 8-cm paddle is suitable for older children.
   - **b.** Electrode interface. Because of the patient's small size, it is relatively easy for a bridge of conductive ointment to form between the individual electrodes. This must be avoided because it will lead to ineffective defibrillation.
   - **c.** The initial defibrillation setting is 2 J per kilogram. If ineffective, this should be doubled and repeated twice. If defibrillation does not occur with higher doses, more aggressive correction of acid-base abnormalities is warranted.
   - **d.** Defibrillation of children on digoxin can result in irreversible cardiac arrest. In these patients, defibrillation should commence with the lowest energy that the defibrillator will deliver and then be cautiously increased.

II. Newborn resuscitation. Resuscitation of the neonate presents unique anatomical as well as physiological concerns. Frequently it is necessary to have three people involved: one to secure the airway and ventilate the patient, one to perform cardiac compressions, and a third to establish IV access, which may be difficult. It is important that a single experienced individual direct the team effort. Modern techniques of fetal monitoring have enabled us to predict neonates who have the greatest risk of requiring resuscitation. Thus, in many circumstances, it will be possible to prepare beforehand and approach the situation with readiness.

A. Temperature regulation

1. Although all neonates are subject to heat loss, asphyxiated neonates are particularly vulnerable to hypothermia.
2. To minimize heat loss, the delivery suite should be kept warm. In addition, all neonates should be:
   - **a.** Completely dried of amniotic fluid
   - **b.** Placed under a radiant warmer

B. Assessment of the newborn. The initial preparation and evaluation of the newborn should be systematic.

1. The oropharynx should be suctioned with a bulb-type suction by the obstetrician at the time of delivery.
2. Place the baby under a radiant warming device.
3. Repeat oropharyngeal suctioning. If the amniotic fluid is meconium stained, manage as described in **V.5.a–d.**
4. Dry the head, torso, and extremities.
5. Determine Apgar score.

C. Apgar score

1. Newborns are assessed at 1 and 5 minutes after delivery using an objective scoring system consisting of five categories: **a**ppearance, **p**ulse, **g**rimace, **a**ctivity, and **r**espiration. A score of 0–2 is possible in each category; thus, a perfect score is 10. However, few newborns achieve a 10 since all have some degree of acrocyanosis. The 1-minute

Apgar score correlates well with intrapartum asphyxia, and the 5-minute score appears to correlate with eventual neurologic outcome. The Apgar score is summarized in Table 27-4.

2. Neonatal depression is usually due to uteroplacental insufficiency, maternal medication (e.g., opiates), or neonatal disease.

D. Intervention based on Apgar score

1. **Apgar score 8–10.** These infants require no specific treatment. Monitoring must be performed for at least 5 additional minutes to be certain that hypoventilation does not occur, and care must be taken to prevent hypothermia.
2. **Apgar score 5–7.** These infants have had minor asphyxia during birth and require stimulation and an oxygen-enriched environment. Stimulation can be accomplished by vigorous rubbing of the baby's back or by gentle slapping on the soles of the feet. Oxygen can be supplied from a Mapleson-type resuscitation bag: Ambu bags deliver oxygen only during positive-pressure ventilation and thus are ineffective for this purpose.
3. **Apgar score 3–4.** Bag and mask ventilation should be started if stimulation does not establish adequate respiration or if the heart rate decreases to fewer than 100 beats per minute. If the heart rate drops to fewer than 60 to 80 beats per minute despite ventilation with 100% oxygen, CPR should be started.
4. **Apgar score 0–2.** These infants require immediate initiation of CPR.

E. Specific resuscitative measures

1. **Airway**
   a. Suctioning is important because blood, mucus, or meconium can obstruct the airway. A bulb and syringe suction device is most appropriate since it is not dependent on external sources of power. In addition, descent into the hypopharynx is limited. Following suction of the oropharynx, each nare should be suctioned to ensure patency because neonates are obligate nose breathers.
   b. Suctioning should be limited to 10-second intervals, and ventilation with 100% oxygen (either spontaneously or with assistance) should be done between attempts.
   c. Monitoring of the heart rate is necessary because suctioning can cause bradycardia secondary to vagal reflex or hypothermia.
   d. If airway obstruction is below the level of the vocal cords, intubation and suctioning should be performed. Suction only as the catheter is being withdrawn to minimize damage to the tracheal mucosa.

Table 27-4. Apgar score

	Points assigned		
Clinical sign	0	1	2
Appearance	Cyanotic	Acrocyanotic	Pink
Pulse (determined by auscultation of the precordium or by palpation of the umbilical artery)	< 60	60-100	> 100
Grimace or reflex Irritability to oropharyngeal suctioning	No response	Weak cry	Vigorous
Activity or muscle tone	Flaccid	Weak	Good
Respiratory effort	Apnea	Irregular	Regular

e. The presence of watery or thin meconium does not mandate routine endotracheal intubation. However, meconium aspiration has probably occurred if there is **thick, particulate, meconium-stained amniotic fluid.** In such cases, patients should be treated as follows:
   (1) Immediate suctioning after delivery of the head by the obstetrician
   (2) Laryngoscopy is performed and the trachea intubated. Suction is applied directly from the wall suction to the ETT as it is being withdrawn.
   (3) Repeat (2) until meconium is no longer obtained from the ETT.
   (4) The heart rate should be monitored during endotracheal suctioning either with a stethoscope or by palpation of the apical or umbilical artery pulsation. **Suctioning should not be carried to the point of severe bradycardia or cardiac arrest.**

2. **Breathing**
   a. **Bag and mask ventilation.** Ventilatory rate of 30–40 breaths per minute at an airway pressure of 20–30 cm H_2O should provide adequate minute ventilation. Higher inflation pressure, however, may be required in asphyxiated infants. Adequacy of ventilation is assessed by symmetrical chest expansion and equal breath sounds in the midaxillary line. A variety of face mask sizes should be available: size 0 for premature infants (<2,500 g) to size 1 for the full-term neonates.
   b. **Endotracheal intubation.** Types and sizes of endotracheal tubes are summarized in Table 27-3. Cole tubes, which have tapered ends, are to be avoided since the distal ends are readily occluded with secretions.

3. **Technique of endotracheal intubation**
   a. Place the neonate in the sniffing position and perform laryngoscopy with a Miller blade (size 1 for full-term infants and size 0 for preterm infants). The tip of the blade is placed in the vallecular, although occasionally it is necessary to elevate the epiglottis directly to expose the glottic opening.
   b. A stylet will provide rigidity to the ETT and facilitate intubation; however, care must be taken to keep the stylet within the ETT to avoid damage to the trachea.
   c. **Endotracheal tube position.** In full-term neonates, the distance from the glottis to the carina is 5 cm. The ETT should be 2.4 cm below the level of the cords. Most tubes are marked for this purpose.
   d. In premature infants, the distance from the glottis to the carina is less than 5 cm. In these patients, limit the ETT length to 1–1.5 cm below the cords. Remember that these small distances make neonates particularly vulnerable to extubation or endobronchial intubation during resuscitation, mandating added vigilance.

4. **Cardiac compressions.** If the heart rate decreases to fewer than 80 beats per minute and does not respond to ventilation with 100% oxygen, external cardiac compressions should be started. The preferred approach in neonates is the **chest encircling technique** with overlapping thumbs compressing in the midline one finger breadth below the nipple line. With larger infants, adequate compressions may require three fingers, with the opposite hand supporting the back. The sternum is depressed $\frac{1}{2}$–$\frac{3}{4}$ inch at a rate of 120 compressions per minute, while lung inflation is at a rate of 40 per minute, to yield a ventilation : compression ratio of 1 : 3 (Table 27-3). As in pediatric CPR, a pause for an effective programmed breath is allowed to coordinate ventilations and compressions. If no response occurs within 30 seconds, appropriate drug therapy should be started.

5. Drugs and fluids can be administered through the umbilical vein, peripheral veins, or ETT. The umbilical vein is the preferred route because it is easily located and accessed. Peripheral vein cannulation of either scalp or extremity veins may be difficult particularly during resuscitation. Epinephrine, atropine, and lidocaine can be given via ETT. The **technique of umbilical vein cannulation** follows:

a. The umbilical cord stump and surrounding skin are aseptically prepared and draped.

b. A sterile umbilical tape is placed at the base of the umbilical stump but is not tightened.

c. The cord is trimmed with a scalpel 1 cm above the skin attachment, while firmly holding the base to prevent bleeding.

d. The umbilical vein is identified. There are two umbilical arteries and one vein. The arteries have thick, muscular walls; the umbilical vein is the thin-walled, largest vessel.

e. An umbilical catheter (size 5F for full-terms and 3.5F for prematures), flushed with heparinized saline and connected to a three-way stopcock to eliminate air, is inserted to a distance sufficient to gain access to the central circulation. If resistance is encountered or if there is no free flow of blood, insert the catheter 2.5–5 cm beyond the end of the cord.

f. Obtain a blood sample for pH determination and attach a syringe to the stopcock for administration of drugs.

g. Strict attention must be paid to prevention of an air embolus, which can be fatal in neonates with a patent foramen ovale.

h. If bleeding occurs, the tie at the base of the cord stump is tightened.

i. Hypertonic solutions such as 25–50% dextrose in water, undiluted $NaHCO_3$, or $CaCl_2$ should not be administered via this route because they may cause parenchymal damage to the liver.

j. The catheter is usually removed following resuscitation if the infant is stable because of the dangers of infection and portal vein thrombosis.

k. Epinephrine atropine and lidocaine may be administered through the ETT.

6. Neonatal ALS drugs

a. Epinephrine is indicated when there is bradycardia or asystole. Use an initial dose of 0.1–0.3 ml per kilogram of 1 : 10,000 solution IV or by ETT, and repeat q5min.

b. Administration of **$NaHCO_3$** following brief arrests or an episode of bradycardia is not recommended. After prolonged arrest, however, $NaHCO_3$ administration will decrease hydrogen ion load, improve myocardial contractility, and optimize catecholamine action. Since there is an association between $NaHCO_3$ infusion and intraventricular hemorrhage in premature infants related to the high osmolar load, the neonatal preparation (0.5 mEq/ml) should be administered slowly and with adequate ventilation.

(1) Initial dose of 1 mEq/kg, administered over 2 minutes

(2) Subsequent dose of 0.5 mEq/kg IV q10min during the resuscitation

(3) When ABGs are available, subsequent doses are based on the base deficit.

c. Dextrose. Hypoglycemia from diminished glycogen stores is common in asphyxiated infants. Since glucose is the primary metabolic substrate of the neonatal myocardium, hypoglycemia may produce poor myocardial function. Rapid infusion of dextrose will correct unrecognized hypoglycemia; however, determination of blood glucose concentrations should not delay administration of glucose.

(1) Initial dose of 0.5 g per kilogram IV (2 ml/kg of 25% dextrose in water)
(2) Following this, a continuous infusion of 10% dextrose in water should be started at a rate of 4 ml/kg/hour or less.

d. **Calcium and atropine** are no longer recommended during the acute phase of neonatal resuscitation.

e. **Naloxone** is a specific competitive antagonist of narcotics at opiate receptors. It is indicated for neonates with respiratory depression following maternal administration of narcotics. This most commonly occurs when narcotics are administered to the mother within 4 hours of delivery. Initial management of the respiratory depression, however, should be with controlled or assisted ventilation until naloxone can be administered. The duration of action of naloxone is shorter than that of most other narcotics. Continued apnea monitoring is required. In the newborn child of the narcotic addict, naloxone may precipitate acute narcotic withdrawal syndrome.

Initial dose of 0.01 mg per kilogram IV repeated q2–3min. May also be given by ETT or, if perfusion is adequate, intramuscularly or subcutaneously.

7. **Hypovolemia**

a. **Hypovolemia** should be considered as an etiology of arrest in any neonate who requires resuscitation.

b. **Symptoms and signs of hypovolemia**
(1) Pre- or intrapartum hemorrhage
(2) Faint pulses with normal heart rate, tachycardia, bradycardia
(3) Severe asphyxia
(4) Hypotension
(5) Persistent pallor after adequate oxygenation and circulatory support are provided

c. Correction of suspected intravascular volume deficit can be accomplished with the following initial amounts and repeated as necessary.
(1) 10 ml per kilogram of 5% albumin
(2) 10 ml per kilogram of lactated Ringer's solution
(3) 10 ml per kilogram of O-negative whole blood, crossmatched with maternal blood

Selected References

American Heart Association. Standards and guidelines for cardiopulmonary resuscitation (CPR) and emergency cardiac care (ECC). *J. Am. Med. Assoc.* 255:2095, 1986.

American Heart Association. *Textbook of Neonatal Resuscitation.* Dallas: American Heart Association, 1987.

American Heart Association. *Textbook of Pediatric Advanced Life Support.* Dallas: American Heart Association, 1988.

28

Pediatric Cardiopulmonary Resuscitation

Jesse D. Roberts, Jr. and I. David Todres

The basic principles of cardiopulmonary resuscitation are the same regardless of the patient's age. However, the significant developmental and physiological differences presented by pediatric patients affect the responses to such efforts. This chapter stresses these differences within a general approach for successful resuscitation.

I. **Airway management.** Primary cardiac arrest is a rare event in pediatric patients. Fastidious attention to airway management with provision of adequate oxygenation and ventilation is often the extent of resuscitation needed.

A. **Airway differences among newborns, infants, children, and adults**

1. The relative dolichocephaly of newborns and infants promotes neck flexion and airway closure while in the supine position. This is especially problematic in those with malar hypoplasia and micrognathia (e.g., Pierre-Robin and Treacher Collins syndromes).
2. The tongue is relatively large and easily obstructs the upper airway.
3. Newborns are obligate nasal breathers until approximately 3–5 months of age. Congenital or acquired mechanical obstruction of the upper airway can lead to difficulties during breathing.

B. **The primary maneuver for establishment of an airway** is neck extension with placement of the head in an exaggerated sniffing position. In cases where airway obstruction persists, jaw thrusting by anterior displacement of the mandible allows anterior displacement of the tongue off the palate, promoting patency of the airway. Airway appliances aid in tongue displacement and airway establishment.

1. Nasopharyngeal airways may be better tolerated in partially conscious children. Their utility in newborns and infants is hampered by increased airway resistance due to their narrow caliber.
2. Oropharyngeal airways may be helpful for tongue displacement. Attention must be given to airway position and size. Oral airways may promote obstruction by posteriorly displacing the tongue or closing the epiglottis.

C. **Endotracheal intubation** is useful in establishment of a patent airway. Continuation of other resuscitative procedures, however, should not await this.

1. Many different types of laryngoscopes are available. The choice is determined by personal preference and the patient's size (Table 28-1). Straight blades are designed to lift the epiglottis directly, and curved blades are designed to enter the vallecula and lift the epiglottis indirectly. It is important to notice important differences between pediatric and adult anatomy.
   a. The larynx is higher in the neck (C3–C4) and often allows easier visualization in infants and children.

Table 28-1. Cardiopulmonary resuscitation in children

Age	Compression rate	Depth	Ventilation-compression ratios
Newborn	120	0.5–1.0	1:3
Infant	120	0.5–1.0	1:5
Child	100	1.0–1.5	1:5
Adolescent	80	1.0–1.5	1:5
Adult	60	1.5–2.0	1:5

b. The infant epiglottis is angled away from the axis of the trachea and may be more difficult to lift with the tip of the laryngoscope blade.

c. The axis of the vocal cords in the infant is not perpendicular to the axis of the trachea; hence, endotracheal tubes may become caught in the anterior commissure.

2. The proper endotracheal tube allows cannulation of the airway and delivery of adequate ventilatory pressures without significant gas leakage. The narrowest portion of the airway in adults is at the level of the vocal cords; it is at the level of the cricoid cartilage in the infant. An air leak at a delivered pressure of 30 cm H_2O pressure indicates proper fit. In children below 7 years of age, an uncuffed endotracheal tube is generally used.

3. Guidelines for endotracheal tube selection and placement

a. An estimate of internal diameter can be given by the following formula:

$$\text{mm internal diameter} = (\text{age in years}/4) + 4$$

b. When a cuffed endotracheal tube is used, a size 0.5–1 mm smaller than the recommended uncuffed endotracheal tube should initially be tried. Check for leak with the endotracheal cuff uninflated.

c. Endotracheal intubation should be assessed by chest expansion, lack of epigastric distension, presence of tube condensation, and capnography, if available. If there is any question, direct laryngoscopy will confirm tube placement. One should not await a chest x ray.

d. The depth of insertion is best judged by observing symmetric chest expansion and breath sounds. This may not be observed despite adequate positioning in the presence of pneumothorax and airway obstruction. When repositioning the endotracheal tube in unstable patients, it is often prudent to do so under direct laryngoscopy.

D. Transtracheal oxygen is useful in situations where upper airway pathology causes obstruction that cannot be relieved by the procedures already noted.

1. **Percutaneous cricothyroidotomy.** With the neck hyperextended, the trachea may be stabilized between the thumb and long finger of the nondominant hand while the index finger locates the cricothyroid membrane. An appropriately sited IV catheter attached to a 3-ml syringe is advanced posteriorly and slightly caudadly while aspirating through the cricothyroid membrane. Once air is aspirated indicating entry into the trachea, the catheter is advanced, and the 3-ml syringe is placed on the cannula. Aspiration again confirms position. An 8-mm endotracheal tube adapter is placed onto the syringe barrel, facilitating connection to ventilating bags.

2. **Emergent tracheostomy** is best performed by the one most skilled in its method. The neck is hyperextended and prepared in a sterile fashion. A transverse incision is made at the level of the thyroid isthmus. Midline dissection is performed with meticulous attention to hemostasis by spreading the strap muscles vertically. Stay sutures are placed around the second and third or third and fourth cricoid rings lateral to midline; a vertical tracheostomy incision is made between them. The tracheostomy tube is placed, and symmetric ventilation is assessed. The tube is secured in place.

II. **Ventilatory management.** Oxygen consumption is approximately 7 ml/kg/minute in infants. Neonatal oxygen consumption is nearly twice that of adults. This corresponds to a significantly higher carbon dioxide production and ventilatory need. Typical ventilatory rates are shown in Table 28-1.

Table 28-2. Approximate developmental parameters

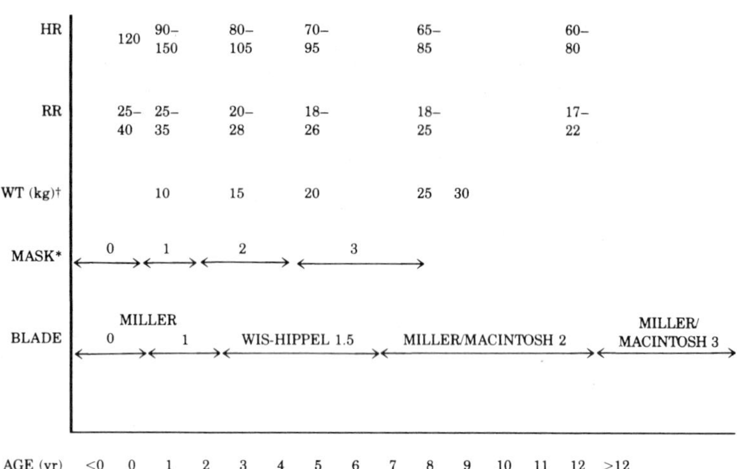

† Approximate 90th per centile values
* Rendell-Baker-Soucek size

Infants and children can tolerate apnea for a much shorter time than adults because of a reduced ratio of functional residual capacity to alveolar ventilation. Table 28-2.

A. Oxygen can be provided using many different appliances, such as a face tent or mask. For provision of adequate controlled ventilation, a properly applied face mask is necessary. Lifting the jaw into the mask provides for the greatest control of the nonintubated airway.

B. Resuscitation bags. Self-inflating bags fill independently of gas flow and utilize valves to provide ventilatory support. They are easy to master but have a number of significant disadvantages. They may fill with entrained air as well as delivered oxygen. Because the proportion of entrained air is dependent on the relative size of the bag reservoir, the inflowing gas rate, and the minute ventilation, a maximum of approximately 50–60% F_{IO_2} will be delivered even with maximal gas flow of 100% oxygen.

III. Circulation. Delivery of oxygen to vital organs is dependent on uptake of inspired gas, the cardiac output, and blood flow distribution. In newborns and infants, the heart is relatively noncompliant, limiting stroke volume reserve. In the absence of hypovolemia, cardiac output is directly dependent on heart rate and may be assessed noninvasively.

A. Heart rate and pulse character may be assessed by palpating great arteries. In newborns, the brachial and femoral arteries may be readily felt.

B. The location of chest compressions to augment cardiac output varies with the size of the pediatric patient. The location is at the infant's midsternum in order to avoid laceration of the spleen and liver by the ribs. For older children, as in adults, the lower sternum is the preferred location. The rate and depth of compressions are shown in Table 28-1.

IV. **Drugs.** Delivery of drugs and fluids can be a problem in the pediatric population.

A. Many drugs can be delivered via the endotracheal tube with rapid uptake and minimal effects on gas exchange or the pulmonary parenchyma.

B. In newborns, medications may be delivered via the umbilical vein. Hypertonic solutions should not be administered via the umbilical vein because of their potential to injure the liver parenchyma. External jugular, saphenous, internal jugular, subclavian, and peripheral veins may also provide routes of venous access.

C. Intraosseous cannulation of the tibia with a 18- or 16-gauge hypodermic or styletted spinal needle may provide a route for drug and fluid administration. It should enter the bone below the tibial tuberosity and be directed inferiorly to avoid the epiphyseal plate.

D. **First-line drugs**

1. **Oxygen.** Because a majority of cardiopulmonary arrests in the pediatric population are secondary to hypoxia, delivery of oxygen via an adequate airway often resolves the problem.
2. **Epinephrine.** Because the most common pediatric arrhythmias are bradycardia and asystole, epinephrine is useful for increasing heart rate and blood pressure. A dose of 0.01 mg per kilogram may be repeated every 5 minutes. Of a 1 : 10,000 dilution (0.1 mg/ml), 0.1 ml per kilogram may be used by an endotracheal, IV, or intraosseous route.
3. **Atropine** is used to treat bradycardia accompanied by hypotension and poor perfusion. It is especially useful in the treatment of bradycardia secondary to vagal stimulation. Low doses of atropine may be accompanied by paradoxical bradycardia in infants. Dose is 0.02 mg per kilogram. A minimum dose of 0.1 is recommended. The dose may be repeated every 5 minutes to a maximum of 1.0 mg in the child and 2.0 mg in the adolescent by the endotracheal, IV, or intraosseous route.
4. **Sodium bicarbonate** is used in the treatment of metabolic acidosis. Administration of sodium bicarbonate is associated with hypernatremia, hyperosmolar states, and, in newborns, intraventricular hemorrhages. Data suggest that intracellular acidosis may be increased by bicarbonate administration. This occurs because the liberated carbon dioxide diffuses intracellularly more rapidly than the ionized form. Dose is guided by arterial pH and $PaCO_2$ or 1 mEq per kilogram initially via an IV or intraosseous route. If an umbilical venous line is used, make sure the catheter tip is not in the liver parenchyma.
5. **Calcium chloride** is useful in the treatment of hypocalcemia, hyperkalemia, and hypermagnesemia. Dose is calcium chloride 10 mg per kilogram or calcium gluconate 30 mg per kilogram. Both are available as 10% solutions. Hence, the dose is CaCl 0.1 ml per kilogram and calcium gluconate 0.3 ml per kilogram. The dose may be repeated every 10 minutes as guided by measured calcium deficiency. Rapid infusion is associated with decreased heart rate. The patency of the IV should be checked prior to infusion because severe tissue damage is associated with interstitial infusion.
6. **Glucose** should be administered if hypoglycemia is present. Rapid infusions of hypertonic glucose solutions are associated with intraventricular hemorrhages in newborns. Glucose supplementation should be administered slowly in newborns. Dose for neonates is 200 mg per kilogram (2 cc/kg of 10% dextrose in water), repeated as

needed. For continued hypoglycemia, start infusion of 3–5 mg/kg/minute glucose. In older patients, 0.5–1 g of dextrose (1–2 cc/kg of 50% dextrose diluted with an equal volume of sterile water).

E. **Second-line drugs.** Following the establishment of adequate oxygenation and ventilation, the following agents may promote circulation. Intravenous infusion solutions can be made according to the following formula:

Amount of agent (mg) diluted to 100 ml with D_5W = 6 × wt (kg) × (desired mμ/kg/minute infusion rate)/(infusion rate in ml/hour)

1. **Dopamine.** Agonist at alpha-, beta-receptors in a dose-dependent manner. Specific dopaminergic receptors are found in the mesenteric and renal beds. Depending on the dosage, dopamine may promote renal perfusion and maintain blood pressure. It may be dysrhythmogenic. Dose is dependent on the individual response and should be observed and titrated to effect.
2. **Epinephrine** is a mixed agonist.
3. **Norepinephrine** is a mixed agonist with predominantly alpha activity. Dose is 0.05–1 μg/kg/minute.
4. **Isoproterenol** is a beta-adrenergic agonist. Dose is 1 μg/kg/minute.

V. **Treatment of arrhythmias.** Arrhythmias should be treated emergently only if they compromise cardiac output or degenerate into pathological rhythms. The optimal energy level and electrode sizes in the pediatric population are unknown. The electrode size should allow the greatest chest wall contact over the entire area of the paddle. Saline-soaked gauze or electrolytic gel ensures electrical conductivity. One paddle is placed in the left midaxillary line at the level of the xiphoid process, and the other is positioned on the right anterior chest below the clavicle.

A. **Sinus bradycardia and sinus node arrest with junctional escape** are the most common terminal arrhythmias in children with cardiopulmonary arrests. These arrhythmias often respond to the treatments outlined in **IV.D.1.**

B. **Supraventricular tachycardia (SVT).** The heart rate varies with age. It may be difficult to differentiate from ventricular tachycardia caused by other pathologic processes. In general, the rate is greater than 230 in infants. Rarely does aberrant conduction occur with this arrhythmia. Synchronized cardioversion is the treatment of choice. Initially 0.5–1.0 J per kilogram is used; if not successful, increase to 2.0 J per kilogram. The use of verapamil has been associated with irreversible cardiac collapse and should be used with great caution, if at all, in this age group.

C. **Ventricular tachycardia (VT).** Heart rate may be above 400 in this arrhythmia. With higher ventricular rates, the QRS complex may appear narrow, and differentiation from SVT may be difficult. Nevertheless, initially cardioversion is recommended: 0.5–1.0 J per kilogram is used; if not successful, increase to 2.0 J per kilogram. Lidocaine (1 mg/kg IV bolus) may be useful in improving cardioversion success if given prior to subsequent attempts. Lidocaine infusion of 20–40 μg/kg/hour may be useful for preventing recurrent ventricular arrhythmias.

D. **Ventricular fibrillation (VF)** is a very uncommon terminal arrhythmia in the pediatric population. Cardioversion may be aided by an epinephrine bolus prior to attempting defibrillation. The optimal dose for defibrillation has not been established. A nonsynchronized dose of 2 J per kilogram may be used initially; if this is not successful, the dose should be doubled and attempted again up to two times. If again unsuccessful, reconsider other correctable causes.

E. **Environment.** With loss of the thermoregulatory reflexes during cardiopulmonary collapse and increased heat loss during resuscitative attempts, body temperature can rapidly drop and lead to significant alterations in cardiopulmonary and metabolic function. It is important to facilitate passive warming until endogenous thermogenic systems are able to resume.

Selected References

American Heart Association. *Textbook of Pediatric Advanced Life Support.* Dallas: American Heart Association, 1988.

Coté C. J., and Todres, I. D. The Pediatric Airway. In *A Practice of Anesthesia for Infants and Children.* New York: Grune & Stratton, 1986.

Levin, D. L. (ed.). *A Practical Guide to Pediatric Intensive Care* (2d ed.). Toronto: C. V. Mosby, 1984.

McIntyre, K. M., and Lewis, A. J. (eds.). *Textbook of Advanced Cardiac Life Support.* Dallas: American Heart Association, 1981.

Coté, C. J., and Todres, I. D. The Pediatric Airway. In J. F. Ryan, I. D. Todres, C. J. Coté, and N. G. Goudsouzian (eds.). *A Practice of Anesthesia for Infants and Children.* Orlando, FL: Grune & Stratton, 1986:35–57.

29

Pharmacology in the Intensive Care Unit

Richard Fine and William Paganelli

c. Nitroglycerin
d. Nitroprusside
3. Ganglionic blockers
VI. Calcium channel blockers
A. Overview
B. Indications for use
C. Effects common to all CCBs
1. Vasodilation
2. Depressed myocardial contractility
3. Myocardial ischemia
4. Cardiac impulse conduction
a. Verapamil (Calan, Isoptin)
b. Nifedipine (Procardia, Adalat)
c. Nicardipine (Cardene)
d. Diltiazem (Cardizem)
VII. Cardiac arrhythmias
A. Mechanisms by which cardiac arrhythmias arise
B. Categorization by degree of urgency
C. General therapeutic principles
1. Ventricular fibrillation (VF)
2. Ventricular tachycardia (Vtach)
3. Bradyarrhythmias (symptomatic)
4. Premature ventricular contractions (PVCs)
5. Supraventricular tachycardia (SVT)
6. Atrial fibrillation (Afib)
D. Drugs used in the therapy of cardiac dysrhythmias
1. Adenosine (Adenocard)
2. Amiodarone
3. Atropine
4. Bretylium (Bretylol)
5. Disopyramide (Norpace)
6. Edrophonium (Tensilon)
7. Encainide (Enkaid)
8. Flecainide (Tambocor)
9. Lidocaine
10. Mexiletine (Mexitil)
11. Phenytoin (Dilantin)
12. Procainamide (Pronestyl)
13. Quinidine
14. Tocainide (Tonocard)

Patients in the ICU commonly require the administration of vasoactive and inotropic drugs to support their circulation. This chapter reviews the drugs that are currently in use, their clinical indications, pharmacodynamics, modes of administration, and potential side effects. While rational use of these substances requires a knowledge of the different adrenergic receptors and the actions of medications, personal preference and institutional bias may play a significant role in the decision process.

I. **Adrenergic receptor pharmacology.** Sympathomimetic agents have different potencies and dosages for each physiologic response observed. These may vary greatly from patient to patient. The understanding of receptors and the function of different binding sites enables the physician to predict the response of most drugs.

A. **Receptor regulation.** Tremendous variability exists for the dose and physiologic effect that the drug produces. This is the result of many factors.

1. **Pharmacokinetics** of a drug relate to its availability at the receptor site. This is governed by modes of molecular transport across membranes, protein binding, circulation to certain vascular beds, lipid solubility, and the speed and extent of the drug's metabolism.
2. **Pharmacodynamics** of a drug deal with the effects that result from the interaction with a specific site of action. The effect of a drug can be altered by changes in the receptor population.
   a. Decreased receptor stimulation results in an increased number of receptors. This up regulation occurs, for example, in chronic beta-blockade, producing an increased number of beta-adrenergic receptors. This is why sudden withdrawal of beta-blockade may result in myocardial ischemia secondary to tachycardia and hypertension.
   b. Increased receptor stimulation will result in a decreased number of receptors. Chronic beta stimulation as a mode of antiasthmatic therapy will result in a reduced number of beta-adrenergic receptors.
   c. The agonist-receptor interaction is the initial step in developing a physiologic response. From this point on, the development of the anticipated effect is dependent on many factors, including the presence of calcium and magnesium, activation of adenyl cyclase, and avoidance of acidosis and hypoxemia.

B. **Adrenergic receptor subtypes** (Tables 29-1 and 29-2)

1. **Alpha-1 receptors** are located on the postsynaptic membrane on vascular smooth muscle and on the myocardium. They mediate vasoconstriction and positive inotropy.
2. **Alpha-2 receptors** are found on the presynaptic membrane on vascular smooth muscle and also postsynaptically. The presynaptic receptors inhibit sympathetic outflow. These receptors regulate norepinephrine release by inhibiting outflow when there is a high concentration of catechols at the nerve terminal. The receptors found postsynaptically may cause direct smooth muscle relaxation and, therefore, vasodilation.
3. **Beta-1 receptors** involve myocardial and electrophysiologic functions. Through their positive inotropic and chronotropic effect, beta-1 stimulation increases ventricular ejection rate and decreases ejection time. Electrophysiologically, there is increased automaticity, increased conduction velocity and decreased refractoriness of the atrioventricular node. Other effects of beta-1 stimulation include increased renin release and lipolysis.
4. **Beta-2 stimulation** results in peripheral vasodilation, coronary arte-

Table 29-1. Catecholamine receptor responses

Receptor	Site	Action
Alpha-1	Postsynaptic on vascular smooth muscle; coronary systemic arterioles and veins	Vasconstriction
	Myocardium	Increase contractility
Alpha-2	Presynaptic on vascular smooth muscle	Vasodilation
Beta-1	SA node	Increase heart rate
	Atria	Increase contractility and conduction velocity
	A-V node His-Purkinje system	Increase automaticity and conduction velocity
	Ventricular myocardium	Increase contactility, conduction velocity, and automaticity
	Kidney	Increase renin release
Beta-2	Bronchiolar smooth muscle	Relaxation
	Coronary arterioles	Dilatation
	Pulmonary and systemic arterioles and veins	Dilatation
	Pancreas	Increase insulin
	Uterus	Relaxation
Dopamine	Kidney	Vasodilation

riolar dilation, insulin release, and gluconeogenesis and uterine relaxation. Presynaptic beta-2 receptor stimulation results in an increased release of norepinephrine.

5. **Dopaminergic receptor** stimulation regulates renal and mesenteric vasodilation. This is associated with an increase in glomerular filtration rate, renal blood flow, and sodium excretion.

II. Beta-adrenergic blocking drugs

A. Actions. Beta-blockers have three principal actions that affect the cardiovascular system: receptor subtype selectivity, intrinsic sympathomimetic activity (ISA), and membrane stabilizing activity. These actions result in a decrease in heart rate (HR), contractility, BP, AV conduction, and automaticity. At the same time, one may see an increase in systemic vascular resistance (SVR) if the drug does not have ISA, which would stimulate the peripheral beta-2 receptors.

B. Advantages

1. **Decrease myocardial oxygen consumption** (MVO_2) by decreasing (prevent increase) left ventricular (LV) systolic pressure, decreasing (prevent increase) HR, and decreasing (prevent increase) contractile state.
2. **Increase myocardial blood flow** by increasing diastolic filling time.
3. **Provides antiarrhythmic action**; prevents supraventricular arrhythmias.
4. **Prevents reflex tachycardias** caused by vasodilators.
5. **Decrease inotrophy and ejection velocity** in patients with aortic dissection or idiopathic hypertrophic subaortic stenosis.
6. **Antihypertensive**
7. Can be **continued by mouth** (PO) preoperatively and **continued IV** until the patient is capable of taking PO postoperatively.

Table 29-2. Drugs acting at adrenergic receptors

Receptor	Agonists	Antagonists
Alpha-1	Ephedrine Dopamine (Inotropin) Metaraminol (Aramine) Methoxamine (Vasoxyl) Phenylephrine (Neo-Synephrine)	Chlorpromazine (Thorazine) Droperidol (Inapsine) Labetalol (Trandate) Phenoxybenzamine (Dibenzyline) Prazocin (Minipress)
Alpha-2	Clonidine (Catapres) Guanabenz (Wytensin) Methyldopa (Aldomet)	Yohimbine
Alpha-1	Epinephrine (Adrenalin)	Phenotolamine (Regitine)
Alpha-2	Norepinephrine (Levophed)	Tolazoline (Priscoline)
Beta-1	Metaraminol (Aramine) Norepinephrine (Levophed) Epinephrine	Acebutalol (Sectral) Atenolol (Tenormin) Esmolol (Brevibloc) Metoprolol (Lopressor)
Beta-2	Albuteral (Ventolin) Metaproterenol (Metaprel) Terbutaline (Brethine, Brincanyl)	
Beta-1	Ephedrine	Labetalol (Trandate)
Beta-2	Epinephrine Dopamine (Inotropin) Dobutamine (Dobutrex) Isoproterenol (Isuprel)	Nadolol (Corgard) Pindolol (Visken) Propranolol (Inderal) Timolol (Blocadren)
Dopamine	Dopamine (Inotropin)	Chlorpromazine (Thorazine) Droperidol (Inapsine) Metoclopramide (Reglan)

C. Disadvantages

1. Administration of beta-blockers **may cause severe bradycardia,** especially in patients on digoxin.
2. **Heart block**
3. **Exacerbation of bronchospastic disease**
4. May potentiate **congestive heart failure**
5. **Blunt the sympathetic response** associated with hypoglycemia (except sweating)
6. **Inhibition of beta-2 receptors** may increase peripheral vascular resistance. May be a consideration in patients with severe peripheral vascular disease.
7. **Vasospasm** in the coronary circulation may be caused by unopposed alpha stimulation.

D. Clinical use (Table 29-3)

1. The IV dose is always much smaller than the PO dose because it is not affected by first-pass hepatic extraction.
2. Always begin with small doses and increase slowly (i.e., Inderal 0.5–1.0 mg IV to start and use same increment every 2–5 minutes until desired effect is achieved). Electrocardiogram, BP, and pulmonary function should be monitored during administration. Initial maximum dose is 0.1 mg per kilogram.
3. Selective beta-1 agonists should be used in patients with hyperactive airway disease. If available, a short-acting drug such as esmolol should be used initially to assess the degree of pulmonary dysfunction

Table 29-3. Beta-adrenergic blocking drugs

	Propranolol (Inderal)	Timolol[a] (Blocadren)	Nadolol (Corgard)	Metoprolol (Lopressor)	Atenolol (Tenormin)	Pindolol (Visken)	Labetalol (Trandate)	Esmolol (Brevibloc)
Bioavailability[b]	33	75	20	50	55	>90	25	NA
Beta half-life[c]	3.5–6.0 hr	3–4 hr	14–24 hr	3–4 hr	6–9 hr	3–4 hr	3–8 hr	9 min
Elimination	H	H (80%) R (20%)	R (75%)	H	R (85%)	H (60%) R (40%)	H	Blood
Active metabolites	Yes	No	No	No	No	No	No	No
Beta-1 selectivity	No	No	No	Yes	Yes	No	No	Yes
ISA	No	No	No	No	No	Yes	No	No
Alpha antagonist	No	No	No	No	No	No	Yes	No
IV use	Yes	No	No	Yes	No	No	Yes	Yes
Relative PO potency[d]	1.0	6.0	1.0	1.0	1.0	6.0	0.3	
Initial PO dose (mg)[e]	10–20 bid–qid	5–15 qd–bid	40 qd	50 qd	50 qd	5 bid	100 bid	NA
Maximum PO dose (mg)[e]	80 qid	30 bid[f]	320 qd[f]	200 bid[f]	100 qd[f]	30 tid[f]	1200 bid	NA
Maximum usual IV dose (mg)[g]	4–8 in 0.5- to 1.0-mg increments	No	No	15 in 5-mg increments	No	No	20 load, then 40–80 q10min to max 300	0.25–0.5 mg/kg/min for 1 min then 50–200 μg/kg/min as a constant infusion

NA = not applicable
H = hepatic elimination; R = renal elimination.
[a] Timolol eye drops can produce systemic beta blockade.
[b] In percent after oral dose.
[c] Half-life may not be predictive of clinical duration of action.
[d] Ratio of potency when compared with propranolol: 1.0 indicates that drug is equipotent with propranolol.
[e] Usual dosages for adults.
[f] Decrease dosage in renal failure.
[g] IV doses must be given in small, divided doses with careful monitoring. Adult dosages are given.
Source: Modified from D. R. Larach, and W. A. Kofke. Cardiovascular Drugs. In W. A. Kofke and J. H. Levy (eds.), *Postoperative Critical Care Procedures of the Massachusetts General Hospital*. Boston: Little, Brown, 1986. p. 469. With permission.

caused by the beta-blockade. This is highly recommended because esmolol has only a 9-minute half-life. Bronchospasm can be treated with a beta-mimetic such as albuterol.

4. Overdoses leading to profound bradycardia or heart block may be treated with isoproterenol, pacing if available, calcium, and glucagon.
5. An appropriate dose of a beta-blocker in the ICU producing adequate beta-blockade may not suffice on the floor as patients begin to ambulate and exert themselves. Beta-blockade should be increased until the patient does not manifest an increase in HR associated with exercise.
6. Depending on a drug's receptor selectivity, one may anticipate less beta effect from a vasoactive substance that has both alpha- and beta-agonist activity.
7. Selectivity of a beta-blocker is not an all-or-none phenomenon. Beta-1 selective drugs possess more activity at beta-1 receptors but still possess activity at beta-2 receptors. Despite this selectivity, these drugs may still cause bronchospasm or an increase in SVR when administered. For this reason, one must always be extremely cautious when giving an asthmatic patient a beta-blocker.
8. The intrinsic sympathomimetic activity of some beta-blockers tends to be a very confusing property. The drugs with ISA mildly activate the same receptors that are being blocked. This is a direct action on the receptor and has nothing to do with the blockade of catecholamines activating the receptor. The ISA will cause a higher resting HR and a lower SVR, thereby maintaining an increased cardiac output (CO). At the same time, however, these patients should not have a change in HR associated with exercise. A theoretical concern is that a pure agonist such as isoproterenol will have a diminished effect because the ISA will competitively inhibit it.

III. Sympathomimetic drugs

A. Naturally occurring catecholamines

1. Epinephrine (Adrenalin)

a. General. Epinephrine is the prototypical sympathomimetic drug produced by the adrenal medulla through the methylation of norepinephrine. As a natural catecholamine, this drug directly stimulates alpha-1, alpha-2, beta-1, and beta-2 receptors to produce effects on cardiac contractility and HR, vascular tone, pulmonary bronchiolar tone, glucose metabolism, gastrointestinal and genitourinary smooth muscle, and the blood coagulation system.

b. Indications

(1) Cardiac arrest, resuscitation (asystole, VF, electromechanical dissociation)
(2) Inotropic and pressor support of the circulation (heart failure, shock, sepsis, trauma)
(3) Therapy of severe allergic reactions (anaphylaxis)
(4) Treatment of bronchospasm
(5) Admixture with local anesthetics to prolong duration and reduce systemic absorption

c. Physiology

(1) Epinephrine is a potent agonist at alpha, beta-1, and beta-2 receptors. At low doses of 1–2 μg per minute, beta-2 receptors are preferentially stimulated, leading to vasodilation in skeletal muscle beds. Concomitant beta-1 stimulation produces increases in inotropy, HR, and CO, although mean BP may not rise due to the beta-2 vasodilation. At doses of 2–10 μg per minute, combined alpha, beta-1, and beta-2 receptor activation leads to variable changes in SVR and increased HR, CO, and

BP. High-dose epinephrine (10–20 μg/minute) produces marked alpha vasoconstriction, especially of skin and renal circulations, and may lead to severe hypertension, tachycardia, cardiac arrhythmias, stroke, and myocardial ischemia.

(2) Epinephrine is a potent inotrope due to beta-1 receptor stimulation.

(3) This drug is more active than norepinephrine in stimulating alpha receptors. At lower doses, however, beta-2-mediated vasodilation in skeletal muscle beds offsets this effect.

(4) Renal blood flow is reduced more by epinephrine than by norepinephrine.

(5) Since epinephrine is a direct-acting catecholamine, tachyphylaxis to its effects is not seen in contrast to the reduced effects on multiple dosing seen with indirect-acting agents.

(6) Renin release by the kidney is augmented by epinephrine.

(7) Epinephrine is an excellent bronchodilator. Given IV or subcutaneously (SQ), it will reverse bronchospasm due to anaphylaxis or severe asthma.

(8) During cardiopulmonary resuscitation (CPR), epinephrine in resuscitation doses (0.5–1.0 mg IV bolus) raises coronary perfusion pressure and may change fine to coarse ventricular fibrillation (VF).

(9) Beta-1 receptor stimulation by epinephrine increases glycogenolysis and lipolysis, while alpha stimulation inhibits insulin release. These effects may lead to hyperglycemia.

(10) Epinephrine causes a leukocytosis and can accelerate blood coagulation due to increased factor V activity.

(11) Epinephrine may produce deleterious effects on a number of organ systems.

(a) Myocardial ischemia may occur due to increases in HR, inotropy, and afterload. Conversely, improved cardiac function, lower ventricular end-diastolic pressures, and increased diastolic coronary perfusion due to epinephrine may ameliorate ischemia in some patients.

(b) Renal perfusion may be compromised, leading to oliguria. Care should be taken to monitor urinary output during epinephrine infusions. Vasodilators such as nitroprusside may be used to counteract these effects.

(c) Epinephrine can cause pulmonary hypertension and right ventricular failure. Pulmonary vasodilators such as nitroglycerin or prostaglandin E may be used to lower pulmonary vascular resistance in this situation.

(d) Arrhythmias may accompany epinephrine therapy due to increased automaticity of ventricular tissue.

(e) Extravasation of epinephrine given via a peripheral IV can lead to severe vasoconstriction and local tissue necrosis. Infiltration of alpha-blocking agents such as phentolamine may reverse this. Epinephrine should be given through a central line if possible.

d. **Metabolism.** Epinephrine is rapidly removed from the circulation by uptake back into postganglionic sympathetic nerve endings. In addition, epinephrine is metabolized with great speed by the enzymes monoamine oxidase (MAO) and catechol-O-methyltransferase (COMT).

e. **Dose**

(1) Epinephrine may be given SQ or IV, via an endotracheal tube or by intracardiac injection (only if other routes of administration have failed or are unavailable). Oral administration is ineffective due to metabolism by gastrointestinal enzymes.

(2) For anaphylactic reactions or bronchospasm, SQ administration in a dose of 10 μg per kilogram (maximum 0.4 mg + 0.4 cc of 1 : 1,000 epinephrine) is recommended.

(3) IV administration

(a) To support the circulation, epinephrine may be infused at 1–20 μg per minute (mix 1–4 mg/250 cc 5% dextrose in water [D_5W]). Boluses of 2–16 μg IV may also be effective.

(b) Pediatric dose, 0.05–0.5 μg/kg/minute.

(c) Cardiac arrest dose. Adult: 0.5–1.0 mg IV, intratracheal, intracardiac. Pediatric: 5–15 μg per kilogram IV, intratracheal, intracardiac.

(d) Beware excessive vasoconstriction, tachycardia, or arrhythmias secondary to epinephrine. Monitor cardiac filling pressures, ECG, and urine output.

(4) Concomitant vasodilator therapy may ameliorate peripheral vasoconstriction caused by epinephrine.

(5) Caution should be exercised when epinephrine is given to patients receiving nonselective beta-blockers. Blockade of beta-2 vasodilation may lead to exaggerated hypertension in this setting.

2. Norepinephrine (Levophed)

a. General. Norepinephrine is a direct-acting, natural catecholamine that serves as the endogenous neurotransmitter released from postganglionic sympathetic nerve terminals. It too, like epinephrine, is a potent beta-1 agonist; however, norepinephrine does not stimulate beta-2 receptors at clinical doses. This drug produces intense alpha-mediated arterial and venous vasoconstriction.

b. Indications

(1) Therapy of hypotension, especially in the setting of low total peripheral vascular resistance (e.g., septic shock, postcardiopulmonary bypass vasodilation, postligation of pheochromocytoma blood supply)

(2) Situations requiring inotropic effect and vasoconstriction

(3) Emergency therapy of hypovolemia until blood volume is normalized

c. Physiology

(1) Produces intense vasoconstriction of skeletal muscle, liver, kidneys, and skin. Blood flow is redirected to perfuse vital coronary and cerebral circulations.

(2) Elevates systolic, diastolic, and mean BP. Heart rate may decrease due to baroreceptor-reflex response to increased BP or may increase with beta-1 stimulation. Cardiac contractility increases; CO may increase, although excessive rise in afterload due to vasoconstriction may actually diminish stroke volume.

(3) Peripheral vasoconstriction may reduce tissue blood flow enough to cause ischemia and produce a metabolic acidosis.

(4) Extravasation of norepinephrine can produce severe local vasoconstriction and tissue destruction. Administration via central line is recommended.

(5) Pulmonary vascular resistance is increased by norepinephrine.

(6) In cases of severe right heart failure, pulmonary vasodilators such as prostaglandin E_1 may beneficially reduce pulmonary resistance. However, accompanying systemic vasodilation may cause serious hypotension. In this case, infusion of norepinephrine into the left atrium can raise systemic resistance without effect on the pulmonary circuit.

d. **Metabolism**
   (1) Norepinephrine is rapidly metabolized by MAO and COMT. Its biologic actions, however, are terminated principally by uptake into sympathetic nerve terminals.
   (2) Norepinephrine is efficiently removed from the blood during passage through the lungs. In contrast, epinephrine and dopamine are not.

e. **Dose**
   (1) Norepinephrine is given by IV infusion at a rate of 0.5–20 μg per minute (mix 1–4 mg/250 cc D_5W = 4–16 μg/cc) and titrated to effect.
   (2) As with epinephrine, close attention should be paid to urine output.
   (3) Concomitant vasodilator therapy may ameliorate vasoconstrictor activity (lowering afterload), while beta-1 stimulation increases CO.

3. **Dopamine (Intropin)**

a. **General.** Dopamine is a catecholamine precursor of norepinephrine that serves as a central and peripheral nervous system neurotransmitter. This drug can stimulate dopaminergic (type 1 and 2), beta (1 and 2), and alpha receptors. At low doses of 1–2 μg/kg/minute, dopamine stimulates dopaminergic renal vascular receptors to produce renal vasodilation with increased renal blood flow; glomerular filtration rate, sodium excretion, and urine output are also increased. Higher rates of infusion of 2–10 μg/kg/minute stimulate beta-1 receptors, which cause an increase in cardiac contractility, HR, and CO; beta-2-mediated vasodilation may occur. Above 10 μg/kg/minute, alpha-mediated vasoconstriction increases systemic and renal resistance and may diminish CO through effects of excessive afterload. Tachycardia and arrhythmias often occur at these doses.

b. **Indications**
   (1) For therapy of severe heart failure and cardiogenic shock
   (2) Treatment of oliguria and renal failure
   (3) Hypotension related to shock, hypovolemia, or trauma, especially with low urine output

c. **Physiology**
   (1) Dopamine's activity is partially a result of release of norepinephrine from peripheral nerve endings.
   (2) At low doses, renal blood flow and urine output increase due to direct stimulation of renal dopaminergic receptors. This effect is not blocked by propranolol (beta-2 blocker) but is abolished by dopamine receptor antagonists such as droperidol.
   (3) At higher doses (above 10 μg/kg/minute), alpha-mediated renal vasoconstriction overrides dopaminergic vasodilation, leading to renal ischemia and decreased urine output. Constriction of splanchnic and cutaneous vessels can lead to necrosis.
   (4) Dopamine may cause cardiac dysrhythmias by stimulating release of norepinephrine from cardiac sympathetic nerve endings. However, dopamine is less arrhythmogenic than epinephrine and causes less of a tachycardia than isoproterenol.
   (5) It increases mesenteric blood flow at the expense of muscle vascular bed.
   (6) Dopamine may increase the pulmonary artery occlusion pressure despite its beneficial effects on contractility. Vasodilator therapy (nitroglycerin) can counteract this effect. At high doses, pulmonary vascular resistance may increase due to alpha effects on lung vessels.

(7) Similar to epinephrine and norepinephrine, extravasated dopamine can lead to skin necrosis, which should be treated by local infiltration of phentolamine.

(8) Hyperglycemia may result from dopamine inhibition of insulin secretion.

(9) Dopamine may be a less potent inotrope when cardiac catecholamine stores are depleted (congestive heart disease [CHD], reserpine treatment).

d. **Metabolism.** Dopamine is not effective orally due to breakdown in the GI tract. In the bloodstream, dopamine is rapidly removed by neural uptake and metabolism by MAO and COMT. Therefore, it must be given by continuous IV infusion.

e. **Dose**

(1) Mix 200–800 mg in 250 cc D_5W (800–3,200 μg/ml).

(2) Infuse at 1–20 μg/kg/minute.

(3) Add vasodilator to optimize CO and systemic vascular resistance.

B. Synthetic catecholamines

1. Dobutamine (Dobutrex)

a. **General.** Dobutamine is a synthetic catecholamine that resembles dopamine with the addition of a large aromatic ring substituent on the amino group. The pharmacological effects of dobutamine are due to direct stimulation of beta-1 and beta-2 adrenergic receptors and to alpha-1 receptor stimulation.

b. **Indications**

(1) Treatment of low CO states following cardiac surgery

(2) Congestive heart failure

(3) Cardiogenic shock, especially in patients with elevated peripheral and pulmonary vascular resistance

c. **Physiology**

(1) Dobutamine is a beta-1 agonist that increases cardiac contractility. Heart rate may increase, but inotropic effects are more prominent. Heart rate does not increase as much as with isoproterenol. Cardiac output increases, while total peripheral resistance remains relatively unchanged, reflecting the counterbalancing effect of alpha-1 vasoconstriction and beta-2 vasodilation. Blood pressure may increase, stay the same, or decrease (if beta-2 stimulation predominates). Pulmonary vascular resistance decreases and may be beneficial in cases of right ventricular failure.

(2) Dobutamine increases stroke volume and lowers atrial filling pressures, which may decrease myocardial oxygen demand. This effect is similar to that seen with isoproterenol or dopamine plus nitroprusside.

(3) Beta-2 vasodilation may lower after load sufficiently **to decrease blood pressure,** despite an increase in CO.

(4) This drug does not enhance sinus node automaticity as much as isoproterenol. Atrioventricular nodal conduction is enhanced, however, and may lead to marked increases in ventricular rate in patients with atrial fibrillation (Afib).

(5) Renal blood flow is improved as a consequence of increased CO; dobutamine does not activate renal dopaminergic receptors.

(6) High doses of dobutamine (greater than 10 μg/kg/minute) may cause tachycardia and arrhythmias, although this is less of a problem than with dopamine since dobutamine does not indirectly release norepinephrine from sympathetic nerve endings on the heart.

(7) Hypovolemic patients treated with dobutamine may develop significant hypotension since this drug is more of an inotrope than a pressor.
(8) In patients with a history of hypertension, exaggerated increases in BP and HR may occur, necessitating reduction in the dobutamine infusion rate.
(9) Myocardial infarct size may be increased if myocardial oxygen demand is increased by dobutamine. In addition, coronary steal may be provoked.

d. Metabolism

(1) Dobutamine is rapidly metabolized by COMT and conjugated in the liver. Its half-life is about 2 minutes; onset of action is very rapid, and, as a result, no loading dose is required.
(2) Absence of metabolism by MAO may make this a preferred drug for use in patients on MAO inhibitors.

e. Dose

(1) Dobutamine is prepared in 5% dextrose to avoid breakdown in alkaline solutions.
(2) Generally, 250 mg is diluted in 50–250 cc D_5W to yield 500–1,000 μg per cubic centimeter.
(3) Intravenous infusion rates run from 2–20 μg/kg/minute.
(4) It may be given peripherally given low risk of skin necrosis (minimal alpha effects).
(5) Dobutamine often acts like a combination of dopamine or epinephrine plus a vasodilator such as nitroprusside.
(6) Tolerance may develop if dobutamine is infused over a period of more than a few days.

2. Isoproterenol (Isuprel)

a. General. Isoproterenol is the most potent sympathomimetic beta-1 and beta-2 agonist. At clinical doses, it causes almost no alpha vasoconstriction. Infusion of this drug leads to beta-2-mediated vasodilation, primarily in skeletal muscle but also in renal and mesenteric vascular beds, which decreases peripheral vascular resistance. Mean BP is reduced, associated with a marked reduction in diastolic BP. Systolic pressure may remain unchanged or increase. Beta-1-mediated increases in HR, contractility, and cardiac automaticity occur; CO is increased by the combination of increased inotropy, chronotropy, and lowered peripheral vascular resistance.

b. Indications

(1) To increase HR in atropine-resistant bradycardia or heart block until temporary pacing measures are instituted
(2) Treatment of severe bronchospasm (such as status asthmaticus)
(3) Situations requiring a potent inotrope and chronotrope with vasodilator properties
 (a) Right heart failure and elevated pulmonary vascular resistance
 (b) Postcardiac transplantation
 (c) Postrepair of pediatric congenital heart disease
(4) Beta-blocker overdose

c. Physiology

(1) Direct-acting, nonselective beta agonist with essentially no alpha effects
(2) Increases CO at expense of tachycardia and increased inotropy, which may lead to myocardial ischemia (increased oxygen demand and diminished coronary perfusion pressure). Isoproterenol has potentially deleterious effects in patients with

coronary artery disease (CAD) or myocardial infarction and should be used with caution in these patients.

(3) Isoproterenol can cause cardiac dysrhythmias and should not be used in patients with preexisting tachydysrhythmias, especially those due to digitalis toxicity. Caution should be exercised when hypokalemia is present.

(4) This drug is an excellent bronchodilator, which relaxes almost all varieties of smooth muscle when tone is elevated, especially in the bronchial tree. Additionally, in asthma, isoproterenol may inhibit antigen-mediated release of histamine.

(5) Coronary steal may occur.

(6) Hyperglycemia may be produced by isoproterenol infusion, although this is less of a problem than with epinephrine.

(7) Isoproterenol is not a pressor; hypotension may lead to hypoperfusion of vital organs.

(8) Increases in automaticity may unmask rapidly conducting accessory pathways with resulting tachydysrhythmias.

d. Metabolism

(1) Isoproterenol is rapidly metabolized in the liver and other tissues by COMT.

(2) There is a little uptake by sympathetic neurons and little metabolism by MAO since isoproterenol is a poor substrate for this enzyme.

e. Dose

(1) Isoproterenol is given IV and occasionally PO or as an inhaled mist (for bronchospasm).

(2) Mix 1–2 mg in 250 cc 5% dextrose or normal saline (4–8 μg/cc) for IV infusion.

(3) IV dose

(a) Adult: 0.5–20 μg per minute

(b) Pediatric: 0.05–0.50 μg/kg/minute

(4) Titrate dose according to HR and rhythm response.

(5) Isoproterenol may be given by peripheral IV since it will not cause skin necrosis if extravasated (no alpha effects).

C. Synthetic noncatecholamines

1. Ephedrine

a. General. Ephedrine is a synthetic noncatecholamine that directly stimulates alpha and beta-1/beta-2 receptors. Indirect release of norepinephrine also contributes to alpha and beta-1 effects of this drug. Ephedrine's cardiovascular effects mimic those of epinephrine, although it is much less potent. Intravenous administration leads to increased HR, BP, and CO. Peripheral vascular resistance is variably increased due to offsetting effects of alpha and beta-2 stimulation.

b. Indications

(1) Treatment of hypovolemia until vascular volume is normalized

(2) Therapy of regional anesthesia-induced hypotension

(3) Especially useful to restore maternal BP following epidural or spinal anesthesia since uterine blood flow is maintained

(4) Therapy of myocardial depression and hypotension due to general anesthetics

(5) May be used orally to treat bronchial asthma

c. Physiology

(1) Blood pressure–elevating response to ephedrine resembles that produced by epinephrine, except it is less intense and lasts up to 10 times longer.

(2) Heart rate increases are usually modest. Patients on MAO inhibitors may have greatly exaggerated response due to indirect norepinephrine release.

(3) Tachyphylaxis to ephedrine occurs due to depletion of norepinephrine stores and to persistent effects of the drug at alpha receptors.
(4) It does not produce hyperglycemia.
(5) Central nervous system stimulation may occur although to a lesser degree than with amphetamine.

d. Metabolism

(1) Since ephedrine lacks a 3-hydroxyl group, it is not degraded by COMT.
(2) Up to 40% of a dose is excreted as unchanged drug in the urine.
(3) There is some deamination by MAO in the liver, followed by conjugation and excretion.
(4) Prolonged duration of action of ephedrine (5–10 minutes) is due to slow inactivation and dependence on renal excretion.
(5) Ephedrine is resistant to metabolism by MAO in the GI tract and is thus effective following oral administration.
(6) Intramuscular (IM) absorption is adequate since modest local vasoconstriction does not hinder systemic absorption.

e. Dose

(1) May be given IV, IM, PO, or SQ
(2) IV bolus: 5–25 mg
(3) Dose may be repeated and should be titrated to response.
(4) Remember the increased sensitivity due to MAO inhibitors.
(5) Convenient-to-prepare solution with 5–10 mg per milliliter in a syringe for quick IV bolus until an infusion drip of another vasoactive drug is prepared

2. Metaraminol (Aramine)

a. General. Metaraminol is a synthetic noncatecholamine with cardiovascular actions similar to ephedrine and norepinephrine. It acts on alpha- and beta-adrenergic receptors via direct and indirect mechanisms (stimulates norepinephrine release from sympathetic nerve terminals). Metaraminol enters sympathetic nerve endings, where it acts as a weak false neurotransmitter.

b. Indications

(1) Treatment of low peripheral vascular resistance states such as sepsis, overdose of alpha-blockers, and regional anesthesia
(2) Hypotension associated with hypovolemia until intravascular fluid volumes are restored
(3) Therapy of paroxysmal atrial tachycardia

c. Physiology

(1) Produces prominent direct alpha-mediated vasoconstriction with a lesser increase in myocardial contractility and systolic and diastolic BP increase. Heart rate may increase or decrease (baroreceptor-induced bradycardia). Cardiac output may be reduced by increased SVR and by reflex-bradycardia.
(2) Blood flow to cerebral and coronary circulations is preserved; muscle, renal, mesenteric, and skin perfusion decrease and may result in tissue ischemia.
(3) Sudden withdrawal of metaraminol may lead to severe hypotension due to norepinephrine depletion from sympathetic nerve endings. Infusion of this drug should be tapered slowly.
(4) Beware of administration to patients taking MAO inhibitors, since this drug indirectly releases norepinephrine.
(5) May increase systemic vascular resistance in cases where other vasoconstrictors have been ineffective

d. Metabolism

(1) Metaraminol is not metabolized by MAO or COMT.

(2) Onset in 1–2 minutes IV
(3) Offset in 20–60 minutes by tissue uptake

e. **Dose**
(1) May be given IV, IM, or SQ
(2) IV bolus: 100–500 μg, in extremis 0.5–5 mg. IV infusion: 100 mg in 250–500 cc D_5W or normal saline (NS) run at 20–500 μg per minute. IM and SQ: 2–10 mg
(3) Titrate dose to BP effects

3. **Methoxamine (Vasoxyl)**

a. **General.** Methoxamine is a synthetic noncatecholamine that acts as a selective alpha-adrenergic agonist. This drug is not a beta-adrenergic receptor agonist.

b. **Indications**
(1) Hypotension in the setting of low SVR, sepsis, or regional anesthesia
(2) Therapy of hypotension associated with hypovolemia until blood volume can be restored
(3) Treatment of paroxysmal atrial tachycardia

c. **Physiology**
(1) Methoxamine produces intense alpha-mediated arterial vasoconstriction that leads to increased systolic and diastolic BP, reflex bradycardia, and a fall in CO.
(2) There is little venoconstriction.
(3) Methoxamine is a potent renal vasoconstrictor. Renal blood flow is reduced more by this drug than it is by norepinephrine.
(4) Coronary blood flow is generally improved due to the rise in diastolic perfusion pressure and the increased diastolic filling time due to reflex bradycardia.
(5) Methoxamine has a modest antiarrhythmic effect.
(6) There is no CNS excitation associated with this drug.

d. **Metabolism**
(1) Longer acting than phenylephrine due to the absence of metabolism by MAO or COMT
(2) Peak effect in 0.5–2 minutes when given IV
(3) Duration of action following IV dose 10–15 minutes
(4) Intramuscular peak effect in 15–20 minutes; duration approximately 1.5 hours
(5) Pressor effect of methoxamine may be potentiated by MAO inhibitors, tricyclic antidepressants, vasopressin, or ergot alkaloids.

e. **Dose**
(1) Adult: IV, 1–5 mg as a slow bolus; IM, 10–20 mg
(2) May give IV dose to correct hypotension rapidly and then an IM dose to maintain BP over a more extended time
(3) Difficult to titrate due to long half-life and slow onset (especially IM)

4. **Phenylephrine (Neo-Synephrine)**

a. **General.** Phenylephrine is a synthetic noncatecholomine that directly activates alpha-adrenergic receptors. There is also a small indirect effect to release norepinephrine from sympathetic nerve terminals. This drug has minimal effects on beta-receptors. It is also fairly selective for alpha-1 receptors.

b. **Indications**
(1) Therapy of hypotension due to low SVR states (sepsis, regional anesthesia)
(2) Treatment of SVT (reflex increase in vagal tone)
(3) Temporary therapy of hypovolemia until blood volume can be restored

c. **Physiology**
(1) Produces intense arteriolar and venoconstriction. Blood pressure (systolic and diastolic) increases. Heart rate slows, and cardiac output may fall.
(2) Renal, splanchnic, and cutaneous blood flows are reduced. Cerebral and coronary blood flow increase. Pulmonary arterial pressure is elevated by phenylephrine.
(3) This drug is quite effective in treating vasodilation due to regional anesthesia or injected or inhaled anesthetics.
(4) Phenylephrine usually has a beneficial effect on coronary myocardial oxygen supply without increasing oxygen consumption.
(5) Often it is used to increase BP during cardiac surgery, carotid endarterectomy, or in patients with aortic stenosis.
(6) Topically applied phenylephrine is a good nasal decongestant and produces mydriasis without cycloplegia.
(7) Phenylephrine can overcome vasodilation due to calcium channel blockers such as nifedipine or verapamil.
(8) Combined with nitroglycerin, phenylephrine is an optimal therapy for hypotension-induced cardiac ischemia.
(9) Tachyphylaxis to the effects of phenylephrine does not occur.

d. **Metabolism**
(1) Metabolized by MAO; lack of 4-hydroxyl group prevents degradation by COMT
(2) Duration of action is 5–15 minutes IV and up to 50 minutes after SQ injection.

e. **Dose**
(1) Adult: IV bolus: 50–100 μg; may need 1–2 mg for refractory vasodilation. IV infusion 20–500 μg per minute.
(2) Pediatric: 1 μg per kilogram IV bolus
(3) Mix 10–30 mg in 250 cc D_5W (40–120 μg/ml).

IV. Nonsympathomimetic drugs

A. Amrinone (Inocor)

1. **General.** As a noncatecholamine inotropic agent, amrinone inhibits cellular phosphodiesterase and stimulates myocardial contractility by increasing cyclic adenosine monophosphate (cAMP). This increase stimulates myocardial contractility and peripheral vasodilation by relaxation of vascular smooth muscle.
Actions:

1. Cardiac index: increase
2. Heart rate: no change
3. SVR: decrease
4. Pulmonary capillary wedge pressure: decrease
5. Mean arterial pressure: decrease

2. **Metabolism.** Conjugated and excreted by the liver. The half-life is 3–5 hours. In patients with congestive heart failure (CHF), the half-life is prolonged to 5–8 hours.
3. **Physiology and indications.** A positive inotrope and vasodilator that is very useful in patients with CHF or in hypertensive patients with decreased CO. It has a minimal effect on HR (but should be used with caution in patients with a history of SVT or those on digoxin). It has been shown to have both additive and synergistic effects in patients on dobutamine to increase their CO. **One of the disadvantages of amrinone** is that due to vasodilation, patients may require alpha stimulation after amrinone is infused. Another is that thrombocytopenia may occur after 24 hours of infusion (in 3% of patients).
4. **Dose.** Amrinone is administered IV with an initial bolus followed by an IV infusion. The initial bolus is recommended to be 0.75–3.0 mg per kilogram over 10–15 minutes. A bolus toward the upper end of the

spectrum usually requires the addition of an alpha agent to prevent profound vasodilation. Because of its long half-life, one may intermittently bolus with more conservative doses and observe the effects on the peripheral resistance but obtain the additive effects on inotropy. At the same time an infusion of 5–10 μg/kg/minute should be started. The concomitant administration of drugs with vasodilator properties should be monitored very carefully (e.g., disopyramide and vancomycin). The maximum daily dose is 10 mg/kg/day.

B. Calcium

1. **General.** Calcium is an inorganic substance critical for excitation-contraction coupling and electrical conduction in myocardial cells. It is physiologically active only in its ionized state (Ca 2+). Approximately 50% is ionized, and the other 50% is bound to proteins and anions. Diminished calcium ion concentration can be associated with myocardial depression and loss of peripheral resistance. These changes lead to hypotension and a low CO state. It is also very important in the normal response to many vasoactive drugs, including catecholamines. Ionized calcium is decreased by alkalosis and by citrate infusion during rapid blood transfusion. An increase in ionized calcium occurs during acidosis. A normal serum value is 1.0–1.5 mmol per liter. It has been shown in vitro that heparin binds to ionized calcium and may therefore cause hypotension.
2. **Indications.** Calcium should be administered to patients who are symptomatic from hypocalcemia. Critically ill patients may be hypotensive from hypocalcemia secondary to decreased myocardial contractility. Calcium will also reverse the effects of hyperkalemia (i.e., AV block, ventricular dysrhythmias, and myocardial depression). Calcium administration may be effective in electromechanical dissociation, some arrhythmias, and, rarely, asystole. It may be used to reverse the effects of hypermagnesemia. During massive blood transfusion, the citrate in the blood may bind significant amounts of calcium to create a hypocalcemic state. This may also occur with fresh-frozen plasma (FFP) transfusion due to binding of calcium by the components of FFP.
3. **Physiology.** The physiologic effects of calcium are related to the initial calcium level prior to its administration. If hypocalcemia is the baseline condition, one can expect increased myocardial contractility without a change in HR. This will increase the CO, stroke volume, and BP. Continued administration after normalization of the ionized calcium will result in an increase in SVT and a gradual decrease in CO to baseline. The effects on preload are dependent on how the calcium affects CO. Calcium is commonly used to wean a patient from bypass. This is because hypocalcemia commonly occurs during bypass. I recommend administering only after the heart has been reperfused. In the ICU, its positive inotropic effects without an increase in HR can be used to reverse the myocardial depression of calcium channel blockers, halogenated anesthetics, hypocalcemia, and beta-blockers. It can also be used to reverse the cardiotoxicity of hyperkalemia that may be manifested by arrhythmias, heart block, and negative inotropy. Rarely, asystole may respond to a calcium bolus. **The disadvantages of calcium administration** are severe bradycardia (vagal effect seen predominantly in children), potentiation of digitalis effect (ventricular arrhythmias, AV block, asystole), and potentiation of hypokalemia.
4. **Metabolism.** Calcium is incorporated into bone and muscle and is excreted though the kidneys.
5. **Dose.** Calcium may be given in two forms: calcium chloride or calcium gluconate. The usual dose of calcium chloride is 5–10 mg per kilogram IV slowly. Calcium gluconate may be given at up to three

times this dose. These doses raise the ionized calcium approximately the same amount. It has been reported that critically ill patients may require infusions of calcium chloride of up to 1.5 mg per kg IV slowly. The calcium gluconate may be given at up to three times this dose.

C. Digoxin

1. **General.** Digoxin is the most commonly administered cardiac glycoside and differs pharmacokinetically from the other preparations but is very similar in clinical use. It may be given PO, IV, or IM. Absorption by all of these routes may be significantly altered by metabolic function. Therefore, it is very important to measure digoxin levels. Digoxin inhibits sodium–potassium–adenosine triphosphate. This inhibition in the myocardial cells leads to sodium accumulation within the cells. This leaves more intracellular sodium available for exchange with extracellular calcium. The increase in intracellular calcium from the sarcoplasm results in increased inotropy from the digoxin.
2. **Indications**
   - **a.** Congestive heart failure, especially secondary to ischemic heart disease; usually in combination with diuretics and angiotensin-converting enzyme inhibitors
   - **b.** Afib with a rapid ventricular response
   - **c.** Supraventricular tachyarrhythmias except Wolf-Parkinson-White (WPW) syndrome with anterograde conduction though an accessory AV pathway. Since digoxin may increase atrial automaticity, WPW patients may convert from an accelerated supraventricular rhythm to ventricular tachycardia (Vtach) or fibrillation.
   - **d.** Ventricular dysfunction
   - **e.** Prophylactic digoxin may be used to prevent postoperative SVTs in coronary artery bypass graft (CABG) and pneumonectomy patients.
3. **Physiology.** The physiologic effects of digoxin differ markedly in the normal and the dysfunctional heart due to the direct inotropic action of the drug and the resulting effects on autonomic reflexes. In the failing heart when digoxin increases contractility, the increase in dP/dT results in an attenuation of baroreceptor-mediated sympathetic outflow. Therefore, digoxin causes a direct increase in ventricular function with a decrease in left ventricular end-diastolic pressure (LVEDP) and a decrease in HR and indirectly lowers SVR and venous tone. The slower HR is due to decreased sympathetic tone and to a vagal and direct effect at the AV node. Patients with normal ventricular function experience a rise in SVR and no change in CO. The etiology of this effect is uncertain. The net result in the patient with CHF is a decrease in HR, SVR, and MVO_2 and an increase in stroke volume. **The electrophysiologic effect** is also a result of direct and indirect actions. The sino-atrial (SA) node changes (lower rate in the failing heart) are primarily from decreased automaticity. An increase in atrial conduction velocity is a result of vagotonic action from the drug. At the AV node, there is lower conduction velocity and an increased refractory period—the result of both direct and vagal effects of digoxin. There is both an increase in automaticity and a decrease in ventricular conduction velocity. The effects on the ventricle are seen at toxic levels. **The disadvantages of digoxin** are its long half-life, low therapeutic index (20% incidence of toxicity), and variable interpatient therapeutic response. The long half-life makes the drug difficult to titrate, knowing that a toxic level will be sustained for a period of time. The toxicity of the drug may initially present with changes in the electrophysiology of the heart. This may be difficult to recognize because just about any known rhythm may occur as a result. That

includes the exact arrhythmia that the physician may be attempting to treat. WPW should not be treated with this drug.

4. **Metabolism.** Digoxin is eliminated primarily through the kidneys and has an elimination half-life of 1.6 days. In anephric patients, this may be as long as 4–5 days.
5. **Dose**
   a. In the adult with normal renal function, a loading dose IV or IM of 0.25–0.5 mg with incremental doses of 0.25 mg up to 1–1.25 mg over the first 24 hours is recommended. The daily maintenance dose is based on the clinical effect and drug level. In the pediatric population, the digitalizing dose ranges from 15–50 μg per kilogram, depending on age. The maintenance dose is approximately one-third of the digitalizing dose. There should be decreased maintenance dosages in patients with renal insufficiency. The onset of action is gradual over 15–30 minutes and has a peak effect in 1–5 hours. Administration is cautioned in patients receiving beta-blockers, calcium channel blockers, or calcium. The physician should be aware of factors that potentiate toxicity: hypokalemia, hypercalcemia, alkalosis, hypomagnesemia, glucose and/or insulin infusion, acidosis, quinicine therapy, hypothyroidism, and renal insufficiency.
   b. The treatment of digoxin toxicity consists of raising the serum potassium level, treating ventricular arrhythmias with phenytoin or lidocaine, and treating atrial arrhythmias with phenytoin. Some refractory arrhythmias may respond to propranolol, but pacing may be required if AV block develops. Antidigoxin antibodies may be administered.
   c. Digoxin levels are considered therapeutic between 0.5–2.5 ng per milliliter. Toxicity may occur at these levels if any of the factors that potentiate toxicity exist (see **b**).

D. Glucagon

1. **General.** Glucagon is a polypeptide hormone produced by the alpha cells of the pancreas.
2. **Indications.** Glucagon has been shown to improve myocardial function in patients with acute dysfunction who are receiving beta-blockers. This has also been shown in patients with cardiogenic shock secondary to an acute myocardial infarction. **Other indications for glucagon administration** include sphincter of Oddi spasm and hypoglycemia (patients without IV access may receive glucagon IM).
3. **Physiology.** Intravenous administration of glucagon results in an increase in MVO_2 and a corresponding increase in myocardial blood flow. It also increases automaticity in the SA and AV nodes without increasing ventricular automaticity. It is believed that glucagon activates membrane adenyl cyclase by binding to its own receptor. For this reason, patients who are receiving beta-blockers are not refractory to glucagon therapy to improve myocardial dysfunction. The risk in this approach is that glucagon may cause an increase in HR with detrimental effects on myocardial oxygen supply and demand. Glucagon may increase catecholamine release from a pheochromocytoma. Other side effects include nausea, vomiting, hyperglycemia, and possibly hypokalemia secondary to insulin release and intracellular shift of potassium. Anaphylaxis may occur.
4. **Metabolism.** Glucagon is broken down by proteolysis in the liver, kidney, plasma, and tissue receptor sites.
5. **Dose.** To achieve cardiovascular effects, the drug may be given as a bolus of 1–5 mg slowly IV or as an infusion of 2–5 mg per hour. The onset of action is in 3–5 minutes and lasts 20–30 minutes. It is sometimes used in the operating room to reverse sphincter of Oddi

spasm in patients who have received narcotics. The dose in this situation is 1 mg IV. The utilization of glucagon is rare in modern clinical practice.

V. **Vasodilators** (Table 29-4)

A. **Overview.** Vasodilators are a diverse group of compounds that have in common the ability to relax arterial and/or venous smooth muscle. These drugs act through a variety of mechanisms: direct smooth muscle dilatation, blockade of alpha-1 adrenergic receptors, ganglionic blockade, alpha-2 agonist effects, and inhibition of the renin-angiotensin system. Clinical indications for the use of vasodilator drugs include:

1. **Hypertensive patients** in whom control of increased SVR and BP is important. Arterial or mixed vasodilators are most helpful in this setting.
2. **Normotensive patients** in whom controlled hypotension must be produced (e.g., in patients with dissecting aortic aneurysms or those who are bleeding where lowered BP might reduce blood loss)
3. **Patients with acute or chronic valvular insufficiency,** such as rheumatic mitral regurgitation, where afterload reduction may improve forward CO
4. **Patients with congestive heart failure** in whom venous and arterial vasodilators may reduce elevated filling pressures and lower afterload, thereby improving myocardial function and CO

B. **Drug therapy**

1. **Alpha-blockers**

a. **Chlorpromazine (Thorazine)**

(1) **General:** phenothiazine-type drug that produces alpha-1 adrenergic blockade and decreased SVR

(2) **Physiology:** clinically a major tranquilizer and antipsychotic that produces hypotension and may be profound and unpredictable in the higher-dose ranges

(3) **Metabolism.** Chlorpromazine is metabolized in the liver. Duration of action is around 8 hours with a half-life of 10–30 hours. Beware the development of extrapyramidal symptoms due to blockade of dopaminergic receptors.

(4) **Dose.** Doses of 1–2 mg IV may be used every 2 minutes and titrated to effect with a maximum of 25 mg.

b. **Clonidine (Catapres)**

(1) **General:** an alpha-2 agonist that decreases sympathetic nervous system output from the CNS and reduces peripheral norepinephrine release

(2) **Physiology:** generally used outside the ICU setting in the treatment of chronic hypertension. In the ICU, it may be useful in the treatment of severe hypertension or hypertensive crisis. In addition, clonidine may be given as a premedicant to produce sedation and blunting of sympathetic reflexes prior to and during surgery. It also has analgesic properties. Clonidine can produce severe rebound hypertension if it is withdrawn suddenly. A dosage taper over 2–4 days is recommended. Alternatively, the drug may be continued until immediately preoperatively and then restarted postoperatively via nasogastric tube, orally, or by transdermal patch.

(3) **Metabolism:** renally excreted (60%) with a half-life of approximately 12 hours

(4) **Dose:** dose range is 0.2–0.8 mg per day PO with a maximum effective dose of 2.4 mg per day; effective transdermal doses, 0.2–0.6 mg per day

c. **Droperidol (Inapsine)**

(1) **General:** a butyrophenone relative of haloperidol and a neuro-

Table 29-4. Vasodilators

Type	Site of action	Site of excretion	Duration	Dose
Direct				
Nifedipine	Arterial	Hepatic	1.5–5.0 hr	10–20 mg SL 10–40 mg PO
Verapamil	Arterial	Hepatic/renal	5–30 min IV 3–10 hr PO	5–10 mg IV 5 μg/kg/min IV 40–80 mg PO
Nicardipine	Arterial	Hepatic/renal	4–12 hr	20–40 mg PO tid
Diazoxide	Arterial	Hepatic/renal	3–12 hr	1–3 mg/kg to 150 mg 7.5–30 mg/min
Hydralazine	Arterial	Hepatic	2–6 hr	2.5–20 mg IV
Minoxidil	Arterial	Hepatic/renal	2–5 days	2.5–25 mg PO
Nitroglycerin	Venous/arterial	Hepatic/smooth muscle	10 min	0.1–7 μg/kg/min 50–200 μg IV bolus
Nitroprusside	Arterial/venous	Renal/hepatic	2–4 min	0.1–8 μg/kg/min
Alpha-blockers				
Chlorpromazine	Arterial/venous	Hepatic	8 hr	1–2 mg IV bolus
Droperidol	Arterial/venous	Hepatic/renal	3–30 min for alpha block effects	1.25–5.0 mg IV/IM
Labetalol	Arterial/venous	Hepatic	3–8 hr	2.5–20 mg
Phentolamine	Arterial/venous	Hepatic/renal	20 min	1–5 mg IV bol. 1–20 μg/kg min
Prazocin	Arterial/venous	Hepatic	2–24 hr	2–20 mg/day PO divided doses
Clonidine	Arterial/venous	Renal	8 hr	0.2–0.8 mg/day PO
Methyldopa	Arterial/venous	Renal	10–16 hr	0.25–1.0 gm IV over 30–60 min
Ganglionic blockers				
Trimethaphan	Autonomic Ganglia	Renal	5–10 min	0.5–20 mg IV bol. 0.5–6.0 mg/min
Angiotensin converting enzyme inhibitors				
Captopril	Decreased angiotensin II	Hepatic/renal	2–6 hr	12.5–50 mg PO TID
Lisinopril	Decreased angiotensin II	Renal	6–24 hr	10–40 mg/day PO

leptic major tranquilizer. Droperidol blocks postsynaptic dopamine receptors and produces alpha-1 adrenergic blockade and reduction in SVR.

(2) **Physiology**

(a) It is a potent antiemetic that sedates patients, making them appear outwardly calm; patients may actually feel dysphoric and anxious but will not volunteer this information.

(b) Droperidol is a cerebral vasoconstrictor and as such may be an undesirable medication in patients with cerebral vascular disease. It is a cardiac antidysrhythmic and protects against epinephrine-induced arrhythmias. Conduction of cardiac impulses along accessory pathways is also depressed by droperidol (e.g., WPW syndrome).

(c) Ventilation and carbon dioxide responses are not changed by droperidol and may actually augment ventilatory responses to hypoxemia.

(d) Extrapyramidal reactions may occur in up to 1% of patients, a side effect that may be treated with IV diphenhydramine.

(3) **Metabolism.** Droperidol is hepatically metabolized.

(4) **Dose.** Droperidol dosages range from 0.625–5 mg IV or IM, with effects lasting 3–8 hours.

d. Labetalol (Normodyne)

(1) **General.** A unique combination alpha- and beta-adrenergic blocker selective for alpha-1 and nonselective for beta-1 and beta-2 receptors

(2) **Physiology**

(a) About one-half as potent as phentolamine as an alpha-blocker and one-fourth as potent as propranolol as a beta-antagonist. It lacks intrinsic sympathomimetic activity.

(b) Used IV to lower BP acutely, to produce deliberate controlled hypotension. The oral form may be used chronically to treat essential hypertension. Labetalol lowers BP through reductions in PVR and CO.

(c) Orthostatic hypotension is its major side effect, along with dry mouth, nausea, and diarrhea.

(3) **Metabolism.** Labetalol is metabolized in the liver with an elimination half-life of 5–8 hours, which is prolonged by liver disease and unchanged by renal dysfunction.

(4) **Dose.** Oral doses start at 100 mg PO bid. Intravenous labetalol is effective with a starting dose of 20 mg followed by 40–80 mg q10min to a maximum of 300 mg. An infusion of 2 mg per minute may also be used.

e. Methyldopa (Aldomet)

(1) **General:** a central-acting antihypertensive. It is converted to alpha-methyl norepinephrine in the brain, where it stimulates inhibitory alpha-2 receptors in the vasomotor center, which reduces sympathetic nervous system activity. Peripheral vascular tone and BP are reduced by the mechanism and possibly by displacement of norepinephrine from peripheral nerve terminals.

(2) **Physiology**

(a) Methyldopa reduces peripheral resistance, while CO and HR are minimally changed. Myocardial, cerebral, and renal blood flows are preserved. In older patients, preload may diminish secondary to venodilation, which can reduce CO in some cases.

(b) Side effects of methyldopa include sedation, postural hypotension, depression, increased liver enzymes, Coombs-positive hemolytic anemia, rebound hypertension, a lupuslike syndrome, salt and water retention, and false-positive tests for pheochromocytoma.

(3) **Metabolism.** Methyldopa is eliminated by the kidneys, with duration of response lasting 12–24 hours.

(4) **Dose.** It has a slow onset of action, with peak effects occurring 6–8 hours after PO or IV administration. Adult doses are 0.25–1.0 g IV over 30–60 minutes and 0.25–1.0 g bid PO. The pediatric dose is 5–10 mg per kilogram q6h (maximum 65 mg/kg or 3 g daily, whichever is less).

f. Phentolamine (Regitine)

(1) **General:** an imidazole derivative that nonselectively blocks alpha-1 and alpha-2 receptors and directly dilates vascular smooth muscle. Phentolamine is used to treat hypertensive emergencies, such as with manipulation of a pheochromocytoma; local infiltration is also used to treat extravasated catecholamines (e.g., epinephrine or norepinephrine).

(2) **Physiology**

(a) Blood pressure is reduced within 2 minutes and remains lower for 10–15 minutes after doses of 10–20 μg per kilogram.

(b) Phentolamine causes reflex cardiac stimulation with increased HR and CO. Angina and arrhythmias may result.

(c) It can cause diarrhea, increased peristalsis, and abdominal pain.

(3) **Metabolism.** Elimination is by hepatic metabolism with some renal excretion.

(4) **Dose**

(a) Intravenous bolus 1–5 mg; IV infusion 1–20 μg/kg/minutes

(b) Infiltrate 5–10 mg in 10 cc normal saline into skin affected by extravasated norepinephrine.

g. Prazosin (Minipress)

(1) **General.** A quinazoline derivative that produces selective postsynaptic alpha-1 adrenergic blockade and peripheral vasodilation. Prazosin is useful in the therapy of essential hypertension and may be of value in reducing afterload in patients with CHF. Since prazosin does not affect presynaptic alpha-2 receptors, inhibitory norepinephrine release mechanisms remain intact, and this may contribute to the lack of compensatory tachycardia seen with this drug.

(2) **Physiology**

(a) Prazosin has a higher affinity for alpha-receptors in veins.

(b) It has been associated with the so-called first-dose phenomenon whereby severe orthostatic hypotension and syncope occur 30–90 minutes after an initial dose. Consequently, prazosin is initially dosed before bedtime.

(i) Prostaglandin inhibitors may abolish the antihypertensive effects of prazosin.

(ii) Other side effects include vertigo and fluid retention.

(iii) Prazosin is useful in the preoperative preparation of patients with pheochromocytoma.

(3) **Metabolism.** Hepatic metabolism accounts for a 3-hour elimination half-time, 4–6-hour duration of action, and unaltered dosing in renal failure.

(4) **Dose.** The initial dose of prazosin is 1 mg PO, 2–3 times per day, with maximal effective dose of 20 mg per day.

2. Direct vasodilators

a. Hydralazine (Apresoline)

(1) **General.** Hydralazine is a phthalazine derivative that reduces

BP by directly dilating arteriolar smooth muscle. There is little venodilation.

(2) **Physiology**

(a) Hydralazine produces a somewhat selective dilation of coronary, splanchnic, cerebral, and renal vascular beds compared with muscle or skin; TPR is reduced, and HR, stroke volume, and CO increase.

(b) Uterine blood flow is maintained in the absence of hypertension.

(c) Orthostatic hypotension is minimized due to the lack of venodilation.

(d) Exaggerated increases in HR may occur. Concurrent beta-blocker therapy may limit these HR increases and prevent development of myocardial ischemia.

(e) Hydralazine can induce a lupuslike syndrome in 10–20% of chronically treated patients. Symptoms occur most often in slow acetylators, who have been treated for more than 6 months with doses above 400 mg per day.

(f) Other side effects include fluid retention, vertigo, drug fever, urticaria, peripheral neuropathies, and pancytopenia.

(g) Hydralazine can produce enhanced defluorination of enflurane, possibly leading to nephrotoxicity.

(3) **Metabolism.** Hydralazine is acetylated in the liver, with only a small fraction (<15%) appearing unchanged in the urine.

(4) **Dose.** Clinically, hydralazine is an effective antihypertensive in the operating room and ICU. Doses of 5–10 mg IV lead to BP reductions in 15 minutes, with effects lasting 3–4 hours. Pediatric dose of hydralazine is 0.2–0.5 mg per kilogram q4–6h, slow IV. Hydralazine may be used to supplement other antihypertensive agents, such as nitroprusside, nitroglycerin, or trimethaphan. Combined therapy often allows a reduced dosage of these drugs with a lower risk of side effects.

b. Diazoxide (Hyperstat)

(1) **General.** Diazoxide is a direct-acting vasodilator of the benzothiadiazine class.

(2) **Physiology**

(a) It produces arteriolar dilation with little effect on venous tone. Cardiac output is increased, and HR is often elevated. Blood pressure is rapidly reduced by this drug, making it suitable for the rapid treatment of severe hypertension.

(b) This drug is a potent relaxer of uterine smooth muscle.

(c) It can increase LV dP/dT, making it a poor choice in the treatment of hypertension associated with dissecting aortic aneurysms.

(d) Diazoxide can produce coronary steal and myocardia ischemia.

(e) Side effects of this drug include salt and water retention, hyperglycemia, and stimulation of catecholamine release. The last effect prohibits use of this drug in treating patients with pheochromocytoma.

(f) This drug is often difficult to titrate to effect. Too rapid administration may produce excessive hypotension, whereas slow IV injection may have reduced effects.

(3) **Metabolism**

(a) Diazoxide is principally excreted as unchanged drug by the kidneys.

(b) Rapid injection leads to reduction in systolic and diastolic BP within 1–2 minutes that lasts 3–15 hours.

(4) **Dose**

(a) Adult: IV, 1–3 mg per kilogram (max 150 mg); may repeat q5–15 min. Infusion 7.5–30 mg per minute. Pediatric: 1–3 mg per kilogram IV in increments

c. **Nitroglycerin**

(1) **General.** An organic nitrate that primarily dilates venous capacitance vessels, epicardial coronary arteries, and, to a lesser extent, arteriolar smooth muscle. Increased venous capacitance leads to reduced venous return, lower cardiac filling pressure, and decreased ventricular wall tension. Because of these effects, nitroglycerin is used to treat angina pectoris and coronary vasospasm and is used for production of controlled hypotension.

(2) **Physiology.** Nitroglycerin has a number of salutory effects on the heart.

(a) Lower LV preload and wall tension decreases myocardial oxygen consumption and increases diastolic coronary blood flow. There may be redistribution of blood flow to ischemic myocardium with increased endocardial to epicardial flow ratio. At higher doses, nitroglycerin can reduce peripheral vascular resistance.

(b) This drug may improve cardiac performance in patients with acute valvular insufficiency (e.g., mitral regurgitation) through its preload and afterload reducing effects.

(c) Nitroglycerin raises the VF threshold in ischemic myocardium.

(d) This drug is effective in the therapy of acute pulmonary edema.

(e) It can limit infarct size in ischemic hearts.

(f) Nitroglycerin can be used to produce controlled hypotension, although its effects are somewhat dependent on the volume status of the patient. It is less potent in this regard than nitroprusside, although nitroprusside is more likely to produce myocardial ischemia when BP is lowered.

(g) Nitroglycerin relaxes smooth muscle in the biliary tract and often relieves opioid-induced biliary spasm. It can relax uterine smooth muscle and may be useful in treatment of the hypertonic uterus. Nitroglycerin also relieves esophageal spasm.

(h) Acute hypertension in the parturient may be safely treated with nitroglycerin, given concern over the possible adverse effects on the fetus of maternal nitroprusside or trimethaphan therapy.

(i) Nitroglycerin is effective in reducing pulmonary artery pressure in the treatment of pulmonary hypertension and right heart failure.

(3) **Side effects**

(a) Nitroglycerin prolongs bleeding time but does not alter platelet aggregation.

(b) If BP falls, coronary perfusion pressure is reduced and baroreceptor-mediated tachycardia and increased contractility may ensue, with detrimental increase in myocardial oxygen consumption.

(c) May cause methemoglobinemia at doses greater than 7–10 μg/kg/minute for prolonged periods. Treat with methylene blue 1–2 mg per kilogram IV over 5 minutes to convert methemoglobin back to hemoglobin.

(d) Nitroglycerin can blunt hypoxic pulmonary vasoconstriction.
(e) The drug may increase intracranial pressure.
(f) Tolerance to nitroglycerin develops after chronic exposure to high doses. This may diminish the hemodynamic response to acute administration of the drug.
(g) Headache frequently accompanies nitroglycerin therapy, presumably stemming from dilatation of cerebral vessels.
(h) Polyvinyl chloride tubing absorbs nitroglycerin, thereby reducing the effective dose administered. Special plastic tubing sets are available that do not absorb this drug.

(4) **Metabolism:** hepatic reductive hydrolysis with a half-life of 1–3 minutes.

(5) **Dose**
(a) Sublingual: 0.15–0.6 mg q5min, up to 3 doses
(b) IV: 50–100 μg bolus versus infusion of 0.1–7 μg/kg/minute
(c) Topical: 2% ointment 0.5–2 inches applied to skin q4–8h; transdermal patch 5–10 mg q24h
(d) Concentrated nitroglycerin solutions contain appreciable ethanol.
(e) Nitroglycerin is best stored in glass bottles rather than plastic bags and is light stable, unlike nitroprusside.

d. Nitroprusside

(1) **General.** Nitroprusside is a direct-acting arterial and venous vasodilator. This drug lowers BP by relaxing arteriolar smooth muscle, which decreases SVR, and through venous pooling, which diminishes venous return and cardiac filling pressures. Nitroprusside has a rapid onset and short duration of action, which necessitates continuous infusion to maintain a therapeutic effect and close monitoring of arterial pressure. Nitroprusside is indicated for the acute management of severe hypertension, for the production of controlled hypotension, and for reducing arterial impedance to improve CO in cases of CHF or cardiac valvular regurgitation.

(2) **Physiology.** Administration of nitroprusside produces nitric oxide, which stimulates guanylate cyclase, resulting in increased cyclic guanosine monophosphate and relaxation of smooth muscle in arteries and veins. This drug causes the following effects on the cardiovascular system:
(a) Blood pressure is reduced through decreases in SVR and preload.
(b) Myocardial contractility and HR increase via an arterial baroreflex-mediated response to hypotension. This tends to counteract reductions in CO due to decreased venous return. Beta blockade may blunt this response.
(c) Coronary steal may occur with nitroprusside due to diversion of blood flow to nonischemic, newly vasodilated vascular beds. These effects may increase tissue damage associated with myocardial infarction. Conversely, treatment of severe hypertension with nitroprusside may lower myocardial oxygen consumption, which may reduce or prevent ischemia.
(d) Administration of nitroprusside may increase release of renin from the kidneys. Rebound hypertension following cessation of nitroprusside therapy may be due to increased levels of angiotension II generated by higher renin levels. Beta blockade, angiotensin blockade, or slow tapering of nitroprusside infusion can prevent this rebound hypertensive response.

(e) This drug directly dilates cerebral vessels, leading to increased cerebral blood flow and blood volume. This effect may increase intracranial pressure (ICP) in patients at risk for intracranial hypertension. Slow administration of nitroprusside in the presence of hypocarbia as opposed to rapid infusion, may not increase ICP.

(f) Hypoxic pulmonary vasoconstriction is blunted by nitroprusside. This can lead to hypoxemia through increased ventilation-perfusion (V/Q) mismatch, especially in patients with pulmonary disease or in those with atelectasis. Positive end-expiratory pressure (PEEP) may help overcome this effect.

(g) Nitroprusside acts rapidly, and its effects last 1–3 minutes.

(h) The pulmonary vascular bed is effectively dilated by this drug.

(3) **Metabolism**

(a) Nitroprusside reacts with erythrocyte hemoglobin to produce cyanmethemoglobin, nitric oxide, and free cyanide ions (CN^-). Cyanide ion binds to and inhibits cytochrome oxidase, which blocks aerobic metabolism and causes tissue hypoxia.

(b) Normally, at low infusion rates, cyanide is converted to thiocyanate, in a reaction requiring thiosulfate, by the action of rhodanese, an enzyme found in liver and kidney. Thiocyanate is much less toxic than cyanide ion, although it too has toxic effects if levels are chronically elevated.

(c) Cyanide may combine with hydroxocobalamin to form cyanocobalamin (vitamin B_{12}).

(d) The risk of cyanide toxicity is increased by:

(i) Initial infusion rates more than 2–3 μg/kg/minute

(ii) Maximal infusion rates more than 8 μg/kg/minute for more than 3 hours

(iii) Risk of thiocyanate toxicity increases for infusions over 24–48 hours, especially in patients with renal dysfunction

(iv) Presence of Leber's optic atrophy or tobacco amblyopia

(v) Total dose more than 1 mg per kilogram over 12–24 hours

(4) **Toxicity**

(a) Signs of cyanide toxicity

(i) Tachyphylaxis to increasing dosages of nitroprusside

(ii) Development of metabolic acidosis with elevated mixed venous PO_2 reflecting impaired tissue oxygen utilization and anaerobic metabolism

(b) Signs of thiocyanate toxicity include fatigue, nausea, anorexia, toxic psychosis, miosis, hyperreflexia, and seizures. Rarely, iodine uptake by the thyroid may be inhibited with resulting hypothyroidism.

(5) **Therapy.** When signs of cyanide toxicity (**4.a**) are detected, prompt discontinuation of nitroprusside therapy is mandatory.

(a) Mild toxicity is treated with sodium thiosulfate 150 mg per kilogram IV over 15 minutes.

(b) In severe cases with extreme metabolic acidosis (base deficit more than 10) and unstable hemodynamics, either sodium nitrate, 5 mg per kilogram IV, is slowly administered or amyl nitrite, 1 ampule, is placed in a breathing bag and inhaled. These therapies convert hemoglobin to methemoglobin, which binds cyanide to produce cyanmethemoglobin. In addition, sodium thiosulfate should be administered as for mild toxicity.

(c) During therapy of cyanide toxicity, high FIO_2 should be maintained, and bicarbonate should be used to treat metabolic acidosis.

(d) Hydroxocobalamin, which reacts with cyanide to form cyanocobalamin, has also been recommended.

(e) Thiocyanate may accumulate in patients with renal dysfunction, and levels should not be allowed to exceed 0.1 mg per milliliter. However, dialysis readily removes thiocyanate from the circulation.

(6) Clinical dosing

(a) Nitroprusside is generally mixed by adding 50 mg to 250 ml IV fluid (200 μg/ml). In some institutions, more concentrated solutions are utilized to accommodate various drip rates.

(b) Automated infusion pumps facilitate accurate dosing and prevent inadvertent overdoses.

(c) Nitroprusside solutions are photosensitive and are generally protected from light by foil wrapping. It is not necessary to wrap the IV tubing.

(d) Dose range: 0.1–8.0 μg/kg minute IV, titrated to BP response

(e) Nitroprusside is most often administered into a central venous line. An arterial line should be used, and Swan-Ganz monitoring of filling pressures is often recommended.

(f) Concurrent therapy with beta-blockers and/or other vasodilators will decrease the amount of nitroprusside required to achieve a given BP reduction.

3. Ganglionic blockers: Trimethaphan camsylate (Arfonad)

a. General. This drug is a peripheral vasodilator and autonomic ganglionic blocker with rapid onset of action and brief duration. It lowers BP by reducing systemic vascular resistance and CO (through decreased venous return and blunting of cardiovascular reflexes). This combination of effects makes it an effective hypotensive agent. In contrast to nitroprusside, plasma catecholamine and renin levels do not increase in response to decreases in BP produced by trimethaphan due to its ganglionic blocking effects. In this regard, trimethaphan is well suited for control of BP in patients with dissecting **aortic aneurysms.** It is also useful in high doses in the treatment of **autonomic hyperreflexia.** In this case, a complete ganglionic blockade interrupts in the spinal reflexes responsible for triggering severe hypertension in patients with cervical or high thoracic spinal cord lesions. Trimethaphan can be used to blunt sympathetically mediated hypertensive and tachycardic responses to endotracheal intubation. This is especially useful in hypertensive patients who cannot tolerate a further rise in BP, such as parturients with eclampsia or preeclampsia. Trimethaphan is a useful adjunct to other hypotensive agents, such as nitroprusside. Combination therapy can lower the amount of either drug required and reduce side effects.

b. Physiology. Trimethaphan produces a number of effects that may diminish its overall usefulness.

(1) It reduces GI motility and may lead to paralytic ileus.

(2) Pupillary dilation (mydriasis) may interfere with the neurologic examination of neurosurgical patients.

(3) There may be urinary retention.

(4) Trimethaphan does not increase ICP as much as nitroprusside does for a given degree of induced hypotension.

(5) Histamine release following trimethaphan infusion can stimulate catecholamine release, which may be deleterious in patients with pheochromocytoma.

(6) This drug inhibits plasma pseudocholinesterase, which may prolong the action of succinylcholine in patients.

(7) High doses (100–300 mg) may have persistent effects (>1 hour).

c. **Metabolism.** Trimethaphan may be metabolized by plasma pseudocholinesterase. It is a quaternary amine and does not penetrate the blood-brain barrier. Duration of action is 5–10 minutes, with onset of effect in 1–2 minutes.

d. **Dose.** Trimethaphan is administered as an IV bolus of 0.5–20 mg or as a continuous infusion of 10–200 μg/kg/minute. Bolus doses may be repeated every minute.

VI. Calcium channel blockers

A. **Overview.** Calcium channel blockers (CCBs) are a structurally diverse group of compounds that share the distinctive feature of blocking slow inward calcium currents across cell membranes. These slow calcium channels are controlled by voltage-sensitive and cAMP-dependent gates that normally regulate calcium inflow. The CCBs interfere with these gates, thereby blocking calcium influx. Calcium influx is responsible for the plateau phase of the cardiac action potential, an important element in excitation-contraction coupling in cardiac muscle and vascular smooth muscle, as well as for depolarization of sinoatrial and atrioventricular nodal tissue. Inhibition of this influx leads to decreased **myocardial contractility,** decreased **heart rate, slowed conduction** through the **AV node,** and **relaxation of vascular smooth muscle.** Each of the clinically available CCBs has a different spectrum of effects depending on its relative potency of action on myocardial cells, conducting tissue, or vascular smooth muscle. Nifedipine and nicardipine produce more specific vascular smooth muscle relaxation, whereas diltiazem and verapamil have greater effects on AV conduction and cardiac contractility. Verapamil and diltiazem also block fast sodium channels responsible for phase 0 and phase 1 of the cardiac action potential. This explains why these two drugs have local anesthetic activity as well.

B. **Indications for use.** The principal uses of CCBs are in the treatment of:

1. Angina pectoris
2. Coronary vasospasm
3. Supraventricular tachydysrhythmias
4. Essential hypertension
5. Cerebral vasospasm
6. Esophageal spasm
7. Hypertrophic cardiomyopathy
8. Other potential applications: cerebral or myocardial cellular protection during potentially ischemic periods, production of controlled hypotension

C. **Effects common to all CCBs**

1. **Vasodilation.** All CCBs produce arterial vasodilation. There is little if any venodilation. Preload is generally unaffected; there is no venous pooling, and afterload reduction generally improves ventricular performance, offsetting negative inotropic effects of these drugs. Most vascular beds (renal, mesenteric, coronary, pulmonary, cerebral, hepatic, and muscle) are dilated by CCBs. The coronary vasculature is particularly sensitive, and coronary vasospasm can be relieved by small doses of CCBs that do not produce significant negative inotropic effects.

2. **Depressed myocardial contractility.** Calcium channel blockers have variable effects on the strength of cardiac contraction based on their individual properties and degree of preexisting ventricular dysfunction. The dihydropyridine CCBs (nifedipine, nicardipine, nimodipine) produce minimal cardiac depression at usual clinical dosages. Conversely, verapamil and diltiazem may diminish contractility at usual clinical doses that lower BP. In the setting of poor ventricular function, nifedipine may improve CO by decreasing afterload and by baroreflex-mediated rise in sympathetic outflow to the heart. Conversely, verapamil, through its direct negative inotropic and chronotropic effects, may worsen myocardial depression in hypodynamic hearts.
3. **Myocardial ischemia.** All CCBs tend to improve the myocardial oxygen supply-demand ratio. In terms of oxygen supply, they relieve coronary spasm, dilate large coronary arteries and arterioles, and possibly increase flow through collateral channels. On the oxygen consumption side, CCBs lower contractility and HR (diltiazem, verapamil) and decrease wall stress (lower afterload), which reduces myocardial oxygen requirements.
4. **Cardiac impulse conduction.** Sinoatrial rate and atrioventricular node conduction are depressed by verapamil and diltiazem; nifedipine and nicardipine exert minimal effects on these automatic tissues. Verapamil has proved to be of great value in the treatment of a variety of AV nodal reentrant tachyarrythmias due to its marked ability to inhibit the AV node. Concomitantly, excessive AV block may complicate the use of verapamil in the treatment of hypertension or angina, especially within the setting of prior beta-blockade. Diltiazem slows sinus node rates to a greater degree than verapamil, while nifedipine often provokes a reflex HR increase.

   a. **Verapamil (Calan, Isoptin)**

      (1) **General.** A papaverine derivative, verapamil has two optical isomers and is supplied as a racemic mixture. The dextro isomer blocks fast sodium channels, and the levo isomer blocks slow calcium channels. Clinically, verapamil lowers BP through reductions in SVR (major effect) and contractility (minor, except in severe LV dysfunction). Heart rate is slightly decreased, and AV conduction is slowed.

      (2) **Indications.** Therapy of SVT, ventricular rate control in Afib or flutter, angina pectoris (classic and vasospastic), and hypertension (including hypertensive crises)

      (3) **Physiology**

         (a) This drug is effective in treating a wide range of tachydysrhythmias:

            (i) In SVT, it terminates the reentrant tachycardia in up to 90% of cases.

            (ii) In Afib/flutter, verapamil slows the ventricular rate more rapidly and effectively than digoxin.

            (iii) Verapamil reduces ventricular arrhythmias associated with halothane-epinephrine anesthesia.

            (iv) Antiarrhythmic doses of this drug produce modest cardiac depression and vasodilation.

         (b) Verapamil is useful as an antianginal agent in the treatment of coronary vasospasm and typical atherosclerotic coronary insufficiency. In the latter case, myocardial oxygen requirements are reduced secondary to afterload reduction, depressed myocardial contractility, and decreased HR. Oxygen supply is increased through prolongation of diastolic coronary perfusion time and by coronary vasodilation (plus possible improved coronary collateral blood flow).

(c) Verapamil is a less potent vasodilator than nifedipine and is less likely to produce a marked decrease in BP, which could lead to myocardial ischemia. Due to its negative chronotropic and inotropic effects on the heart, verapamil blunts reflex sympathetic stimulation of the myocardium. This effect makes verapamil (or diltiazem) a good drug to use in combination with nitrates in the therapy of angina since verapamil will prevent reflex increases in HR, which may result from nitrate-induced vasodilatation.

(d) Verapamil should be used with caution in patients receiving beta-blocker therapy. Additive depression of the myocardium and AV conduction could lead to severe AV block, profound bradycardia, and LV failure.

(e) Patients with preexisting poor ventricular function and CHF may exhibit exaggerated depression of LV contractility and acute heart failure following IV verapamil.

(f) Verapamil and other CCBs are ideal drugs for the management of angina and hypertension in patients with asthma or chronic obstructive airway disease since they do not cause bronchospasm.

(g) Verapamil can cause an increase in plasma digoxin levels, although this effect rarely leads to toxicity.

(h) This drug is contraindicated in the therapy of accessory pathway arrhythmias such as WPW syndrome when anterograde aberrant conduction exists. Verapamil does not slow accessory pathway conduction and may increase the ventricular rate or lead to VF during Afib in these patients.

(i) This drug should be avoided in patients with sick sinus syndrome or preexisting AV block.

(4) **Metabolism.** Verapamil is hepatically metabolized and principally excreted in the urine (70%) and bile (15%). The elimination half-time is 2–7 hours, which may be prolonged in patients with liver disease. Norverapamil, which is the principal active metabolite, can accumulate in renal failure. Verapamil is highly protein bound and can be displaced by lidocaine, diazepam or propranolol.

(5) **Dose**

(a) Adults: IV 75–150 μg per kilogram (5–10 mg). Administer slowly in increments to unstable patients. After bolus loading, 5 μg/kg/minute may be infused continuously to achieve prolonged effects. The infusion should be decreased after 30–60 minutes. PO: 40–160 mg q6–8h.

(b) Pediatrics: IV: 75–200 μg per kilogram in increments

(c) Excessive hypotension from verapamil may be treated with phenylephrine (50–100 μg) or calcium gluconate (100 mg, although 1–2 g may be required) infusion. Bradycardia and AV block may respond to atropine (1 mg) or B agonists such as isoproterenol.

(d) Peak hemodynamic effects occur within 5 minutes after IV dose and are over within 10–15 minutes. Arterioventricular nodal effects take 10–15 minutes to reach a maximum and last for up to 6 hours.

b. Nifedipine (Procardia, Adalat)

(1) **General.** Nifedipine is a dihydropyridine derivative that produces mainly peripheral arteriolar vasodilation. Heart rate and myocardia contractility are reflexly increased, AV conduction is improved, and there is little change in venous capacitance.

(2) **Indications.** This drug is used to treat coronary vasospasm, essential hypertension, and acute and chronic angina pectoris.

(3) **Physiology**

(a) At usual clinical doses, nifedipine produces little or no direct myocardial depression or AV block. It can thus be combined with a beta-blocker or digoxin with little risk of conduction disturbance. Use in patients with LV dysfunction is possible with close hemodynamic monitoring.

(b) Nifedipine may reflexly increase HR and contractility, which could increase myocardial oxygen consumption. Combined with significant hypotension, this could exacerbate myocardial ischemia. Prompt therapy to increase BP and substitution of another antianginal are indicated in this situation.

(c) Nifedipine is extremely light sensitive and is available only in a PO formulation (the capsule may be swallowed or the contents delivered sublingually [SL] or intranasally).

(d) Some patients develop peripheral edema; others suffer GI upset.

(e) Severe hypotension may result from therapy with nifedipine. High dosages of an alpha-agonist such as phenylephrine may be required to counteract this effect.

(f) Occasional glucose intolerance and hepatic dysfunction have been reported.

(4) **Metabolism.** This drug is well absorbed after PO/SL administration and has detectable effects in 20 minutes. Nifedipine is almost completed metabolized in the liver to inactive by-products, which are excreted in the urine (80%) and bile. Elimination half-life is 4–6 hours.

(5) **Dose**

(a) Usual dose is 10–40 mg PO tid.

(b) Sublingual dose is 10–20 mg (puncture capsule at both ends with a needle and squeeze contents under tongue or intranasally; after SL administration, absorption occurs in 1–5 minutes).

c. **Nicardipine (Cardene)**

(1) **General.** Nicardipine is a dihydropyridine derivative with a basic structure related to nifedipine. Its pharmacologic properties are similar to those of nifedipine in that it produces vasodilation, especially of the coronary bed, without significant negative inotropic effects.

(2) **Indications.** Nicardipine is indicated for the treatment of chronic stable angina. It may be used concomitantly with beta-blockers and oral nitrates. Nicardipine reduces the number of anginal episodes and increases exercise tolerance. This drug is a more potent coronary vasodilator than nifedipine, although its beneficial effects during myocardial ischemia may result more from its beneficial effects on afterload and myocardial oxygen consumption.

(3) **Physiology**

(a) Nicardipine is an effective antihypertensive. In response to nicardipine-induced decreases in BP, HR and contractility are reflexly increased. These effects, together with the fall in afterload, often lead to an increase in CO.

(b) This drug has been shown to cause marked cerebral vasodilation and may increase cerebrospinal fluid pressure, although to a lesser degree than nitroglycerin.

(c) Renal blood flow is increased in conjunction with decreased renovascular resistance.
(d) Nicardipine has been used to treat perioperative hypertension and to induce controlled hypotension, where it is more effective than nitroprusside. In contrast to nitroprusside, rebound hypertension following therapy has not been observed with nicardipine.
(e) There may be fewer negative inotropic effects on the myocardium from nicardipine when compared with nifedipine.
(f) Nicardipine is not light sensitive, so unlike nifedipine, an IV preparation is available.
(g) There may be a role for nicardipine in the treatment of cerebral vasospasm associated with subarachnoid hemorrhage.
(h) Nicardipine may improve diastolic relaxation in patients with CAD.
(i) **Cautions**
   (i) Nicardipine is contraindicated in patients with advanced aortic stenosis since it may lower diastolic BP sufficiently to worsen myocardial oxygen supply balance.
   (ii) Careful dose titration must be observed when treating patients with severe renal or hepatic dysfunction.
   (iii) Nicardipine has been associated with an increase in angina, although coronary steal may not be involved.

(4) **Metabolism**
(a) Completely absorbed following PO administration
(b) Peak plasma levels between 30 minutes and 2 hours
(c) Extensive first-pass hepatic metabolism with renal (60%) and fecal (35%) elimination
(d) Elimination half-life: 2–4 hours

(5) **Dose**
(a) 20–40 mg PO tid; allow 3 days between dose increases to ensure steady state.
(b) 0.5–10 mg IV titrated
(c) Infusion for therapy of subarachnoid hemorrhage 0.01–0.15 mg/kg/hour

d. Diltiazem (Cardizem)

(1) **General.** Diltiazen is a benzothiazepin derivative that produces cardiovascular effects similar to those of verapamil.

(2) **Indications.** This drug causes selective coronary vasodilation and is effective in the treatment of vasospastic and classic angina. Like other CCBs, it causes peripheral arterial vasodilation and can be used in the therapy of hypertension. Since its electrophysiologic properties mimic those of verapamil, diltiazem may be useful in prophylaxis or acute treatment of supraventricular tachyarrhythmias.

(3) **Physiology**
(a) Diltiazem is well tolerated with fewer side effects than the other CCBs.
(b) This drug often decreases the resting HR, a beneficial effect in patients with CAD. Occasionally, severe sinus bradycardia may occur, however, necessitating discontinuation or a lower dose.
(c) In hypertrophic cardiomyopathy, diltiazem may improve diastolic function.
(d) By prolonging AV conduction, diltiazem improves ventricular rate control in patients with Afib who take digoxin.
(e) Although it seems to have a lesser negative inotropic effect

than verapamil, diltiazem may produce significant LV dysfunction, especially in patients with preexisting CHF or those on beta-blockers.

(f) High-grade AV block may complicate therapy with diltiazem.

(g) Diltiazem may increase serum digoxin levels.

(h) Abdominal discomfort and constipation are potential side effects.

(4) **Metabolism.** Diltiazem is well absorbed orally and is metabolized in the liver. Onset of action is within 15–30 minutes, with peak effects at 1–2 hours. Desacetyl diltiazem is a major metabolite that has half the vasodilating potency of the native compound and accumulates with chronic therapy. Excretion of metabolites is 60% in the bile and 35% in the urine. Elimination half-life is 4–7 hours.

(5) **Dose:** 30–90 mg PO qid to total dose maximum of 360 mg. Sustained release form may be given tid.

VII. Cardiac arrhythmias. Therapy of cardiac arrhythmias requires the ability to recognize the various types of arrhythmias (such as atrial or ventricular) and a knowledge of the therapeutic drugs available to treat a specific disorder.

A. Mechanisms by which cardiac arrhythmias arise

1. **Disturbances in automaticity**
   - **a.** Sinus tachycardia or bradycardia
   - **b.** Premature beats (atrial, AV junctional, ventricular)
   - **c.** Atrial or Vtach
2. **Disturbances in conductivity**
   - **a.** Atrioventricular block
   - **b.** Accessory pathway conduction (Wolff-Parkinson-White)
3. **Combinations of disordered automaticity and conductivity**
   - **a.** Atrial flutter with AV block 3:1 or greater
   - **b.** Premature auricular contraction (PAC) with first-degree block

B. Categorization by **degree of urgency**

1. Fatal arrhythmias if untreated
   - **a.** Ventricular fibrillation
   - **b.** Sustained Vtach producing severe hypotension
   - **c.** Bradyarrhythmias with compromised CO leading to severe hypotension (asystole, complete heart block, severe atrial, or idioventricular bradycardia)
2. Potentially dangerous arrhythmias
   - **a.** Premature ventricular contractions (frequent, coupled, multifocal, "RonT" phenomenon)
   - **b.** Supraventricular tachycardias
     - (1) Sinus tachycardia
     - (2) Afib/flutter
     - (3) Junctional
     - (4) Atrial
     - (5) Accessory pathway (Wolff-Parkinson-White, Lown-Ganong-Levine syndromes)
3. Generally benign rhythms
   - **a.** Sinus bradycardia (in absence of hypotension or premature venticular contractions [PVC])
   - **b.** Isolated atrial premature beats
   - **c.** Sinus arrhythmias

C. General therapeutic principles

1. **Ventricular fibrillation (VF)**
   - **a.** Precordial thump
   - **b.** Initiate CPR, advanced cardiac life support (ACLS)

c. Unsynchronized dc countershock (200–360 J) as soon as possible since CO is zero in absence of cardiac rhythm
d. Bretylium may occasionally convert VF to stable rhythm. In the absence of defibrillation or while awaiting its arrival, administer 5 mg per kilogram IV. If defibrillation is unsuccessful, the dose may be increased to 10 mg per kilogram.
e. Other drugs such as epinephrine, lidocaine, and procainamide may be useful. Correction of acid-base abnormalities along with effective CPR is also important.

2. **Ventricular tachycardia (Vtach)**
   a. If the patient is hemodynamically stable, drug therapy with lidocaine, bretylium, or procainamide should be instituted.
   b. If the patient is unstable, **synchronized** dc cardioversion should be attempted. The synchronization circuit detects the patient's QRS complex and times the delivery of the defibrillator discharge so that it occurs immediately after inscription of the QRS complex. It is important to use an EKG lead with an adequate R-wave height to trigger the synchronizing circuit. If the synchronizer circuit is unable to lock on the QRS or if the patient is in VF, the defibrillator will not fire. Rhythms suitable for synchronized cardioversion include:
      (1) Vtach
      (2) Afib/flutter
      (3) Supraventricular tachycardia
   c. Of note, emergency cardioversion is not recommended for termination of arrhythmias related to digitalis toxicity.
   d. If defibrillation is unsuccessful, drug therapy (lidocaine, bretylium, procainamide) or overdrive pacing may be useful in terminating the arrhythmia.

3. **Bradyarrhythmias (symptomatic)**
   a. Drug therapy to increase HR is preferable in this situation since CPR may induce VF.
   b. Atropine, isoproterenol, calcium chloride, and epinephrine may be useful in this setting.
   c. Definitive therapy involves ventricular pacing with a temporary pacing wire (transvenous or transthoracic).
   d. What appears to be asystole may be very fine VF, which requires dc countershock.

4. **Premature ventricular contractions (PVCs)** may be benign in patients without heart disease, in which case therapy may be unnecessary. They may be harbingers of myocardial ischemia, disordered blood gases, or electrolytes, in which case the potential for progression to Vtach or fibrillation exists. Prompt therapy of PVCs should start with IV lidocaine. Other drugs that may be used include quinidine, procainamide, diphenylhydantoin, propranolol, disopyramide, and digitalis. Overdrive pacing may inhibit PVCs; atropine can be used to increase slow HRs, which may be predisposing to PVCs.

5. **Supraventricular tachycardia (SVT)**
   a. Therapy of SVTs depends on the patient's hemodynamic status. If angina, pulmonary edema, or hypotension is present, synchronized cardioversion is the therapy of choice. Generally, low energy levels (e.g., 50–100 J) are sufficient. Start with a low initial energy, and double with each successive cardioversion attempt.
   b. In stable patients, vagal maneuvers or drug therapy should be tried initially to convert the SVT.
      (1) Carotid sinus massage (unilateral)
      (2) Valsalva maneuver
      (3) Alpha-receptor stimulation with phenylephrine to increase BP

by 30–40 mm Hg should increase vagal tone and slow or convert the SVT. Careful monitoring of BP is essential. Mix 10–30 mg of phenylephrine in 250 cc D_5W and titrate to effect.

(4) Cholinomimetic stimulation with edrophonium. Start with 1 mg IV, wait 1 minute, and administer up to 10 mg IV to produce an effect. Beware bronchospasm.

(5) Other drug therapy options
- (a) Propranolol 1 mg IV q5min up to 5 mg
- (b) Verapamil 75–150 μg per kilogram over 1–3 minutes
- (c) Procainamide 1.5 mg per kilogram (max 1 g)
- (d) Digoxin load with 1 mg over 24 hours
- (e) Adenosine (Adenocard) is a recently released drug that has been used for the acute termination of SVT.
  - (i) Adult dose is 6 mg given by rapid IV push. If the SVT does not terminate after 30 seconds, incremental doses of 9 and 12 mg may be given 1–2 minutes apart.
  - (ii) Pediatric dose is 37.5 μg per kilogram with increments of 37.5 μg per kilogram to a maximum of 350 μg per kilogram.

6. Atrial fibrillation (Afib)

a. Afib may result from excitation of multiple ectopic areas within the atria.

b. Unstable patients (myocardial ischemia, pulmonary edema) should be cardioverted starting at 50 J.

c. In a less acute setting, drug therapy generally starts with digoxin loading 0.25–0.50 mg increments to a total of 1.0–1.25 mg (10–15 μg per kilogram) over 24 hours, followed by 0.125–0.25 mg per day.

d. Quinidine

(1) A PO regimen is recommended. Intravenous quinidine has a high incidence of serious side effects.
- (a) Adult: sulfate 200–600 mg q6–8h; gluconate 324–648 mg q8–12h
- (b) Pediatric: Quinidine sulfate 3–6 mg/kg q3h

(2) Intravenous for emergencies: 4–10 mg per kilogram at a rate of no more than 0.3–0.4 mg/kg/minute, to a maximum of 600 mg

D. Drugs used in the therapy of cardiac dysrhythmias

1. Adenosine (Adenocard)

a. General. Adenosine is a purine nucleoside involved in regulation of the microcirculation, especially in coronary and renal beds and in modulation of autonomic nervous system activity. In pharmacologic doses, it produces marked slowing of the sinus node rate and atrioventricular nodal conduction. At the highest doses, transient, high-degree AV block is produced, which accounts for its ability to terminate SVTs.

b. Indications. This drug is indicated for the acute termination of narrow complex SVT, perhaps as a first-line agent supplanting verapamil.

c. Physiology

(1) Compared with verapamil, efficacy 90%, adenosine is capable of slightly better results, terminating more than 95% of junctional reentrant tachycardias. In addition, adenosine has fewer side effects and contraindications. It can be used safely in patients with LV dysfunction, those on beta-blockers, infants under 1 year, and patients with WPW syndrome.

(2) It has been suggested that adenosine may be a valuable diagnostic tool in the differentiation of SVT with aberration from sustained Vtach.

(3) Adenosine has modest and very transient side effects (due to an ultra-short half-life measured in seconds).

(a) Hypotension is rare.
(b) Bradycardia after cardioversion of SVT is short-lived.
(c) Transient atrial or ventricular premature contractions may occur but are immediately self-terminated.
(d) Cutaneous flushing, dyspnea, and chest pain have been reported in up to 20% of patients; however, these effects are quite short-lived and pose no clinical problem, especially if the patient is forewarned.

(4) Patients taking dipyridamole should be given much lower doses of adenosine since this drug inhibits adenosine uptake by cells.
(5) Theophylline and other methylxanthines competitively inhibit adenosine's effects; patients taking these drugs are refractory to conventional doses and should not receive adenosine.
(6) Relative contraindications
(a) In asthmatics, adenosine has the potential to cause bronchoconstriction and so should be used with caution.
(b) Patients with severe sinus node dysfunction (sick sinus syndrome) should receive adenosine only if they have a functioning ventricular pacemaker.

(7) Adenosine will not convert Afib/flutter or reentrant atrial tachycardia.

d. Metabolism
(1) Adenosine is rapidly taken up and inactivated in cells. Its half-life is measured in seconds.
(2) Extravasation does not lead to local irritation.

e. Dose
(1) Adults: 1 vial (6 mg) IV given as a very rapid bolus. Adenosine must be given over as short a time period as possible since its antiarrhythmic effect depends on a high plasma concentration reaching atrial tissue. Slower administration would result in low plasma levels due to rapid metabolism. Half of all patients who respond to adenosine will do so within 30 seconds of the first injection. If no response occurs after 30 seconds, additional incremental doses of 9 and 12 mg, respectively, may be given 1–2 minutes apart.
(2) Pediatric: 37.5 μg per kilogram with successive increments of 37.5 μg per kilogram to a maximum dose of 350 μg per kilogram.

2. Amiodarone

a. General. Amiodarone is a benzofuran derivative that resembles thyroxine. It prolongs the duration of the action potential of atrial and ventricular muscle without changing the resting membrane potential. Repolarization is delayed, and the effective refractory period is increased. Amiodarone slows AV nodal conduction and sinus node automaticity.

b. Indications. This drug is used in the treatment of:
(1) Recurrent Vtach or fibrillation
(2) Wolff-Parkinson-White syndrome to prevent recurrent paroxysmal supraventricular tachydysrhythmias (e.g., Afib)

c. Physiology
(1) Prolongs action potential duration, QRS, QT, and PR intervals
(2) May inhibit arrhythmias that do not respond to any other therapy
(3) Coronary vasodilator with antianginal effects. Peripheral vasodilation may lead to hypotension.
(4) Acts as a noncompetitive inhibitor of alpha- and beta-adrenergic receptors

(5) Produces HR slowing, which is resistant to atropine
(6) During general anesthesia, profound cardiovascular depression may occur with sinus arrest, AV block, hypotension, and decreased CO as the manifestations. Halothane and lidocaine may increase the risk of sinus arrest by accentuating the effects of amiodarone. Isoproterenol and temporary pacing may be required in these patients.
(7) Amiodarone may exacerbate or induce arrhythmias and may lead to torsade de pointes.
(8) Patients may develop severe diffuse pulmonary fibrosis, proximal skeletal muscle weakness, gait abnormalities, tremor, and peripheral neuropathies as a result of therapy.
(9) Hypo- and hyperthyroidism occur in 2–4% of patients.
(10) Other side effects: transaminase elevations, fatty liver, corneal microdeposits, and photosensitivity. Some patients may exhibit a persistent cyanotic facial discoloration even after cessation of drug therapy.
(11) Amiodarone increases plasma concentration of digoxin and other drugs through displacement from protein binding sites.

d. **Metabolism.** Amiodarone is extensively protein bound and has a very high lipid solubility, which results in significant tissue uptake and binding. As a result, the half-life is on the order of 25 days, and the drug is almost exclusively eliminated by the liver.

e. **Dose.** Adult daily dose 3–5 mg per kilogram PO; patients may be loaded with a higher initial dose over 1–3 weeks and then tapered to a reduced maintenance level. After oral dosing, onset of action is slow, with full effects not occurring for several days. An IV dose of 5 mg per kilogram given over 2–5 minutes will produce prompt effects lasting up to 4 hours. After chronic oral therapy, pharmacologic effects may persist for greater than 45 days. Therefore, systemic toxicity may be quite prolonged despite drug discontinuation.

3. **Atropine**

a. **General.** Atropine is a belladonna derivative that competitively antagonizes the effects of acetylcholine at muscarinic cholinergic receptors.

b. **Indications** for clinical uses
(1) Treatment of bradyarrhythmias
(2) Use as a premedicant to protect the heart from vagal reflexes during anesthesia
(3) Antisialogogue effect
(4) Bronchodilation in patients with asthma or chronic bronchitis
(5) Concomitant administration with anticholinesterase drugs used to reverse neuromuscular blockade to block their muscarinic effects

c. **Physiology**
(1) Atropine increases HR by blocking vagal cholinergic effects on the heart. These actions may be useful in treating hemodynamically compromised patients with slow HRs produced by ventricular asystole, second- and third-degree heart block, and severe sinus bradycardia.
(2) Tachycardia produced by atropine may lead to myocardial ischemia.
(3) Atropine may increase intraocular pressure in patients with narrow-angle glaucoma. Simultaneous application of a cholinomimetic drug, such as pilocarpine, will offset these effects.
(4) Similar to scopolamine, atropine can produce sedation. At-

ropine may produce symptoms of the central anticholinergic syndrome, which is characterized by restlessness, hallucinations, somnolence, and unconsciousness. Physostigmine, 15–60 μg per kilogram IV, is a specific treatment for this syndrome since this tertiary amine anticholinesterase crosses the blood-brain barrier.

(5) Atropine may produce urinary retention through relaxation of the bladder fundus and increase in vesical sphincter tone.

d. **Metabolism.** Atropine is approximately 50% metabolized by the liver, the other half being excreted unchanged in the urine. Plasma half-life is 15–30 minutes when given IV and approximately 4 hours after IM, SQ, or PO administration.

e. **Dose.** Atropine has the advantage that it may be given via many routes—IV, IM, SQ, and through an endotracheal tube. Administration PO leads to unpredictable absorption. In adults, the IV dose is 0.4–1.0 mg (may be repeated).

4. **Bretylium (Bretylol)**

a. **General.** Bretylium is a class III antiarrhythmic that prolongs action potential duration and refractory period in Purkinje and ventricular muscle fibers. It is a bromobenzyl quaternary ammonium compound.

b. **Indications.** Bretylium is generally used to treat refractory VF or tachycardia. In some instances, bretylium has converted VF to a normal rhythm without cardioversion.

c. **Physiology**

(1) This drug initially causes release of norepinephrine from adrenergic nerve terminals, which can cause a transient increase in HR and BP. Subsequently, it prevents release of norepinephrine and induces bradycardia. Patients should remain supine during therapy.

(2) Bretylium elevates the VF threshold and facilitates the electrical conversion of ongoing fibrillation.

(3) It is possibly contraindicated in treatment of dysrhythmias related to digitalis toxicity.

(4) Nausea and vomiting may accompany too-rapid IV infusion in the awake patient.

d. **Metabolism.** Bretylium is almost completely eliminated by the kidneys as the unchanged drug. There is no hepatic metabolism. The average elimination half-time is 13.5 hours, and duration of action is 8–24 hours. Accumulation will occur.

e. **Dose**

(1) Emergency use in setting of VF/VT

(a) Rapid IV injection 5 mg per kilogram. Electrical defibrillation must be attempted again after the bretylium is given because bretylium is administered to facilitate conversion of VF by dc countershock.

(b) Repeat doses of 10 mg per kilogram may be given q15–30min as needed to a total 30 mg per kilogram if VF persists.

(c) In this setting, use undiluted bretylium (50 mg/ml).

(d) Onset of effect should be within a few minutes.

(2) For refractory or recurrent Vtach

(a) Dilute 500 mg (10 ml) bretylium to 50 ml and administer 5–10 mg per kilogram over 8–10 minutes.

(b) If the arrhythmia persists, a second dose of 5–10 mg per kilogram can be given in 1–2 hours, and thereafter the same dose can be given every 6–8 hours. Alternatively, an infusion of 2 mg per minute may be used.

(c) Onset of effect in therapy of VT may be delayed for 20 minutes or more.

5. **Disopyramide (Norpace)**
   a. **General.** This drug is a member of the class IA antiarrhythmics and as such has properties similar to quinidine and procainamide. It is useful in the therapy of atrial and ventricular arrhythmias by virtue of its ability to slow phase 0 depolarization and to slow conduction velocity in Purkinje fibers. In general, HR is unchanged, and changes in cardiac conduction intervals (P-R, QRS, and Q-T) are less than seen with quinidine. Because it possesses significant anticholinergic activity, disopyramide does not cause depression of AV nodal conduction and may be used in patients with preexisting conduction problems such as bundle branch block.
   b. **Indications.** Disopyramide is used to suppress and prevent:
      (1) Unifocal PVCs
      (2) Multifocal PVCs
      (3) Paired PVCs (couplets)
      (4) Episodic Vtach
      (5) In Europe, disopyramide has been effective in treating paroxysmal SVT.
   c. **Physiology**
      (1) Disopyramide shortens sinus node recovery time, lengthens the effective refractory period of the atrium, and slows conduction in accessory pathways.
      (2) This drug rarely causes significant changes in BP except in patients with CHF. Intravenous disopyramide may lower BP and CO.
      (3) Anticholinergic side effects are prominent with therapy; disopyramide can aggravate glaucoma and myasthenia gravis and cause urinary retention. Disopyramide has about 10% of the cholinergic blocking activity of atropine.
      (4) Negative inotropic effects of this drug may induce or aggravate heart failure in some patients.
      (5) Hypoglycemia may rarely accompany use of disopyramide.
   d. **Metabolism.** About 50% of disopyramide is excreted unchanged by the kidney, with another 20% eliminated in the urine as the dealkylated metabolite (10% of the activity of the parent drug). After PO administration, peak plasma levels are reached in 1–2 hours, and elimination half-time is 7–8 hours.
   e. **Dose.** A loading dose of 300 mg may be given to expedite antiarrhythmic effects when rapid control is desired. Subsequently, 100–200 mg PO qid is the recommended maintenance dose. Lower doses should be used in patients under 40 kg, those with cardiomyopathy or CHF, and those with impaired renal function.

6. **Edrophonium (Tensilon)**
   a. **General.** This is a quaternary ammonium anticholinesterase drug that reversibly inhibits acetylcholinesterase.
   b. **Indications.** Edrophonium may be used to terminate SVT. It acts, presumably, through enhancement of vagal acetylcholine action on the AV node to block AV nodal reentry.
   c. **Physiology**
      (1) This drug may cause sinus arrest or third-degree heart block. Atropine should be available to counteract these effects. Edrophonium should be given only with continuous ECG monitoring.
      (2) High doses can lead to cholinergic crisis with muscle weakness, abdominal cramps, salivary hypersecretion, loss of bladder and rectal control, apnea, confusion, and seizures. Atropine (35–70

μg/kg) and pralidoxime (15 mg/kg) may be used to counteract these effects.

d. **Metabolism.** Renal excretion is responsible for about 75% of the elimination of edrophonium. There is some hepatic metabolism leading to production of edrophonium glucuronide. Onset of action is rapid (1–2 minutes); duration of effect is 60 minutes, with an elimination half-time of close to 2 hours. Low doses of edrophonium produce much shorter duration of effects—on the order of 5–10 minutes.

e. **Dose.** For termination of SVT, a test dose of 1 mg IV may be delivered followed by 9 mg IV.

7. **Encainide (Enkaid)**

a. **General.** Encainide is a local anesthetic antidysrhythmic drug that blocks fast Na^+ channels. It combines the properties of quinidine and lidocaine. Its ability to suppress ventricular arrhythmias is quite similar to that of flecainide. At therapeutic concentrations, encainide causes a substantial increase in the P-R interval and the QRS duration.

b. **Indications**

(1) Encainide is indicated for treatment of life-threatening ventricular arrhythmias.

(2) Recent evidence suggests that encainide increases the risk of sudden death in patients who have had a previous myocardial infarction and are being treated for asymptomatic, nonsustained ventricular arrhythmias. For this reason, this drug is no longer recommended for the therapy of benign or **only potentially malignant ventricular ectopy.**

c. **Physiology**

(1) Proarrhythmic effects occur in 8–15% of patients with malignant ventricular dysrhythmias.

(2) Unlike flecainide, encainide does not depress myocardial contractility, so this drug may be used (with caution) in patients with CHF.

(3) In contrast to quinidine, encainide does not consistently lower peripheral vascular resistance, so BP does not decrease after oral administration.

(4) Encainide can potentiate sinus node dysfunction.

(5) Cimetidine increases plasma levels of encainide.

(6) Visual disturbances (blurred or double vision) are not uncommon.

(7) Other side effects include headache, dizziness, ataxia, and nausea.

(8) Encainide is not very effective in the treatment of sustained Vtach.

d. **Metabolism**

(1) Extensive first-pass hepatic metabolism

(2) Metabolites account for the majority of clinical effects except in the 10% of the population who are deficient in cytochrome P450 system. In these patients, the half-life is markedly prolonged, and it is the parent drug that is the clinically important compound.

(3) Peak concentrations in plasma within 30–90 minutes

(4) Elimination half-life 3–12 hours

(5) Renal failure prolongs half-life and leads to accumulation of metabolites.

e. **Dose**

(1) Initial PO dose is 25 mg tid; may be increased every 3–5 days to a maximum of 50 mg qid.

(2) Adjust dosage in patients with renal or hepatic disease.

8. **Flecainide (Tambocor)**
   a. **General.** Flecainide is a fluorinated local anesthetic analog of procainamide, which is in the IC antiarrhythmic group and has properties similar to encainide. Flecainide prolongs the PR and QRS intervals and is effective in suppressing ventricular dysrhythmias.
   b. **Indications**
      (1) Treatment of life-threatening ventricular arrhythmias
      (2) Recent evidence suggests that flecainide increases the risk of sudden death and cardiac arrest in patients who have had a previous myocardial infarction and are being treated for asymptomatic nonsustained ventricular arrhythmias. For this reason, this drug is no longer recommended for the therapy of **benign** or **only potentially malignant ventricular ectopy.**
   c. **Physiology**
      (1) Flecainide has a proarrhythmic effect similar to that of encainide, and its use in the treatment of sustained Vtach should be instituted in hospital.
      (2) This drug usually does not alter HR and may have negative inotropic effects. It should be given with caution in patients with LV dysfunction.
      (3) Flecainide may cause sinus arrest in patients with sick sinus syndrome; AV block may occur also.
      (4) This drug increases serum digoxin levels. Cimetidine increases flecainide levels. Amiodarone can cause a doubling of plasma flecainide.
      (5) Caution should be exercised when coadministering other negative inotropic antiarrhythmics (disopyramide, verapamil) with flecainide.
      (6) This drug may increase endocardial pacing thresholds and should be used with caution in patients dependent on permanent or temporary pacemakers.
      (7) Side effects include vertigo and difficulty with visual accommodation.
   d. **Metabolism**
      (1) Approximately 25% of flecainide is excreted unchanged by the kidney. The rest is excreted as weakly active metabolites. Renal failure prolongs the plasma half-life.
      (2) There is no significant first-pass hepatic metabolism.
      (3) Peak concentrations occur in plasma within 3 hours.
      (4) The elimination half-time is about 11 hours.
      (5) Alkaline urine PH slows flecainide elimination.
   e. **Dose**
      (1) Initial dose is 100 mg PO bid. This may be increased in increments of 100 mg per day every 4 days to a maximum of 400–600 mg per day in 2–3 doses.
      (2) Plasma concentrations should be followed. Therapeutic levels are 0.2–1.0 μg per milliliter.

9. **Lidocaine**
   a. **General.** Lidocaine is a tertiary amine local anesthetic that slows inward Na^+ currents. This drug is a class IB antiarrhythmic, which increases the VF threshold and decreases Purkinje fiber automaticity, especially in ischemic tissue. Lidocaine causes almost no change in the duration of the action potential in atrial fibers and decreases the AV nodal refractory period, which explains its lack of beneficial effect on atrial dysrhythmias. The ECG is essentially unchanged.

b. Indications

(1) Suppression of reentry dysrhythmias such as PVCs and Vtach
(2) Aids in conversion of VF by dc countershock
(3) Not useful in management of SVT and other atrial arrhythmias

c. Physiology

(1) Lidocaine is a very safe drug for the heart with a good toxic-to-therapeutic ratio.
(2) Lidocaine has beneficial effects on many types of ischemia-related ventricular ectopy through improvements in conduction or by converting uni- to bidirectional block.
(3) Although lidocaine does not generally depress the conduction system, heart block or depressed sinus node discharge may occur in patients with underlying conduction disturbances.
(4) Compared to quinidine and procainamide, lidocaine has a faster onset and more rapid metabolism, making it more easily titrated to effect.
(5) Lidocaine does not alter autonomic nervous system function.
(6) Principal side effects are on the CNS. Mild overdose may produce excitation with accompanying confusion or seizures. Severe overdose produces sedation apnea and cardiac arrest. The lidocaine convulsive threshold is decreased by hypoxia, hyperkalemia, or acidosis.
(7) Toxic levels of lidocaine (5–10 μg/ml) produce peripheral vasodilation and direct myocardial depression.

d. Metabolism. Lidocaine is metabolized by the liver to mainly inactive metabolites. Intravenous bolus produces antidysrhythmic effects for 15–60 minutes. Short duration is due to rapid tissue uptake and hepatic breakdown. Factors that decrease hepatic blood flow such as shock, CHF, general anesthesia, or liver disease significantly reduce lidocaine breakdown.

e. Dose

(1) May be given IV, IM, and through an endotracheal tube
(2) Loading dose 1–1.5 mg per kilogram IV; a second bolus 0.5–1.0 mg per kilogram may be given within 10–30 minutes, depending on the clinical situation.
(3) Maintenance dose 15–60 μg/kg/minute (usually 1–4 mg/minute)
(4) Therapeutic levels 1–5 μg per milliliter

10. Mexiletine (Mexitil)

a. General. Mexiletine is an orally active, type IB antiarrhythmic and local anesthetic related to lidocaine. This drug shortens the action potential duration and refractory period. It does not alter the QRS duration.

b. Indications

(1) Mexiletine is used for the oral treatment of ventricular arrhythmias.
(2) This drug can suppress Vtach in patients who have not responded to quinidine or other class IA antiarrhythmics.

c. Physiology

(1) Responsiveness to lidocaine is quite often predictive of a good response to mexiletine.
(2) This drug is available only in oral form.
(3) It has little effect on atrial arrhythmias.
(4) No significant autonomic nervous system effects occur.
(5) Mexiletine may be proarrhythmic and can reduce conduction velocities in sinus node, AV node, and ventricular tissues, leading to sinus arrest or heart block.

(6) Central nervous system symptoms are not infrequent side effects with this drug, and dizziness, tremor, and lightheadedness occur. Gastrointestinal upset (nausea, vomiting, and anorexia) is common.

d. **Metabolism**

(1) This drug is eliminated after hepatic metabolism.

(2) Approximately 10% of a dose is excreted unchanged in the urine.

(3) The half-life is about 10 hours.

(4) Hepatic metabolism may be accelerated by rifampin or phenytoin, with resultant lower mexiletine blood levels.

e. **Dose**

(1) Usual dose is 100–400 mg PO tid (maximum 1,200 mg/day).

(2) Reduce dosage in hepatic failure.

(3) Plasma drug levels should be monitored.

11. **Phenytoin (Dilantin)**

a. **General.** Phenytoin is a member of the class IB antiarrhythmics. It is also an antiepileptic drug that is structurally related to the barbiturates. Its effects on cardiac impulse conduction resemble those of lidocaine. Phenytoin decreases automaticity, excitability, and duration of action potential in ventricular tissue without change in the QRS duration or PR interval.

b. **Indications**

(1) Phenytoin is particularly effective in the suppression of ventricular arrhythmias associated with digitalis toxicity.

(2) This drug is useful in treating multiform and complex PVCs and Vtach.

(3) Phenytoin is relatively ineffective against atrial flutter, Afib, and SVT.

c. **Physiology**

(1) Similar to lidocaine, phenytoin has little effect on the ECG; AV nodal conduction is improved, but activity of the sinus node may be depressed.

(2) Small doses of phenytoin may be quite effective in treating atrial tachycardia with AV block induced by digitalis.

(3) Rapid IV administration can lead to hypotension, myocardial and respiratory depression, cardiac arrhythmias, and VF.

(4) Intramuscular absorption is too unpredictable to treat cardiac arrhythmias.

(5) Signs of CNS toxicity are the most prominent drug side effects related to phenytoin therapy of arrhythmias. Nystagmus, sedation, and ataxia commonly indicate that plasma phenytoin concentration has exceeded 20 μg per milliliter.

(6) Hyperglycemia, glycosuria, osteomalacia with hypocalcemia, and systemic lupus erythematosus may be seen with chronic therapy.

d. **Metabolism**

(1) Phenytoin is hydroxylated and conjugated with glucuronic acid in the liver and excreted in bile and in urine, mainly as the parahydroxyphenyl derivative, which is inactive.

(2) Plasma half-life ranges from 6–24 hours and increases as plasma levels rise due to saturation of the enzymatic pathways.

(3) Oral absorption of phenytoin is slow and variable.

(4) Plasma levels should be monitored during therapy.

(5) Coumadin and cimetidine can increase phenytoin levels.

e. **Dose**

(1) Phenytoin is administered IV in a dose of 1.5 mg per kilogram every 5 minutes until the arrhythmia is suppressed or a

dose of 10–15 mg per kilogram has been reached (1,000 mg maximum).

(2) Infusion rate should not exceed 50 mg per minute to avoid hypotension and other side effects.

(3) Phenytoin is not compatible with D_5W.

(4) **Maintenance** dose is on the order of 3–5 mg/kg/day (300–500 mg/day) in adults given in divided doses.

(5) **Pediatric**: 5–20 mg per kilogram IV as a loading dose given slowly (1–3 mg/kg/minute), followed by 4–8 mg/kg/day in divided doses

(6) Therapeutic levels 7.5–20.0 μg per milliliter

12. **Procainamide (Pronestyl)**

a. **General.** Procainamide is an analog of the local anesthetic procaine, which is useful in the treatment of atrial and ventricular dysrhythmias. This drug is a group IA membrane stabilizer with electrophysiologic properties similar to quinidine. Procainamide decreases automaticity and excitability, increases action potential duration and effective refractory period, and lengthens the QRS interval. Group IA drugs are capable of converting unidirectional to bidirectional block, thus terminating reentrant arrhythmias.

b. **Indications**

(1) Treatment of PVCs, paroxysmal Vtach

(2) Supraventricular tachycardias, Afib, APCs

(3) Accessory pathway tachydysrhythmias, such as WPW syndrome

c. **Physiology**

(1) The drug is comparable to quinidine in effectiveness against atrial arrhythmias and has a broader spectrum than lidocaine against SVT.

(2) Rapid IV administration can cause hypotension.

(3) High plasma concentrations can cause direct myocardial depression, which is exacerbated by hyperkalemia.

(4) Excessive plasma levels may cause ventricular dysrhythmias.

(5) Digitoxic patients with heart block may have ventricular asystole or VF induced by procainamide.

(6) A syndrome resembling systemic lupus erythematosus may develop following chronic, but not acute, therapy. Slow acetylators may be more prone to develop this syndrome; discontinuation of therapy leads to symptom resolution.

(7) Other side effects include development of agranulocytosis and drug fever. Central nervous system effects are less common than with lidocaine but can manifest as confusion and seizures.

(8) Procainamide may cause significant cardiac conduction delay in patients with preexisting conduction disease.

(9) This drug does not have alpha-adrenergic blocking properties, and anticholinergic effects are less than with quinidine.

(10) Procainamide can induce torsade de pointes, especially in patients with QT prolongation.

(11) Patients in Afib/flutter should be digitalized prior to starting procainamide to prevent the paradoxical ventricular rate increase that can occur with this drug.

d. **Metabolism**

(1) This drug is eliminated by a combination of hepatic metabolism (50%) and renal excretion as unchanged drug (50%).

(2) The principal hepatic metabolite is *N*-acetyl procainamide (NAPA), which has antiarrhythmic properties and is also renally excreted. In renal failure, NAPA levels may become dangerously elevated, especially in slow acetylators.

(3) The *N*-acetyl transferase enzyme has a genetically determined activity level. In fast acetylators, elimination half-time is 2.5 hours compared to 5 hours in slow acetylators.

e. **Dose**

(1) Loading dose

(a) IV: 1.5 mg per kilogram over 1–2 minutes, repeated q5min until dysrhythmia is controlled or total dose reaches 15 mg per kilogram (never more than 1,000 milligram)

(b) IM: 6–12 mg per kilogram

(c) Pediatric: IV 3–6 mg per kilogram slowly infused

(2) **Maintenance** in adults: IV: 2 mg/kg/hour; IM: 6 mg per kilogram q3–8h; PO: 250–1,000 mg q3h

(3) Plasma levels of 4–12 μg per milliliter result in therapeutic antidysrhythmic effects. Levels above 8 μg per milliliter are often associated with increased side effects.

(4) Discontinue loading infusion if QRS is prolonged over 50%, PR interval increases, or marked hypotension occurs.

(5) Due to its multiple side effects, procainamide should be used only if other antiarrhythmics (e.g., lidocaine) have not been effective.

13. Quinidine

a. **General.** Quinidine is the dextrostereoisomer of quinine and one of a number of alkaloids isolated from cinchona bark. It is a class IA antiarrhythmic drug, which:

(1) Decreases phase 4 depolarization slope (thus suppressing arrhythmias due to enhanced automaticity)

(2) Slows impulse conduction through atrial and ventricular tissue (abolishing reentry arrhythmias by conversion of one-way to two-way conduction blockade)

(3) Increases the fibrillation threshold in atrial and ventricular tissue

(4) Prolongs atrial refractory period

(5) Prolongs the P-R and Q-T intervals and QRS complex at higher drug concentrations

b. **Indications**

(1) Effective in the treatment of acute and chronic supraventricular dysrhythmias (Afib/flutter, PSVT)

(2) Suppresses premature ventricular complexes

(3) Treats tachydysrhythmias associated with the WPW syndrome

c. **Physiology**

(1) Quinidine is effective in slowing the atrial rate in Afib/flutter and often will lead to conversion to sinus rhythm in one-third of patients.

(2) It is common to administer digitalis prior to treating patients with quinidine to prevent a possible paradoxical increase in the ventricular rate. This may be due to a decrease in AV node concealed conduction brought on by lower atrial rate and/or anticholinergic effects.

(3) Quinidine may increase plasma digoxin concentration.

(4) Intramuscular injection is not recommended due to associated pain and unpredictable absorption.

(5) Quinidine has a low therapeutic ratio; side effects are predictable at higher levels. Above 2 μg per milliliter, the P-R interval and QRS complex are prolonged. A greater than 50% increase in QRS length requires a dosage reduction, or heart block may ensue. Patients with preexisting Q-T prolongation or AV block should not be treated with quinidine. Ventricular arrhythmias and torsade de pointes may be induced, especially in patients with hypokalemia.

(6) This drug can cause significant hypotension, reflecting peripheral vasodilation from alpha-adrenergic blockade. High concentrations can cause direct myocardial depression. Intravenous administration accentuates these effects and should be reserved for the most special circumstances (i.e., it is not recommended).
(7) Tachycardia may result due to an atropinelike anticholinergic effect.
(8) Other important side effects include nausea, vomiting, diarrhea, development of cinchonism (tinnitus, blurry vision, decreased auditory acuity), drug fever, and thrombocytopenia.
(9) Quinidine may accentuate the actions of neuromuscular blocking drugs and exacerbate myasthenia gravis.

d. **Metabolism**
(1) Quinidine is well absorbed when taken PO, and peak levels are reached in 60–90 minutes for the sulfate form and 3–4 hours for the gluconate.
(2) The drug is hepatically metabolized to inactive by-products (80%), which are excreted in the urine along with unchanged drug (20%).
(3) Induction of hepatic enzymes will shorten duration of action.
(4) Plasma half-life is around 6 hours.
(5) Hepatic or renal failure or CHF may prolong this half-life.

e. **Dose**
(1) **Intravenous administration is not recommended.** If IV dosing must be used, dose is 4–10 mg per kilogram (as quinidine gluconate), given at 0.3–0.4 mg/kg/minute with vigilant ECG monitoring. Infusion should be stopped for hypotension, significant QRS prolongation (25–50%), loss of P waves, or arrhythmia termination.
(2) **PO dose**
(a) **Adult:** 200–600 mg tid to qid (sulfate); 324–648 mg bid to tid (gluconate)
(b) **Pediatric:** 3–6 mg per kilogram q3h, maximum 12 mg per kilogram (sulfate)
(3) **Intramuscular administration not recommended.**

14. **Tocainide (Tonocard)**

a. **General.** Tocainide is an orally active, local anesthetic analog of lidocaine used for the suppression of ventricular arrhythmias. Like lidocaine, it is a group IB antiarrhythmic.

b. **Indications:** symptomatic ventricular dysrhythmias

c. **Physiology**
(1) Tocainide has a spectrum of activity similar to lidocaine. The amide group decreases first-pass hepatic metabolism, making this an orally effective drug.
(2) This drug has a modest negative inotropic effect and may aggravate CHF in patients with poor ventricular function.
(3) Central nervous system side effects are not infrequent and include headache, tremor, paresthesias, dizziness, confusion, and seizures.
(4) Combination with propranolol may lead to psychosis.
(5) Gastrointestinal upset occurs.
(6) Agranulocytosis and bone marrow depression have been reported. Complete blood counts should be performed weekly during the first 3 months of therapy.

d. **Metabolism**
(1) It is rapidly absorbed from the GI tract.
(2) Peak levels in plasma are reached in 1–2 hours.

(3) Forty percent of unchanged drug is excreted in the urine; the remainder undergoes hepatic breakdown to inactive compounds.
(4) Therapeutic plasma levels are 3–10 μg per milliliter.
(5) Plasma half-life is 11–15 hours, and this may be doubled in patients with renal or hepatic disease.

e. **Dose**

(1) **By mouth dose** is 400–600 mg q8h to a maximum of 2,400 mg per day.
(2) Because of the risk of bone marrow suppression, tocainide should be used only when other drugs have proved ineffective in the management of ventricular ectopy.

Selected References

Barnhardt, E. R. *Physicians Desk Reference.* Montvale, New Jersey: Medical Economics Company, 1991.

D'Ambra, M. N., LaRaia, P. J., Philbin, D. M., et al. Prostaglandin E1 (PGE1): A new therapy for refractory right heart failure and pulmonary hypertension after mitral valve replacement. *J. Thorac. Cardiovasc. Surg.* 89:567, 1985.

Disesa, V. J. The rational selection of inotropic drugs in cardiac surgery. *J. Cardiovasc. Surg.* 89:385, 1987.

Firestone, L. L., Lebowitz, P. W., and Cook, C. E. (eds.). *Clinical Anesthesia Procedures of the Massachusetts General Hospital.* Boston: Little, Brown, 1988.

Gilman, A. G., Rall, T. W., Nies, A. S., and Taylor, P. *The Pharmacological Basis of Therapeutics.* New York: Pergammon Press, 1990.

Hensley, F. A., and Martin, D. E. *The Practice of Cardiac Anesthesia.* Boston: Little, Brown, 1990.

Kaplan, J. A. (ed.). *Cardiac Anesthesia,* Vol. 1. Philadelphia: Saunders, 1987.

Kofke, W. A., and Levy, J. H. *Postoperative Critical Care Procedures of the Massachusetts General Hospital.* Boston: Little, Brown, 1986.

McIntyre, K. M., and Lewis, A. J. (eds.). *Textbook of Advanced Cardiac Life Support.* Dallas: American Heart Association, 1981.

Opie, L. H. (ed.). *Drugs for the Heart* (2d ed.). Philadelphia: Saunders, 1987.

Pinski, S. L., and Maloney, J. D. Adenosine: A new drug for acute termination of supraventricular tachycardia. *Cleve. Clin. J. Med.* 57:383, 1990.

Stoelting, R. K. *Pharmacology and Physiology in Anesthetic Practice.* Philadelphia: Lippincott, 1987.

Turlapaty, P., Vary, R., and Kaplan, J. A. Nicardipine, a new intravenous calcium antagonist: A review of its pharmacology, pharmacokinetics and perioperative applications. *J. Cardiothorac. Anesth.* 3:344, 1989.

30

Endocrine Disorders

David J. Fish

I. Adrenal disorders

A. Acute adrenal insufficiency

1. **Background.** There are two major hormones secreted by the adrenal glands: cortisol and aldosterone.
   a. Cortisol is controlled through the hypothalamic-pituitary axis. Corticotropin-releasing hormone from the hypothalamus causes release of adrenocorticotropic hormone (ACTH) from the pituitary. The ACTH causes adrenal secretion mainly of cortisol and, to a lesser extent, aldosterone.
   b. Aldosterone is primarily under the control of the renin-angiotensin system.
   c. Deficiency of both hormones can be a primary process (i.e., direct involvement of the adrenal glands leads to inadequate production of all adrenal products) or secondary process (i.e., hypothalamic-pituitary disease or suppression leads to a decrease in cortisol products). Aldosterone secretion is thus relatively normal in secondary deficiency.
2. **Etiology**
   a. Primary adrenal insufficiency is most commonly caused by an autoimmune process with circulating adrenal antibodies (similar to Hashimoto's thyroiditis or pernicious anemia). The adrenal glands can also be destroyed by tuberculosis, infiltrative diseases (e.g., amyloidosis, hemochromatosis), hemorrhage, adrenal vein thrombosis, and bilateral adrenalectomy.
   b. Secondary adrenal insufficiency is most commonly caused by iatrogenic suppression following exogenous steroid administration or by hypopituitarism due to a pituitary tumor, infarction, or infiltration. The hypothalamic-pituitary axis may be suppressed for as long as 1 year following steroid therapy of a few weeks' to months' duration.
3. **Clinical features**
   a. Primary adrenal insufficiency is usually more striking in presentation than secondary adrenal insufficiency. However, the overlap of signs is wide. Weakness, weight loss, failure to thrive, hypotension, increased pigmentation, and gastrointestinal complaints are frequent. Secondary insufficiency is characterized by absence of hyperpigmentation and a lower frequency of hypovolemia. Acute insufficiency is usually superimposed on chronic insufficiency. Shock may be present as well.
   b. Laboratory findings include hyponatremia, hyperkalemia, hyperchloremic metabolic acidosis, and hypoglycemia. The electrolyte abnormalities are more common in primary insufficiency, because of the lack of aldosterone.
4. **Diagnosis**
   a. **History.** A high degree of suspicion is most helpful in a rapidly decompensating patient. A history of chronic insufficiency or steroid administration will suggest the diagnosis.
   b. **Diagnostic evaluation.** Laboratory tests are useful for subsequent evaluation but have no effect on initial therapy. The following tests can be performed:
      (1) **Serum cortisol.** Blood for this test should be drawn prior to any steroid administration. It is the only test used when the patient's condition demands immediate steroid therapy.
      (2) **One-hour ACTH stimulation test** is usually reliable. Blood for the baseline serum cortisol level is drawn. Then synthetic ACTH (Cortrosyn), 0.25 mg (25 units) is injected IV or IM. Serum cortisol level is then drawn again 60 minutes later. With

normally reactive adrenal glands, cortisol will rise 60 minutes after synthetic ACTH administration by 7 μg per dl over the baseline to a level greater than 18 μg per dl.

(3) **Three-day ACTH stimulation test** can also be utilized. It gives a better yield than the 1-hour test.

(4) **Serum ACTH levels** will help distinguish primary from secondary insufficiency (high in the former).

5. **Therapy**

a. **Steroid replacement** is crucial. Because hydrocortisone has both gluco- and mineralocorticoid effects, it is the steroid of choice. An IV dose of 100 mg immediately, then every 6–8 hours, is adequate and will duplicate the maximum output of normal adrenal glands. Simultaneous administration of fludrocortisone (Florinef) or desoxycorticosterone (Percorten) for mineralocorticoid effect is probably not necessary. As clinical improvement occurs, the daily steroid replacement can be reduced to approach normal daily output, approximately 20 mg hydrocortisone (or its equivalent). Preparations with variable potency, mineralocorticoid effect, and half-life can be substituted (Table 30-1). Mineralocorticoid replacement is necessary for primary, but not secondary, adrenal insufficiency.

b. **Fluid administration.** Because of pronounced hypovolemia and hyponatremia, saline and glucose solutions should be vigorously administered. Central venous pressure monitoring may be required to guide rehydration.

c. **Treatment of the precipitating event.** The decompensation of adrenal function is usually the result of some other disease process such as infection or infarction. The underlying dysfunction should be sought and treated.

d. **Long-term steroid therapy**

(1) **Primary and secondary adrenal insufficiency.** Chronic daily glucocorticoid administration equal to 20 mg of hydrocortisone is necessary and must be increased in anticipation of physiologic stresses.

(2) In deciding whether to administer steroids for surgery or other physiologic stresses, the following considerations apply:

(a) If steriods were administered for longer than 1 month during the prior 12 months, the patient should be treated as

Table 30-1. Steroid preparations

Drug	Glucocorticoid potency	Mineralocorticoid potency	Equivalent doses (mg)
Short acting			
Hydrocortisone sodium succinate (Solu-Cortef)	1	1	20
Cortisone (Cortone)	0.8	1	25
Intermediate acting			
Prednisone (Meticorten)	4	0.8	5
Prednisolone (Meticortelone)	4	0.8	5
Triamcinolone (Aristocort)	5	0	4
Long acting			
Dexamethasone (Decadron)	25	0	0.75

having relative adrenal insufficiency and be given stress doses of steroids (100 mg hydrocortisone every 6–8 h).

(b) If steroids were given for less than 1 month, recovery of the hypothalamic-pituitary axis generally follows within 1–2 weeks (Christy, 1984).

(3) Recovery is considered adequate when there is a normal 1-hour ACTH stimulation test.

(4) If the clinical situation is equivocal, steroid administration before and during a period of stress is the safest course.

(5) Alternate day therapy gives satisfactory coverage for maintenance administration and may minimize hypothalamic-pituitary axis suppression. Other complications of steroid administration, however, are probably not affected by this method of administration.

B. Cushing's syndrome

1. **Etiology.** Glucocorticoid excess is most often due to exogenously administered steroids. Endogenous causes of hypercortisolism (with normal to high ACTH levels) include pituitary-dependent adrenal hyperplasia, which is most commonly caused by pituitary microadenoma or loss of sensitivity for feedback control of either the hypothalamic corticotropic releasing hormone or ACTH. Microadenoma accounts for up to two-thirds of all endogenous Cushing's syndromes, the remainder consisting of adrenal adenoma, adrenal carcinoma, and ectopic ACTH-secreting tumors.
2. **Clinical features.** Truncal obesity (sparing of extremities), hypertension, hyperglycemia (with a decreased glucose tolerance), menstrual dysfunction, hirsutism, striae, myopathy, osteoporosis, and mental status changes (steroid psychosis) are among the complications of cortisol excess. Immunosuppression can also occur and may be the primary reason for seeking therapy in a critically ill patient.
3. **Diagnosis.** There are several maneuvers to diagnose the presence of Cushing's syndrome and to differentiate the causes.
   a. **Overnight dexamethasone suppression test.** After drawing blood for a serum cortisol level, dexamethasone, 1 mg, is given at midnight, and serum cortisol is again checked at 8 A.M. The morning cortisol, due to suppression, normally will be lower than the midnight cortisol. Dexamethasone is used because it does not cross-react with the agents used to identify cortisol. The specificity of the test is not good during stress or depression.
   b. **Urine metabolites.** A 24-hour measurement of urinary 17-hydroxy-corticosteroids (metabolities of cortisol) or urinary-free cortisol may give a better yield.
   c. **Plasma cortisol** can be obtained, in order to detect loss of normal diurnal variation.
   d. **Other tests** to differentiate the causes of Cushing's syndrome are available but are beyond the scope of this chapter.
4. **Therapy.** There is rarely a need for emergency intervention (except perhaps because of immunosuppression). Management modalities include surgery, irradiation, and drugs that interfere with steroid synthesis (metyrapone, aminoglutethimide, and mitotane). These therapies are best utilized after endocrinologic consultation. Awareness of the syndrome and its complications is paramount in the ICU setting.

C. Pheochromocytoma

1. **Background.** These tumors of neuroendocrine origin arise primarily in the adrenal gland, usually unilaterally, although they can be bilateral in other tissues of chromaffin origin. Only 10% are malig-

nant. Norepinephrine is the major catecholamine released from a pheochromocytoma, although epinephrine can also be secreted in varying proportions, especially from those of adrenal origin.

2. **Clinical features.** Overstimulation of alpha- (and sometimes beta-) adrenergic receptors causes the classic sympathomimetic findings.
   a. **Hypertension** is probably the most common sign and can be paroxysmal or sustained, occasionally discovered only during surgery for a unrelated disorder.
   b. **Paroxysmal attacks** occur, associated with headache, diaphoresis, arrhythmias, and gastrointestinal complaints. These episodes can be triggered by a variety of events, which can include postural changes, abdominal palpation, micturition, exercise, drugs, anesthesia, and surgery.
   c. **Glucose intolerance** is frequent, due to the hypermetabolic state.
   d. **Catecholamine-induced cardiomyopathy** can result in ventricular dysfunction with hypotension.
3. **Diagnosis.** Urinary metabolites of catecholamines are good indicators of presence of pheochromocytoma. A short 4-hour or traditional 24-hour collection of urine for metanephrine or vanillylmandelic acid (VMA) is usually sufficient. The diagnosis is suggested if concentrations of these metabolites are high. Methyldopa or monoamine oxidase inhibitor use will interfere with the assay.
4. **Therapy**
   a. **Surgery** is definitive if the entire tumor can be excised.
   b. **Medical therapy** is otherwise required to stabilize the patient who is perioperative or is not an operative candidate. The goal is to block alpha- and (sometimes) beta-adrenergic receptors.
      (1) **Alpha-adrenergic blockade** can be accomplished usually with phenoxybenzamine, a long-acting oral medication (given over several weeks prior to an elective procedure). A starting dose of 10–12 mg daily is increased 10 mg every other day until adequate BP control is achieved. For a prompt effect, 5–10 mg of phentolamine can be administered IV and will last about 1 hour.
      (2) **Beta-adrenergic blockade** may be required because of the effects of epinephrine from the tumor and unopposed beta-adrenergic effects after alpha-adrenergic blockade. Propranolol is the standard medication. It can be given orally, 20–40 mg, or IV, 1–2 mg, the dosage being titrated as tolerated and indicated.
      (3) **Adequate hydration** is required to prevent orthostatic hypotension. There is usually a sustained intravascular volume contraction prior to therapy. Thus with alpha-adrenergic blockade, systemic BP may decrease.
   c. **Postoperative management**
      (1) With the removal of the catecholamine source and the continued activity of long-acting alpha-adrenergic antagonists, hypotension is possible. Norepinephrine infusion should be started and subsequently weaned as volume repletion and stabilization occur.
      (2) Continued uncontrolled hypertension suggests incomplete removal of the tumor, in which case alpha- and beta-adrenergic blockade should be continued. If hypertensive crisis occurs at any point despite seemingly appropriate alpha-adrenergic blockade, IV nitroprusside infusion, starting at 0.1–0.5 μg/kg per minute, and propranolol in 1-mg IV increments can control the BP.

II. Management of the diabetic patient

A. General considerations.

A. General considerations. Tight blood sugar control in a diabetic patient may be the goal in the non-ICU setting. However, in the critically ill or postoperative diabetic patient, this is rarely possible and probably not necessary. Appropriate attention to blood glucose control will circumvent the severe metabolic derangements associated with diabetes and thereby smooth the perioperative course. Mild hyperglycemia may interfere with white cell function or induce an osmotic diuresis but causes little other harm. On the other hand, the long-standing effects of poor diabetic management and associated complications of the disorder should be considered. Small vessel diseases, heart diseases, nephropathy, and autonomic neuropathy are some of the major concerns in the diabetic patient. Less than tight control of blood glucose in the ICU will not affect these chronic sequelae. However, recent evidence suggests avoiding hyperglycemia in the setting of neuronal ischemia. Hypoglycemia associated with insulin therapy should be avoided.

B. Routine postoperative blood glucose management

1. **Non-insulin-dependent diabetes** (type II)
   - **a. Diet controlled.** This group may sustain a marked elevation of blood glucose with the stress of surgery. It usually returns to near normal with resolution of the stress. However, small dosages of IV insulin may be needed to control a rising blood sugar if the stress is prolonged or if the rise is high enough to anticipate complications (e.g., diuresis, acidosis).

     The response of these patients to low dosages of insulin (6–10 units/L of maintenance IV fluid) can be dramatic, since many of them have never "seen" insulin before. Frequent measurement of blood glucose is required when administering insulin to these non-insulin-dependent diabetics.
   - **b. Oral agent controlled.** If the oral agent was stopped the day of or before surgery, hypoglycemia is possible because of the long half-life of some of these agents (Table 30-2). These patients tend to need insulin when critically ill. Like the diet-controlled patient, they also can be very sensitive to insulin. The patient's oral agent is not useful for blood sugar control in the ICU, where fluxes in the patient's status can occur, and absorption is frequently uncertain.
2. **Insulin-dependent diabetes** (type I)
   - **a.** Many different approaches to preoperative and intraoperative management have been advocated. Thus, the patient may arrive in the ICU having received an earlier subcutaneous dosage of neutral protamine Hagedorn (NPH) or regular insulin or a continuous IV infusion of regular insulin (Table 30-3). A wide range of blood glucose levels results, and therapy should start immediately postoperatively. Accordingly, assessment of the blood glucose should be done promptly on arrival in the ICU.
   - **b.** Frequent blood glucose measurements may subsequently be required.

Table 30-2. Oral hypoglycemic drugs

Drug	Half-life
Tolbutamide (Orinase)	6–8 h
Chlorpropamide (Diabinese)	≥36 h
Acetohexamide (Dymelor)	12–18 h
Tolazamide (Tolinase)	10–12 h

Table 30-3. Insulin kinetics and subcutaneous administration (normal skin perfusion)

Insulin type	Peak	Duration
Crystalline (regular)	2–4 h	5–7 h
NPH (Lente)	6–12 h	24–28 h
Protamine zinc	16–24 h	36 h

(1) Hypoglycemia can occur with some insulin regimens. Thus, unless a patient is ketoacidotic, dextrose-containing solutions should be given if insulin is being or has been recently administered. In addition, decreases in stress, removal of septic sites, and changing nutritional status may further contribute to variability in insulin requirements and thus a higher potential for hypoglycemia.

(2) Urine ketone and dextrose spillage are simple **outpatient** methods of following blood glucose levels. They depend on the renal threshold and can be several hours behind in reflecting blood glucose. Although they may be worthwhile for correlating with blood glucose levels for future non-ICU management of the diabetes, there is no substitution for measurement of blood glucose in the ICU. Bedside glucometers utilizing glucose-reagent paper and self-contained colorimetric devices are also useful and closely approximate laboratory-derived values.

c. **Insulin administration schemes.** Three basic approaches can be utilized: subcutaneous, intermittent IV, and continuous IV. The last offers the best control.

(1) **Subcutaneous insulin administration.** This scheme combines a prior knowledge of the patient's dosage requirements with an estimate of current needs. This method is often unsatisfactory in the critically ill patient. First, the patient's usual dosage is not adequate in the face of increased physiologic stress. Second, and more important, is the unreliable absorption of subcutaneous insulin when relative hypoperfusion exists, as with hypotension, use of vasoconstricting drugs, or hypothermia. Subcutaneous administration, however, can be useful after the patient has stabilized in preparation for transfer out of the ICU.

(2) **Intermittent IV dosing.** Adequate control of blood glucose can sometimes be achieved with IV boluses of regular insulin every 1–2 hours. The doses are determined empirically from frequent blood glucose determinations. Five to 10 units are usual doses and may be increased or decreased as indicated by the response. This approach can be unsatisfactory in many circumstances, however. Rapid uptake by insulin receptors with rapid degradation may be a major reason for the difficulties. Stable control may be achieved slowly, and hypoglycemia can occur. Sometimes IV boluses are helpful as an adjunct to continuous infusion techniques to gain better immediate control.

(3) **Continuous IV infusion.** This method generally provides the smoothest control of blood glucose in the critically ill. Regular insulin can be infused with a dextrose-containing solution, 10–16 units per liter initially, or by a separate pump-controlled infusion, initially at 0.1–0.2 units/kg per hour, subsequently being adjusted as indicated by blood glucose level. Both

methods are relatively safe. Control is occasionally achieved in several hours, although a longer time is usually required.

If closely monitored, the patient will not have episodes of hypoglycemia, and the blood sugar will come into reasonable range with adjustment of either the infusion rate or the concentration of insulin. Insulin infusion can thus be altered (decreased or increased) until the patient is ready for subcutaneous administration.

Blood glucose should be checked every 3–4 hours until desired levels are achieved and have stabilized. The previously reported problems of insulin absorption into the IV tubing do not appear to be of clinical importance. Flushing the IV line with the insulin-containing solution is advisable (and adequate) prior to administering the infusion.

C. **Diabetic ketoacidosis** (DKA)

1. **Background.** This major complication of diabetes results from a profound relative insulin deficiency. In the face of an increasing insulin requirement, catabolic processes are induced. The metabolic apparatus accelerates lipolysis, resulting in ketone body generation such that the body is overwhelmed by the ketone load. Concomitantly, the glucose load continues to increase by hepatic gluconeogenesis. Severe metabolic acidosis results, with a marked depletion of both salt and water and the consequent electrolyte imbalances. The precipitating factors include physiologic stresses such as infection, trauma, and myocardial infarction, in addition to improper insulin administration.

2. **Clinical features**

a. **History.** A variety of complaints may be offered. However, many patients will be ketoacidotic as a result of some other major insult on which much of the history will be based. Vomiting, thirst, polyuria, recent weight loss, abdominal pain, and weakness (i.e., the usual outpatient signs and symptoms of DKA) can also be seen and may be a clue to the metabolic abnormality after an operation.

b. **Presentation.** A spectrum of signs is usually observed and includes the following:

(1) **Kussmaul's respirations,** rapid and deep breathing, are a result of significant metabolic acidemia. In addition, the breath may smell like acetone.

(2) **Hypovolemia** may be evident from low central venous or pulmonary arterial pressures or hypotension. Oliguria usually is not present until the end stage of DKA.

(3) **Temperature dysautoregulation.** Although many patients develop DKA from an infectious process, only a minority will have fever. Hypothermia is more common.

(4) **Mental status alterations** with loss of consciousness are frequent but variable. Coma is not usual.

c. **Laboratory findings.** Suspicion of DKA should be raised in the critically ill patient with an unexplained anion gap, metabolic acidosis, and hyperglycemia.

(1) **Hyperglycemia** will usually be present, usually between 500 and 1000 mg per dl; however, glucose levels may be much lower or much higher.

(2) **Ketonemia** will increase from the normal 0.15 mmol per liter to as high as 30 mmol per liter. Semiquantitative analysis is performed with nitroprusside reagent tablets. They can be crushed and serum dropped into them, starting with 1 ml of serum that is diluted with saline to a 1 : 2 dilution. If this test is positive, it is repeated at a 1 : 4 dilution. This can subsequently

be repeated until the highest positive dilution is found and thus can provide an approximation of the degree of ketonemia. This reagent measures mostly acetoacetate. However, with the altered redox state of DKA, mostly beta-hydroxybutyrate is produced. This does not necessarily negate the diagnostic assistance of the tablets. However, as the redox state becomes more favorable with treatment, the beta-hydroxybutyrate will be converted to acetoacetate and thus lead to an erroneous conclusion of increasing ketone bodies. Therefore, this analysis is best utilized to assess response to therapy in conjunction with serial blood glucose measurements.

(3) **Lactic acidosis** may also contribute to the acidemia. Thus, the arterial blood acid-base state and the electrolyte concentrations will demonstrate a severe metabolic acidosis with an anion gap (see Chap. 21).

(4) **Potassium** may be high or low and is difficult to interpret because although serum potassium concentration is frequently elevated secondary to the acidemia, there is usually depletion of total body stores of potassium.

(5) **Hypophosphatemia** may result from urinary losses.

(6) **Pseudohyponatremia** may be present secondary to the hyperglycemia.

3. **Therapy.** There are no formulas. A therapeutic plan must be chosen initially and then be altered as indicated by patient response.

a. **Fluid administration.** The fluid deficit in these patients can be as much as 5–10 liters. Isotonic solutions without glucose are best used initially. One liter infused rapidly and then 1 liter per hour for the first few hours is frequently needed. The rate and type of fluid can then be adjusted according to the laboratory and clinical picture. Half normal saline solution can subsequently be introduced and alternated with normal saline. Glucose should be added to IV fluids when the blood glucose decreases to the 250–300 mg per dl range. Central venous or pulmonary artery pressure may be useful, especially in the fragile cardiac patient or postoperative patient with major fluid shifts.

b. **Insulin.** There are a variety of approaches: low dose versus high dose, IV versus IM. All require frequent glucose monitoring (every 2 h until stable) to avoid hypoglycemia. The following are recommendations in the ICU:

(1) **A low-dose continuous IV insulin infusion** offers a reasonable and reliable technique. Doses as low as 5 units per hour produce plasma levels of insulin sufficient to inhibit lipolysis, retard ketone production, and decrease hepatic glucose production. An infusion of insulin in saline should be run at 6–12 units per hour, titrated to produce a decrease in blood glucose of about 60–100 mg/dl per hour. The rate of infusion can then be titrated upward for stubborn cases. The problem of insulin absorption into plastic tubing and glassware is insignificant.

(2) **Intramuscular insulin** can alternatively be given, 5–20 units per hour, using a needle long enough to reach muscle. The IM route gives good absorption, peaking in about 1 hour; however, it can be difficult to titrate precisely. There is no role for subcutaneous insulin administration in DKA.

c. **Potassium.** Because of acidemia, the potassium level may be high, although it is likely that there is a significant total body deficit. Insulin administration and correction of the acidosis will decrease plasma levels of potassium as intracellular stores are repleted. It is thus best to obtain frequent potassium determinations after treatment of DKA starts. Replacement of potassium should then begin when the potassium concentration is within the normal range. The rate of potassium administration (usually 40 mEq/L) can be as fast as 40 mEq per hour. It should be moderated if oliguria is present and subsequently titrated as indicated by further potassium determinations. The potassium may be given as either a chloride or phosphate salt.

d. **Bicarbonate**
   (1) Unless the pH has dropped to 7.1 or lower or supervening problems such as arrhythmia or shock occur, administration of bicarbonate is not usually necessary.
   (2) Complications of too rapid correction of pH with bicarbonate include paradoxic central nervous system acidosis (bicarbonate is slow to cross the blood-brain barrier), leftward shift of the oxyhemoglobin dissociation curve, and hypokalemia. Thus, infusion rather than bolus therapy is usually better tolerated. One hundred mEq of sodium bicarbonate added to 1 liter of 0.25 normal saline results in an isotonic solution that can be used for volume replacement (see Chap. 21).

e. **Phosphate.** There is often a phosphate deficit as a result of the diuresis. However, the need for immediate replacement is controversial and rarely urgent. A phosphate level is the best guidance for replacement.

f. **Treatment of the precipitating event** is of utmost importance in treating DKA.

D. Alcoholic ketacidosis

1. The usual setting for this is an alcoholic who has stopped most or all oral intake (including alcohol) and has been vomiting.
2. The presentation includes variable blood glucose levels, although they usually are less than 200 mg per dl. Ketoacidosis (again more beta-hydroxybutyrate than acetoacetate), lactic acidosis, and dehydration are salient presenting abnormalities.
3. Management is directed at the fluid deficit, electrolyte and acid-base imbalances, thiamine deficiency, and the assorted disorders that afflict the chronic alcoholic.

E. Hyperosmolar nonketotic coma (HNC)

1. **Etiology** is typically a problem of non-insulin-dependent diabetics with mild or formerly undiagnosed diabetes. A variety of physiologic stresses (e.g., infection, surgery, or drugs such as steroids, phenytoin, or diuretics) can lead to the syndrome. Decreased water intake due to impaired mental status can further exacerbate the dehydration. While similar to DKA, it differs in that there is enough endogenous insulin present to prevent lipolysis and ketogenesis.
2. **Clinical features**
   a. **Hyperglycemia** induces an inappropriate diuresis, which produces dehydration with worsening of the physiologic stress and **hyperosmolarity.**
   b. **Dehydration with hyperosmolarity** is thus the major clue to HNC. Laboratory data will support this with an elevated glucose and blood urea nitrogen (BUN) with increased calculated or measured osmolarity.

$$\text{Calculated osmolarity} = 2 \times (\text{Na} + \text{K}) + (\text{BUN} \div 2.8) + (\text{glucose} \div 18)$$

   The osmolarity is usually 330 mOsm per liter or greater in HNC.

   c. An **altered mental status,** ranging from confusion to coma, is possible. There may also be focal deficits, including seizure activity. All of these will usually resolve with treatment of the metabolic disorder and thus control of the hyperosmolar state.

3. **Therapy**
   a. **Rehydration** with a hypotonic solution (half normal saline) is the most urgent and major intervention. Because there is a major free-water deficit, isotonic solutions are not the first choice. The first liter can be given rapidly, followed by a liter per hour for several hours. Subsequently, replacement should be guided by central venous or pulmonary artery pressure. Frequent neurologic assessment should be performed because of the possibility of cerebral edema with too rapid a decrease in osmolarity.
   b. **Insulin** administration should be done gingerly. Although the blood glucose may be very high, the patients are highly sensitive to exogenous insulin. Blood glucose can fall precipitously. Therefore, low-dose regimens can be followed. Because of the theoretic concern of cerebral edema from too rapid and too large a decrease in glucose, stabilization of blood glucose at 250–300 mg per dl is the goal. Decreasing the blood sugar by 60–100 mg/dl per hour is reasonable. The approach is similar to that described for DKA, but because of the possible insulin sensitivities, lower dosages should be used.

F. **Hypoglycemia**
1. **Etiology**
   a. **Insulin induced.** In an ICU, hypoglycemia is often seen in the "overtreated" (with insulin) diabetic. In the setting of changing clinical status and thus varying insulin requirements, blood sugars may decrease unexpectedly as stress levels decrease, infections abate, caloric intake changes, or renal status deteriorates.
   b. **Sulfonylurea induced.** This is more common as an emergency presentation resulting from oral agent overdose. A relative overdose of oral hypoglycemic drug can occur, for example, because of decreasing oral intake (e.g., NPO order or gastroenteritis) or drug interactions that increase the amount of free sulfonylurea (e.g., coumadin, sulfonamide, salicylates, alcohol). Because of the prolonged half-life of some of these agents (see Table 30-2), prolonged therapy may be required.
   c. **Alcohol induced.** Typically, this is seen in the chronic alcoholic with little or no food intake associated with vomiting. Because alcohol inhibits hepatic gluconeogenesis, glycogen depletion ultimately leads to hypoglycemia.
   d. **Other causes.** Etiologies not commonly seen as a cause of hypoglycemia in the ICU include insulinoma, adrenal insufficiency, hypothalamic pituitary deficiency, malnutrition, and hereditary enzyme abnormalities.
2. **Clinical features**
   a. The range of signs and symptoms includes increased sympathetic tone (e.g., tachycardia, systolic hypertension, sweating, arrhythmias), headache, hypothermia, and altered mental status (e.g., clouded sensorium, coma, focal deficits, or seizures).
   b. The adrenergic response may be blunted or masked entirely by concurrent administration of beta-blockers or residual general anesthesia.
   c. The blood glucose may be below 50 mg per dl. Alternately, a rapid fall of blood sugar in a diabetic patient may present with hypoglycemic responses, even though the blood glucose is well above the usual hypoglycemic definition.
3. **Therapy.** Raising the blood glucose level with IV glucose solution is the most logical and efficient mechanism. Some patients require treatment before glucose levels are known and should have a blood glucose level drawn before therapy.

a. **A 50% glucose bolus** is the most widely used method for quick treatment and diagnosis (by virtue of the response). A 50-ml dose of 50% glucose usually raises the blood glucose concentration by 100 mg per dl and thus solves most problems. It is a hypertonic solution and can cause local phlebitis. It is most useful in situations when quick reversal of the signs and symptoms is necessary (e.g., coma, confusion), as well as for simultaneous diagnostic considerations. Repeat dosages may be needed on occasion if constant infusion is not utilized.

b. **A 5–20% dextrose solution** is most useful for the patient who is mildly symptomatic or who has just undergone treatment with 50% dextrose. The concentration chosen for constant infusion is selected on the basis of severity of the hypoglycemia and the likelihood of recurrence. If an inadequate amount or concentration is given, hypoglycemic symptoms may recur.

c. **Glucagon.** One unit either IM or SQ will elevate the blood sugar in 5–10 minutes. Alcohol-induced hypoglycemia is typically refractory to this method. It is more costly than dextrose but can be lifesaving in the face of no immediate IV access for dextrose administration.

d. **Diazoxide,** usually used for hypertensive emergencies, can also raise the blood sugar adequately in refractory cases of a prolonged nature (e.g., sulfonylurea overdose or insulinomas). Unlike the IV bolus form used for hypertension, a slow infusion can be used.

III. Calcium and magnesium disorders

A. Hypercalcemia

1. **Background.** About 99% of total body calcium (1.0–1.5 kg) is found in bones and teeth, 0.5% in other cells, and 0.1% in extracellular fluid. Calcium is needed for many metabolic functions, including muscle contraction, neurotransmission, and enzyme actions. The level of calcium is regulated by the individual and combined effects of parathyroid hormone and vitamin D on intestines, bone, and kidney. Most extracellular calcium is bound to albumin, and thus the levels will decrease 0.8 mg per dl for each drop of 1 g per dl of albumin. Ionized calcium may more accurately reflect the physiologically important level.

2. **Etiology**

   a. Significant hypercalcemia is seen in neoplasms as a result of bony metastasis or humoral factors (e.g., parathyroid hormone, osteoclastic activating factor, prostaglandins) that appear to cause osteoclastic reabsorption. If causing hypercalcemia, the malignancies are seldom occult.

   b. Less severe hypercalcemia can be seen in hyperparathyroidism, sarcoidosis, Paget's disease (with immobilization), endocrinopathies (thyrotoxicosis, adrenal insufficiency, pheochromocytoma), vitamin A intoxication, milk-alkali syndrome, and thiazide and lithium ingestion.

3. **Clinical features**

   a. Central nervous system manifestations include lethargy, coma, or psychiatric disturbances.

   b. Gastrointestinal manifestations include nausea, vomiting, constipation, pancreatitis, or anorexia.

   c. Genitourinary manifestations include diminished renal concentrating capacity, nephrocalcinosis, or renal stones.

   d. Soft tissue calcifications can also occur.

4. **Therapy**

   a. **Fluid administration.** Hypovolemia is usually coexistent with hypercalcemia. Administration of **isotonic solutions** for volume expansion should be the first maneuver. Center pressure measurements may be needed to guide fluid replacement if hemodynamic status is unstable. When a satisfactory urine output occurs with fluid administration, furosemide, 20–40 mg IV, should be given to maintain urine output at 100–200 ml per hour. This diuretic (not a thiazide) assists additionally by increasing calcium excretion. This combination of furosemide and normal saline administration will lower serum calcium by excretion and dilution. The clinician must be alert to the complications of congestive heart failure or hypovolemia (which will increase calcium), as well as hypokalemia, hypomagnesemia, and hypophosphatemia.

b. **Mithramycin** is effective in lowering calcium levels at dosages much less than its antineoplastic dosage. The onset of osteoclastic activity is 24–36 hours after administration, peaking several days later.

c. **Phosphate therapy** is safe and effective orally, usually as a chronic management technique. Parenteral phosphate is hazardous, however, because it can cause metastatic calcifications, hypocalcemia, renal failure, and cardiovascular problems. However, in emergency situations refractory to other therapy, this can be cautiously used. Neutral phosphate, 100 mmol, can be administered to a rehydrated patient over 6–8 hours.

d. **Steroids** can reduce calcium levels in certain situations such as sarcoidosis, hypervitaminoses, lymphoma, and myeloma but can take several days to be effective. Therefore, this is not a generally useful technique in the ICU.

e. **Dialysis,** either by peritoneal or hemodialysis, can acutely decrease calcium in patients with significant renal insufficiency.

f. **Calcitonin** is not usually a good choice in the ICU. Despite a rapid onset of action (2 h), its effectiveness is usually limited.

B. Hypocalcemia

1. **Etiology.** The causes include iatrogenic problems (e.g., surgical hypoparathyroidism), renal failure, hypomagnesemia, pancreatitis, vitamin D deficiencies and resistances, and fluoride intoxication.

2. **Clinical features**

a. Central nervous system signs include lethargy, decreased mental status, irritability, or hallucinations.

b. Muscle irritability with Chvostek's and Trousseau's signs, twitching, and seizures are all possible.

c. The laboratory level of calcium must be corrected for hypoalbuminemia. Magnesium level should be checked.

3. **Therapy**

a. **Calcium infusion** is the keystone. Elemental calcium, 100–200 mg, is given over 15 minutes. (A 10-ml ampule of calcium chloride is equivalent to 272 mg of elemental calcium; 5 ml of calcium gluceptate and 10 ml of calcium gluconate are equivalent to 90 mg of elemental calcium.) Calcium chloride should be diluted to prevent venous sclerosis. The initial therapy can be followed by 500–1500 mg of elemental calcium per liter, given as a constant infusion, initially about 1 dl per hour titrated as indicated by subsequent calcium determinations and clinical response.

b. **Magnesium replacement.** Hypomagnesemia inhibits release and peripheral action of parathormone. Magnesium replacement will return calcium levels to normal (see **C.3**).

c. **Chronic therapy** should provide as oral calcium 1–3 g of elemental calcium per day. The forms include calcium citrate and calcium glubionate.

d. **Vitamin D** may be necessary in some states (e.g., vitamin D deficiency, renal failure, hypoparathyroidism). Various forms are available: calciferol, dihydrotachysterol, and 1,25 dihydroxy D_3.

C. Hypomagnesemia

1. **Etiology.** Causes include decreased oral intake secondary to starvation or chronic alcohol intake, increased gastrointestinal losses (e.g., malabsorption syndrome, vomiting, diarrhea, gastric drainage), and excessive renal excretion of magnesium (e.g., diuretics, aminoglycosides, cisplatinum, renal tubular dysfunction).
2. **Clinical features.** The signs and symptoms resemble those of hypocalcemia: lethargy, confusion, and muscle irritability.
3. Therapy
   a. **Initial replacement** can be by IV or IM routes with 500–600 mg elemental magnesium (magnesium sulfate contains 98 mg or 8.1 mEq/g; 10 ml of a 50% solution contains 490 mg of elemental magnesium). It should be infused IV over 3–4 hours.
   b. **Follow-up replacement** requires 500–600 mg elemental magnesium each day. Oral therapy can be utilized for chronic therapy (500–2000 mg elemental magnesium divided into four dosages).
   c. The cause should be treated if possible.

D. Hypermagnesemia

1. **Hypermagnesemia** is often seen with renal failure, increased (or normal) magnesium administration, or inability to excrete magnesium. The most common surgical situation where this occurs is in the patient with renal failure who is given the standard magnesium-containing antacids or is prepared for a barium enema with magnesium citrate.
2. **Clinical features** include hypotension, nausea, and vomiting, which can occur with levels of 3–9 mEq per liter. With between 5 and 10 mEq per liter, myocardial conduction disturbances, hyporeflexia, and muscle weakness occur. Respiratory depression and asystole are seen at levels above 15 mEq per liter.
3. **Therapy** includes discontinuation of exogenous magnesium and, where necessary for acute emergent problems, parenteral calcium administration. This will reverse the effects of severe hypermagnesemia. Calcium gluconate, 10 ml (90 mg elemental calcium), should be sufficient. Definitive therapy requires removal of magnesium. Hemodialysis or peritoneal dialysis can be used for crisis situations. If renal function is adequate, furosemide, 20–40 mg IV, can be given with replacement of urine volume with half-normal saline. Adding calcium gluconate (1 ampule/L) will facilitate urinary calcium excretion and, therefore, magnesium excretion as well.

IV. Thyroid disorders

A. Normal thyroid function

1. **Thyroid hormones**
   a. Thyroxine (T4): about 80 μg is produced daily.
   b. Triiodothyronine (T3) is three to four times more active than T4, most of it being produced peripherally by monodeiodination of T4. Monodeiodination can also lead to reverse T3 (a relatively inactive form of T3 that tends to increase with critical illness).
2. **Laboratory tests**
   a. **Total T4** is a good indicator used in conjunction with T3 uptake.
   b. **Uptake of T3** measures the relative saturation of T4-binding protein since many disorders can cause increases (e.g., pregnancy, contraceptives, porphyria) or decreases in these proteins (e.g., steroids, cirrhosis, nephrotic syndrome, systemic illness). It also helps distinguish if T3 is high due to high unbound T3 or increased concentration of binding protein. The **free T4 index** is derived from the product of T4 and T3 uptakes. By itself, T3 uptake is not useful and should therefore be used only in conjunction with T4.
   c. The **T3** measurement is similar to the T4 measurement. It mea-

sures only the absolute T3 level, which may be useful in T3 thyrotoxic states.

d. **Thyroid-stimulating hormone (TSH)** is the pituitary hormone that usually increases with primary hypothyroidism and decreases with hyperthyroidism.

e. **Thyrotropic-releasing hormone (TRH) stimulation.** When given IV, TRH will raise TSH levels within 30 minutes. Lack of a rise indicates an abnormal control mechanism in thyroid function. Response to TRH is probably the most sensitive indication of hyperthyroidism.

B. Hyperthyroidism

1. **Background.** The range of disorders varies from mild hyperthyroid states that require minimal intervention to thyroid storm—a severe, life-threatening multisystem problem. The clinical findings are more significant than the actual laboratory numbers in determining the severity.

2. **Etiology.** Common causes include Graves' disease, multinodular goiter, autonomous thyroid nodules, Hashimoto's thyroiditis, subacute thyroiditis, and iatrogenic causes (overdosage of thyroid medication).

3. Clinical features

a. Common **signs and symptoms** include palpitations, anxiety, tremor, diaphoresis, heat intolerance, weight loss, diarrhea, goiter, exophthalmus, lid lag, atrial fibrillation, muscle wasting, and hyperreflexia.

b. In **thyroid storm,** the signs and symptoms also include fever, tachycardia, nausea and vomiting, arrhythmias, possible ventricular dysfunction, and altered mental status. (Note that this spectrum of clinical findings may be indistinguishable from malignant hyperthermia presentation in the perioperative period. See Chap. 27.) This condition tends to be precipitated by surgery, systemic illness, infection, severe metabolic dysfunction (e.g., DKA), or cardiovascular events.

4. **Therapy**

a. **Nonemergent therapy**

(1) **Beta-adrenergic blockade** will block the effects of beta-adrenergic activity seen in hyperthyroidism. While not influencing the levels of thyroid hormones (except for the peripheral conversion of T4 to T3), appropriate titrated dosages will lead to symptomatic improvement.

(2) **Propylthiouracil or methimazole** will block the pathways of thyroid hormone synthesis and will help control symptoms by directly lowering hormone levels. Propylthiouracil will additionally interfere with peripheral conversion of T4 to T3.

(3) **Iodine solutions** (e.g., Lugol's solution, SSKI) will block the release of T4 from the thyroid and may also inhibit the peroxidase enzyme system.

b. **Thyroid storm**

(1) **Supportive measures** must be carried out while instituting antithyroid medication. These include cooling the patient, maintaining intravascular volume, and appropriate management of heart failure if present.

(2) The drugs noted in **a** all play a role.

(a) **Propranolol** is started immediately, 1–10 mg IV (cautiously administered to the patient in congestive heart failure).

(b) **Propylthiouracil** is administered enterally, 1000–1200 mg per day in divided doses. It should precede iodide administration by at least 1–2 hours.

(c) **Sodium iodide** (for parenteral use) can be given IV 1–2 g per day.

(d) **Steroids** are of possible efficacy and may inhibit T4 secretion and peripheral conversion.

C. Hypothyroidism and myxedema coma

1. Etiology

a. The most common cause of spontaneous hypothyroidism is Hashimoto's chronic lymphocytic thyroiditis. Other nonhereditary causes include iatrogenic ablation surgery, radiation, antithyroid drugs, hypopituitarism, and hypothalamic disorders.

b. Nonthyroid illness can induce euthyroid-sick syndrome. While the patient is clinically normal, laboratory data show a decreased T4.

2. Clinical features include lethargy, weight gain, coarse skin features, menorrhagia or secondary amenorrhea, cold intolerance, hypothermia, or hyponatremia.

3. Diagnosis is made by showing decreased T4 and free T4 index. Confirmation is made by demonstrating an elevated TSH (except in the case of hypopituitarism or hypothalamic disease).

4. Therapy. Replacement of thyroid hormone is the keystone. Various products are available, ranging from desiccated thyroid to levothyroxin (T3). Thyroid-stimulating hormone should fall into low-normal range with adequate medication. Replacement should be done cautiously in patients with significant cardiac disease.

5. Myxedemic coma

a. This form of decompensated hypothyroidism has a poor prognosis. Precipitating causes include cold exposure, drugs (e.g., phenothiazines, narcotics), and infection.

b. Presenting signs include respiratory depression, increased sensitivity to respiratory depressants, hypothermia, hypotension, hypoglycemia, altered mental status (possibly coma), and hyporeflexia.

c. Diagnosis can be very difficult in the critically ill elderly patient. The usual thyroid tests will document the deficiency state; however, the results are rarely available quickly. Thus, replacement therapy may need to be done presumptively.

d. Therapy

(1) **Thyroid-hormone.** Levothyroxin (Synthroid), 200–500 μg IV, as a loading dose with 50–100 μg per day IV. It should be administered with caution to the cardiac patient.

(2) **Corticosteroids** are of questionable value but usually are given because of the coexistent possibility of adrenal insufficiency (100 mg hydrocortisone IV q8h).

(3) **Supportive measures** may be needed to treat hemodynamic, respiratory, metabolic, and infectious problems.

(4) **Central pressure measurements** will help guide fluid management.

Selected References

Axelrod, L. Glucocorticoid therapy. *Medicine* 55:39, 1976.

Christy, N. P. HPA failure and glucocorticoid therapy. *Hosp. Pract.* 19:77, 1984.

Gordon, E., and Kabadi, U. The hyperglycemic hyperosmolar syndrome. *Am. J. Med. Sci.* 271:253, 1976.

Hershman, J. (ed.). *Management of Endocrine Disorders*. Philadelphia: Lea & Febiger, 1980.

Sönkson, P. H., and Lowy, C. (eds.). Endocrine and metabolic emergencies. *Clin. Endocrinol. Metab.* 9:1, 1980. (See all of Vol. 9.)

Appendix: Hyperglycemia and Neuronal Ischemia

Recent work has examined the role of hyperglycemia in exacerbating ischemic neurologic injury. Myers and Yamaguchi reported in 1977 that monkeys who had received dextrose infusions prior to asystole had a far poorer outcome than fasted monkeys who had not received intravenous glucose.

Hyperglycemia contributes to the development of ischemic injury by supplying the brain with an increased supply of glucose. The augmented glucose stores are available to the ischemic brain and perform anaerobic glycolysis during hypoperfusion. As a consequence of anaerobic metabolism, increased amounts of lactate are produced. Intracellular lactate may be responsible for increased injury to neural tissue.

Although the majority of reports demonstrating the detrimental effects of hyperglycemia have been in animal models, Pulsinelli et al. have retrospectively examined outcome in patients admitted to hospital with ischemic stroke. They noted an increase in adverse outcomes in those patients with a history of diabetes mellitus.

Although much work remains to be done in this area, prudence dictates careful regulation of the blood glucose concentration in those patients at increased risk for neuronal ischemia.

Myers, R. and Yamaguchi, S. Nervous system effects of cardiac arrest in monkeys, *Arch Neurol* 34:65–74, 1977

Drummond, J., and Moore, S. The influence of dextrose administration on neurologic outcome after temporary spinal cord ischemia in the rabbit, *Anesth.* 70:64–70, 1989

Pulsinelli, W., Levy, D., Sigsber, B., et al. Increased damage after ischemic stroke in patients with hyperglycemia with or without established diabetes mellitus, *Am J Med* 74:540–543, 1983

Appendix

Perioperative Procedures

William H. Frist

This appendix discusses procedures commonly needed in surgical patients.

I. Pacemakers

A. Description

1. A pacemaker is a device composed of a lead, an energy source, and an electronic circuit that is capable of modifying the electrical activity of the heart. Transcutaneous pacing is also employed.
2. Pacemakers may be classified as either permanent or temporary.
   a. **Temporary pacing.** A temporary transvenous electrode, inserted either blindly or under direct fluoroscopic visualization, or a temporary transthoracic electrode is attached to an external pulse generator. Transcutaneous pacing is also employed.
   b. **Permanent pacing.** A permanent transvenous or epicardial electrode is attached to a pulse generator implanted under the skin. The transvenous route is more common than the epicardial route because of ease of insertion and lower associated morbidity.
3. **Types of pacing.** Pacing systems available for both temporary and permanent use include the following:
   a. **Asynchronous.** The stimulation rate is independent of the electrical or mechanical cardiac activity.
   b. **Ventricular inhibited** (or ventricular demand). The pulse generator delivers an impulse in the absence of intrinsic activity and suppresses its output in response to intrinsic ventricular activity. This type comprises the majority of currently implanted pacemakers.
   c. **Ventricular synchronous** (or ventricular-triggered). The pulse generator delivers an impulse synchronously with the intrinsic ventricular activity.
   d. **Atrioventricular (AV) synchronous.** A double-electrode system controls the stimulation of the pulse generator such that the atrial electrode senses atrial contractions and initiates an impulse to the ventricular electrode at an appropriate P–R interval. This type is especially useful for physically active individuals in whom rate increase in response to physiologic stress is important.
   e. **Atrioventricular sequential.** Both the atrium and ventricle are actively stimulated at a designated P–R interval by atrial and ventricular electrodes. This type of pacing is most commonly used when the contribution of atrial contraction to cardiac performance is crucial. It may improve cardiac output by 15–20%.
   f. **Rapid atrial pacing.** Stimulation of the atrium at rates of 200–600 impulses per minute may be useful in conversion of rapid regular supraventricular tachyarrhythmias.
4. **A five-position pacemaker code** defines each pacemaker's function as depicted in Table A-1. For example, a DDDMO pacemaker can stimulate the atrium and ventricle (first D for double) and sense each chamber (second D). It has a dual sensing function and thus after a sensed atrial event can trigger the ventricular stimulus or inhibit atrial or ventricular impulses (third D). It is multiprogrammable (M) and has no antitachyarrhythmic function (O).

B. Indications for pacemaker insertion

1. **Permanent pacemaker**
   a. **Clinical** conditions that may require permanent pacemaker implantation
      (1) Acquired conditions
         (a) Bradyarrhythmias or tachyarrhythmias associated with palpitations, syncope, near syncope, congestive heart failure, or low-output syndromes

Table A-1. Five-position pacemaker codes

Position number	Function	Possible codes
1	Chamber(s) paced	A, V, D
2	Chamber(s) sensed	A, V, D, O
3	Mode of response(s)	I, T, D, R, O
4	Programmable functions	P, M, C, O
5	Special tachyarrhythmia functions	B, N, S, E, O

A = atrium; B = burst stimuli; C = multiprogrammable with telemetry; D = double; E = externally controlled; I = inhibited; M = multiprogrammable; N = normal rate competition; O = none; P = simple programmable (rate and/or output); R = reverse; S = scanning; T = triggered; V = ventricle.

- **(b)** Complete heart block after an acute anterior myocardial infarction
- **(c)** Anginal syndrome with bradycardia
- **(2)** Congenital conditions, either familial or nonfamilial block
- **(3)** Other conditions. After cardiac surgery if block is observed or anticipated or after some types of antiarrhythmia surgery

b. Electrocardiographic conditions that may require permanent pacemaker implantation

- **(1)** Supraventricular dysrhythmias
  - **(a)** Sick sinus syndrome (e.g., sinus bradycardia, sinoatrial block, sinus arrest or pause)
  - **(b)** Other sinus bradycardia (e.g., carotid sinus sensitivity)
  - **(c)** Supraventricular tachycardia
  - **(d)** Accelerated conduction syndromes (for prevention of reentrant tachycardias)
- **(2)** Abnormal AV conduction
  - **(a)** Atrioventricular blocks (fixed or intermittent)
    - **(i)** Prolonged P–R interval
    - **(ii)** Mobitz block types I and II
    - **(iii)** Bifascicular and trifascicular blocks
    - **(iv)** Complete heart block
  - **(b)** Accelerated conduction and reentrant tachycardias
  - **(c)** Atrial fibrillation with persistent slow ventricular response
- **(3)** Special tachyarrhythmias (self-propagating)
- **(4)** Drug-resistant ventricular irritability (which may be suppressed with pacing)

2. Temporary pacemaker. Conditions that may require a temporary pacemaker include:

a. Symptomatic sinus bradycardia (e.g., complicating acute inferior myocardial infarction, sick sinus syndrome, AV block, digitalis toxicity, or permanent pacemaker dysfunction)

b. Complete heart block with episodes of asystole, ventricular bradycardia, or ventricular tachycardia-fibrillation

c. Incomplete heart block with syncopal attacks or prolonged asystolic intervals

d. Threatened complete heart block

- **(1)** Acute anterior myocardial infarction complicated by Mobitz block type II or complete heart block
- **(2)** Inferior myocardial infarction with unstable Mobitz block type I
- **(3)** Stokes-Adams attacks with trifascicular block

e. **Cardiopulmonary arrest with asystole.** Basic CPR always takes precedence over pacing. Ventricular fibrillation does not respond to cardiac pacing.

f. **Other uses**

(1) Diagnosis and treatment of symptomatic arrhythmias. Intracardiac tracings may aid arrhythmia interpretation when surface ECGs fail to do so. Appropriate therapeutic pacing may then be implemented (e.g., overdrive of ventricular irritability or conversion of atrial arrhythmias by rapid atrial stimulation).

(2) After cardiac surgery for heart block, suppression of ventricular irritability, or rhythm analysis

(3) As a temporizing step, prior to implantation of a permanent pacemaker

C. Pacemaker insertion technique

1. Pacemaker equipment

a. Pacing pulse generators

(1) **Permanent**

(a) Lithium cells, with an iodine or copper sulfide cathode, are the most common energy sources.

(b) A wide variety of programmable features exists, including rate, output, refractory period, input sensitivity, threshold, mode, antitachycardia features, and hysteresis (the capacity to have two separate escape and pacing intervals).

(c) It is not possible to predict an absolute longevity for any particular device. Patients are followed at 3–6-month intervals with ECG confirmation of pacemaker performance.

(2) **Temporary.** A self-contained battery-powered pacemaker (Medtronic 5375) that provides demand (R-wave inhibited) or asynchronous (fixed-rate) external single-chambered pacing is commonly used.

b. Pacing wires

(1) The **lead** conducts the pacemaker stimulus to the heart and detects spontaneous cardiac depolarizations by a sensing amplifier. The **electrode** is that portion of the lead that actually contacts the heart.

(2) Electrodes attach to the heart in one of two ways:

(a) **Passively.** The electrode tip is manipulated into the ventricular trabeculations or is sutured directly onto the epicardium.

(b) **Actively.** The integrity of the endocardium is invaded by an electrode with bristles, screw tip, helical cord, or hooks.

(3) **Polarity of leads**

(a) Unipolar refers to the presence of the cathode in the intracardiac position and the anode (or indifferent lead) in a remote position (frequently, the metallic case of the pulse generator).

(b) Bipolar refers to the presence of both cathode and anode in contact with myocardium. A bipolar lead may be constructed in a side-by-side or a coaxial arrangement.

(c) For temporary transvenous pacing, flexible bipolar leads are commonly used, whereas for permanent pacing, unipolar leads are most common.

(4) **Size.** Pacing leads range in size from 4F to 6F.

2. Emergency temporary pacemaker insertions. A temporary pacemaker may be inserted via either a **transvenous** or a **transthoracic** approach. The principal indication for transthoracic lead placement is the situation in which pacing is urgently required and transvenous lead placement has been unsuccessful due to either difficult venous access or inability to position the electrode. Transthoracic pacing carries a higher risk of hemothorax, pneumothorax, hemopericardium, and unstable pacing.

a. **Transvenous** insertion
   (1) Equipment
      (a) Semifloating (or balloon-tipped) flexible bipolar pacing electrode (USCI intracardiac electrode, 4F, 115 cm) with insertion cannula
      (b) Pacemaker pulse generator (Medtronic 5375)
      (c) Electrocardiograph machine, oscilloscopic monitor, and alligator clip
      (d) Skin preparation materials (e.g., povidone-iodine [Betadine] solution, sterile sponges)
      (e) Sterile field equipment (e.g., towels, gloves, mask, cap, gown)
      (f) Local anesthetic materials (lidocaine 1%, 10 ml; 25- and 22-gauge needles; 10-ml syringe)
      (g) Skin sutures (3-0 silk) and needle holder
      (h) Sterile dressing materials (e.g., povidone-iodine ointment, sponges, tape)
   (2) Procedure
      (a) If life-threatening bradycardia is present, atropine, 0.5–2.0 mg; isoproterenol, 1–10 μg per minute; or epinephrine, 1–10 μg per minute is used to accelerate an idioventricular pacemaker while temporary pacing equipment is obtained and the electrode positioned.
      (b) The ECG is monitored continuously for arrhythmias and pacemaker capture.
      (c) The patient is positioned in slight Trendelenburg (or lower extremities are elevated). A cylindrical support is placed longitudinally between the scapulae to abduct the shoulders.
      (d) **Approach.** A preferred approach for emergency insertion is the **left subclavian vein.** The smooth anatomic curve from the skin entrance through the superior vena cava, right atrium, and tricuspid valve into the right ventricle facilitates unimpeded passage of the lead. Moreover, the anatomic landmarks are easily palpable and relatively constant. The **right internal jugular vein** provides a satisfactory alternative approach and is associated with a lower incidence of pneumothorax.

         Other approaches may be used if necessary. When the **external jugular vein** is visible, the electrode may be introduced via needle puncture or simple cutdown. The **femoral vein** provides access outside the immediate field of CPR. However, passage across the tricuspid valve is difficult without fluoroscopy, displacement is likely in ambulatory patients, and thrombosis of the inferior vena cava is a risk if the lead remains for more than 5 days. The **brachial vein** may be the best approach for patients with bleeding tendencies, although risk of dislodgment with upper extremity motion and unpredictable success with catheter passage through the axillary region limit its usefulness.
      (e) The field is prepared and draped widely.
      (f) After local anesthetic infiltration, the subclavian vein is identified with the 22-gauge needle. The insertion cannula

is then placed with a larger needle (14-gauge Angiocath). Venous blood is aspirated to ensure proper placement in the subclavian vein.

(g) The needle is withdrawn, and the pacing lead is introduced through the cannula, with care taken to avoid air embolization.

(h) The electrode is advanced either with ECG monitoring or blindly, depending on presence or absence of intrinsic ventricular activity. When the patient has **spontaneous ventricular activity,** the external end (i.e., distal electrode, inactive pole) of the pacing wire is attached to a precordial lead of the ECG machine via a double-ended alligator clip, with the limb leads placed in the standard manner. The electrode is advanced slowly through the right atrium where large intraatrial deflections (large, spiked P waves) will be apparent on the intracavitary ECG. The position at which intraventricular potentials (large, intracavitary QRS complexes) are first recorded is noted. The electrode is then advanced another 2–4 cm. When the electrode is in optimal pacing position, an injury current (S–T-segment deflection) will be obtained.

When **little or no intrinsic electrical activity** is present, the lead is immediately advanced the estimated distance to the superior vena cava. An external pacing pulse generator is attached and set at maximum output (usually 20 mA) and a rate of 70 beats per minute. The lead is advanced blindly while monitoring the ECG for evidence of ventricular pacing. If more than 45 cm of lead has been inserted and capture has not been achieved, the lead is withdrawn slowly to approximately the level of the superior vena cava because the electrode may have passed into the inferior vena cava or coiled in the atrium. The insertion procedure is then repeated, rotating the lead as it is advanced. Multiple rapid trials may be necessary.

(i) The pacing generator is attached to the external end of the lead, and pacing is begun at 5 mA and a rate of 70 beats per minute. The mode (asynchronous versus demand) selected depends on the specific rhythm disorder and intrinsic rate.

(j) The pacing threshold is determined by slowly decreasing the output of the generator until capture is intermittent or absent. Output is then set at approximately twice that level.

(k) A 12-lead ECG is obtained to document pacing and confirm left bundle-branch block pattern.

(l) The cannula in the subclavian vein is carefully withdrawn without dislodging the lead from the right ventricle, and the lead is anchored securely to the skin. A sterile dressing is applied.

(m) A chest radiograph (posteroanterior and lateral) is obtained to confirm electrode position and exclude a pneumothorax.

b. Transthoracic insertion

(1) Equipment

(a) Equipment for transvenous pacing (see **(1)(a)**)

(b) Transmyocardial pacing kit, commercially packaged and sterilized (Electro-Catheter). This includes a placement needle with 6-inch, 18-gauge steel cannula and obturator, electrical connector, and a bipolar pacing stylet.

(c) Pacemaker pulse generator

(2) Procedure
  (a) The ECG is monitored continuously.
  (b) The anterior left chest is prepared and draped widely.
  (c) The needle cannula is inserted with the obturator into the fourth intercostal space, 2 cm to the left of the sternal border, in a direction perpendicular to the skin. Alternately, a subxiphoid approach can be used, inserting the needle at a 45-degree angle along the left side of the xiphoid process, aiming toward the midpoint of the right clavicle.
  (d) The obturator is removed, a syringe attached, and the needle slowly withdrawn as negative pressure is maintained on the syringe until blood flows freely to confirm placement inside the ventricular cavity.
  (e) The syringe is removed, and the pacing wire stylet is inserted through the needle cannula. The cannula is withdrawn over the pacing stylet carefully so as not to dislodge the stylet from the heart.
  (f) The terminals are attached to the pacemaker generator.
  (g) The pacing stylet is withdrawn gently until resistance is encountered, indicating that it is in contact with the endocardial wall of the ventricle.
  (h) Pacing is begun at 5 mA at a rate of 70 beats per minute. Once capture is achieved, the threshold is determined, and the output is set to approximately twice the threshold.
  (i) A transvenous or permanent pacemaker should be placed as soon as it is practical.
  (j) The catheter should be anchored to the skin and a sterile dressing applied.

3. **Permanent pacemaker insertion.** The fundamental principles of permanent pacemaker implantation are outlined below.
  a. **Transvenous implantation.** Access via direct subclavian vein puncture has become increasingly popular. The lead is introduced by a modified Seldinger technique, in which a disposable plastic sheathed dilator is passed over a guide wire. The dilator and guide wire are withdrawn with the sheath left in place, the electrode lead is inserted into the vein through the sheath, and the sheath is split and withdrawn. The permanent pacemaker is then usually placed in a subcutaneous pocket through an incision overlying the deltopectoral groove. The threshold of stimulation, amplitude of the ECG, and lead impedance are measured and recorded.
  b. **Transthoracic epicardial implantation.** Less than 10% of all permanent leads placed today are epicardial leads. Epicardial leads may be placed through a subxiphoid or left chest incision. Leads are secured directly on the epicardium of the left ventricle. Epicardial leads may be used under the following circumstances:
    (1) At the time of thoracotomy for other procedures (e.g., aortic valve replacement)
    (2) If equipment or technical skill needed for transvenous placement is not available
    (3) For pacing in small children
    (4) If unencumbered upper extremity mobility is required
    (5) If repeated attempts at transvenous electrode placement have been unsuccessful

4. Technical problems with pacemaker insertion
  a. **Cannulation difficulty** is related to problems with central vein puncture. Potential complications include arterial puncture, pneumothorax, phlebitis, wound infection, and air embolism (see Chap. 5).

b. **Failure to capture** is most commonly due to
   (1) Poor positioning of the electrode with blind insertion of the catheter lead
   (2) Electrode displacement from the apex of the ventricle after initial seating of the electrode
   (3) Contact of the electrode to a region of scarred endocardium
   (4) Myocardial perforation
   (5) Faulty equipment (e.g., generator not charged, electrode fractured)
   (6) Poor connection between electrode and pacemaker generator

c. Transient **ventricular irritability** is common during electrode insertion, but significant persistent dysrhythmias are unusual. Catheter repositioning may be required.

d. **Myocardial perforation** is more common than generally thought. Findings may include new pericardial friction rub, diaphragmatic or intercostal muscle twitching, failure to capture, and failure to sense appropriately. Pericardial tamponade seldom occurs in the absence of anticoagulant therapy. The use of flexible, soft catheters and gentle catheter advancement minimizes this complication. If perforation occurs, the catheter must be repositioned.

e. **Diaphragmatic stimulation** may occur with either perforation of the right ventricle and direct pacing of the diaphragm or transmitted pacing of the phrenic nerve. The patient may complain of rhythmic, forceful muscular movements. Diagnosis is confirmed by palpation of left upper quadrant or with fluoroscopy. Spontaneous resolution does not occur; the electrode must be repositioned.

D. **Pacemaker emergencies and complications**

1. **Cessation of pacing** is the most common serious emergency in a patient with a pacemaker. The first priority is to reestablish a satisfactory cardiac rate and rhythm. Loss of pacing may be due to the following:
   a. **Pulse generator failure** is usually manifested by slowing of basic pacing rate, loss of the demand function, failure to sense spontaneous beats or capture the ventricle, or a combination of these. Depletion of the power source tends to be slow, whereas electronic failure of the pulse-forming circuit may be sudden and catastrophic.
   b. **A malfunctioning lead system** should be tested for five factors from which the etiology can be determined: voltage, current threshold, impedance, amplitude, and rate. Etiology includes partial or incomplete fracture, insulation failure, displacement or poor position of the electrode, failure of the connector between lead and pulse generator, and poor sensing.
   c. **Physiologic alterations** may be due to development of fibrosis around the electrode, which raises pacing threshold.

2. **Runaway pacemaker** is defined as the electronic current instability causing a rapid rate of more than 120 beats per minute. Despite manufacturers' attempts to eliminate this malfunction, it still occasionally occurs and is probably the most dangerous of all pacemaker malfunctions.
   a. It must be differentiated from an intrinsic ventricular tachycardia.
   b. The pacing circuit should be immediately interrupted. This may require emergency electrode transection.

3. **Catheter migration** may be due to inadequate initial positioning of the electrode tip, excessive length of catheter allowing redundancy, or slippage of the cutaneous catheter at the insertion site. It usually occurs within the first 24 hours of placement.

4. **Interference by electromagnetic phenomena**
   a. A temporary lead system is a direct, low-resistance conductor to the heart. Minuscule alternating currents may induce ventricular fibrillation. If possible, attachment of line-powered monitoring devices to the pacemaker terminals is avoided. When an ECG is recorded from the endocardial lead, the patient should not be otherwise grounded; all other connections to electrical equipment should be removed.
   b. The effect of external interference is greatly reduced by the bipolar lead's filtering circuitry and built-in shielding. Very strong interference, including electrocautery equipment, diathermy, and microwave ovens, may temporarily inhibit a demand pacemaker.
   c. Many pacemaker manufacturers recommend that at least one lead be disconnected from the pacemaker during cardioversion.
5. **Infection** may complicate pacing. Temporary pacing, often established under less than ideal conditions, may be associated with wound or electrode infection. This requires careful documentation and replacement with another system under appropriate antibiotic coverage. Infection of a permanent pacemaker requires removal of the entire assembly.

II. Cardioversion and defibrillation

A. Description

1. Cardioversion is accomplished with a **synchronized direct-current (DC) shock;** the discharge is synchronized to occur within 20 milliseconds of the peak of the R wave on the ECG. Synchronization ensures avoidance of discharge during the period of ventricular vulnerability at the peak of the T wave. All excitable fibers are depolarized, the reentrant circuits are interrupted, and the sinoatrial node is allowed to reinitiate normal cardiac rhythm.
2. Cardioversion is most effective for arrhythmias caused by continuous reentry and is much less effective for tachyarrhythmias due to increased intrinsic automaticity.
3. In acute atrial fibrillation or flutter, the drugs of choice for conversion or control of heart rate are digitalis, beta-blockers, or calcium-channel blockers. If they are unsuccessful, electrical cardioversion may then be considered. Conversion is successful in restoring sinus rhythm, at least transiently, in more than 85% of patients with atrial flutter, paroxysmal supraventricular tachycardia, and ventricular tachycardia.

B. Indications

1. Urgent cardioversion is indicated with the following:
   a. Atrial fibrillation, flutter, or other supraventricular arrhythmias associated with hemodynamic deterioration or ischemia on the ECG
   b. Ventricular tachycardia unresponsive to antiarrhythmic drugs. Any underlying hypoxemia, acidosis, or electrolyte disturbances should be aggressively sought and treated.
2. Elective cardioversion
   a. **Indicated** with recent onset (<6 mo) of atrial fibrillation or atrial flutter that has not responded to pharmacologic treatment or control of the underlying cause
   b. **Relatively contraindicated** with long-term atrial fibrillation (>6 mo), recent systemic embolization, massively dilated left atrium, underlying heart block, uncontrolled thyrotoxicosis, decompensated chronic obstructive pulmonary disease (COPD), and left ventricular dysfunction
   c. **Contraindicated** in the presence of digitalis toxicity because of the risk of precipitating more serious arrhythmias
3. Urgent defibrillation is indicated with ventricular fibrillation

C. Cardioversion technique

1. Equipment
   - **a. Synchronized** DC cardioverter with electrode paddles, ECG machine, and monitor
   - **b.** Electrode jelly
   - **c.** Drugs for sedation (e.g., diazepam, thiopental, methohexital) and emergency cardiovascular support
   - **d.** Intravenous infusion set
   - **e.** Oxygen (with self-inflating resuscitation bag) and intubation equipment
2. Procedure
   - **a.** For supraventricular arrhythmias
     - **(1)** The patient should be positioned on a firm surface in the event that CPR is required.
     - **(2)** An IV infusion is established.
     - **(3)** The patient is connected to the input mode of the cardioverter. The ECG is monitored continuously.
     - **(4)** The patient is sedated as required.
     - **(5)** Paddles are precoated with electrode paste.
     - **(6)** Energy level is set to 50 watt-seconds for atrial arrhythmias.
     - **(7)** Paddles are positioned such that one is anterior to the heart and the other posterior at the angle of the left scapula. Alternately, both may be placed anteriorly, with one to the right of the sternum in the second intercostal space and the other lateral to the left nipple in the midaxillary line.
     - **(8)** The synchronization switch is activated, and the current is delivered. An ECG is then recorded.
     - **(9) If cardioversion is unsuccessful,** energy settings are increased in 50-watt-second increments.
     - **(10)** If necessary, ventricular irritability is treated with lidocaine.
   - **b.** For ventricular tachycardia and fibrillation
     - **(1)** Lidocaine, 100 mg IV, is given.
     - **(2)** The patient is connected as in **a.(3),** but the synchronizing switch is turned off.
     - **(3)** Sedation is administered, if necessary.
     - **(4)** The paddles are coated with electrode gel or covered with saline-soaked gauze sponges.
     - **(5)** The energy level is set at 200 watt-seconds for ventricular tachycardia and 300–400 watt-seconds for ventricular fibrillation.
     - **(6)** Paddles are positioned as in **a.(7),** and the current is administered directly (without synchronization). If the first discharge fails, the discharge is repeated at the same energy level one more time and then is increased incrementally until successful.
     - **(7)** Continuous IV lidocaine may be required after cardioversion or defibrillation.

D. Problems and complications of cardioversion

1. **Current is not discharged.** Proper synchronization mode should be checked ("off" for ventricular fibrillation), and the cardioverter should be examined to confirm charge.
2. **Cutaneous burns** result from arcing between skin and paddle. Electrode gel or saline-soaked sponges should be used to ensure satisfactory contact.
3. **Significant arrhythmias** occasionally occur after DC electrical shock. They are usually brief and require no treatment. However, ventricular fibrillation may also occur. If the synchronization mode is off, the discharge may be delivered during the T wave, and fibrillation may ensue. In addition, ventricular tachyarrhythmias may result if

significant dosages of digitalis preparations have been recently administered. To treat cardioversion-induced ventricular fibrillation, the energy level should be reset to the highest output, the synchronizer turned off, and the charge delivered. Intravenous lidocaine or phenytoin may be administered.

4. Other potential complications include **myocardial injury** due to energy content of the shock, **pulmonary edema** or worsening of left ventricular failure after conversion of atrial fibrillation, and **systemic embolization** of intracardiac thrombus.

III. Extracorporeal membrane oxygenation (ECMO)

A. Description

1. Extracorporeal membrane oxygenation is the process by which venous blood is drained from the circulation via a partial venoarterial or venovenous bypass system, pumped through a membrane oxygenator, and returned to the systemic circulation of the patient.
2. Extracorporeal membrane oxygenation is effective in temporarily correcting hypoxemia and hypercapnia and reduces pulmonary blood flow and right-to-left shunts, thereby allowing lower ventilatory pressures and inspired oxygen concentrations.

B. Limitations. For practical purposes, ECMO remains **investigational.** It has been shown **not** to increase the probability of long-term survival in patients with irreversible acute respiratory failure. Although ECMO can support respiratory gas exchange and thereby provides favorable conditions for the lung to heal, its clinical usefulness is limited by the irreversibility of the underlying pulmonary pathology.

IV. Intraaortic balloon pump (IABP)

A. Description

1. The IABP is an intraarterial circulatory assist device that raises aortic diastolic pressure and lowers left ventricular systolic pressure in synchrony with the heart's contraction.
2. The balloon is rapidly inflated with helium in diastole and deflated just before systole to produce the desired hemodynamic effects.
3. Beneficial effects
   a. Reduction of cardiac work (the integral of pressure and flow) by reducing afterload and myocardial oxygen requirements
   b. Enhancement of coronary perfusion by augmenting diastolic pressure
   c. Support of mean aortic pressure by increasing diastolic pressure

B. Indications and contraindications to IABP therapy

1. Indications
   a. **Unstable angina** with persistent ECG changes, persistent pain that is not responsive to pharmacologic therapy, or both
   b. **Cardiogenic shock.** Patients in cardiogenic shock who fail to respond to optimal fluid management, correction of acidosis and arrhythmias, and administration of vasoactive agents are candidates for IABP. The IABP can be an efficacious therapeutic device for the management of cardiogenic shock, although mortality remains high.
   c. **Refractory left ventricular failure after cardiopulmonary bypass**
   d. **Specific postmyocardial infarction complications,** including ventricular septal defect, acute mitral regurgitation, and ventricular ectopic activity uncontrollable with pharmacologic agents and overdrive pacing.
2. Relative contraindications
   a. Aortic regurgitation
   b. Aneurysmal or severe obstructive femoral, iliac, or aortic arterial disease or recent aortic surgery (transthoracic IABP inserted di-

rectly into the aorta may be considered in cases of severe peripheral vascular disease)

c. An irreversible underlying pathophysiologic process (e.g., end-stage cardiomyopathy)

C. Technique

1. Equipment

a. **Catheters.** There are a wide variety of balloon catheters available, all of which consist of a long, flexible catheter with a cylindrical balloon attached to one end. They are commercially packaged and include introducers, J-tip wires, dilators, and sheaths.

b. **Pump.** The pump console regulates inflation and deflation of the balloon to achieve the desired intraaortic pressure changes.

c. **Monitoring equipment.** The intraarterial pressure, ECG, rhythm, pulmonary capillary wedge pressure, and cardiac output are monitored.

2. Catheter insertion procedure

a. **Percutaneous** technique

(1) The percutaneous balloon is tightly wrapped as directed for the specific balloon catheter selected.

(2) The femoral pulse is palpated, and the insertion site is anesthetized. Generally, the leg with the stronger femoral pulse in a nonoperated groin will be chosen.

(3) The common femoral artery is penetrated by Seldinger technique with an introducer. Heparin is given after intravascular access is achieved. A J-tip wire is passed through the introducer, and the introducer is removed.

(4) A No. 8 dilator is passed over the wire into the artery and then removed. A No. 12 dilator with balloon sheath is then introduced over the wire, and the wire is removed.

(5) The No. 12 dilator is removed, leaving the sheath in place. The balloon with internal wire is inserted through the sheath. The internal wire is advanced through the balloon. The wire and balloon are then threaded into the thoracic aorta, the wire subsequently being withdrawn. The balloon tip is positioned just distal to the subclavian artery.

(6) The balloon is unwound, and the catheter is connected to the pump.

(7) The catheter is securely anchored to the skin with a heavy silk suture.

b. Open **surgical** technique

(1) Under local anesthesia, a skin incision is made parallel to common femoral artery in the groin with the strongest pulse.

(2) Heparin IV is given.

(3) With appropriate proximal and distal control of the common femoral artery, a longitudinal arteriotomy is made.

(4) The balloon catheter is inserted through a 10-mm (3/8-inch) prosthetic vascular graft and into the artery. It is advanced retrograde to the point at which the tip lies just distal to the left subclavian artery.

(5) Pumping is begun.

(6) The prosthetic graft is sutured end to side to the common femoral artery and is secured around the catheter with several heavy silk ligatures.

(7) The wound is closed over the prosthetic graft.

D. Complications of IABP

1. Ischemia of the lower extremity is usually secondary to severe peripheral atherosclerosis or insertion into the superficial rather than common femoral artery.

2. Femoral, iliac, or aortic dissection
3. Distal clot embolus as the catheter is removed
4. Wound problems, including infection, lymph fistula, and neuralgia

E. Management of IABP

1. Anticoagulation is continued to prevent clotting and platelet aggregation. In the postoperative patient, low-molecular-weight dextran (Rheomacrodex) rather than heparin is administered to avoid major bleeding.
2. The balloon is phased so inflation occurs on the downslope of the radial artery pressure curve, and deflation occurs just before the onset of ventricular systole.
3. The balloon should never remain totally motionless (i.e., not pumping) in the aorta.
4. Distal extremity vascular supply should be monitored regularly.

V. Pericardiocentesis

A. Description

1. Pericardiocentesis is the process by which fluid is removed from the pericardial space. The most urgent indication is acute tamponade.
2. When fluid accumulates in the pericardial sac, intrapericardial pressure increases and restricts atrial and ventricular filling, thus impairing coronary blood flow and ventricular function.
3. The diagnosis of pericardial tamponade is suggested by the following:
   - **a.** Hypotension and pulsus paradoxus (a decrease in systolic BP on spontaneous inspiration of >10 mm Hg)
   - **b.** Narrow pulse pressure
   - **c.** Elevated venous pressure (jugular and peripheral), Kussmaul's sign (elevation of central venous pressure with spontaneous inspiration), or both
   - **d.** Diminished heart sounds
   - **e.** Equalization of right- and left-sided intracardiac pressures
   - **f.** The clinical situation (e.g., chest trauma)
4. A portable chest radiograph is rarely useful in the diagnosis of **acute** pericardial tamponade; however, a large pericardial silhouette on chest radiograph is frequently associated with chronic causes of tamponade. Portable echocardiography may be helpful in diagnosing pericardial effusion (in patients who are stable).

B. Indications

1. Urgent relief of **acute tamponade** with hemodynamic deterioration. Pericardiocentesis is performed on the basis of reasonable clinical suspicion.
2. Diagnostic tap of a pericardial effusion
3. Evacuation of a chronic pericardial effusion

C. Technique

1. Equipment
   - **a.** Skin preparation materials, sterile field equipment, sterile dressing materials
   - **b.** Local anesthetic materials
   - **c.** Syringes (10 and 50 ml)
   - **d.** Three-way stopcock with connecting tube
   - **e.** Needle-over-catheter assembly (e.g., subclavian catheter kit with metal-hubbed No. 14 needle)
   - **f.** Spinal needle (18-gauge)
   - **g.** Alligator clip
2. **Procedure** (Fig. A-1)
   - **a.** The head of the bed is elevated approximately 30 degrees.
   - **b.** The ECG arm leads are placed on the patient. The ECG, BP, and central venous pressure are monitored.

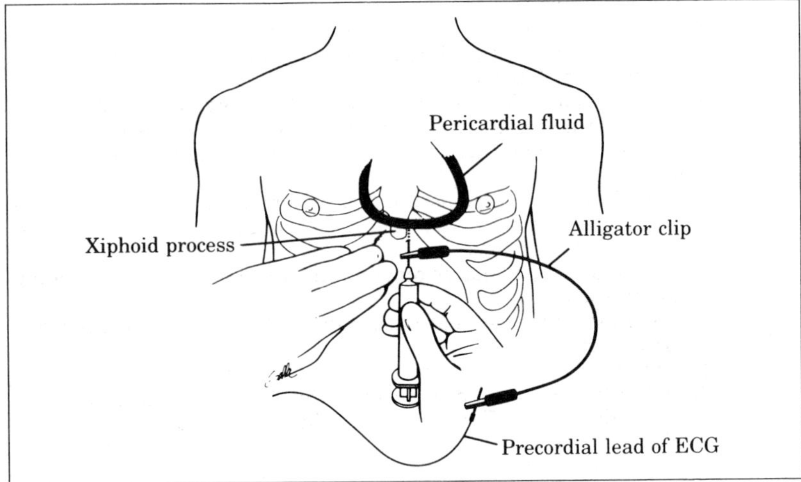

Fig. A-1. Pericardiocentesis technique.

- **c.** The upper abdomen and chest are prepared and draped widely.
- **d.** Local anesthetic is infiltrated between the xiphoid cartilage and left costal margin.
- **e.** The metal 14-gauge (or 16-gauge) needle is attached to the precordial lead of the ECG with an alligator clip. (For diagnostic pericardiocentesis, the 18-gauge spinal needle may be used.) Under urgent circumstances, it may be necessary to forgo ECG monitoring of the probing needle.
- **f.** The needle-syringe assembly is inserted just left of the xiphoid cartilage and advanced at approximately a 30-degree angle toward the left shoulder, while maintaining constant suction with the syringe.
  - **(1)** The precordial lead is monitored. The ECG will initially appear normal. S–T-segment elevation or extrasystoles suggest contact with ventricular epicardium.
  - **(2)** Intrapericardial position is suggested by
    - **(a)** Aspiration of nonpulsatile, nonclotting blood
    - **(b)** Electrocardiographic evidence of epicardial contact
    - **(c)** A "scratching" sensation as epicardium strikes the needle
- **g.** If epicardial contact is made, the needle is withdrawn a few millimeters to prevent epicardial damage.
- **h.** The syringe is then detached, and the catheter is passed through the needle. The needle is removed, leaving the catheter in place.
- **i.** The 50-ml syringe is attached and fluid withdrawn. Hemodynamic status may dramatically improve with aspiration of as little as 50 ml of blood.
- **j.** If indicated, fluid is sent for appropriate studies (e.g., cell count, protein, cytology, Gram's stain, and culture).
- **k.** If the procedure is unsuccessful in reestablishing hemodynamic stability, a left anterior thoracotomy through the fourth or fifth intercostal space should be performed immediately to relieve the tamponade.

D. Complications of pericardiocentesis

1. **Arrhythmias** may occur secondary to myocardial needle contact. The needle should be withdrawn slightly.

2. **Ventricular perforation** is avoided by careful ECG monitoring coupled with slow advancement and continuous aspiration.
3. **Coronary artery laceration.** An ECG is obtained after the procedure, to identify new myocardial ischemia.

VI. **Thoracentesis**

A. **Description.** Thoracentesis is the process of draining air or fluid from the pleural space by a catheter or needle inserted percutaneously into the chest cavity.

B. The principal **indications** for thoracentesis are to sample a pleural effusion for diagnosis and to remove air or fluid (or both) therapeutically from the pleural space.

1. **Pleural effusions** are of two types.
   a. Free-flowing. A chest radiograph with apical and decubitus views confirms fluid shift.
   b. Loculated. Ultrasound or fluoroscopic assessment may aid diagnosis.
2. **Pleural air (pneumothorax).** The physical signs associated with significant pneumothorax include diminished breath sounds, hyperresonance to percussion, and a prominent but poorly moving hemithorax. A chest radiograph taken during the expiratory phase may be required to reveal a small pneumothorax.
   a. **Tension** pneumothorax
      (1) An air leak through a one-way valve mechanism causes a progressive increase in intrapleural pressure, thereby shifting the mediastinum toward the opposite side and producing hypotension, tracheal deviation, and hyperresonance.
      (2) Decompression is urgently required.
   b. Pneumothorax **without tension**
      (1) If the patient is **asymptomatic,** otherwise healthy, and can be closely observed, one may elect not to treat a small, spontaneous pneumothorax. However, almost all patients at the Massachusetts General Hospital (MGH) with pneumothorax are treated with a chest tube or, more rarely, thoracentesis.
      (2) If the patient is symptomatic, usually reflected by dyspnea, hypoxemia, or both, a chest tube should be inserted, irrespective of the extent of pneumothorax.

C. **Thoracentesis procedure**

1. Equipment
   a. Skin preparation materials, sterile field equipment, local anesthetic supplies, and sterile dressing materials
   b. Syringes (5- and 50-ml)
   c. Needles (22-, 18-, 15-gauge; 14-gauge Intracath [optional])
   d. Three-way stopcock
   e. Two curved clamps
   f. Sterile IV tubing
   g. Specimen tubes, including 1000-ml self-suction evacuation containers (optional)
2. Technique
   a. **Pneumothorax (without tension)**
      (1) Localizing chest radiographs should be obtained if the patient's condition permits.
      (2) The patient should be supine, with the head of bed elevated 30 degrees.
      (3) The anterior and lateral chest on the affected side are prepared and draped.
      (4) The skin, subcutaneous fat, underlying muscles, and pleura are infiltrated with a local anesthetic at the upper border of the third rib (second intercostal space) in the midclavicular line, including the pleura. The needle is kept close to rib.

(5) Aspiration is performed with the anesthetizing needle to confirm pleural penetration and the presence of air.
(6) An 18-gauge thoracentesis needle attached to the stopcock and syringe is inserted along the upper rib margin to avoid the intercostal vessels. It is advanced as constant suction is maintained on the syringe to the approximate depth to which the original anesthetic needle had penetrated the pleura (can be felt as a sudden "give").
(7) A clamp is applied to the needle at the skin to maintain a constant insertion depth as the specimen is aspirated.
(8) The specimen is aspirated via the three-way stopcock.
(9) Although a small pneumothorax may be aspirated in this manner, it is generally more prudent to proceed with chest tube placement after (5) for a significant pneumothorax.
(10) The needle is removed, and a chest radiograph is obtained.

b. **Tension pneumothorax.** A tension pneumothorax must be urgently decompressed by inserting a 15-gauge needle or 16-gauge catheter-over-needle in the second intercostal space in the midclavicular line. A chest tube is subsequently inserted.

c. **Pleural fluid**
(1) The collection is localized with posteroanterior and lateral chest radiographs obtained in the upright position. A free-floating effusion is confirmed with lateral decubitus films.
(2) The approach may be either posterior or midaxillary. The patient should be comfortably seated, leaning forward slightly with forearms resting on an adjustable table. The midaxillary approach is most commonly used for patients who will not tolerate position changes.
(3) The interspace below the fluid level determined by percussion is used, although generally one should use no lower than the eighth intercostal space.
(4) A 15-gauge needle is inserted using the same technique as described in **a.**
(5) **Alternately,** a 14-gauge Intracath needle (Deseret) attached to a 10-ml syringe may be inserted just above the rib. The syringe is removed, rapidly occluding the hub of the needle with a gloved finger, and the flexible catheter (16-gauge, 8-inch) is inserted through the needle into the pleural cavity. The needle is withdrawn with the catheter remaining in the chest, the catheter is attached to a three-way stopcock, and fluid is aspirated with either a 50-ml syringe or a vacuum bottle. It should be noted that flexible catheters may be plugged more easily than large-bore needles.
(6) After removal of approximately 500–1000 ml of fluid, the clinical status of patient should be evaluated before proceeding with further immediate aspiration.
(7) The specimen is sent for appropriate studies (i.e., cell count, Gram's stain, culture-cytology, chemistries, pH).
(8) The needle or catheter is removed, and chest radiograph is obtained to assess residual fluid, pneumothorax, and underlying pathology.

d. Complications of thoracentesis
(1) Lung laceration
(2) Intercostal blood vessel laceration
(3) Penetration of abdominal organs. The costophrenic sulcus is narrow below the eighth intercostal space. A common error is to attempt thoracentesis too low, thereby penetrating the diaphragm. In addition, effusions often obscure the diaphragm, which may be elevated.

(4) Dyspnea and discomfort secondary to excessive mediastinal shift can occur with too rapid or too extensive evacuation of a large effusion.

(5) Pneumothorax, by opening the system to the atmosphere or by puncturing the lung

VII. Chest tubes

A. Description. A chest tube is a drain that evacuates air or liquid from the pleural space.

B. Indications

1. Pneumothorax
2. Pleural effusion
3. Access for administration of sclerosing agents and drainage of empyema

C. Chest tube insertion technique

1. Equipment
   - **a.** Skin preparation materials
   - **b.** Sterile field equipment
   - **c.** Local anesthetic materials
   - **d.** Knife handle with No. 10 scalpel blade
   - **e.** Curved clamps
   - **f.** Chest tube (for pneumothorax, No. 24 French Argyle; for pleural effusion, No. 28 French Argyle)
   - **g.** Three-bottle chest suction equipment or commercial equivalent (Pleur-evac)
   - **h.** Skin suture materials, needle holder, and scissors
   - **i.** Dressing materials (petrolatum gauze, sterile sponges, benzoin, Elastoplast, tape)
2. Site of insertion. There are two basic approaches for chest tube placement:
   - **a.** The **anterior** (midclavicular) approach in the second or third intercostal space is used principally for pneumothorax.
   - **b.** The **lateral** (midaxillary) approach in the sixth or seventh intercostal space is used for fluid and air drainage. It is safer in the hands of the less experienced and may be the preferred approach for cosmetic or technical reasons (e.g., easier insertion in muscular men).
3. For pneumothorax (Fig. A-2)
   - **a.** The patient is advised in detail what to expect during chest tube insertion, including the burning sensation of local anesthesia, transient discomfort at the moment of pleural penetration, and cough as air or fluid is evacuated.
   - **b.** The skin is prepared, and the anterior or lateral chest field is draped.
   - **c.** The site of planned pleural entry is determined. Approximately 2–3 cm inferior to this site, a skin weal is produced with local anesthetic. Liberal infiltration of lidocaine through all layers of the chest wall is continued, directing the needle in a cephalad direction toward the interspace of planned pleural entry. Three milliliters of local anesthetic is injected just inferior to the rib, both anterior and posterior to the site of planned pleural penetration to block the intercostal nerve bundle.
   - **d.** The pleura is infiltrated with local anesthetic and is penetrated to confirm pneumothorax (Fig. A-2A).
   - **e.** A linear skin incision is made at the site of the skin weal. The subcutaneous tissues and intercostal muscles are spread bluntly with the curved clamp, creating a subcutaneous tunnel from the skin to the site of pleural entry.

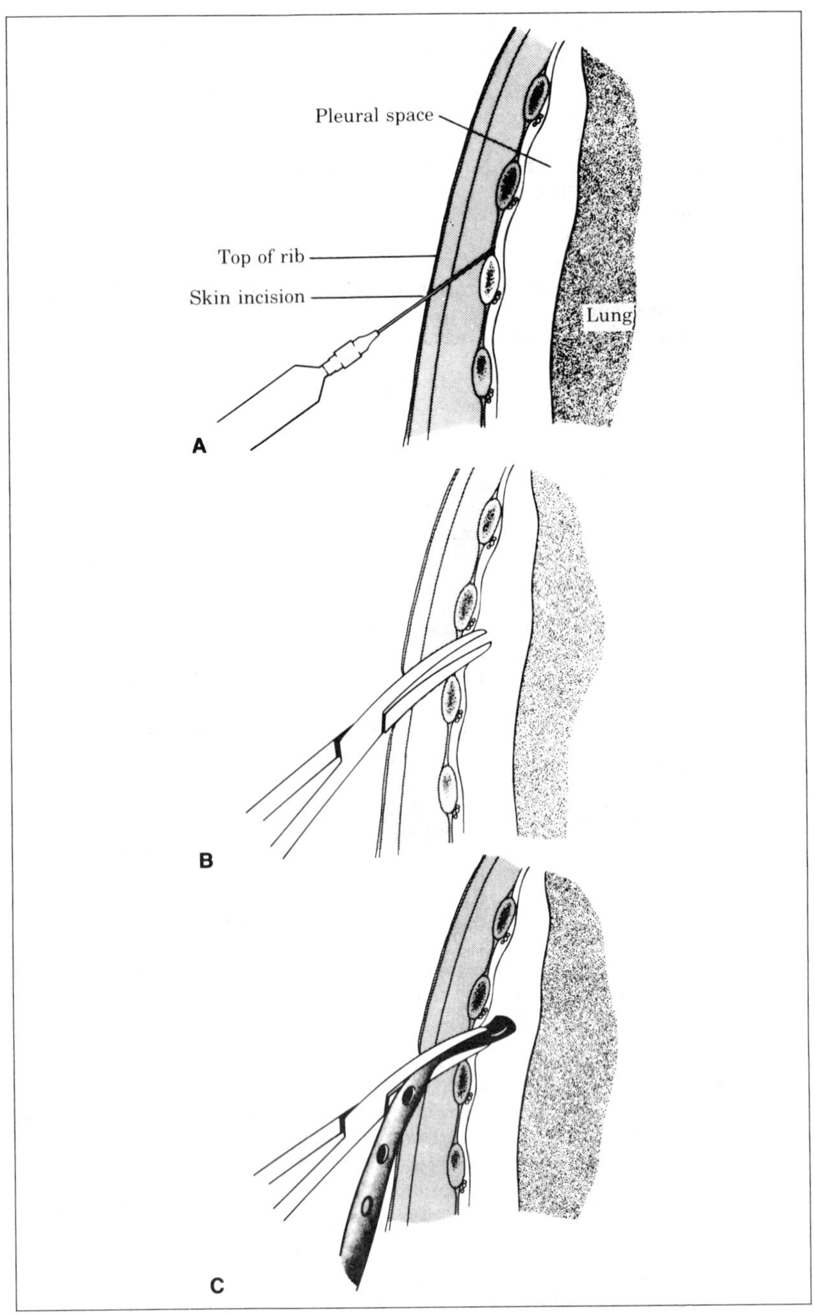

Fig. A-2. Chest tube insertion technique. A. Local anesthetic infiltration and aspiration of pleural air (to confirm pneumothorax). B. Perforation of parietal pleural with a blunt, curved clamp. C. Insertion of chest tube with curved clamp.

f. The curved clamp is firmly grasped in the palm of the hand, such that the index finger will serve as a stop to prevent excessive penetration. The parietal pleura is perforated with the clamp closed, hugging the upper border of the rib and climbing over the rib margin as firm force is applied (Fig. A-2B). The clamp is then spread to widen the hole. The patient should be forewarned that the moment of pleural perforation will be transiently uncomfortable.

g. A free pleural space is confirmed by exploring the wound with a gloved digit.

h. The end of the chest tube is grasped with the curved clamp and inserted into the pleural space (Fig. A-2C). The tube is advanced toward the apex, ensuring that all side holes are within the pleural cavity.

i. The chest tube is connected to a three-bottle drainage system, which is placed on 15-cm water suction.

j. The wound is sutured and the chest tube secured with a No. 1-0 silk suture.

k. An airtight dressing is applied using benzoin, petrolatum gauze, sponges, and Elastoplast.

l. A chest radiograph is obtained to document the position of tube.

4. For hemothorax

a. The chest tube should be placed in the sixth or seventh interspace in the midaxillary line.

b. The procedure is otherwise the same as that for pneumothorax (see **3**).

c. A large chest tube (28F) is used.

D. Management of chest tubes

1. Chest tubes are connected by a tapered adapter to either of the following:

a. Waterseal, if minimal air or fluid drainage is expected

b. Suction, if significant drainage is expected

2. The drainage apparatus most commonly used is a three-bottle system or commercial equivalent. This sealed system allows for suction regulation and removal of air and fluid from the pleural space. The first bottle collects drainage fluid, the second bottle provides an underwater seal with a low-resistance valve for air removal, and the third bottle regulates the degree of suction. The modern commercial drainage units operate on the same principle as the three-bottle system, with added reservoirs and valves that make them safer and easier to use (Fig. A-3A, B).

3. The entire system must be checked extensively to be certain the water seal is intact and fluctuates with respirations, the suction control bottle bubbles continuously at the proper level, and dependent loops in the drainage tubing are avoided. All connections should be fixed securely with tape in such a way that visualization of the integrity of the connection is not obscured.

4. "Never clamp a chest tube" is a prudent rule of thumb followed at the MGH with only two exceptions. The first is to locate the source of an air leak when bubbling occurs in the water-seal bottle, and the second is to replace the drainage unit when necessary.

5. Before concluding that there is an ongoing intrapleural air leak, all connections should be checked, and the intrathoracic position of all chest tube holes should be confirmed. If an air leak in the water-seal chamber persists when the chest tube is transiently occluded, there is a discontinuity in the drainage system.

6. Patients will typically be maintained on suction (15 cm water) until

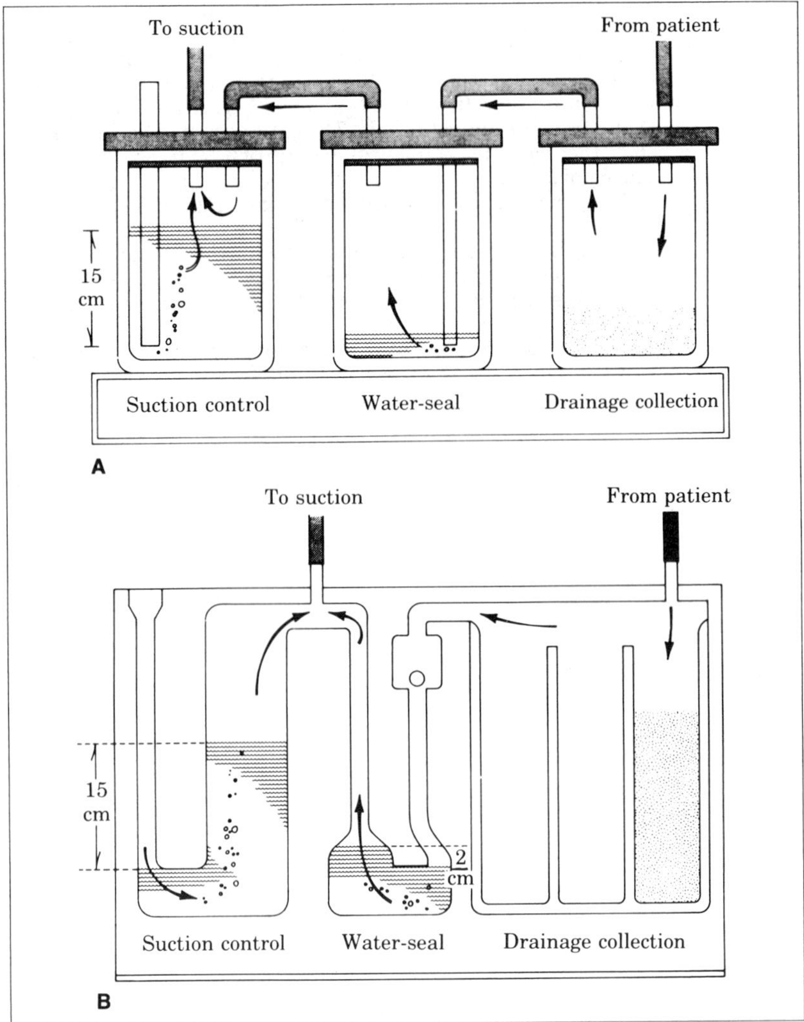

Fig. A-3. Chest tube drainage apparatus. A. Traditional three-bottle collection system. B. Commercial equivalent to three-bottle collection system.

chest radiograph shows a fully inflated lung, there is no air leak, and drainage is less than 150 ml in 24 hours.

7. Chest tube removal
    a. A petrolatum gauze dressing is prepared, and the anchoring suture is removed.
    b. The patient is instructed to hold a deep breath (or Valsalva maneuver). To increase intrathoracic pressure, the petrolatum gauze dressing is applied securely to the insertion site with one hand, and the tube is rapidly withdrawn. The dressing is taped to the chest wall with Elastoplast for 24 hours.
    c. A chest radiograph is obtained after removal.

E. **Complications of chest tubes**

1. **Bleeding** may be caused by laceration of intercostal or internal mammary vessels. This usually requires exploration for repair.
2. **Lung laceration** is prevented by careful aspiration before chest tube placement, avoiding trocars, and grasping the clamp to prevent excessive penetration into the chest.
3. **Subcutaneous emphysema** may be caused by either inadequate decompression of a pneumothorax with dissection of air around the tube into the subcutaneous space or malposition of the most proximal chest tube hole such that it lies subcutaneously.

VIII. **Emergency open thoracotomy**

A. **Description.** Emergency thoracotomy implies that chest cavity exposure is urgently required, usually without the convenience of a fully equipped operating room, in order to relieve pericardial tamponade, resuscitate the heart, or control bleeding.

B. **Indications**

1. Unsuccessful pericardiocentesis with **acute pericardial tamponade.** This situation may arise if there is rapid reaccumulation of pericardial fluid after pericardiocentesis or if pericardiocentesis has not adequately restored hemodynamic stability.
2. **Ineffective closed chest massage** for CPR. This may occur in situations of reverse pectus excavatum or barrel chest.
3. **Penetrating wound** to the heart or major vessels. If a patient arrives at the hospital in shock from a hemothorax and does not respond satisfactorily to aggressive resuscitative measures, immediate thoracotomy is indicated.
4. Postcardiac surgery, in situations in which **excessive postoperative bleeding** and acute pericardial tamponade make emergency surgical evacuation mandatory

C. **Technique**

1. Equipment
   a. Scalpel
   b. Rib spreader
   c. Scissors
   d. Forceps
   e. Aortic cross clamp
   f. Sternal saw or cast cutter (optional)
   g. Lung retractor
   h. Skin preparation materials and sterile field equipment
2. Procedure
   a. The entire anterior and lateral chest is rapidly prepared and draped.
   b. The skin and all subcutaneous tissues are incised in the left inframammary crease, and the fourth or fifth intercostal space is entered.
   c. The incision may be readily extended into the right chest by transecting the sternum with a cast cutter or sternal saw and gaining control of the internal mammary vessels after division of the sternum. This allows exposure of the right atrium and intrapericardial venae cavae. The incision may be extended laterally for exposure of the descending aorta, if required.
   d. The rib spreader is placed and opened widely.
   e. For pericardial tamponade or exposure to the heart directly for open cardiac massage, the pericardium is widely incised parallel to the phrenic nerve. If the patient is explored for massive hemothorax, blood clots are evacuated, and the source of bleeding is sought. If possible, the bleeding should be controlled with pressure

until the blood volume is replaced and hemodynamic stability has been achieved.

f. Closure is carried out in the operating room.

Selected References

Behrendt, D. M., and Austen, W. G. *Patient Care in Cardiac Surgery.* Boston: Little, Brown, 1980.

Bing, O. H. L., McDowell, J. H., Hantman, J., and Messer, J. V. Pacemaker placement by electrocardiographic monitoring. *N. Engl. J. Med.* 287:651, 1972.

Furman, S. Pacemaker emergencies. *Med. Clin. North Am.* 63:113, 1979.

Kirsh, M., and Sloan, H. *Blunt Chest Trauma: General Principles of Management.* Boston: Little, Brown, 1977.

Krikorian, J. G., and Hancock, E. W. Pericardiocentesis. *Am. J. Cardiol.* 65:808, 1978.

Ream, A. K., and Fogdall, R. P. *Acute Cardiovascular Management: Anesthesia and Intensive Care.* Philadelphia: Lippincott, 1982.

Rosenberg, A. S., Grossman, J., Escher, E. J. W., et al. Bedside transvenous cardiac pacing. *Am. Heart J.* 77:696, 1969.

Vander Salm, J., Cutler, B., and Wheeler, H. B. *Atlas of Bedside Procedures.* Boston: Little, Brown, 1979.

Wilkins, E. W., Jr., Dineen, J. J., Moncure, A. C., and Gross, P. L. *Massachusetts General Hospital Textbook of Emergency Medicine.* Baltimore: Williams & Wilkins, 1983.

Zapol, W. M., Snider, M. T., Hill, J. D., et al. Extracorporeal membrane oxygenation in severe acute respiratory failure. *J.A.M.A.* 242:2193, 1979.

Index

Note: Figures are indicated by f; *tables are indicated by* t.